DSM-5-TR® Made Easy

Also from James Morrison

Diagnosis Made Easier:
Principles and Techniques for Mental Health Clinicians, Second Edition

The First Interview, Fourth Edition

Interviewing Children and Adolescents:
Skills and Strategies for Effective DSM-5® Diagnosis, Second Edition
with Kathryn Flegel

The Mental Health Clinician's Workbook:
Locking In Your Professional Skills

When Psychological Problems Mask Medical Disorders:
A Guide for Psychotherapists

For more information, see *www.guilford.com/morrison*

DSM-5-TR® Made Easy

The Clinician's Guide to Diagnosis

James Morrison

THE GUILFORD PRESS
New York   London

Copyright © 2023 The Guilford Press
A Division of Guilford Publications, Inc.
370 Seventh Avenue, Suite 1200, New York, NY 10001
www.guilford.com

Printed in the United States of America

This book is printed on acid-free paper.

Last digit is print number: 9   8   7   6   5   4   3   2   1

The author has checked with sources believed to be reliable in his efforts to provide
information that is complete and generally in accord with the standards of practice
that are accepted at the time of publication. However, in view of the possibility of
human error or changes in behavioral, mental health, or medical sciences, neither the
author, nor the editor and publisher, nor any other party who has been involved in
the preparation or publication of this work warrants that the information contained
herein is in every respect accurate or complete, and they are not responsible for any
errors or omissions or the results obtained from the use of such information. Readers
are encouraged to confirm the information contained in this book with other sources.

Library of Congress Cataloging-in-Publication Data is available from the publisher.

ISBN 978-1-4625-5134-7 (hardcover)

DSM-5-TR is a registered trademark of the American Psychiatric Association. The
APA has not participated in the preparation of this book.

For Mary, always my sine qua non

For Mary, always my sine qua non

About the Author

James Morrison, MD, is Affiliate Professor of Psychiatry at Oregon Health and Science University in Portland. His long career includes extensive experience in both the private and public sectors. With his acclaimed practical books—including *Diagnosis Made Easier, Second Edition; The First Interview, Fourth Edition;* and others—Dr. Morrison has guided hundreds of thousands of mental health professionals and students through the complexities of clinical evaluation and diagnosis.

Acknowledgments

This book was created on the backs of so many people.

My editor, Kitty Moore, a keen and wonderful critic, helped develop the original concept, and has been a mainstay of the enterprise for this new edition as for every one preceding it.

I want especially to thank my excellent first readers. They include Mary Morrison, who has been there for me from the beginning. My brilliant international (UK) first readers, Dave Morrison and Fiona Morrison, have over and again saved me from myself. Thank you, all.

I also deeply appreciate the many other editors and friends at The Guilford Press, notably Editorial Project Manager Anna Brackett, who helped shape and speed this book into print; my meticulous and valued copy editor, Deborah Heimann; Senior Copy Manager Katherine Lieber; Editorial and Contracts Administrator Carolyn Graham; and Editorial Technology Coordinator William Meyer. And always, my friend Seymour Weingarten.

Late in the editing process, DSM-5-TR changes were announced that profoundly affected how we code neurocognitive disorders. To assist with my understanding, I reached out to several people. I want to express my profound thanks to my old friend Marc A. Schuckit, MD, and to two new friends, Ann M. Eng and Susan K. Schultz, MD. You are all stars!

To each of these, and to the countless patients who have provided the clinical inspiration for this book, I am profoundly grateful.

Contents

Frequently Needed Tables

Introduction

The summer after my first year in medical school, I visited a classmate at his home near the mental institution where his parents both worked. One afternoon, walking around the vast, open campus, we fell into conversation with a staff psychiatrist who told us about an interesting patient.

This young woman had been admitted a few days earlier. While attending college nearby, she had suddenly become agitated—speaking rapidly and rushing in a frenzy from one activity to another. After she impulsively sold her nearly new Corvette for $500, her friends had brought her for evaluation.

"Five hundred dollars!" exclaimed the psychiatrist. "That kind of thinking, that's schizophrenia!"

Now, my friend and I had had just enough exposure to mental health diagnosis to recognize that this young woman's symptoms and course of illness were far more consistent with an episode of mania than with schizophrenia. We were too young and callow to challenge the diagnosis of an experienced clinician, but as we went on our way, we each expressed the fervent hope that this patient's care would be less flawed than her assessment.

For decades, the memory of that blown diagnosis has haunted me, in part because it is by no means unique in the annals of mental health. Indeed, it wasn't until many years later that the first diagnostic manual to include specific criteria (DSM-III) was published. That book has since morphed into the enormous fifth edition of the *Diagnostic and Statistical Manual of Mental Disorders,* now a text revision (DSM-5-TR) published by the American Psychiatric Association.

Anyone who evaluates and treats mental health patients must understand the latest edition of what has become the world standard for evaluation and diagnosis. But getting value from DSM-5-TR requires a great deal of concentration. Written by a committee with the goal of providing standards for research as well as clinical practice in a variety of disciplines, it covers nearly every conceivable subject related to mental health. But you could come away from it not understanding how diagnostic criteria translate to an actual patient.

I wrote *DSM-5-TR Made Easy* to make mental health diagnosis more accessible to clinicians from all mental health professions. In these pages, you will find descriptions of every mental disorder, with emphasis on those that occur in adults. With its careful use, today's readers would be unlikely to mistake that young college student's manic symptoms for schizophrenia.

What Have I Done to Make DSM-5-TR Easy?

Quick Guides. Opening each chapter is a summary of the diagnoses to be found therein—and other disorders that might afflict patients who complain about similar problems. It also provides a useful index to the material in that chapter.

Introductory material. Each section begins with a brief description designed to orient you to the diagnosis. There might be a discussion of the major symptoms, perhaps a little historical information, and some of the demographics—who is likely to have this disorder, and in what circumstances. Here, I've tried to include the details that I would want to know if I were just starting out as a student.

Essential Features. OK, this is the name I've given the defining symptoms in *DSM-5-TR Made Easy*, but they're also known as *prototypes*. I've used them in hopes that they will make the official criteria more accessible. For years, working clinicians have known that when we evaluate a new patient, we don't grab a list of emotional and behavioral attributes and start ticking off boxes. Rather, we compare the data we've gathered to the mind's eye picture we've formed of the various mental and behavioral disorders. When the data fit an image, we have an "aha!" moment and pop that diagnosis into our list of differential diagnoses. (From long experience and conversations with countless other experienced clinicians, I can assure you that this is exactly how it works.)

Some years ago, a study of mood and anxiety disorders* found that clinicians who make diagnoses by rating their patients against prototypes perform at least as well as, and sometimes better than, other clinicians who adhere to strict criteria. That is, it can be shown that prototypes have validity even greater than that of some DSM diagnostic criteria. Moreover, prototypes are reported to be usable by clinicians with a relatively modest level of training and experience; you don't need 20 years of clinical work to succeed with prototypes. Clinicians also report that prototypes are less cumbersome and more clinically useful. (However—and I hasten to underscore this point—the prototypes used in the studies I have just mentioned were generated from the diagnostic criteria inherent in the DSM criteria.) The bottom line: Sure, we need criteria, but we can adapt them so they work even better for us.

---

*DeFife JA, Peart J, Bradley B, Ressler K, Drill R, Westen D: Validity of prototype diagnosis for mood and anxiety disorders. *JAMA Psychiatry* 2013; 70(2): 140–148.

Once you've collected the data and read the prototypes, you can assign a number to indicate how closely your patient fits the ideal of any diagnoses you are considering. Here's the accepted convention: 1 = little or no match; 2 = some match (the patient has a few features of the disorder); 3 = moderate match (there are significant, important features of the disorder); 4 = good match (the patient meets the standard—the diagnosis applies); 5 = excellent match (a classic case). Obviously, the vignettes I've provided will always match at the 4 or 5 level (if not, why would I use them as illustrative examples?), so I haven't bothered to grade them on the 5-point scale. But, if you wish, you can do just that with each new patient you interview.

There may be times you'll want to turn to the official DSM-5-TR criteria. For example, when you're just starting out, DSM-5-TR will give you a picture of the exact numbers of each set of criteria that officially count the patient as "in." You'll also refer to it when doing clinical research, where you must be able to report that participants were all selected according to a scientifically studied, reproducible standard. Even as an experienced clinician, I return to the actual criteria from time to time. Perhaps it's just to have fresh in my mind the complete information that allows me to communicate with other clinicians; sometimes it is related to my writing. (As you read through the discussions of the patients presented in this book, you will find that the evaluations are couched in terms of the official DSM-5-TR criteria.) But mostly, whether I am with patients or talking with students, I stick to the prototype method—just like nearly every other working clinician.

The Fine Print. Most of the diagnostic material in these sections is what I call *boilerplate*. I suppose that sounds pejorative, but each Fine Print section contains one or more important steps in the diagnostic process. Think of it this way: The prototype is useful for purposes of inclusion, whereas the boilerplate is useful largely for the also important exclusion of other disorders and delimitation from normal. The boilerplate verbiage includes several sorts of stereotyped phrases and warnings, which as an aid to memory I've dubbed *the D's*. (I started out by using "Don't disregard the D's" or similar phrases, but soon got tired of all the typing; so, I eventually adopted "the D's" as shorthand.) In any event, this boilerplate stuff is important: It forms part of the diagnostic requirements for the condition in question. Do not gloss over it.

> *Differential diagnosis.* Listed here are all the disorders to consider as alternatives when evaluating symptoms. In most cases, this list starts off with substance use disorders and general medical disorders, which despite their relative infrequence you should always place first on the list of disorders competing for your consideration. Next I put in those conditions that are most treatable, and hence should be addressed early. Only at the end do I include conditions that have a poor prognosis, or that you can't do very much to treat. I call this the *safety principle* of differential diagnosis.
>
> There are some disorders that DSM-5-TR lists right in the diagnostic criteria

themselves. These, I have emphasized with **bold print.** Conditions mentioned in the text I have also mentioned, but not emphasized.

Distress or disability. Most DSM-5-TR diagnostic criteria sets require that the patient experience distress or some form of impairment (for work, social interactions, interpersonal relations, or something else). The purpose is to ensure that we discriminate people who are patients from those who, while diagnostically normal, perhaps have lives with interesting aspects.

The word *distress* is explained exactly once in all of DSM-5-TR. DSM-IV didn't define the term anywhere; Campbell's *Psychiatric Dictionary* doesn't even list it. The DSM-5-TR sections on trichotillomania and excoriation (hair-pulling and skin-picking disorders, respectively) both describe distress as including negative feelings such as embarrassment and forfeiture of control. It's unclear, however, whether the same definition is employed anywhere else, or what might be the dominant thinking throughout the manual. But for me, some combination of pain, anxiety, and suffering works pretty well as a definition.

Duration. Many disorders require that symptoms be present for a certain minimum length of time before they can be ruled in. Again, this is to ensure that we don't go around indiscriminately handing out diagnoses. For example, nearly everyone will feel blue or down at one time or another. To qualify for a diagnosis of a depressive disorder, however, symptoms must last for at least a couple of weeks.

Demographics. A few disorders are limited to certain age spans, genders, or cultural groups.

Definitions. I have tried to provide definitions of all the terms needed to evaluate and diagnose patients with mental disorders. Mostly, those definitions are sprinkled into the text as needed. In the index I use *italicized* page numbers to locate those definitions—a sort of distributed glossary.

Specifiers. Many DSM-5-TR diagnoses aren't content to sit there by themselves; they want us to modify them in some way when we write them down. They indicate ways in which we clinicians, after settling on a diagnosis, must make further judgments about a patient's symptoms or course of illness, to cram as much information as possible into the final diagnostic product. Don't worry: After you've read a few, you'll get the idea.

Coding Notes. Many of the Essential Features sections conclude with guidance on coding, which supplies additional information about specifiers, subtypes, severity, and other subjects relevant to the disorder in question. I've occasionally included a signpost pointing to a discussion of principles you can use to determine that a disorder is caused by using substances.

Sidebars. To underscore or augment what you need to know, I have sprinkled additional bits of information throughout the text (such as the sidebar about *distress* that you just read). Some of these merely highlight information that will help you make a diagnosis quickly. Some contain historical information and other sidelights about diagnoses that I've found interesting. Many include editorial asides—my opinions about patients, the diagnostic process, and clinical matters in general.

Vignettes. I have based this book on that reliable device, the clinical vignette. As a student, I found that I often had trouble recalling the features of disorders. But once I had evaluated and treated a patient, I always had a mental image to help me remember important points about symptoms and differential diagnosis. I hope that the more than 130 patients described in *DSM-5-TR Made Easy* will do the same for you.

Evaluation. This section summarizes my thinking for each patient I've written into a vignette. I explain how the patient fits the diagnostic criteria and why I think other diagnoses are unlikely. Sometimes I suggest that additional history or medical or psychological testing should be obtained before a final diagnosis is given. The conclusions stated here allow you to compare your thinking to mine. There are two ways you can do this. One is by picking out from the vignette the Essential Features I've listed for each diagnosis. But so that you can follow the thinking of the folks who wrote the actual DSM-5-TR, I've also included references (in parentheses) to the official criteria. If you disagree with any of my interpretations, I hope you'll email me (*morrjame@ohsu.edu*).

Final diagnosis. Code numbers can be assigned by clinicians or support staff. To guide staff on how to proceed, we need to put all the diagnostic material that seems relevant into language that conforms to the approved format. The final diagnoses included in the book not only explain how I'd code each patient, but also provide models to use in writing up the diagnoses for your own patients.

Tables. I've included several tables to provide an overall picture of certain topics—specifiers that apply across different diagnoses, a list of physical disorders that can produce emotional and behavioral symptoms, and more. Tables that are of principal use in a given chapter appear in that chapter. A few, which apply more generally throughout the book, you'll find in the Appendix. Some of these tables are complicated, but they consolidate into one place information that you'd have to read page after page in DSM-5-TR to unearth.

My writing. Throughout, I've tried to use language that is clear and simple. Clinically relevant information is written in declarative sentences that describe what you need to know in diagnosing a patient. My goal has been to make the material sound as though it was written by a clinician to use for patients, not by a lawyer to brandish in court. Wherever I've failed, I hope you will email me to let me know. I'll try to put it right in a future edition.

Structure of *DSM-5-TR Made Easy*

The first 18 chapters* of this book contain descriptions and criteria for the major mental diagnoses and personality disorders. Chapter 19 comprises information concerning other terms that you may find useful. Many of these are Z-codes, which are conditions that are not mental disorders but may require clinical attention anyway. Most noteworthy are the problems people with no actual mental disorder have in relating to one another. (Occasionally, you might even list a Z-code as the reason a patient was referred for evaluation.) Also described here are codes that indicate medications' effects, malingering, and the need for more diagnostic information.

Chapter 20 contains a very brief description of diagnostic principles, followed by some additional case vignettes, which are generally more complicated than those presented earlier in the book. I've annotated these cases to help you review the diagnostic principles and criteria covered previously. Of course, I could include only a fraction of all DSM-5-TR diagnoses in this section.

Quirks

Here are comments regarding some of my idiosyncrasies.

Abbreviations. I can think of two disorders that are sometimes abbreviated CD and four that are sometimes (though not all by me) abbreviated SAD, so always watch for context.

And, I'll cop to manufacturing nonstandard abbreviations, especially for the names of disorders. For example, BPsD (for brief psychotic disorder) isn't something you'll read elsewhere, certainly nowhere official. I've used it and others for the sake of shortening things up just a bit, and perhaps reducing ever so slightly the amount of time it takes to read all this stuff. I generally use these ad hoc abbreviations just in the sections about specific disorders, so don't worry about having to remember them when you are elsewhere in the book. A couple of exceptions: PTSD, OCD, and ADHD are so familiar they beg to be abbreviated in any context.

My thirst for brevity has also extended to chapter titles. In the service of seeming inclusive, DSM-5-TR has sometimes overcomplicated these names, in my view. So, you'll find that I've occasionally (but not always—I've got *my* obsessive–compulsive disorder under control!) shortened them up a bit for convenience. You shouldn't have any problem knowing where to turn for sleep disorders (which DSM-5-TR calls *sleep–wake disorders*), mood disorders (*bipolar and related disorders* plus *depressive disorders*), psychotic (*schizophrenia spectrum and other psychotic*) disorders, cognitive (*neurocog-*

---

*OK, I cheated a little. DSM-5-TR actually has 19 chapters, but for ease of description, I combined the two mood disorder chapters into one (which is how DSM-IV presented them). However, no confusion should result: DSM-5-TR doesn't number its chapters.

nitive) disorders, substance (*substance-related and addictive*) disorders, eating (*feeding and eating*) disorders, and various other categories from which I've simply dropped *and related* from the official titles. Similarly, I've often dropped the */medication* from *substance/medication-induced* [*just about anything*].

{Curly braces}. I've used these in the Essential Features and in some tables to indicate two mutually exclusive specifier choices, such as {with}{without} good prognostic features (for schizophreniform disorder). Again, I do this just to shorten things up a bit.

Prevalence. Wow!—prevalence figures are all over the map. Sometimes we're given 12-month prevalence, sometimes lifetime; figures may be given for different age groups; sometimes they are broken down by age, gender, race, nationality, and ethnic group. I've tried to provide the best consensus ballpark figures I can muster, but if you want finer detail, consult texts and research studies.

Severity specifiers. One of my issues with DSM-5-TR is its use of complicated severity specifiers that differ from one chapter to another, and sometimes from one disorder to the next. Some of these are easier to use than others.

For example, for the psychoses, we are offered the Clinician-Rated Dimensions of Psychosis Symptom Severity, which asks us to rate on a 5-point scale, based on the past 7 days, each of eight symptoms (the five psychosis symptoms of schizophrenia [p. 58] plus impaired cognition, depression, and mania); there is no overall score, only the eight individual components, which we are encouraged to rate again every few days. My biggest complaint about this scale, apart from its complexity and the time required, is that it tells us little about overall functioning—only the degree to which the patient experiences each of the eight symptoms. Helpfully, DSM-5-TR informs us that we are allowed to rate the patient "without using this severity specifier," an option that many clinicians will surely rush to embrace.

Evaluating functionality. Whatever happened to the Global Assessment of Functioning (GAF)? In use from DSM-III-R through DSM-IV-TR, the GAF was a 100-point scale that reflected the patient's overall occupational, psychological, and social functioning—but not physical limitations or environmental problems. The scale specified symptoms and behavioral guidelines to help us determine our patients' GAF scores. Perhaps because of the subjectivity inherent in this scale, its greatest usefulness lay in tracking changes in a given patient's level of functioning across time. (Another problem: It was a mash-up of severity, disability, suicidality, and symptoms.)

However, the GAF is now GONE, eliminated for several reasons (as described in a 2013 talk by Dr. William Narrow, who was then research director for the DSM-5 Task Force). Dr. Narrow accurately pointed out that the GAF mixed concepts (psychosis with suicidal ideas, for example) and that it had problems with interrater reliability. Furthermore, what's really wanted is a disability rating that helps us understand how well a patient can fulfill occupational and social responsibilities, as well as generally participate in society. For that, the Task Force recommends the World Health Organization Disability Assessment Schedule, Version 2.0 (WHODAS 2.0), which was developed for use with clinical as well as general populations and has been tested worldwide. DSM-5-TR gives it beginning on page 856; it can also be found online (*www.who.int/classifications/icf/whodasii/en*). WHODAS 2.0 is scored as follows: 1 = none, 2 = mild, 3 = moderate, 4 = severe, and 5 = extreme. Note that scoring systems for the two measures are reciprocal; a high GAF score equates with a low WHODAS 2.0 rating.

After quite a bit of experimentation, it appears to me that the WHODAS 2.0 is so heavily weighted toward physical abilities that it poorly reflects the qualities mental health clinicians are interested in. Some of the most severely ill mental patients received a moderate WHODAS 2.0 score; for example, Velma Dean (p. 91) would score 20 on the GAF but 1.6 on the WHODAS 2.0. In addition, calculating the WHODAS 2.0 score depends on the answers given by the patient (or clinician) to 36 questions—a burden of data collection that many busy professionals will not be able to fulfill. And, because these answers cover conditions over the previous month, the score cannot accurately represent patients with rapidly evolving mental disorders.

So, I've decided not to recommend the WHODAS 2.0 after all. (Anyone interested in further discussion can write to me; I'll be happy to send along a chart comparing the GAF with the WHODAS 2.0 for most of the patients mentioned in this book.) Rather, here's my fix for evaluating function and severity, and it's the final quirk I'll mention: Go ahead and use the GAF. Nothing says that we can't, and sometimes I find it useful for tracking a patient's progress through treatment. It's quick, easy (OK, it's *still* subjective), and free. You can specify the patient's current level of functioning, or the highest level in any past time frame. You'll find the GAF in the Appendix of this book.

Using This Book

There are several ways in which you might use *DSM-5-TR Made Easy*.

Studying a disorder. Of course, you can go about this in several ways, but here's how I'd do it. Scan the introductory information for some background, then read the vignette. Next, compare the information in the vignette to the Essential Features, to assure yourself that you can pick out what's important diagnostically. If you want to see how well the vignettes fit the actual DSM-5-TR criteria, read through the vignette evaluations where I touched upon each of the important diagnostic points. In each evaluation section, you'll also find a discussion of the differential diagnosis, as well as some other conditions often found in association with the disorder in question.

Evaluating a patient whose diagnosis you think you know. Read through the Essential Features, then check the information you have on this patient against the prototype. If you wish, you can assign a 1–5 score, using the key given earlier (p. 3). Carefully consider the D's to make sure you've thought about all disqualifying information and relevant alternative diagnoses. If all's well and you've hit the mark, you might then read through the evaluation section of the relevant vignette, just to make sure you've understood the criteria. Then you could check the introductory material for background.

Evaluating a new patient. Follow the sequence just given, with one exception: After identifying one of several areas of clinical interest as a diagnostic possibility—let's say it's an anxiety disorder—you could start with the Quick Guide in the relevant chapter. There you will find capsule statements (too brief even to be called summaries) that point to one or more disorders to consider further. Some patients will have problems in several areas, so you might need to explore several chapters to select all of the right diagnoses. Chapter 20 provides some additional pointers on diagnostic strategy.

Getting the broader view. Finally, there are a lot of disorders out there. Many will be familiar to you, but for others your information may be a little sketchy. So just reading through the book to hit the high points (perhaps sampling the vignettes) may load your quiver with a few new diagnostic arrows. I hope that eventually you'll read the entire book. Besides introducing you to a lot of mental disorders, you'll also gain a feel for how a diagnostician might approach an array of clinical problems.

Whatever course you take, I recommend that you limit your reading to a few disorders at a time. I have done my best to simplify the criteria and to explain the reasoning behind them. But if you overload yourself with too many diagnoses, they'll probably begin to run together in your mind.

Code Numbers

The current coding system is that of the tenth edition of the *International Classification of Diseases* or ICD-10.* These codes are much more complete than was true for previous iterations. That serves us well for accurate identification, retrieval of data for research, and other informational purposes. But it increases the number of, well, numbers we must be familiar with. Mostly, I've tried to include what you need to know along with the diagnostic information associated with each disorder discussed. Some of this information is so extensive and complex that I have condensed it into one or two

---

*Technically, this ICD version is called ICD-10-CM (the CM stands for *clinical modification*). I'll use the CM version here, but for the sake of simplicity, I refer to it as just ICD-10. You can find this information online at *www.icd10data.com/ICD10CM/Codes*.

tables. Most notable is Table 15.2 in Chapter 15, which gives the ICD-10 code numbers for substance-related mental disorders. I've now updated coding and other material to reflect ICD-10 and DSM-5-TR usage as of 2022.

Using the DSM-5-TR Classification System

After decades of using five axes on which to record the biopsychosocial assessment of our patients, DSM-5 took a bold step and reversed course. Now all mental, personality, and physical disorders are recorded in the same place, with the principal diagnosis mentioned first. (The *principal diagnosis* is the one most responsible for the current outpatient visit or hospital admission.) When you've made a "due to" diagnosis (such as catatonic disorder due to tuberous sclerosis), the ICD convention is to list first the physical disease process. The actual reason for the visit comes second, with the parenthetical statement (reason for visit or principal diagnosis) appended. I'm not sure just how often clinicians will adhere to this convention. Many will reason, I suspect, that this is a medical records issue for support staff to address and pay it no further mind. In any event, here is how you can write up the diagnosis.

Obviously, you need to record every mental diagnosis. Nearly every patient will have at least one of these, and many will have two or more. For example, imagine that you have a patient with two diagnoses: bipolar I disorder and alcohol use disorder. (Note, incidentally, that I've followed DSM-5-TR's refreshing style, which is to abandon the practice of capitalizing the names of specific diagnoses.)

First list the diagnosis most responsible for the current evaluation. Suppose that, while evaluating the social anxiety disorder, you discover that your patient has also been drinking enough alcohol to qualify for a diagnosis of mild alcohol use disorder. Then the diagnosis should read:

F40.10   Social anxiety disorder
F10.10   Alcohol use disorder, mild

In this example, the first diagnosis will have to be social anxiety disorder (that's why the patient sought treatment). Of course, if the alcohol use is what prompted the evaluation, you'd reverse the positions of the two diagnoses.

DSM-IV required a separate location (the notorious Axis II) for personality disorders and what back then was called mental retardation. The purpose was to give special status to these lifelong attributes and to help ensure that they would not be ignored as we deal with our patients' often more pressing major pathology. But though the motive was noble, the logic was not impeccable, and the rest of the world was moving on. So, DSM has let the axes fall, so to speak. Personality disorders and intellectual developmental disorder are included right along with all other diagnoses, mental and physical. Overall, I think this is a good thing, but it also means that we must now place material such as a patient's GAF score (or WHODAS 2.0 rating) and general medical disorders in the body of a summary statement.

An Uncertain Diagnosis

When you're not sure whether a diagnosis is correct, consider using the DSM-5-TR qualifier *(provisional)*. This term may be appropriate if you believe that a certain diagnosis is correct, but you lack sufficient history to support your impression. Or perhaps it is still early in your patient's illness, and you expect that more symptoms will develop shortly. Or you may be waiting for laboratory tests to confirm the presence of another medical condition that you suspect underlies the mental illness. Any of these situations could warrant a provisional diagnosis. Three DSM-5-TR diagnoses—schizophreniform psychosis, brief psychotic disorder, premenstrual dysphoric disorder—should have *(provisional)* appended if the course is not yet clear. But you could use this term in just about any situation where it seems that safe diagnostic practice warrants it.

What about a patient who comes very close to meeting full criteria, who has been ill for a long time, who has responded to treatment appropriate for the diagnosis, and who has a family history of the same disorder? Such a patient deserves a definitive diagnosis, even though the criteria are not quite met. (Hey, even DSM-5-TR, in its introductory material, acknowledges that we will need to give a diagnosis to some patients who fall a little short of meeting full requirements, if symptoms are severe and persistent.)

So, for these and other reasons, I've gone over to the use of prototypes. After all, diagnoses are not decided by the criteria; diagnoses are decided by clinicians, who use criteria as guidelines. That's *guidelines,* as in "help you," not *shackles,* as in "restrain you."

DSM-5-TR provides another way to list a diagnosis that seems uncertain: "Other specified [name of] disorder." This allows you to write down the name of the category along with the specific reason the patient doesn't meet criteria for the diagnosis. For example, a patient who has a massive hoard of useless material in the house, but who has suffered no distress or disability, could be recorded as "other specified hoarding disorder, lack of distress or impairment."

I'll bet we'd both be interested to learn just how often this option gets exercised.

Indicating Severity of a Disorder

DSM-5-TR includes specific severity specifiers for many diagnoses. They are generally self-explanatory, and I've usually tried to boil them down just a bit, for the sake of your sanity and mine. In one or two places (I'm talking about you, Schizophrenia Spectrum and Other Psychotic Disorders), I've recommend against using specific severity schemes that seem too cumbersome.

Other Specifiers

Many disorders include specifiers indicating a wide variety of information—with (or without) certain defined accompanying symptoms; current degrees of remission; and course features such as early (or late) onset or recovery, either partial or full. Some of these specifiers require additional code numbers; some are just additional tacked-on verbiage. Add as many of these as seem appropriate. Each could help the next clinician understand that patient just a little better.

Physical Conditions and Disorders

Physical illness may have a direct bearing on the patient's mental diagnoses; this is especially true of the cognitive disorders. In other cases, physical illness may affect (or be affected by) the management of a mental disorder. An example would be hypertension in a patient with psychosis who believes that the medication has been poisoned. (Some of this stuff is formalized in the diagnosis of psychological factors affecting other mental conditions; p. 270.) In any event, whereas physical disorders used to have their own axis, that's no longer the case, either. In fact, the ICD-10 recording scheme requires that when a mental disorder is due to a physical condition, list first the physical condition itself.

Psychosocial and Environmental Problems

You can report certain environmental or other psychosocial events or conditions that might affect the diagnosis or management of your patient. These may have been caused by the mental disorder, or they may be independent events. DSM-5-TR requires that we use the ICD-10 Z-codes for this sort of problem. In Chapter 19 I've given a reasonably complete list of available Z-codes. When stating them, be as specific as possible. You'll find plenty of examples scattered throughout the text.

Just What Is a Mental Disorder?

There are many definitions of *mental disorder,* none of them both accurate and complete. Perhaps this is because no one yet has adequately defined the term *abnormal.* (Does it mean that the patient is uncomfortable? Then many patients with manic episodes are not abnormal. Is abnormal that which is unusual? Then people with genius-level intelligence are abnormal.)

The authors of DSM-5-TR provide the definition of mental disorder they used to help them decide whether to include a diagnosis in their book. Paraphrased, here it is:

> A *mental disorder* is a clinically important collection of symptoms (these can be behavioral, emotional, or psychological) that usually causes the person distress or disability in social, personal, or occupational functioning.

The symptoms of any disorder must be more than an expected reaction to an everyday event, such as the death of a relative. Behaviors that primarily reflect a conflict between the individual and society (for example, fanatical religious or political ideology) are not usually considered mental disorders.

I'd like to add these further points about the criteria for mental disorders:

1. Mental disorders describe processes, not people. This point is made explicit to address the fears of some clinicians that by using the criteria, they are somehow pigeonholing people. Patients with the same diagnosis will differ from one another in many important aspects, including symptoms, personality, other diagnoses they may have, life experiences, and the many other distinctive aspects of their personal lives that may have nothing at all to do with their emotional or behavioral condition.

2. To a degree, some of what's abnormal, and of course far more that isn't, is shaped by an individual's culture. For example, in *nervios* ("nerves"), often found in Latinx cultures in the Americas, people experience themselves as vulnerable to a variety of physical and emotional symptoms (such as problems of anxiety, mood, and somatic symptoms). Increasingly, we are learning to take such cultural background into account when defining disorders and evaluating patients. Indeed, DSM-5-TR provides enhanced emphasis on culture throughout the text.

3. Don't assume always to find sharp boundaries between disorders, or between any disorder and so-called normality. For example, the criteria for bipolar I and bipolar II disorders clearly set these two disorders off from one another and from people who have neither. But in reality, all bipolar conditions (and probably lots of others) will likely fit somewhere along a continuum. With our criteria (Essential Features) and with our experience, we do our best to determine which patients require which diagnosis.

4. The essential difference between a physical condition such as pneumonia or diabetes, and mental disorders like schizophrenia and bipolar I disorder, is that we know what causes pneumonia and diabetes. However, either of those two mental disorders could turn out to have a tangible basis; perhaps we just haven't found it yet. In operational terms, the difference between physical disorders and mental disorders is that the former are the subjects of neither DSM-5-TR nor *DSM-5-TR Made Easy*.

5. Basically, DSM-5-TR follows the medical model of illness. By this, I don't mean that it recommends the prescription of medication; rather, I mean that it is a descriptive work derived (largely) from scientific studies of groups of patients who appear to have a great deal in common, including symptoms, signs, and life course of their disease. Inclusion is further justified by follow-up studies show-

ing that members of these groups have a predictable course of illness months, or sometimes years, down the road.

6. With a few exceptions, DSM-5-TR makes no assumptions about the etiology of most of these disorders. This is the famous "atheoretical approach" that has been much praised and criticized. Of course, most clinicians would agree about the cause of some mental disorders (neurocognitive disorder due to Huntington's disease and PTSD come to mind). The descriptions of the majority of DSM-5-TR diagnoses will be well accepted by clinicians whose philosophical perspectives include social and learning theory, psychodynamics, and psychopharmacology.

Some Warnings

In defining mental health disorders, several warnings seem worth repeating:

1. The fact that the manual omits a disorder is no indication that it doesn't exist. Right up to the present, the number of listed mental disorders has increased with each new edition of the DSM. Depending on how you measure these things, DSM-5-TR may appear to be an exception. On the one hand, it contains close to 600 codable conditions—nearly double the number included in DSM-IV.* On the other hand, DSM-5-TR contains, by my count, 156 main diagnoses, an overall reduction of about 9%; this feat was achieved by lumping conditions under one title (as occurred, for example, in the sleep–wake disorders chapter). However, there are undoubtedly still more conditions out there, waiting to be discovered. Prepare to invest in DSM-6 and *DSM-6 Made Easy*.

2. Diagnosis isn't for amateurs. Owning a set of prototypes is no substitute for professional training in interview techniques, evaluation, and the many other skills that a mental health clinician needs. DSM-5-TR states—and I agree— that diagnosis consists in more than just ticking the boxes on a bunch of symptoms. It requires education, training, patience, and yes, patients (that is, the experience of evaluating many mental health patients).

3. DSM-5-TR may not be uniformly applicable to all cultures. These criteria are derived largely from studies of North American and European patients. Although the DSMs have been widely used with great success throughout the world, it is not assured that mental disorders largely described by North American and European clinicians will translate perfectly to other languages and

---

*To be fair, the vast bulk of the increase is due not to new disorders, but to ever-thinner slices of the original pie, served up with new codes that reflect DSM-5-TR's—and ICD-10's—finer diagnostic distinctions. Especially well represented are the now nearly 300 variations on "substance/medication-induced this or that."

other cultures. We should be wary of diagnosing pathology in patients who express beliefs that may be widely held in ethnic or other subcultures but are unfamiliar to a clinician whose background is different from theirs. An example would be a belief in witches once prevalent among certain Native Americans— not to mention early American settlers. Beginning on page 859 of DSM-5-TR, you'll find a list of specific cultural syndromes.

4. DSM-5-TR doesn't have the force of law. Its authors recognize that the definitions used by the judicial system are often at odds with scientific requirements. Thus, having a DSM-5-TR mental disorder may not exempt a patient from punishment or other legal restrictions on behavior.

5. This information isn't set in stone. During the final editing process, an update was issued detailing many changes in how we label and code the cognitive disorders, so I scrambled to rewrite Chapter 16. We need to be alert for similar changes that may occur in the future.

6. Finally, the diagnostic manual is only as good as the people who use it. Late in his career, George Winokur, one of my favorite professors in medical school (and my first boss after I completed training), co-wrote a brief paper* that discussed how well the DSM (at that time, it was DSM-III) assured consistency of diagnosis. Even among clinicians at the same institution with similar diagnostic approaches, it turned out, there were problems. Winokur et al. especially called attention to the amount of time expended on making a mental health diagnosis, to systematic misinterpretations of criteria, and to nonsystematic misreadings of the criteria. They concluded, "The Bible may tell us so, but the criteria don't. They are better than what we had, but they are still a long way from perfect." In DSM-5-TR, those statements remain true.

The Patients

Some of the patients I've described in the vignettes are composites of several people I have known. But most, frankly, I just made up to illustrate a diagnosis. In every instance (except the very few in which I have used historical persons with documented backgrounds), I have tweaked the vital information to protect identities, to provide additional details, and sometimes just to add interest. Of course, the vignettes do not present all of the features of the diagnoses they are meant to illustrate, but then, hardly any patient does. Rather, my intention has been to convey the flavor of each disorder.

Although I have provided over 130 vignettes and other descriptions to cover most mental disorders, you'll notice some omissions. For one thing, to illustrate every possible substance-related mood, psychotic, and anxiety disorder would require a book

---

*Winokur G, Zimmerman M, Cadoret R: 'Cause the Bible tells me so. *Arch Gen Psychiatry* 1988; 45(7): 683–684.

twice the length of this one. For disorders that begin in early life (Chapter 1), I have included vignettes and discussion only for those conditions likely also to be encountered in an adult. Specifically, these are intellectual developmental disorder, attention-deficit/hyperactivity disorder, autism spectrum disorder, and Tourette's disorder. However, you will find prototypes and brief introductory discussions for all disorders that begin during the neurodevelopmental period. *DSM-5-TR Made Easy* therefore contains diagnostic material pertinent to all DSM-5-TR mental disorders.

And Finally...

On my website I will try to keep up with the changes in DSM-5-TR criteria and coding. Visit *www.jamesmorrisonmd.org* for more information.

CHAPTER 1

Neurodevelopmental Disorders

Prior to DSM-5, the name of this chapter was even more of a mouthful: "Disorders Usually First Evident in Infancy, Childhood, or Adolescence." With the focus on the individual during the formative period of the nervous system, the name *neurodevelopmental* seems logical and appropriate. However, *DSM-5-TR Made Easy* emphasizes the evaluation of older patients—later adolescence to maturity and beyond. For that reason, I've taken some liberties in arranging the conditions discussed in this chapter—placing at the beginning those to be discussed at length and listing later those where I provide just prototypes and limited discussion.

Of course, many of the disorders considered in subsequent chapters can be first encountered in children or young adolescents; anorexia nervosa and schizophrenia are two examples that spring to mind. Conversely, many of the disorders discussed in this chapter can continue to cause problems for years after a child has grown up. But only a few commonly preoccupy clinicians who treat adults. For the remainder of the disorders DSM-5-TR includes in its first chapter, I provide introductions and Essential Features, but no illustrative case example.

Quick Guide to the Neurodevelopmental Disorders

In every Quick Guide, the page number following each item refers to the point at which discussion begins. Also mentioned below, just as in any other competent differential diagnosis, are various conditions arising in early life that are discussed in other chapters.

Autism Spectrum and Intellectual Developmental Disorder

Intellectual developmental disorder. This condition usually begins in infancy; people with it have low intelligence that causes them to need special help in coping with life (p. 20).

Borderline intellectual functioning. This term indicates persons nominally ranked in the IQ range of 71–84 who do not have the coping problems associated with intellectual developmental disorder (p. 616).

Autism spectrum disorder. From early childhood, the patient has impaired social interactions and communications, and shows stereotyped behaviors and interests (p. 26).

Global developmental delay. Use when a child under the age of 5 seems to be falling behind developmentally but you cannot reliably assess the degree (p. 26).

Unspecified intellectual developmental disorder. Use when a child at least 5 years old cannot be reliably assessed, perhaps due to physical or mental impairment (p. 26).

Communication and Learning Disorders

Language disorder. A child's delay in using spoken and written language is characterized by limited vocabulary, grammatically incorrect sentences, or trouble understanding words or sentences (p. 46).

Social (pragmatic) communication disorder. Despite adequate vocabulary and the ability to create sentences, these patients have trouble with the practical use of language; their conversational interactions tend to be inappropriate (p. 49).

Speech sound disorder. Difficulty producing the sounds of normal speech limits the patient's ability to be understood (p. 47).

Childhood-onset fluency disorder (stuttering). The normal fluency of speech is frequently disrupted (p. 48).

Selective mutism. A child chooses not to talk, except when alone or with select intimates. DSM-5-TR lists this as an anxiety disorder (p. 186).

Specific learning disorder. This may involve problems with reading (p. 50), mathematics (p. 50), or written expression (p. 50).

Academic or educational problems. These Z-codes are used when a scholastic problem (other than a learning disorder) is the focus of treatment (p. 608).

Unspecified communication disorder. Use for communication problems where you haven't enough information to make a specific diagnosis (p. 50).

Tic and Motor Disorders

Developmental coordination disorder. The patient is slow to develop motor coordination; some also have attention-deficit/hyperactivity disorder or learning disorders (p. 43).

Stereotypic movement disorder. Patients repeatedly rock, bang their heads, bite themselves, or pick at their own skin or body orifices (p. 44).

Tourette's disorder. Multiple vocal and motor tics occur frequently throughout the day in these patients (p. 39).

Persistent (chronic) motor or vocal tic disorder. A patient has either motor or vocal tics, but not both (p. 43).

Provisional tic disorder. Tics occur for no longer than 1 year (p. 42).

Other specified, or unspecified, tic disorder. Use one of these categories for tics that do not meet the criteria for any of the preceding (p. 43).

Attention-Deficit and Disruptive Behavior Disorders

Attention-deficit/hyperactivity disorder. In this common condition (usually abbreviated as ADHD), patients are hyperactive, impulsive, or inattentive, and often all three (p. 33).

Oppositional defiant disorder. Multiple examples of negativistic behavior persist for at least 6 months (p. 388).

Conduct disorder. A child persistently violates rules or the rights of others (p. 389).

Disorders of Eating, Sleeping, and Elimination

Pica. The patient eats material that is not food (p. 293).

Rumination disorder. There is persistent regurgitation and chewing of food already eaten (p. 294).

Encopresis. At age 4 years or later, the patient repeatedly passes feces into clothing or onto the floor (p. 300).

Enuresis. At age 5 years or later, there is repeated voiding of urine (it can be voluntary or involuntary) into bedding or clothing (p. 298).

Non–rapid eye movement sleep arousal disorder, sleep terror type. During the first part of the night, these patients cry out in apparent fear. Often they don't really wake up at all. This behavior is considered pathological only in adults, not children (p. 339).

Other Disorders or Conditions That Begin in the Developmental Period

Parent–child relational problem. One of these Z-codes is used when there is no mental disorder, but a child and parent have problems getting along, for example, overprotection or inconsistent discipline (p. 606).

Sibling relational problem. Z62.891 is used for difficulties between siblings (p. 606).

Problems related to abuse or neglect. A variety of Z-codes can be used to cover difficulties that arise from neglect or from physical or sexual abuse of children (p. 613).

Disruptive mood dysregulation disorder. A child's mood is persistently negative between severe temper outbursts (p. 149).

Separation anxiety disorder. The patient becomes anxious when apart from parent or away from home (p. 187).

Posttraumatic stress disorder in preschool children. Children repeatedly relive a severely traumatic event, such as a car accident, natural disaster, or war (p. 218).

Disinhibited social engagement and reactive attachment disorders. There is evidence of pathogenic care in a child who habitually doesn't seek comfort from parents or who fails to show expected reticence in the company of strangers (p. 235).

Gender dysphoria in children. A boy or girl wants to be of the other gender (p. 399).

Factitious disorder imposed on another. A caregiver induces symptoms in someone else, usually a child, with no intention of material gain (p. 273).

Other specified, or unspecified, neurodevelopmental disorder. These categories serve for patients whose difficulties don't fulfill criteria for one of the above disorders (p. 54).

Intellectual Developmental Disorder and Autism Spectrum Disorder

Intellectual Developmental Disorder

Individuals with intellectual developmental disorder (IDD), at one time called mental retardation, have two sorts of problem, one resulting from the other. First, there's a fundamental deficit in their ability to think. This will be some combination of difficulties with abstract thinking, judgment, planning, problem solving, reasoning, and general learning (whether from academic study or from experience). Overall intelligence level, as determined by a standard individual test (not one of the group tests, which tend to be less accurate), will be markedly below average. In practical terms, this generally means an IQ of less than 70. (For infants, we can only subjectively judge intellectual functioning.)

Most people with such a deficit need special help to cope, and this need defines the other major requirement for diagnosis: The patient's ability to adapt to the demands of everyday life—in school, at work, at home with family—must be impaired in some important way. We can break down adaptive functioning into three areas: (1) the conceptual (also referred to as the academic), which depends on language, math, reading, writing, reasoning, and memory to solve problems; (2) the social, which includes deploying such abilities as empathy, communication, awareness of the experiences of other people, social judgment, and self-regulation; and (3) the practical, which includes regulating behavior, organizing tasks, managing finances, and dealing with personal care and recreation. How well these adaptations succeed depends on the patient's education, job training, motivation, personality, support from significant others, and innate intelligence level.

By definition, IDD begins during the developmental years (childhood and adolescence). In most instances the onset is at the very beginning of this period—usually in infancy, often even before birth. If the behavior begins at age 18 or after, it is often called a neurocognitive disorder (NCD), which of course can coexist with IDD. Diagnostic assessment must be done with caution, especially in younger children whose other problems may interfere with accurate assessment. For example, a patient who can overcome a sensory impairment of hearing or vision may no longer appear intellectually challenged.

Various behavioral problems are commonly associated with IDD, but they don't constitute criteria for diagnosis. Among them are aggression, dependency, impulsivity, passivity, self-injury, stubbornness, low self-esteem, and poor frustration tolerance. Gullibility and naïveté can lead to risk for exploitation by others. Some patients with IDD also suffer from mood disorders (which often go undiagnosed), psychotic disorders, poor attention span, and hyperactivity. However, many are placid, loving, pleasant people whom relatives and associates find enjoyable to live with and befriend.

Although many people with IDD bear no evident distinguishing features, others have physical characteristics that even the untrained observer can notice. These include short stature, seizures, hemangiomas, and eyes, ears, and other parts of the face that bear distinctive shapes. A diagnosis of IDD is likely to be made earlier when there are associated physical abnormalities such as those associated with Down syndrome. IDD affects about 1% of the general population. Males outnumber females roughly 3:2.

The many causes of IDD include genetic abnormalities, chemical effects, structural brain damage, inborn errors of metabolism, and childhood disease. An individual's IDD may have biological or social causes, or both. Some of these etiologies (with the approximate percentages of all patients with IDD they represent) are given below. Note that the percentages are only approximate and the categories tend to flow into one another.

Genetic causes (about 5%). Trisomy 21 (Down syndrome), chromosomal abnormalities, Tay–Sachs, tuberous sclerosis.

Early pregnancy factors (about 30%). Maternal substance use, infections (e.g., rubella).

Later pregnancy and perinatal factors (about 10%). Prematurity, anoxia, birth trauma, fetal malnutrition.

Acquired childhood physical conditions (about 5%). Lead poisoning, infections, trauma.

Environmental influences and mental disorders (about 20%). Cultural deprivation, poverty.

No identifiable cause (about 30%).

Though measurement of intelligence no longer figures in the official DSM-5-TR criteria, in the Essential Features below I have included IQ ranges to provide some anchoring for the several severity specifiers. However, remember that the actual diagnosis given to any individual depends on adaptive functioning, not some number on a page.

Even individually administered IQ tests will have a few points of error. That's one reason why patients with measured IQs as high as 75 can sometimes be diagnosed as having IDD: They still have the problems with adaptive functioning that help define the condition. On the other hand, an occasional person with an IQ of less than 70 may function well enough not to qualify for this diagnosis. In addition, cultural differences, illness, and mental set can all affect the accuracy of IQ testing.

Interpretation of intelligence test scores must also consider the possibility of *scatter* (better performance on verbal tests than on performance tests, or the reverse), as well as physical, cultural, and emotional disabilities. These factors are not easy to judge; some test batteries may require the help of a skilled psychometrist. Such factors are among the reasons why definitions of IDD have moved away from relying solely on test results.

Essential Features of **Intellectual Developmental Disorder**

From their earliest years, people with IDD are in cognitive trouble. Actually, it's trouble of two sorts. First, as assessed both clinically and with formal testing, they have difficulty with intellectual tasks such as reasoning, making plans, thinking in the abstract, exercising judgment, solving problems, and learning from formal study or from life's experiences. Second, they experience difficulty modifying their behavior so they can become independent, socially accountable citizens. They require support to function adequately in the conceptual domain (defined below), social interactions, and practical living skills. These patients experience difficulty in at least one of these domains across multiple life areas—family, school, work, and social relations.

The Fine Print

Conceptual (academic) domain: Memory, use of language, reading and writing, mathematical reasoning, solving problems, judgment.

Social domain: Awareness of how others think and feel, ability to communicate, empathy, ability to make friends.

Practical domain: Self-care, workplace responsibilities, managing money, behavioral self-management—and many other factors.

Don't forget the D's: • Duration (from early childhood) • Differential diagnosis (autism spectrum disorder, cognitive disorders, borderline intellectual functioning, specific learning disorders, and communication disorders)

Coding Notes

Specify level of severity (and code numbers) according to descriptions below.

IQ ranges are stated only for points of reference; severity depends on level of adaptive functioning.

F70 Mild. As children, these individuals learn slowly and lag schoolmates, though they can be expected to attain roughly sixth-grade academic skills by the time they are adults. As they mature, deficiencies in judgment and solving problems cause them to require extra help managing everyday situations; personal relationships may suffer. They typically need help with such tasks as paying bills, shopping for groceries, and finding appropriate living accommodations. However, many can work independently, though at jobs that require relatively little cognitive involvement. Memory and the ability to use language can be quite good, but these patients become lost when confronted with metaphor or other examples of abstract thinking. IQ typically ranges from 50 to 70. They constitute 85% of all patients with IDD.

F71 Moderate. When they are small children, the differences these individuals have from nonaffected peers are marked and encompassing. Though they can learn to read, to do simple math, and to handle money, language use is slow to develop and remains relatively simple. Far more than is the case with mildly affected individuals, in early life they need help in learning to provide their own self-care and engage in household tasks. Relationships with others (even romantic ones) are possible, though they often don't recognize the cues that govern ordinary personal interaction. Although they require assistance with making decisions, they may be able to work (with help from supervisors and co-workers) at relatively undemanding jobs, typically in sheltered workshops. IQ will range from the high 30s to low 50s. They represent about 10% of all patients with IDD.

F72 Severe. Though these people may learn simple commands or instructions, communication skills are rudimentary (single words, some phrases). With guidance, they may be able to perform simple jobs. They can maintain personal relationships with relatives but require supervision for all activities; they need help dressing and with personal hygiene. IQs are in the low 20s to high 30s. They make up roughly 5% of the total of all patients with IDD.

F73 Profound. With limited speech and only rudimentary capacity for social interaction, these individuals may communicate largely through gestures. They rely completely on other people for their needs, including activities of daily living, though they may help with simple chores. Even so, they can enjoy relationships with close family and associates. Profound IDD usually results from a serious neurological disorder, which often carries with it sensory or motor disabilities. IQ ranges downward from the low 20s. About 1–2% of all patients with IDD are so profoundly affected.

Grover Peary

Grover Peary was born when his mother was only 15. Mercedes was an obese girl who hadn't realized she was pregnant until she was 6 months along. Even then, she didn't seek prenatal care. Born after 30 hours of hard labor, Grover hadn't breathed right away. After the delivery, Mercedes lost interest in him; he had been reared alternately by his grandmother and an aunt.

Grover walked at 20 months; he spoke his first words at age 2½ years. A pediatrician pronounced him "somewhat slow," so his grandmother enrolled him in an infant school for children with developmental disabilities. At the age of 7, he had done well enough to be mainstreamed at his local elementary school. Throughout the remainder of his school career, he worked with a special education teacher for 2 hours each day; otherwise, he attended regular classes. Individual testing when he was in the 4th and 10th grades pegged his IQ at 70 and 72.

Despite his disability, Grover loved school. He had learned to read by the time he was 8, and he spent much of his free time poring over books about geography and natural science. (He had a great deal of free time, especially at recess and lunch hour. He was clumsy and short for his age, and the other children routinely excluded him from their games.) At one time he wanted to become a geologist, but his teachers steered him into a general curriculum. He lived in a county that provided special education and training for individuals with IDD, so by the time he graduated, he had learned some manual skills and knew by heart the complicated local public transportation system. A job coach helped him to find work washing dishes at a restaurant in a downtown hotel—and to acquire the social skills necessary to maintain that job. The restaurant manager negotiated a bedroom for him in the hotel basement.

Living at the hotel, he didn't need much money—his room and food were covered, and the tiny dish room where he worked didn't require much of a wardrobe. The waitresses often gave Grover a few dollars out of their tips, which he spent on his CD collection and going to baseball games. His aunt, who saw him every week, helped him with grooming and reminded him to shave. She and her husband also took him to the ballpark; otherwise, he would have spent nearly all of his free time in his room, listening to music and reading magazines.

When Grover was 28, an earthquake hit the city where he lived. Badly damaged, the hotel closed without notice. Thrown out of work, Grover's fellow employees were too busy with their own families to think about him. With his aunt out of town on vacation, he had nowhere to turn. It was summertime, so he placed the few possessions he had rescued in a heavy-duty lawn and leaf bag and walked the streets until he grew tired; he then rolled out some blankets in the park. He slept this way for nearly 2 weeks, eating what he could scrounge from other campers. Although FEMA workers had been sent to help those hit by the earthquake, Grover did not realize he could request relief. Finally, a park ranger recognized his plight and referred him to the mental health clinic.

During the interview, Grover's shaggy hair and thin face add years to his appearance. Dressed in a soiled shirt and baggy pants—they look like someone's castoffs—he sits quietly in his chair and gives little eye contact. He speaks hesitantly at first, but he is clear and coherent, and eventually he communicates quite well with the interviewer. (However, much of the background information is obtained later from old school records and from his aunt, when she returns from vacation.)

Grover's mood is surprisingly good, and totally appropriate to the topic of conversation. He smiles when he talks about his aunt but looks serious when he is asked where he plans to stay. He has no delusions, hallucinations, obsessions, compulsions, or phobias. He denies having any panic attacks, though he admits he feels "sorta worried" about sleeping in the park.

Grover scores 25 out of 30 on the Mini-Mental State Exam (MMSE). He is oriented except to month and day of the week; with a great deal of effort subtracting sevens, he finally gets two correct. He can recall three objects after 5 minutes and manages a perfect score on the language section. He recognizes that he has a problem of finding a place to live, but aside from asking his aunt, he hasn't the slightest idea how to begin.

Evaluation of Grover Peary

Before the hotel closed, Grover had a place to live, food to eat, and activities to occupy him. Although his aunt would occasionally have to remind him about shaving and keeping his clothing presentable, had he been evaluated then, he might not have fully met the criteria for IDD. Despite low scores on at least two IQ tests (criterion A in DSM-5-TR), he was functioning pretty well in a highly, if informally, structured environment.

When his support system quite literally collapses, Grover cannot cope with the change. He doesn't make use of the resources available to others who have lost their homes. He is also unable to find work; only through the attentiveness and generosity of others does he manage even to eat—overall, a clear deficit of adaptive functioning (B). Of course, his condition has existed since early childhood (C). Therefore, despite an IQ that hovers in the low 70s, he seems impaired enough to warrant the diagnosis of IDD. Note that Grover comfortably matches the prototype for mild IDD.

The differential diagnosis of IDD includes a variety of learning and communication disorders, which are presented later in this chapter. Major neurocognitive disorder in DSM-5-TR would have been diagnosed if Grover's cognitive issues represented a marked decline from a previous level of functioning. (NCD and IDD sometimes coexist, though they can be difficult to tease apart.) At his intellectual level, Grover might be diagnosed as having borderline intellectual functioning were it not for his obvious difficulties in coping with life.

Youngsters and adults with IDD often have associated mental disorders, which include attention-deficit/hyperactivity disorder and autism spectrum disorder; these conditions can exist concurrently. Mood and anxiety disorders are often present, though clinicians may not recognize them without adequate collateral information. Personality traits such as stubbornness are also sometimes noted. Patients with IDD may have physical conditions such as epilepsy and cerebral palsy. As they approach middle age, people with Down syndrome may be at special risk for developing major neurocognitive disorder due to Alzheimer's disease. Attempted (and completed) suicide is also a risk for some.

Adding in his homelessness (and a GAF score of 45), Grover's diagnosis would be as follows:

F70	Mild intellectual developmental disorder
Z59.0	Homelessness
Z56.9	Unemployed

The various editions of the DSM have recorded more than 200 changes in the names of mental disorders (a figure that doesn't even include new disorders added over the years), but the case of intellectual disability (now intellectual developmental disorder) may be the only time a mental disorder was renamed pursuant to an act of Congress.

During the 2009–2010 legislative session, Congress approved, and President Obama signed, a statute substituting in law the term *intellectual disability* for *mental retardation*. The inspiration was Rosa Marcellino, a 9-year-old girl with Down syndrome who, with her parents and siblings, worked to expunge the words *mentally retarded* from the health and education codes in Maryland, her home state.

Note further that, as it is used in law, the term *developmental disability* is not restricted to people with IDD. The legal term applies to anyone who by age 22 has permanent problems functioning in at least three areas because of mental or physical impairment.

F88 Global Developmental Delay

Use the category of global developmental delay for a patient less than 5 years old who has not been adequately evaluated. Such a child may have delayed developmental milestones. Obviously, fuller assessment will be required later.

F79 Unspecified Intellectual Developmental Disorder

Use the category of unspecified IDD for a patient 5 years of age or older who has additional disabilities (blindness, mental or behavioral disorder) too severe to allow full evaluation of intellectual abilities. Again, reassess later.

F84.0 Autism Spectrum Disorder

Autism spectrum disorder (ASD) is a heterogeneous group of neurodevelopmental disorders with widely varying degrees and manifestations that have both genetic and environmental causes. Typically recognized in early childhood, these conditions continue through to adult life, though the form may be greatly modified by experience and education. The symptoms fall into three broad categories.

Communication. Despite normal hearing, the speech of patients with ASD may be delayed by as much as several years. Their deficits vary greatly in scope and severity, ranging from what we used to call Asperger's disorder (people with this type of ASD can speak clearly and have normal, even superior, intelligence) to patients so severely affected that they can hardly communicate at all. Others may show unusual speech patterns and idiosyncratic use of phrases. They may speak too loudly or lack the prosody (lilt) that supplies the music that underlies speech. They may also fail to use body language or other nonverbal behavior to communicate—for example, the smiles or head nods with which most of us express approval. They may not understand the basis of humor (the concept that the words people use can have multiple or abstract meanings, for instance). Children with ASD often have trouble beginning or sustaining conversation; rather, they may talk to themselves or hold monologues on subjects that interest them, but not other people. They tend to ask questions over and again, even after they've obtained repeated answers.

Socialization. The social maturation of patients with ASD occurs more slowly than for most children, and developmental phases may occur out of the expected sequence. Parents often become concerned in the second 6 months, when their child doesn't make eye contact, smile reciprocally, or cuddle; instead, the baby will arch away from a parent's embrace and stare into space. Toddlers don't point to objects or play with other children. They may not stretch out their arms to be picked up or show age-appropriate anxiety at separation from parents. Perhaps because of frustration at the inability to communicate, ASD can result in tantrums and aggression in young children. With little apparent requirement for closeness, older children with ASD have few friends and seem not to share their joys or sorrows with other people. In adolescence and beyond, this can play out as a nearly absent need for sex.

Motor behavior. The motor milestones of patients with ASD typically arrive on time; it's the types of behavior they choose that mark them as different. These include compulsive or ritualistic actions (called *stereotypies*)—twirling, rocking, hand flapping, head banging, and maintaining odd body postures. Patients with ASD suck on toys or spin them rather than using them as symbols for imaginative play. Their restricted interests lead them to be preoccupied with parts of objects. They tend to resist change, preferring to adhere rigidly to routine. They may appear indifferent to pain or extremes of temperature; they may be preoccupied with smelling or touching things. Many such patients injure themselves by head banging, skin picking, or other repetitive motions.

Apart from the subtype formerly known as Asperger's disorder, ASD wasn't recognized at all until Leo Kanner introduced the term *early infantile autism* in 1943. Since then, the concept has expanded in scope and grown new subdivisions (DSM-IV listed four types plus the ubiquitous *not otherwise specified*). The category has now contracted again into the unified concept presented by DSM-5-TR. Although the degree of disability varies widely, the effect upon the lives of most patients and their families is profound and enduring.

ASD is often associated with intellectual developmental disorder; discriminating between these two disorders can be difficult. Sensory abnormalities occur in perhaps 90% of patients with ASD; some children hate bright lights or loud sounds, or even the prickly texture of certain fabrics or other surfaces. A small minority have cognitive "splinter" skills—special abilities in computation, music, or rote memory that occasionally rise to the level of savantism.

Physical conditions associated with ASD include phenylketonuria, fragile X syndrome, tuberous sclerosis, and a history of perinatal distress. Mental health comorbidity issues include anxiety disorders (especially prevalent) and depression (2–30%), obsessive–compulsive behavior (in about one-third), attention-deficit/hyperactivity disorder (over half), intellectual developmental disorder (about half), and seizures (25–50%). Some patients complain of initial insomnia or a reduced need for sleep; a few even sleep days and remain awake nights. Researchers have recently reported an association of a form of autism with a gene responsible for kidney, breast, colon, brain, and skin cancer. The bottom line: Many patients with ASD will require additional diagnoses to capture the full complexity of their symptoms.

ASD's overall prevalence in the United States is currently stated as a bit above 1% of children; studies from other countries tend to report somewhat lower figures. Numbers have increased in recent years, at least in part due to increased awareness of ASD. ASD affects all cultural and socioeconomic groups, with boys affected two to three times as often as girls. Siblings of patients with ASD have an elevated risk for the same disorder.

Note that ASD's impressive range of severity can be reflected in separate ratings for the social communication and behavioral components. Though the DSM-5-TR definitions for severity levels are a bit fussy, they boil down to *mild, moderate,* and *severe.* That's how I've listed them, though DSM-5-TR hasn't for a practical reason: Some DSM-5 committee members who wrote the criteria worried that a label of *mild* could give an insurance company leverage to deny services. Of course, that reasoning could apply to just about any disorder in the book.

Essential Features of **Autism Spectrum Disorder**

From early childhood, contact with others affects to some extent nearly every aspect of how patients with ASD function. Social relationships vary from mild impairment to an almost complete lack of interaction. Some patients may experience a reduced sharing of interests and experiences, whereas others fail utterly to initiate or respond to the approach of other people. Patients with ASD tend to speak with few of the usual physical signals most people use to communicate emotions and ideas—eye contact, hand gestures, smiles, and nods. Relationships founder, so that those with ASD have trouble adapting their behavior to different social situations; they may lack general interest in other people and make few friends, if any.

Repetition and narrow focus characterize the activities and interests of those with ASD. They may resist even small changes in their routines (perhaps demanding exactly the same menu every lunchtime or endlessly repeating already-answered questions). Some are fascinated with movement (such as spinning) or small parts of objects. Their reaction to stimuli (pain, loud sounds, extremes of temperature) may be either feeble or excessive. Some are unusually preoccupied with sensory experiences: They are fascinated by visual movement or certain smells, or they sometimes fear or reject certain sounds or the texture of particular fabrics. They may use peculiar speech or show stereotypies of behavior, such as hand flapping, body rocking, or echolalia.

The Fine Print

Note that there are varying degrees of ASD, some of which received separate diagnoses and codes in DSM-IV that no longer apply in DSM-5-TR. What was formerly called *Asperger's disorder* is relatively milder; many communicate verbally quite well, yet still lack other skills needed to form social bonds with others.

Deal with the D's: • Duration (from early childhood, though symptoms may appear only later, in response to the demands of socialization) • Distress or disability (work/academic, social, or personal impairment) • Differential diagnosis (ordinary children may have strong preferences and enjoy repetition; consider also **intellectual developmental disorder, global developmental delay,** attention-deficit/hyperactivity disorder, stereotypic movement disorder, obsessive–compulsive disorder, social anxiety disorder, language disorders, social [pragmatic] communication disorder)

Coding Notes

Specify:

> {With}{Without} accompanying intellectual impairment
> {With}{Without} accompanying language impairment
> Associated with a known genetic or other medical condition or environmental factor. [Don't forget to code that factor, too.]
> Associated with a neurodevelopmental, mental, or behavioral disorder
> With catatonia (p. 100)
> Severity (separate ratings are required for social communication and restricted, repetitive behavior)

Social communication

Level 1 (mild). The patient has trouble starting conversations or may seem less interested in them than most people. Code as "Requiring support."

Level 2 (moderate). There are pronounced deficits in both verbal and nonverbal communication. Code as "Requiring substantial support."

Level 3 (severe). Little response to the approach of others markedly limits functioning. Speech is limited, perhaps to just a few words. Code as "Requiring very substantial support."

Restricted, repetitive behaviors

Level 1 (mild). Change provokes some problems in at least one area of activity. Code as "Requiring support."

Level 2 (moderate). Problems in coping with change are readily apparent and interfere with functioning in various areas of activity. Code as "Requiring substantial support."

Level 3 (severe). Change is exceptionally hard; all areas of activity are influenced by behavioral rigidity. Causes severe distress. Code as "Requiring very substantial support."

Temple Grandin

Temple Grandin's career would be noteworthy even had she not been born with ASD. Her life story serves as an inspiration for patients, their families, and for all of us who would offer help. The following information, intended not to present a full picture of her life but to illustrate the features of ASD, has been abstracted from several of her own books.

Born in 1947, Temple began walking shortly after her first birthday. Even as a toddler, she didn't like to be picked up, and would stiffen when her mother tried to hold her. In her autobiographies, she recalls that she would sit and rock for long periods; rocking and spinning helped calm her when she felt overstimulated. Much later, she remembers that being touched by other people caused such sensory overload that she would struggle to escape; hugging was "too overwhelming." She couldn't even tolerate the feel of edges of clothing, such as seams of her underwear.

Temple was alert and well-coordinated, and she had normal hearing; yet she didn't speak until after her fourth birthday. Later, she recalls her frustration at understanding what was said but being unable to respond. For many years thereafter, her voice was toneless and uninflected, without lilt or rhythm. Even as a college student, she would speak too loudly, unaware of the effect her voice was having on others.

As a small child, Temple was taken to a psychiatrist who diagnosed her as having "childhood schizophrenia"; her parents were advised that she might need institutionalization. Instead, she received the benefit of private schooling, where her teachers taught the other students to accept her—and her eccentricities.

For example, she was unable to meet the gaze of others and she lacked the sense of emotion normally attached to personal relationships. She might even hold a cat too tightly, not recognizing the signals of distress it was giving her. Uninterested in playing with other children, she would instead sit and spin objects such as coins or the lids of cans or bottles. She had an intense interest in odors and was fascinated by bright colors and the movement of sliding doors and other objects.

Consistency was balm for Temple. At school age, she resisted change in her routines and would repeatedly ask the same questions. She reacted badly to Christmas and Thanksgiving because they entailed so much noise and confusion. As an older child, she became fixated on issues such as elections—the campaign buttons, bumper stickers, and posters for the governor of her state held special interest for her.

But emotional nuance escaped her. With no internal compass for navigating personal relationships, understanding ordinary social communication was, for her, like being "an anthropologist on Mars." Because she doesn't have the feelings people usually attach to others, her social interactions had to be guided by intellect, not emotion. To communicate, she used lines scripted in advance—she didn't have the instinct to speak in a socially appropriate manner. What she has learned of empathy she attained by visualizing herself in the other person's place.

Although Temple always rejected human contact, she nonetheless craved comfort. She found it one summer she spent on a farm, when she observed that a device used to immobilize cattle so that they could be immunized appeared to calm them. As a result, she designed and built a squeezing machine that applied mechanical pressure to her own body; the result was tranquility she hadn't found by other means. Refined over the years, her invention led to her eventual career in creating devices used in animal husbandry.

As an adult, Temple still has trouble responding to unexpected social situations, and she would have severe panic attacks were they not controlled with a small dose of the antidepressant imipramine. But she became salutatorian of her college graduating class; eventually she earned a PhD and ran her own company. She is world-famous as a designer of machinery that helps calm animals on their road to slaughter. And she is a sought-after speaker on autism. But if someone's pager or cell phone goes off when she's giving a lecture, it still causes her to lose her train of thought.

Evaluation of Temple Grandin

Of course, we should make a solid diagnosis only with multiple sources of information—for Temple, as for any patient. But lacking that, we can garner material from the treasure trove of data in her own books.

Working our way through the diagnostic criteria, I think we can agree that she has persistent problems in social interaction and communication (criterion A). They include social and emotional reciprocity (rejection of being hugged—A1); use of non-verbal behaviors (poor eye contact—A2); and relationships (lacking interest in other children—A3). There must be deficits in each of these three areas for a person to be given a DSM-5-TR diagnosis of ASD.

Temple's restricted behavior and interests include examples of all four symptoms in the criterion B category (only two are required for diagnosis): stereotyped spinning of coins and other objects (she even twirled herself—B1); a rejection of change in routine (dislike of holiday festivities—B2); fixed, restricted interests in, for example, sliding doors and the paraphernalia of political campaigns (B3); and hyperreactivity to sounds and fascination with smells (B4). Temple had symptoms from early childhood (C); her biography and other books richly document the degree to which they have dominated and impaired her everyday functioning (D). However, she eventually surmounted them brilliantly, thereby disposing of the final possible objection (E) that the symptoms must not be better explained by intellectual developmental disorder.

Patients with stereotypic movement disorder will exhibit motor behaviors that do not fulfill an obvious function, but the criteria for that diagnosis specifically exclude ASD. Temple began speaking late and had difficulty communicating verbally, but the criteria for social communication disorder also exclude ASD. Her parents were supportive and sensitive to her needs, eliminating severe psychosocial deprivation as a possible etiology. We'd also need to consider general medical problems such as a hearing deficit, which Temple herself explicitly denies having.

She does have a history of severe anxiety, well controlled with medication, that would probably qualify for a comorbid diagnosis of panic disorder, though it cannot account for most of her past symptoms. (I'm leaving the details of that diagnosis as an exercise for diligent readers.) Although some aspects of her history are reminiscent of obsessive–compulsive disorder, she has many other symptoms that it cannot explain.

Besides panic and other anxiety disorders, ASD can be comorbid with intellectual developmental disorder, attention-deficit/hyperactivity disorder, developmental coordination disorder, specific learning disorders, and mood disorders. I'd judge Temple's childhood GAF score as about 55. Though today she may no longer meet DSM-5-TR's diagnostic standards, she clearly did when young. She is highly intelligent but gives clear indication in her own writings of childhood difficulty with language.

F84.0	Autism spectrum disorder, requiring support, without accompanying intellectual impairment, with accompanying language impairment
F41.0	Panic disorder

With the elimination of Asperger's disorder (and other specific autism diagnoses) from DSM-5-TR, patient support groups have been up in arms. Used since 1944, Asperger's has a history as extensive as autism. It seems to define a group of people who, though clearly burdened by their symptoms, also possess a sometimes remarkable intelligence and range of capabilities that may even be superior. It's tempting to regard Asperger's as a sort of "autism lite." However, that would be a mistake, for patients with Asperger's have many of the same deficits as do other individuals with ASD. Perhaps desiring friends, but lacking the empathy necessary for social interaction, these solitary individuals might like to change but have no idea how to go about it.

The concept of Asperger's has been so useful and is so ingrained in the common usage of patients and professionals alike, that it seems unlikely to disappear—even though it hasn't been blessed by recent DSMs. It is an irony that because of her language delay, DSM-IV criteria would have deemed Temple Grandin ineligible for a diagnosis of Asperger's, though she remains the poster person for that diagnosis. This is a great example in support of the prototype-matching method of diagnosis I describe in the Introduction (p. 2). Using it, I'd rate Temple (when she was a child) a 4 out of 5 for the diagnosis of Asperger's disorder. However, DSM-5-TR, in a nod to voluble statements from the community of patients, does state that those who were formerly diagnosed as Asperger's can still be regarded as having ASD, whether or not they meet current criteria. That's the second irony in one paragraph.

Attention-Deficit/Hyperactivity Disorder

Attention-deficit/hyperactivity disorder (ADHD) has borne a long string of names since it was first described in 1902. Though it is one of the most common behavioral disorders of childhood, only recently—within a few decades, at most—have we recognized the persistence of ADHD symptoms into adult life.

Although this disorder usually isn't diagnosed until the age of 9, symptoms typically begin even before a child starts school. (DSM-5-TR criteria require some symptoms before age 12.) Parents sometimes report that their child with ADHD cried more than their other babies, that they were colicky or irritable, or that they slept less. Some mothers will even swear that their children with ADHD kicked a lot before they were born.

Developmental milestones may occur early; children with ADHD may be described as running almost before they could walk. "Motorically driven," they have trouble just sitting quietly. They may also be clumsy and have problems with coordination. At least one study found that they require more emergency care for injuries and accidental poisonings than do children without ADHD. They often cannot focus on schoolwork; therefore, though intelligence is usually average or better, they may perform poorly in school. They tend to be impulsive, to say things that hurt the feelings of others, to be unpopular.

A competent history is essential: Direct observation may not reveal the typical symptoms, which the stress of close scrutiny or an office visit with a new clinician can drive temporarily underground.

These behaviors typically decrease with adolescence, when many patients with ADHD settle down and become normally active and capable students. But some use substances or develop other forms of delinquent behavior. Adults may have interpersonal problems, alcohol or drug use, or personality disorders. Adults may also complain of trouble with concentration, disorganization, impulsivity, mood lability, overactivity, quick temper, and intolerance of stress.

ADHD affects perhaps 7% of all children, with a male preponderance ratio of 2:1 or greater. DSM-5-TR criteria identify perhaps 2.5% of adults ages 17 and over, though the range reported in various studies is great. The male–female ratio is less among adults, for reasons that are obscure.

The condition tends to run in families: Parents and siblings are more likely than average to be affected; alcoholism and divorce, as well as other causes of family disruption, are common in family backgrounds. There may be a genetic association with antisocial personality disorder and somatic symptom disorder. Also associated with ADHD are learning disorders, especially problems with reading. In adults, look for substance use, mood, and anxiety disorders.

Several disorders are likely to co-occur with ADHD. These include oppositional defiant disorder and conduct disorder, each of which will be present in a substantial minority of people with ADHD. Patients with these comorbidities may be so unhappy that they also fulfill criteria for persistent depressive disorder. Disruptive mood dysregulation disorder, a newly devised condition, may be even more strongly associated. Also look for specific learning disorders, obsessive–compulsive disorder, and tic disorders. Adults may have antisocial personality disorder or a substance use problem.

Essential Features of **Attention-Deficit/Hyperactivity Disorder**

Teachers often notice and refer for evaluation children with ADHD, who are forever in motion, disrupting class by their restlessness or fidgeting, jumping out of their seats, talking endlessly, seeming unable to play quietly or take turns, intruding on or interrupting others—perhaps even answering questions before they are fully asked. However, hyperactivity/impulsivity is only half the story. Such children also have difficulty paying attention when spoken to directly or maintaining focus on their work or play—the inattentive feature. Readily distracted (and therefore disliking and avoiding sustained mental effort such as homework), they neglect details and make careless errors. Their poor organization habits lead to messy work or lost assignments or other materials and an inability to follow through with chores or other responsibilities.

These behaviors plague many aspects of their lives, including school, family relations, and social life away from home. Although the behaviors associated with ADHD may be somewhat attenuated with increasing age, they can affect these individuals through the teen years and beyond.

The Fine Print

Determine the D's: • Duration and demographics (6+ months; onset before age 12) • Disability (work/educational, social, or personal impairment) • Differential diagnosis (intellectual developmental disorder, **anxiety** and **mood disorders,** autism spectrum disorder, **dissociative disorder,** conduct disorder, substance intoxication disorders, oppositional defiant disorder, reactive attachment disorder, PTSD, intermittent explosive disorder, specific learning disorders, cognitive disorders, disruptive mood dysregulation disorder, **psychotic disorders,** or **other mental disorders, personality disorders, substance intoxication** or **withdrawal**)

Coding Notes

Specify (for the past 6 months):

> **F90.0 Predominantly inattentive presentation.** Inattentive criteria met, but not hyperactive/impulsive criteria.
>
> **F90.1 Predominantly hyperactive/impulsive presentation.** The reverse of F90.0.
>
> **F90.2 Combined presentation.** Both criteria sets are met.

Specify if:

> **In partial remission.** For at least 6 months impairment persists (perhaps into adulthood), but with fewer symptoms so that full criteria are no longer met.

Specify current severity:

> **Mild.** Relatively few symptoms are found, resulting in only minor impairment.
> **Moderate.** Intermediate.
> **Severe.** Many symptoms are experienced, or some are especially severe.

If you read the actual DSM-5-TR criteria carefully, you'll encounter this anomaly: Criterion D specifies that the symptoms "interfere with, or reduce the quality of" the patient's functioning (p. 69), whereas nearly every other disorder in the book specifies "impairment" of functioning. The subcommittee that wrote the criteria apparently decided that "impairment" was too much influenced by culture. This, of course, prompts the question: Why should the diagnosis of ADHD pay more attention to cultural influences than does every other disorder in DSM-5-TR?

The answer is, also of course, that it shouldn't, and neither should we. Stick with the Essential Features: They might just keep you sane.

Denis Tourney

"I think I've got what my son has."

Denis Tourney is a 37-year-old married man who works as a research chemist. Denis has always had trouble focusing his attention on any task at hand, but he is bright and personable, so he has been able to overcome his handicap and succeed at his job for a major pharmaceutical manufacturer.

At home one evening the week before this appointment, Denis was working on plans for a new chemical synthesis. His wife and children were in bed, and it was quiet, but he had been having an unusually hard time keeping his mind on his work. Everything seemed to distract him—the ticking of the clock, the cat jumping up onto the table. Besides, his head was beginning to pound, so he grabbed what he thought were two aspirin tablets and washed them down with a glass of milk.

"What happened next seemed like magic," he tells the clinician. "It was as if somebody had put my brain waves through a funnel and squirted them onto the paper I was working on. Within half an hour I had shut out everything but my work. In 2 hours, I accomplished what would ordinarily take a day or more to get done. Then I got suspicious and looked at the pill bottle. I had swallowed two of the tablets that were prescribed last month for Randy."

Denis's son is 8, and until a month ago he was the terror of the second grade. But after 4 weeks on Ritalin, he has become less driven, his grades have improved, and he has become "almost a pleasure to live with."

For years, Denis has suspected that he himself might have been hyperactive as a child. Like Randy, during the first few grades of elementary school he had been unable to sit still in his seat—bouncing up to use the pencil sharpener or to watch a passing ambulance. His teacher had once written a note home complaining that he talked constantly and that he "squirmed like a bug on a griddle." It was part of the family mythology that he "crawled at 8 months, ran at 10." On questioning, Denis admits that as a kid he was always on the go and could hardly tolerate waiting his turn for anything ("I felt like I was going to climb right out of my skin").

He was almost stupifyingly forgetful. "Still am. I really can't recall much else about my attention span when I was a kid—it's too long ago," he says. "But I have the general impression that I didn't listen very well, just like I am today. Except when I took those two tablets by mistake."

The remainder of Denis's evaluation is unremarkable. He is in excellent physical health, and he has had no other mental health problems. Apart from some fidgeting in his chair, his appearance, speech, and affect are all completely ordinary, and he earns a perfect score on the MMSE.

Denis was born in Ceylon, where his parents were both stationed as career diplomats with the Foreign Service. His father drank himself into an early grave, but not before divorcing his mother when their only child was 7 or 8. Because he was its subject, Denis vividly remembered their last major argument. His mother pleaded to have Denis's behavioral problems evaluated, but his father banged his fist and swore that no kid of his was "going to see some damn shrink." Not long afterward, his parents split up for good.

Denis feels he has learned a lot from his father's example—he doesn't drink, has never tried drugs, and doesn't argue with his wife; he had readily agreed when she suggested having Randy evaluated. "You always dream that your kids will have what you never did," he says. "In our case, it's Ritalin."

Evaluation of Denis Tourney

As a child, Denis undoubtedly had several symptoms of ADHD. It is easier for him to remember the problems relating to his activity level (the A2 criteria). Those include the childhood symptoms of squirming (A2a), inability to remain seated (A2b) or wait his turn (A2h), always being on the go (A2e), excessive running (A2c), and excessive talking (A2f). (For children, DSM-5-TR requires six of these symptoms—but, because they tend to be poorly remembered years later, only five for patients ages 17 and above. The same numbers and rationale hold for symptoms of inattention.) Denis thinks that his attention span was also problematic, though he is less clear about the details.

His symptoms were present when he was a small child, certainly before age 12 (B); we have only anecdotal "clear evidence" that they interfered with the quality of his schoolwork, but at this remove, it seems to be enough. His clinician should ascertain that he had had difficulties in more than one setting (such as school and at home, C). But even 3 decades later, he remembers enough hyperactivity/impulsivity symptoms to justify the childhood diagnosis. As adults, many such patients recognize restlessness as their predominant symptom. It would be a good idea for the clinician to verify what Denis thought he remembered, perhaps by obtaining old school records.

In children, several other conditions make up the differential diagnosis. (Note that in a clinician's office, many children with ADHD can sit still and focus attention well; the diagnosis often hinges on the history.) Those with intellectual developmental disorder learn slowly and may be overly active and impulsive, but patients with ADHD, once their attention is captured, are able to learn normally. Unlike children with autism spectrum disorder, patients with ADHD communicate without undue difficulty. Depressed patients may be agitated or have a poor attention span, but the duration is not usually lifelong. Many patients with Tourette's disorder are also hyperactive, but those who only have ADHD will not show motor and vocal tics.

Children reared in a chaotic social environment may also have difficulty with hyperactivity and inattention; although ADHD can be diagnosed in a child who lives in an unstable social environment, the process requires extra care and thought. Oppositional defiant disorder and conduct disorder may involve behavior that runs afoul of adults or peers, but those behaviors appear purposeful and are not accompanied by the feelings of remorse typical of ADHD behavior. However, many children with ADHD have comorbid conduct, oppositional defiant, or Tourette's disorder.

The differential diagnosis in adults includes antisocial personality disorder and mood disorders (patients with mood disorders can have problems with concentration and agitation). The diagnosis should not be made if the symptoms are better explained by schizophrenia, an anxiety disorder, or a personality disorder.

As a child, Denis might have fulfilled criteria for ADHD, combined type; with the information currently available, however, this would be a tough sell to any coder with a hard nose. Although as an adult he continued to have severe problems concentrating, he overcame them with drive and raw intelligence. Until he compared his usual concentration to the kind of work he could do with medication, he never realized just how disabled he had been.

Although we have some specifics that would constitute a current DSM-5-TR diagnosis (he was distractible—A1b), even with more information we might not be able to dredge up enough detail to make a full adult diagnosis by contemporary standards. As a clinician, I feel more comfortable with the qualifier "in partial remission." A fuller examination, perhaps with added information from his wife (or boss), might justify a different final diagnosis. Oh, and I'd give him a GAF score of 70.

F90.2   Attention-deficit/hyperactivity disorder, combined presentation, in partial remission

---

ADHD is probably underdiagnosed in adults. Although some writers have expressed skepticism about its validity, the evidence of its legitimacy in this age range is increasing. However, the fussiness of their language makes the specifier criteria seem ripe for neglect.

F90.8 Other Specified Attention-Deficit/Hyperactivity Disorder

F90.9 Unspecified Attention-Deficit/Hyperactivity Disorder

Use other specified ADHD or unspecified ADHD for patients with prominent symptoms that don't fulfill the criteria for ADHD proper. Examples would include people whose symptoms begin after age 12 or who have too few symptoms. Remember that, to qualify, the symptoms that are present should be associated with impairment. If you want to specify the reason why ADHD doesn't work for the patient, choose F90.8 and tack on something to the effect of "symptoms first identified at age 13." Otherwise, choose F90.9. See page 11 (sidebar).

Tic Disorders

A *tic* is a sudden vocalization or movement of the body that is unrhythmic, repeated, and rapid—so quick, in fact, that it can occur literally in (and sometimes is) the blink of an eye. Complex tics, which may include several simple tics in quick succession, naturally take longer. Tics are common; they can occur by themselves or as symptoms of Tourette's disorder.

Tics range from the occasional twitch to repetitive motor and vocal outbursts that can occur in clusters that create utter (!) chaos in the classroom. Motor tics first appear in early childhood, sometimes as early as 2 years of age. Classically, they involve the upper part of the face (grimaces and twitching of the muscles around the eyes), though affected children can present with a wide range of symptoms that include abdominal tensing and jerking of shoulders, head, or extremities. Vocal tics tend to begin somewhat later. Simple vocal tics may include barks, coughs, throat clearing, sniffs, and single syllables that may be muttered or called out.

Tics cause children to feel out of control of their own bodies and mental processes, though as they get older, some patients do develop a "tension and release" buildup of the urge to tic that is relieved by the tic itself. Although tics are involuntary, patients can sometimes suppress them for a time; they usually disappear during sleep. Though tic disorders are described as persistent, they do change in intensity with time, perhaps disappearing entirely for weeks at a time. Frequency often increases when a person is sick, tired, or stressed.

Childhood tics are common, occurring in around 10% of boys and 5% of girls. Most of these are motor tics that disappear as the child matures; typically, they don't generate enough concern to warrant an evaluation. When they persist into adulthood, the prevalence is lower, though males still predominate. Adults rarely develop tics de novo; when it does happen, it is often in response to use of cocaine or other street drugs. The tics of adult patients tend to remain the same, varying in intensity though less severe than in childhood. Several factors contribute to a worse prognosis in an adult: comorbid mental conditions or chronic physical illness, lack of support at home, and psychoactive drug use.

Because tics look pretty much the same regardless of diagnosis, I've presented an example only in the context of Tourette's disorder.

F95.2 Tourette's Disorder

Tourette's disorder (TD) was first described in 1895 by the French neurologist Georges Gilles de la Tourette. It entails many tics that affect various parts of the body. Motor tics of the head are usually present; eye blinking is often the first symptom to appear. Some patients have complex motor tics—for example, doing deep knee bends. The location and severity of motor tics in patients with TD typically change with time.

But the vocal tics are what make this disorder so distinctive and bring patients to the attention of professionals—often mental health clinicians rather than neurologists. Vocal tics can include an astonishing variety of barks, clicks, coughs, grunts, and understandable words. A sizeable minority (10–30%) of patients also have *coprolalia*, which means that they utter obscenities or other language that can render the condition intolerable by family and acquaintances. Mental coprolalia (intrusive dirty thoughts) can also occur.

Now acknowledged to be far from rare, TD affects up to 1% of young people, with males outnumbering females 2–3:1. For unknown reasons, it is less common in African Americans than in other racial/ethnic groups. Associated symptoms include self-injury due to head banging and skin picking. TD is strongly familial, with concordance over 50% in monozygotic twins and 10% in dizygotic. There is often a family history of tics or obsessive–compulsive disorder (OCD), so that clinicians suspect a genetic linkage between Tourette's and early-onset OCD.

Typically, TD begins by age 6; most patients reach maximum severity by ages 10–12, after which improvement occurs in perhaps 75%. The rest will continue to have tics that are moderate or worse. Though there may be periods of remission, TD usually lasts throughout life. Maturity, however, can bring reduced severity or even complete disappearance. Most patients have comorbid conditions, especially OCD and ADHD.

Essential Features of Tic Disorders (Compared)

	Tourette's disorder	Persistent (chronic) motor or vocal tic disorder	Provisional tic disorder
Specific tic type	1+ vocal tics & 2+ motor tics (see The Fine Print)	Motor or vocal tics, but *not* both	Motor or vocal tics, or both, in any quantity
Duration	Longer than 1 year; tic-free periods may occur		Less than 1 year
Differential diagnosis	No other medical condition or substance use	No other medical condition or substance use; not TD	No other medical condition or substance use; never TD or persistent motor or vocal tic disorder
Demographics	Must begin by age 18		
Specify if	—	With motor tics only With vocal tics only	—
Tic definition	Abrupt, nonrhythmic, rapid, repeated motor movement or vocalization		

The Fine Print

In TD, motor and vocal tics need not occur in the same time frame.

Essential Features of **Tourette's Disorder**

The first tics of patients with TD are often eye blinks that appear around age 6 years. They are joined by vocal tics, which may initially be grunts or throat clearings. Eventually, patients with TD have multiple motor tics and at least one vocal tic. The best-known tic of all, coprolalia—swear words and other socially unacceptable speech—is relatively uncommon.

The Fine Print

Delve into the D's: • Duration and demographics (1+ years; beginning before age 18, though typically by age 4–6) • Differential diagnosis (OCD, other tic disorders, substance use disorders, and physical disorders)

Gordon Whitmore

Gordon is a 20-year-old college student who comes to the clinic with this chief complaint: "I stopped my medicine, and my Tourette's is back."

The product of a full-term pregnancy and uncomplicated delivery, Gordon's development seemed completely ordinary. But when he was 8½ years old, his mother noticed the first tic. At the breakfast table, she was looking at him across the Post Toasties box he was reading. Every few seconds he would, quite deliberately, blink his eyes, squeezing them shut and then opening them wide.

"She asked me what was wrong, said she wondered if I was having a convulsion," Gordon tells the mental health clinician. He suddenly interrupts his story to yell, "Shit-fuck! Shit-fuck!" As he barks out each exclamation, he twists his head sharply to the right and shakes it so that his teeth actually rattle.

"But I never lost consciousness or anything like that. It was only the beginning of my Tourette's." Unperturbed by his sudden outburst, Gordon continues his story. Gradually throughout his childhood, he accumulated an assortment of facial twitches and other abrupt movements of his head and upper body. Each new motor tic earned renewed taunts from his classmates, but these were mild compared with the abuse he suffered once the vocal tics began.

Not long after he turned 13, Gordon noticed that a certain tension creeps into the back of his throat. He cannot describe it—it doesn't tickle, and it doesn't have a taste. It isn't something he can swallow down. Sometimes a cough will temporarily relieve it, but more often it requires some form of vocalization to ease it. A bark or yelp usually works just fine. But at its most intense, only an obscenity will do.

"Shit-fuck! Shit-fuck!" he yells again. Then, "Cunt!" Gordon shakes his head again and hoots twice.

Halfway through his third year in high school, the vocal tics got so bad that they placed Gordon on "permanent suspension" until he could learn to sit in a classroom without creating pandemonium. The third clinician his parents consulted prescribed haloperidol. This relieved his symptoms completely, except for the tendency to blink when he is under stress.

He remained on this drug until a month ago, when he read an article about tardive dyskinesia and began to worry about side effects. But once he stopped taking haloperidol, the full spectrum of tics rapidly returned. He was recently evaluated by his general physician, who pronounced him healthy. He has never abused street drugs or alcohol.

Gordon is a neatly dressed, pleasant-appearing young man who sits quietly during most of the interview. He really seems quite ordinary, aside from exaggerated blinking, which occurs several times a minute. He sometimes accompanies the blinks by opening his mouth and curling his lips around his teeth. But every few minutes there occurs a small explosion of hoots, grunts, yelps, or barks, along with a variety of tics that involve his face, head, and shoulders. Irregularly, but with some frequency, his outbursts include the expletives quoted above—uttered with more volume than conviction. Afterward, he placidly resumes the conversation.

The remainder of Gordon's mental status is unremarkable. When he isn't having tics, his speech is clear, coherent, relevant, and spontaneous, and he scores a perfect 30 on the MMSE. He worries about his symptoms but denies feeling especially depressed or anxious. He has never had hallucinations, delusions, or suicidal ideas. He also denies having obsessions or compulsions, adding, "You mean like Uncle George. He does rituals."

Evaluation of Gordon Whitmore

Gordon's symptoms began when he was a child (criterion C) and include vocal as well as multiple motor tics (A), which have occurred frequently enough and long enough (B) to qualify him fully for a diagnosis of Tourette's disorder. He is otherwise healthy, so another medical condition (especially a neurological disorder such as dystonia) would not appear to be a likely cause of his symptoms. Other mental disorders associated with abnormal movements include schizophrenia and amphetamine intoxication, but Gordon presents no evidence for either of these (D). The duration and full spectrum of vocal and multiple motor tics distinguish his condition from other tic disorders (persistent motor or vocal tic disorder, provisional tic disorder).

We should also inquire about conditions that may be associated with Tourette's. These include OCD and ADHD of childhood. (Gordon's uncle may have had OCD.) Gordon's diagnosis would therefore be as follows (I'd assign him a GAF score of 55):

F95.2   Tourette's disorder

F95.0 Provisional Tic Disorder

By definition, the tics in provisional tic disorder are transient. Typically, they are simple motor tics that begin somewhere in the 3–10 age range and wax and wane over a period of weeks to months; vocal tics are less common than motor tics. A patient who has been diagnosed with persistent motor or vocal tic disorder can never receive the diagnosis of provisional tic disorder.

F95.1 Persistent (Chronic) Motor or Vocal Tic Disorder

Once tics have been present for a year, they can no longer be considered provisional. Persistent motor tics also wax and wane over a range of severity. However, persistent vocal tics are rare. Even persistent motor tics usually disappear within a few years, though they may recur in an adult who is tired or stressed. Although persistent tics are probably related genetically to TD, patients with TD cannot receive this diagnosis.

F95.8 Other Specified Tic Disorder

F95.9 Unspecified Tic Disorder

Use unspecified tic disorder to code tics that don't fulfill criteria for one of the preceding tic disorders. Or you can specify the reason by using other specified tic disorder. One example would be tics that have apparently begun after age 18.

Motor Disorders

F82 Developmental Coordination Disorder

Developmental coordination disorder (DCD) is perhaps better known by a pejorative label—"clumsy-child syndrome." More or less synonymous with *dyspraxia* (difficulty in performing skilled movements despite normal strength and sensation), DCD remains a focus of some controversy. And it's a big controversy, because DCD affects perhaps 6% of children ages 5–10; a third of these have severe symptoms. By a ratio of around 4:1, boys are affected more often than girls.

Young people with DCD have difficulty getting their bodies to perform as they might wish. Younger children may experience delayed milestones, especially crawling, walking, speaking—even getting dressed. Older children, chosen last for team sports because they don't catch, run, jump, or kick well, may have trouble making friends. Some children have trouble mastering classroom skills such as coloring, printing, cursive, and cutting with scissors.

Although the symptoms often stand on their own, for over half of patients DCD exists as part of a broader problem that includes attention deficits or learning problems such as dyslexia. Autism spectrum disorder has also been linked.

After years of study, the cause is still unknown. In the individual case, a variety of physical conditions must be ruled out: muscular dystrophy, congenital myasthenia, cerebral palsy, central nervous system tumors, epilepsy, Friedreich's ataxia, and

Ehlers–Danlos disease. Obviously, late onset of motor incoordination would weigh heavily against DCD.

Motor skill deficits can persist through adolescence and into adult life, though little is known about the course of DCD in adults.

Essential Features of Developmental Coordination Disorder

Motor skills are so much poorer than you'd expect, given a child's age, that they get in the way of progress in academics, sports, or other activities. The specific motor behaviors involved include general awkwardness; problems with balance; delayed developmental milestones; and slow achievement of basic skills such as jumping, playing catch with a ball, and writing legibly.

The Fine Print

The D's: • Demographics (onset in early childhood) • Disability (work/educational, social, or personal impairment) • Differential diagnosis (**physical conditions** such as **impaired vision, cerebral palsy, muscular dystrophy; intellectual developmental disorder;** autism spectrum disorder; ADHD)

F98.4 Stereotypic Movement Disorder

Stereotypies are behaviors that people seem driven to perform over and again without any apparent goal—repetitive movement for the sake of motion. Such behavior is expected in babies and young children, who will rock themselves, suck their thumbs, and put into their mouths just about anything that will fit. But when stereotypies persist until later childhood and beyond, they may come to clinical attention as stereotypic movement disorder (SMD).

The behaviors include rocking, hand flapping or waving, twiddling of fingers, picking at skin, and spinning of objects. Serious injury can result from biting, head banging, or striking fingers, mouth parts, or other body parts. You'll typically encounter these behaviors in patients with intellectual developmental disorder or autism spectrum disorder, though also in perhaps 3% of otherwise healthy children with ADHD, tics, or OCD.

Just what percentage of adults may be affected isn't known; though, other than in individuals with intellectual developmental disorder, it's probably uncommon. Of 20 adults with SMD in one study, 14 were women; a lifetime history of mood and anxiety disorders was the rule in these patients.

Patients who abuse amphetamines may become fascinated with handling mechanical devices such as watches or radios or picking at their own skin. Some will sort or rearrange small objects such as jewelry or even pebbles—*punding* (from a word popularized by amphetamine abusers), which may be related to excessive dopamine stimulation.

SMD behaviors are associated with blindness (especially when it's congenital), deafness, Lesch–Nyhan syndrome, temporal lobe epilepsy, and postencephalitic syndrome, as well as severe instances of schizophrenia and OCD. It has also been reported in individual patients with Wilson's disease (a disorder of copper metabolism) and brainstem stroke, several with the genetic syndrome *cri du chat* ("cry of the cat," so called because of the characteristic sound the patients make as infants). You may also find SMD behavior in demented elderly patients. Perhaps 10% of people with intellectual developmental disorder who live in a facility have the self-injury type of SMD.

In 1995, *The New Yorker* reported that Bill Gates, then the CEO of Microsoft, rocks when he works. "His upper body rocks down to an almost forty-five-degree angle, rocks back up, rocks down again. His elbows are often folded together, resting in his crotch. He rocks at different levels of intensity according to his mood. Sometimes people who are in the meetings begin to rock with him." Claiming it a holdover from "an extremely young age," Gates told the reporter, "I think it's just excess energy."

Essential Features of **Stereotypic Movement Disorder**

You can't find another physical or mental cause for the patient's pointless, repeated movements, such as head banging, swaying, biting or hitting of self, or hand flapping.

The Fine Print

The D's: • Demographics (begins in early childhood) • Distress or disability (social, occupational, or personal impairment; self-injury can occur) • Differential diagnosis (normal child development, **OCD**, autism spectrum disorder, **trichotillomania,** tic disorders, excoriation disorder, intellectual developmental disorder, **substance use disorders,** and **physical disorders**)

Coding Notes

Specify:

> **{With}{Without} self-injurious behavior** (includes behavior potentially injurious if not prevented)

Specify current severity:

Mild. Symptoms are readily managed behaviorally.
Moderate. Symptoms require behavior modification and specific protective measures.
Severe. Symptoms require continuous watching to avert possible injury.

Specify if:

Associated with a known medical or genetic condition, neurodevelopmental disorder, or environmental factor such as intellectual developmental disorder or fetal alcohol syndrome.

Communication Disorders

Communication disorders are among the most frequent reasons that children are referred for special evaluation. For some children, problems with communication are symptomatic of broader developmental problems, such as autism spectrum disorder and intellectual developmental disorder. Many other children, however, have stand-alone disorders of speech and language.

Disorders of speech include lack of speech fluidity (for example, stuttering); inaccurately produced or appropriately used speech sounds (as in speech sound disorder); and developmental verbal dyspraxias, which result from impaired motor control and coordination of speech organs. Disorders of language comprise problems with formation of words (morphology) or sentences (syntax), language meaning (semantics), and the use of context (pragmatics).

These disorders still are not well understood or (often) well recognized. Whereas they are differentiable, they are also highly comorbid with one another.

F80.2 Language Disorder

Language disorder (LD) is a recently devised category intended to cover language-related problems including spoken and written language (and even sign language) that are manifested in receptive and expressive language ability—though these may be affected to different degrees. Both vocabulary and grammar are typically affected. Patients with LD speak later and less often than most children, ultimately impairing academic progress. Later in life, occupational success may be affected.

The diagnosis should be based on history, direct observation, and standardized testing, though no actual testing results are specified in the criteria. The condition tends to persist, so that affected teens and adults will likely continue to have difficulty expressing themselves. This disorder has strong genetic underpinnings.

Language impairments can also coexist with other developmental disorders, including intellectual developmental disorder, ADHD, and autism spectrum disorder.

Essential Features of **Language Disorder**

Beginning early in childhood, a patient's use of spoken and written language persistently lags age expectations. Compared to peers, patients will have small vocabularies, impaired use of words to form sentences, and impaired ability to employ words and sentences to express ideas.

The Fine Print

The D's: • Demographics (begins in early childhood; tends to chronicity) • Disability (work/educational, social, or personal impairment) • Differential diagnosis (**hearing or other sensory impairment,** autism spectrum disorder, **intellectual developmental disorder, global developmental delay, other medical conditions**—though any of these may coexist with LD)

F80.0 Speech Sound Disorder

Substituting one sound for another or omitting certain sounds completely is the sort of error made by patients with speech sound disorder (SSD), formerly called *phonological disorder.* The difficulty can arise from inadequate knowledge of speech sounds or from motor problems that interfere with speech production. Consonants are affected most often, as in lisping. Other examples include errors in the order of sounds ("gaspetti" for spaghetti). The errors of speech found in those who learn English as a second language are not considered examples of SSD. When SSD is mild, the effects may appear quaint or even cute, but the disorder renders more severely affected individuals hard to understand, sometimes unintelligible.

Although SSD affects 2–3% of preschool children (it's more prevalent in boys), spontaneous improvement is the rule, reducing the prevalence to about 1 in 200 by late teens. The condition is familial and can occur with other language disorders, anxiety disorders (including selective mutism), and ADHD.

Essential Features of **Speech Sound Disorder**

The patient has problems producing the sounds of speech, compromising communication.

The Fine Print

The D's: • Demographics (beginning in early childhood) • Disability (work/educational or social) • Differential diagnosis (**physical disorders** such as **cleft palate** or **neurological disorders; hearing impairment;** selective mutism; **other medical disorders**)

F80.81 Childhood-Onset Fluency Disorder

Although the loss of fluency and rhythm once called *stuttering* (the title was changed to comply with ICD-10) is familiar to every layperson, the stutterer's agonized sense of dyscontrol is not. The momentary panic that ensues may cause people with childhood-onset fluency disorder to take extreme measures to avoid difficult sounds or situations—even such ordinary experiences as using a telephone. Typically, they report anxiety or frustration, even physical tension. You'll notice children clenching their fists or blinking their eyes in the effort to regain control, especially when there is extra pressure to succeed (as when speaking to a group).

Stuttering occurs especially with consonants; the initial sounds of words, the first word of a sentence; and words that are accented, long, or seldom used. It may be provoked by joke telling, saying one's own name, talking to strangers, or speaking to an authority figure. Stutterers often find that they are fluent when singing, swearing, or speaking to the rhythm of a metronome.

On average, stuttering starts at age 5, but it can begin as young as 2. Because young children often have dysfluencies of speech, early stuttering is often ignored. Sudden onset may correlate with greater severity. As many as 3% of young children stutter; the percentage is higher for children with brain injuries or intellectual developmental disorder. Boys outnumber girls at least 3:1. Although reports vary, the prevalence in adults is about 1 in 1,000, of whom 80% are male.

Stuttering runs in families, and there is some evidence of heritability. There are genetic (and some symptomatic) links to Tourette's disorder, which is a dopamine-related disorder; dopamine antagonists have been used to ameliorate the effects of stuttering.

Essential Features of **Childhood-Onset Fluency Disorder (Stuttering)**

These patients have problems speaking smoothly, most notably with sounds that are drawn out or repeated. Entire (monosyllabic) words may be repeated, or there may be pauses in the middle of words. Patients experience marked physical tension while speaking and may substitute easier words for those that are difficult to produce. The result: anxiety about the act of speaking.

The Fine Print

The D's: • Demographics (beginning in early childhood) • Distress or disability (social, academic, or occupational) • Differential diagnosis (**speech motor deficits; neurological conditions** such as **stroke; hearing deficits; other mental** or **medical disorders**)

Coding Note

Stuttering that begins later in life should be recorded as adult-onset fluency disorder and coded F98.5.

F80.82 Social (Pragmatic) Communication Disorder

Social (pragmatic) communication disorder (SCD) describes patients who, despite adequate vocabulary and ability to form sentences, still have problems with the practical use of language. The world of communications calls this *pragmatics,* and it involves several principal skills:

- Using language to pursue different tasks, such as welcoming someone, communicating facts, making a demand, issuing a promise, or making a request.

- Adapting language in accord with the needs of a particular situation or individual, such as speaking differently to children than to adults or in class versus at home.

- Adhering to the conventions of conversation, such as taking turns, staying on topic, using nonverbal (eye contact, facial expressions) as well as verbal signals, allowing adequate physical space between speaker and listener, or restating something that's been misinterpreted.

- Understanding implied communications, such as metaphors, idioms, and humor.

Patients with SCD, whether children or adults, have difficulty understanding and using the pragmatic aspects of social communication, to the point that their conversations can be socially inappropriate. Yet they do not have the restricted interests and repetitive behaviors that would qualify them for a diagnosis of autism spectrum disorder. SCD can occur by itself or with other diagnoses, such as other communication disorders, specific learning disorders, or intellectual developmental disorder.

Essential Features of **Social (Pragmatic) Communication Disorder**

From early childhood, the patient has difficulty with each of these features: using language for social reasons, adapting communication to fit the context, following the conventions (rules) of conversation, and understanding implied communications (such as metaphor, idiom, and humor).

The Fine Print

The D's: • Disability (work/educational, social, or personal impairment) • Demographics (usually first appears around age 4–5) • Differential diagnosis (**physical** or **neurological conditions, autism spectrum disorder, intellectual developmental disorder,** social anxiety disorder, ADHD)

F80.9 Unspecified Communication Disorder

The usual drill applies: Diagnose unspecified communication disorder when a problem with communication doesn't fulfill criteria for one of the previously mentioned conditions yet causes problems for the patient.

Specific Learning Disorder

Specific learning disorder (SLD) is a particular problem in acquiring information—a problem that isn't consistent with a child's age and native intelligence, and that can't be explained by external factors such as culture or lack of educational opportunity. SLD thus comprises a set of discrepancies (in reading, mathematics, and written expression, as well as some not yet specified) between the child's theoretical ability to learn and actual academic achievement.

Before a diagnosis can be affirmed, the criteria require evidence of significant deficit obtained from an individually administered, standardized test that is psychometrically sound and culturally appropriate. Like most DSM-5-TR disorders, SLD cannot be diagnosed unless it affects school, work, or social life. Of course, the child's intellectual level will affect the manifestation, prognosis, and remedy of the SLD.

Except for the descriptive specifier "with impairment in written expression," which can appear a year or two later than the others, SLD usually declares itself by the time the child reaches second grade. Two main groups of affected children have been identified. Most affected children have problems with language skills, including spelling and reading; these stem from a basic difficulty in processing sounds and symbols of language (in other words, they have a phonological processing disability). A smaller number have difficulties solving problems—visuospatial, motor, and/or tactile perceptual problems that manifest as dyscalculia.

In one form or another, SLD affects 5–15% of Americans over the course of their lifetimes; boys are two or three times more often affected than girls. Of course, a child's behavioral and social consequences are proportional to the severity of the impairment and to the available educational remediation and social support. Overall, however, as many as 40% of children formally diagnosed with SLD leave school before completing high school, against a national average of about 6%. These disorders are likely to persist into adult life, where the prevalence is about half that for children. Of the types of SLD, problems with math are the most likely to have an influence on adult functioning.

Children with SLD are also more likely to have behavioral or emotional problems, specifically ADHD (which worsens the mental health prognosis), autism spectrum disorder, developmental coordination disorder, and communication disorders, as well as anxiety and mood disorders.

Specific Learning Disorder with Impairment in Reading (Dyslexia)

The best-studied disorder of this group, the reading type of SLD (aka dyslexia), occurs when a child (or adult, should it persist) cannot read at the level expected for age and intelligence. It can take several forms: difficulty with comprehension or speed when the person is reading silently; with accuracy when the person is reading aloud; with spelling when the person is, well, trying to spell. Normally distributed throughout the population (and occurring at every intelligence level), dyslexia affects about 4% of school-age children, most of them boys.

In the quest for causation, it is interesting to note that children are less likely to have reading problems when their native language has good correspondence between phonemes and graphemes (that is, the words sound generally the way they look). In that sense, English is relatively troublesome, Italian *facile*.

Dyslexia has been attributed to a variety of environmental factors (lead poisoning, fetal alcohol syndrome, low socioeconomic status) and familial causes (inheritance may account for 30% of cases). Especially at risk are socially disadvantaged children, who are less likely to receive the early stimulation that is important to childhood development. Clinicians must rule out vision and hearing problems, behavioral disorders, and ADHD (which is often comorbid).

Prognosis for dyslexia depends on several factors, especially its severity in the individual patient: Reading at two standard deviations below the population mean signifies an especially poor outlook. Other factors include parents' educational levels and the child's overall intellectual capabilities.

Early identification of dyslexia improves outcome. One study showed that 40% of children treated when age 7 could read normally at age 14. However, some news isn't so good: Perhaps 40 million adult Americans are barely literate. Although reading accuracy tends to improve with time, fluency continues to be a problem into maturity. Adults may read slowly, confuse or mispronounce proper names and unfamiliar words, avoid reading aloud (due to embarrassment), or spell imaginatively (and choose words that are easier to spell). They may find reading such a tiring chore that they avoid recreational reading.

Specific Learning Disorder with Impairment in Mathematics (Dyscalculia)

What do we know about the mathematics type of SLD? It's a little hard to figure. People with dyscalculia have difficulty performing mathematical operations—counting, understanding mathematical concepts, and recognizing symbols, learning multiplication tables, performing operations as simple as addition or as complex as story problems—but we don't really know the cause. Perhaps it's part of a larger nonverbal learning disability, or a problem in making a connection between number sense and the representation of numbers.

Whatever the cause, about 5% of schoolchildren are affected. Of course, you won't identify it in very young children. Although it's been shown that even babies have number sense, this condition cannot rear its head until the age at which children are expected to start doing math—sometimes in kindergarten, but more usually by the beginning of second grade.

Gerstmann's syndrome is a collection of symptoms that results from a stroke or other damage to the left parietal lobe of the brain in the region of the angular gyrus. It comprises four main disabilities: writing clearly (agraphia or dysgraphia), understanding the rules for calculation (dyscalculia), telling left from right, and distinguishing fingers on the hand (finger agnosia). In addition, many adults have aphasia.

The syndrome is sometimes reported in children, for whom the cause is unknown; some kids with Gerstmann's syndrome are otherwise quite bright. It is usually identified when a child starts school. Besides the four main symptoms, many children also have dyslexia and cannot copy simple drawings—a disability called *constructional apraxia*.

Specific Learning Disorder with Impairment in Written Expression

Patients with the written expression form of SLD have problems with grammar, punctuation, spelling, and developing their ideas in writing. Children have problems translating information from oral/auditory form to visual/written form; what they write may be too simple, too brief, or too hard to follow. Some have trouble generating new ideas. Note that though handwriting may be indecipherable, you wouldn't make this diagnosis when poor penmanship is the *only* problem.

SLD written expression doesn't usually appear until second grade or later—well after the typical onset of SLD in reading—as writing demands increase. SLD written expression can be due to troubles with working memory (there's a problem with the organization of what the child is trying to say). The diagnosis is generally not appropriate if the patient is poorly coordinated, as in developmental coordination disorder. Perhaps 10% of school-age children are affected; the condition is strongly familial.

Essential Features of **Specific Learning Disorder**

Despite targeted interventions, the patient has problems with reading, writing, or arithmetic, *to wit:*

Reading is slow or requires inordinate effort, or the patient has marked difficulty grasping the meaning.
The patient has trouble with writing content (not the mechanics): There are gram-

matical errors, ideas are expressed in an unclear manner or are poorly organized, or spelling is unusually "creative."
The patient experiences unusual difficulty with math facts, calculation, or mathematical reasoning.

Whichever skill is affected, standardized tests reveal scores markedly less than
expected for age.

The Fine Print

School records of impairment can be used instead of testing for someone 17+ years
of age.

The D's: • Duration and demographics (beginning in early school years, though full
manifestation may come only when demands exceed the person's abilities; lasts at
least 6 months) • Disability (social, academic, occupational) • Differential diagnosis
(**physical disorders** such as **vision** or **hearing impairment,** or motor performance;
intellectual developmental disorder; ADHD; extrinsic factors such as **lack of ability in the language being used in school, lack of educational opportunity, poverty**)

Coding Notes

F81.0 With impairment in reading. Specify word reading accuracy, reading rate
or fluency, reading comprehension.

F81.2 With impairment in mathematics. Specify number sense, memoriza-
tion of arithmetic facts, accurate or fluent calculation, accurate math reasoning.

F81.81 With impairment in written expression. Specify spelling accuracy,
grammar and punctuation accuracy, clarity or organization of written expression.

Specify severity for each affected discipline (with subsets) as a group:

Mild. There are some problems in a skill or two, but (often with support and
accommodation, especially in school) the patient can compensate well
enough to succeed.

Moderate. Difficulties are serious enough to require specialized education;
accommodation and support may also be needed at school, work, and
home.

Severe. Critical problems will be difficult to overcome without intensive remediation throughout the years in school. Even extensive support services may
not be adequate for success.

F88 Other Specified Neurodevelopmental Disorder

Use this category for those patients who have a disorder that appears to begin before adulthood and is not better defined elsewhere, but you can specify a reason. Here are two:

Neurodevelopmental disorder associated with ingestion of lead

Neurodevelopmental disorder associated with prenatal alcohol exposure. Neurodevelopmental disorder associated with prenatal alcohol exposure is the formal name for *fetal alcohol syndrome*, which carries with it a number of developmental disabilities as well as a variety of physical (especially facial) features.

F89 Unspecified Neurodevelopmental Disorder

Use unspecified neurodevelopmental disorder when full criteria are not met or when you lack adequate information.

CHAPTER 2

Schizophrenia Spectrum and Other Psychotic Disorders

Quick Guide to the Schizophrenia Spectrum and Psychotic Disorders

When psychosis is a prominent reason for a mental health evaluation, the diagnosis will be one of the disorders or categories listed below. To facilitate discussion, I have not adhered to the order in which DSM-5-TR presents these conditions.

Schizophrenia and Schizophrenia-Like Disorders

Schizophrenia. For at least 6 months, these patients have had two or more of these five types of psychotic symptom: delusions, disorganized speech, hallucinations, negative symptoms, and catatonia or other markedly abnormal motor behavior. Ruled out as causes of the psychotic symptoms are significant mood disorders, substance use, and general medical conditions (p. 63).

Catatonia associated with another mental disorder (catatonia specifier). These patients have three or more of several characteristics of motor behavior (defined on p. 100). The specifier can be applied to disorders that include psychosis, mood disorders, autistic spectrum disorder, and other medical conditions (p. 104).

Schizophreniform disorder. This category is for patients who have the basic symptoms of schizophrenia but have been ill for only 1–6 months—less than the time specified for schizophrenia (p. 75).

Schizoaffective disorder. For at least 1 month, a patient has had basic psychotic symptoms while at the same time experiencing prominent symptoms of mania or depression (p. 88).

Brief psychotic disorder. For less than 1 month, a patient has had at least one of the basic psychotic symptoms (p. 79).

Other Psychotic Disorders

Delusional disorder. These patients have delusions, but not the other symptoms of schizophrenia (p. 82).

Psychotic disorder due to another medical condition. A variety of medical and neurological conditions can produce psychotic symptoms that may not meet criteria for any of the conditions above (p. 97).

Substance/medication-induced psychotic disorder. Alcohol or other substances (intoxication or withdrawal) can cause psychotic symptoms that may not meet criteria for any of the conditions above (p. 93).

Other specified, or unspecified, schizophrenia spectrum and other psychotic disorder. Use one of these categories for a patient with a psychosis that doesn't seem to fit any of the categories above (p. 106).

Unspecified catatonia. Use when a patient has symptoms of catatonia but there isn't enough information to substantiate a more definitive diagnosis (p. 107).

Disorders with Psychosis as a Symptom

Some patients have psychosis as a symptom of mental disorders discussed in other chapters. These disorders include the following:

Mood disorder with psychosis. Patients with a severe major depressive episode (p. 112) or manic episode (p. 123) can experience hallucinations and mood-congruent delusions.

Cognitive disorders with psychosis. Many patients with delirium (p. 487) or major neurocognitive disorder (p. 503) have hallucinations or delusions.

Personality disorders. Patients with borderline personality disorder may have transient periods (minutes or hours) when they appear delusional (p. 561). Those with schizophrenia may have premorbid schizoid or (especially) schizotypal personality disorder (pp. 551, 554).

Disorders That Masquerade as Psychosis

Patients with some disorders may have symptoms that make them appear psychotic when they are not. These disorders include the following:

Specific phobia. Some phobic avoidance behaviors can appear quite strange without being psychotic (p. 181).

Intellectual developmental disorder. These patients may at times speak or act bizarrely (p. 20).

Somatic symptom disorder. Patients who have a history of multiple somatic symptoms that distress them or cause marked disruption to their daily lives may report pseudo halluci-nations or pseudo delusions (p. 254).

Factitious disorder imposed on self. These patients may feign delusions or hallucinations to obtain hospital or other medical care (p. 272).

Malingering. Some people feign delusions or hallucinations to obtain money (insurance or disability payments), avoid work (such as in the military), or escape from punishment (p. 616).

Whatever happened to *folie à deux* ("madness of two")? For generations, this rarely encountered condition was a staple of mental health diagnostic schemes. It was termed *shared psychotic disorder* in recent DSMs, where it denoted patients who develop delu-sions similar to those held by a relative or other close associate. Often the second patient's delusions cleared up once association with the first patient was severed. There are several reasons why this condition has been excluded from DSM-5-TR.

Through the decades, there has been precious little research that would help us understand shared psychotic disorder. We have case reports, some describing multiple secondary patients dependent on one primary source (*folie à trois, à quatre, à famille*), but not much in the way of data.

Although most of these patients live with someone who has schizophrenia or delu-sional disorder, the phenomenon has also been linked to somatic symptom disorder, obsessive–compulsive disorder, and the dissociative disorders. In other words, *folie à deux* may be better conceptualized as a descriptive syndrome similar to the Capgras phenom-enon (in which patients believe that close associates have been replaced by exact doubles). Many patients who would formerly have been diagnosed as having *folie à deux* (shared psychotic disorder) will fulfill criteria for delusional disorder, which is the label you can give them now. Some, like Miriam Phillips, whom we will meet later in the chapter, you may want to lumber with a very long diagnostic term, "Delusional symptoms in the context of relationship with an individual with prominent delusions," which means the same thing. Just imagine trying to squeeze it into that little box on the insurance form.

Introduction

During the second half of the 20th century, one great leap forward came when mental health professionals began to agree that psychosis can have many causes. This prog-ress can be credited in part to DSM-III and its forebears and successors, which have used research findings to establish diagnostic criteria. To distinguish among the vari-ous types of psychoses, DSM-5-TR uses four classes of information: type of psychotic symptom, course of illness, consequences of illness, and exclusions.

Type of Psychotic Symptom

The presence of psychosis usually isn't hard to determine. The behaviors by which we recognize that a person with psychosis is out of touch with reality (the term that's been used for decades as a short-form definition) are usually pretty obvious, and they often represent a dramatic change from a person's usual behavior. This state of mind can manifest in one or more of five basic symptom types. Collectively, they form DSM-5-TR's "A" criteria for schizophrenia—about which we'll have a lot more to say later.

Delusions

A *delusion* is a false belief that cannot be explained by the patient's culture or education and that the patient cannot be persuaded to reject, despite evidence or the weight of other people's opinions to the contrary. Delusions can be of several types, including these:

> **Erotomanic.** Someone (often of higher social station) is in love with the person.
>
> **Grandeur.** A person is someone of exalted station, such as God or a movie star, or is hugely talented or insightful. Some grandiose people express the idea that they have a special relationship with a prominent person, or even *are* themselves famous.
>
> **Guilt.** An individual has committed an unpardonable sin or grave error.
>
> **Jealousy.** A spouse or partner has been unfaithful.
>
> **Nihilism.** The person is dead, obliterated, perhaps rotted, no longer an existing human being.
>
> **Passivity.** A person is being controlled or manipulated by some outside influence, such as radio waves.
>
> **Persecution.** An individual is being hounded, followed, or otherwise interfered with.
>
> **Poverty.** Contrary to evidence (a job and ample money in the bank), the person faces destitution.
>
> **Reference.** The person interprets the gestures or comments of others or ordinary occurrences in the environment as having special personal meaning; being talked about on TV is an example.
>
> **Somatic.** A person has a dread disease or altered body functions, or offensive body odor.
>
> **Thought control.** Others are putting thoughts or ideas into a person's mind.

Delusions must be distinguished from *overvalued ideas,* which are beliefs that are not clearly false but continue to be held despite lack of proof that they are valid. Examples include belief in the superiority of one's own race, nationality, or gender.

Hallucinations

Hallucinations are false sensory perceptions that occur in the absence of a related sensory stimulus. They are nearly always abnormal and can affect any of the five senses, though auditory and visual hallucinations are the most common. But even these dramatic symptoms do not always mean that the person experiencing them is psychotic.

To count as psychotic symptoms, hallucinations must occur when a person is awake and fully alert. This means that one occurring only during a delirium cannot be taken as evidence of one of the psychotic disorders discussed in this chapter. The same can be said for hallucinatory experiences that occur when someone is falling asleep (*hypnagogic*) or awakening (*hypnopompic*). These common experiences (which are not true hallucinations) are normal; they are better referred to as *imagery*.

Another requirement is that, as with a delusion, the person must lack insight into the unreality of the hallucination. You might think that this would apply to pretty much every hallucination, but you'd be wrong. Consider, for example, the Charles Bonnet syndrome, in which people who have significant loss of vision see complex visual imagery—but with full realization that the experience is unreal.

We must also discriminate hallucinations from *illusions,* which are simply misinterpretations of actual sensory stimuli. They typically occur during conditions of decreased sensory input, such as at night. For example, a person awakens to the impression that a burglar is lurking near the bed; when the light comes on, the "burglar" is only a pile of clothes on a chair. Illusions are common and usually carry no diagnostic weight.

Disorganized Thinking

With or without delusions or hallucinations, a patient with psychosis may have *disorganized thinking* (sometimes also called *loose associations*), in which mental associations are governed not by logic but by rhymes, puns, and other rules not apparent to the observer, or by no evident rule at all. Of course, the only way we can know what someone thinks is to listen to that person's speech. Thought and speech aren't the same, of course, but near enough for most clinical purposes.

Some disorganization of speech is quite common—try reading an exact transcript of a politician's off-the-cuff remarks, for example. That can be annoying, but it's hardly psychotic. And by and large, when those words were spoken, listeners understood perfectly well what was intended. To be regarded as psychotically disorganized, the speech must be so badly impaired that it interferes with communication. The person switches topics without warning (perhaps without even realizing), or two thoughts are run together in what's sometimes called *derailment*. Examples: "He tells me something in one morning and out the other," "Half a loaf is better than the whole enchilada."

Abnormal Behavior

Disorganized behavior, or physical actions that do not appear to be goal-directed—disrobing in public (without theatrical or, perhaps, political intent), repeatedly making religious signs, assuming and maintaining peculiar and often uncomfortable postures—may indicate psychosis. Again, note how hard it can be to identify a given behavior as disorganized. There are plenty of people who do strange things (clowns, political demonstrators), lots of whom aren't psychotic. Many patients whose behavior qualifies as psychotic will have actual catatonic symptoms, each of which I have defined and listed on page 100.

Negative Symptoms

Negative symptoms include reduced range of expression of emotion (flat or blunted affect), markedly reduced amount or fluency of speech, and loss of the will to do things (*avolition*). They are called *negative* because they give the impression that something has been taken away, reducing the apparent textural richness of a patient's personality. However, they can be hard to differentiate from dullness due to depression, drug use, or ordinary lack of interest. They can also be mistaken for the stiffening of affect sometimes caused by antipsychotic medications or physical disease.

Negative symptoms can be hard to pinpoint, unless you ask an informant about a patient's changes in affective lability, volition, or amount of speech. They are more typically found in schizophrenia than in other psychotic disorders.

Course of Illness

The symptoms a person is showing right now (I call these cross-sectional symptoms) are less important to the differential diagnosis of psychosis than is the course of illness. That is, the diagnosis you make will be strongly influenced by the longitudinal patterns and associated features of the disorder. Here are several of these factors:

Duration. How long has the patient been ill? A duration of at least 6 months is required for a DSM-5-TR diagnosis of schizophrenia. This rule was formulated decades ago, in response to the observation that patients who for a long time have been ill with psychosis tend at follow-up to have schizophrenia. Patients with a briefer duration of psychosis may turn out to have some other disorder. For decades, we've operationally defined the time required as 6 months or longer.

Precipitating factors. Severe emotional stress sometimes precipitates a brief period of psychosis. For example, the stress of childbirth precipitates what's called a postpartum (now, officially, peripartum) psychosis. The presence of precipitating factors suggests the likelihood of a course of illness that is not chronic.

Previous course of illness. A prior history of complete recovery (no residual symptoms) from a psychosis suggests a relatively good outcome for a later episode.

Premorbid personality. Good social and job-related functioning before the onset of psychotic symptoms directs our diagnostic focus away from schizophrenia and toward another psychotic disorder, such as a mood disorder with psychosis or a psychosis due to another medical condition or substance use.

Residual symptoms. Once the acute psychotic symptoms have been treated (usually with medication), residual symptoms may persist. These are often milder manifestations of the person's earlier delusions or other active psychotic symptoms: odd beliefs, vague speech that wanders off the point, a reduced lack of interest in the company of others. They augur for the subsequent return of psychosis.

Differentiating the various causes of psychosis can be difficult. Even experienced clinicians cannot definitively diagnose some patients, perhaps even after several interviews, perhaps only in the fullness of time.

Consequences of Illness

Psychosis can seriously affect the functioning of both patient and family. The degree of this effect can help discriminate among the various causes of psychosis. To be diagnosed as having schizophrenia, the patient must have materially impaired social or occupational functioning. For example, many people with schizophrenia never marry and either don't work at all or hold jobs that require a lower level of functioning than is consistent with their education and training. Some of the other psychotic disorders do not require this criterion for diagnosis. In fact, the criteria for delusional disorder even specify that functioning is not impaired in any important way except as it relates specifically to the person's delusions.

Exclusions

Once the fact of psychosis is established, can it be attributed to any mental disorder other than schizophrenia? We must consider at least three sets of possibilities.

The top place in any differential diagnosis belongs to disorders caused by physical conditions. History, physical examination, and laboratory testing must be scrutinized for evidence. For a listing of some of these disorders, see the table "Physical Disorders That Affect Mental Diagnosis" in the Appendix (p. 661).

Next, rule out substance-related disorders. Has the patient a history of abusing alcohol or street drugs? Some of these (alcohol, psychostimulants, hallucinogens) can cause psychotic symptoms that closely mimic schizophrenia. The use of prescription medications (such as adrenocorticosteroids) can also produce symptoms of psychosis. For more information, see the table "Classes (or Names) of Medications That Can Cause Mental Disorders" in the Appendix (p. 665).

Finally, consider mood disorders. Are there prominent symptoms of either mania or depression? The history of mental health treatment is awash in patients whose mood disorders have for years been diagnosed as schizophrenia. Mood disorders should be included early in the differential diagnosis of any patient with psychosis.

Other Features

You should also consider several features of psychosis that are not included in the DSM-5-TR criteria sets. Some of these can help predict outcome. They include the following:

Family history of illness. A close relative with schizophrenia increases your patient's chances of having schizophrenia, too. Bipolar I disorder with psychotic features also runs in families. (However, negative family history is more common than a positive one.) Always learn as much as you can about the family history, so you can form your own judgment; accepting another clinician's opinion about diagnosis can be risky.

Response to medication. Regardless of how psychotic the patient appears, previous recovery with, say, lithium treatment suggests a diagnosis of mood disorder.

Age at onset. Schizophrenia usually begins by a person's mid-20s. Onset of illness after the age of 40 suggests some other diagnosis. It could be delusional disorder, but you should consider a mood disorder. However, late onset does not completely rule out a schizophrenia diagnosis, especially when persecutory delusions are the prominent feature.

Each of these categories (plus a few other features) can help you distinguish schizophrenia, the most common psychotic disorder, from other disorders that include psychosis among their symptoms. The reason for this emphasis is that the differential diagnosis of psychosis very often boils down to schizophrenia versus something that is not schizophrenia. In terms of the numbers of patients affected and the seriousness of implications for treatment and prognosis, schizophrenia is the single most important cause of psychotic symptoms.

For a diagnosis of schizophrenia, earlier DSM versions required only one type of psychotic symptom if it was either a bizarre delusion or hallucinated voices that talk to one another. We can feel pretty clear about the hallucinated voices, but what exactly does *bizarre* mean, anyway? Unfortunately, the definition is neither exact nor constant across different studies. It isn't even consistent across different versions of the DSM, which refer to it with decreasing degrees of certitude: "with no possible basis in fact" (DSM-III), "totally implausible" (DSM-III-R), and "clearly implausible and not understandable and do[es] not derive from ordinary life experiences" (DSM-IV). DSM-5-TR hedges a bit further with "clearly implausible and not understandable to same-culture peers" and not derived from life's ordinary experiences. The assessment of what is and is not bizarre may vary with our emotional distance from those we seek to judge: "I am unique, you are odd, that stranger over there is bizarre."

So, we might as well adopt the original sense that came to us several hundred years ago from the French: *odd* or *fantastic*. Examples of delusions we could call *bizarre* include falling down a rabbit hole to Wonderland, being controlled (in thoughts or actions) by aliens from Halley's comet, or having one's brain replaced by a computer chip. Examples of non-bizarre delusions include being spied upon by neighbors or being betrayed by one's spouse.

The recent weight of opinion is that the quality of bizarreness has little importance when it comes to diagnosis or prognosis. Therefore, in DSM-5-TR, all patients with schizophrenia must have two or more types of psychotic symptom, no matter how fantastic any of them might be.

The Variety of Psychotic Disorders

I have purposely written up the following material in an order different from that used by DSM-5-TR. The stated intention of that manual is to order its material along "a gradient of psychopathology" that clinicians should generally follow, so that they first consider conditions that don't attain full status as psychotic disorders or that affect relatively fewer aspects of a patient's life. That's why DSM-5-TR begins the psychosis chapter with delusional disorder and progresses through brief psychotic disorder and schizophreniform disorder before finally getting to schizophrenia.

As a general principle, I agree that we should evaluate our patients along a safety continuum, beginning with more treatable conditions (such as a substance-induced psychotic disorder) or those that have a relatively better prognosis (mood disorder with psychosis, for example). However, to describe these complicated conditions, I think it works better first to discuss schizophrenia, which involves all the symptoms and features that can characterize psychosis, and then fiddle with variations.

F20.9 Schizophrenia

To achieve precision, the DSM criteria for schizophrenia have become more complicated over the years. But the basic pattern of diagnosis remains straightforward enough to outline briefly.

1. From their earliest years, some patients have a withdrawn or otherwise peculiar personality.

2. For some time (perhaps 3–6 years) before becoming clinically ill, the patient

may have experiences that, while not actually psychotic, portend the later onset of psychosis. This *prodromal* period is characterized by abnormalities of thought, language, perception, and motor behavior that do not rise to the level of psychotic symptoms.

3. The illness proper begins gradually, often imperceptibly. At least 6 months before a diagnosis is made, behavior begins to change. Right from the start, this may involve delusions or hallucinations; or it may be heralded by increasing symptoms of the prodromal period.

4. During those 6 months, the patient has been frankly psychotic for at least 1 month. There have been two or more of the five basic symptom types described at the start of this chapter; at least one of those two must be hallucinations, delusions, or disorganized speech.

5. The illness causes important problems with work and social functioning. Lack of insight into the fact of being ill can lead to eventual nonadherence to treatment recommendations.

6. The clinician can exclude other medical disorders, substance use, and mood disorders as probable causes.

7. Although most patients improve with treatment, relatively few recover so completely that they return to their premorbid state.

There are several reasons why it is so important to diagnose schizophrenia accurately:

Frequency. Up to 1% of the general adult population will contract this disorder. For unknown reasons, males become symptomatic several years younger than do females.

Chronicity. Most patients who develop schizophrenia continue to have symptoms throughout their lives.

Severity. Although most patients do not require months or years of hospitalization, as was the case before antipsychotic medications were developed, incapacity for social and work functioning can be profound. Psychotic symptoms can vary in their degree of severity (see sidebar, p. 74).

Management. Adequate treatment almost always means using antipsychotic drugs, which, despite the risk of side effects, often must be taken lifelong.

Although we all do it, it is probably incorrect to speak of schizophrenia as a single disease. It is almost certainly a collection of several underlying etiologies, resulting in the same basic diagnostic pattern. It is also important to note that many symptoms in addition to the formal criteria are often found in patients with schizophrenia. Here are a few:

Cognitive dysfunction. Distractibility, memory deficits, or other cognitive problems are often noted, though the symptoms of schizophrenia are classically described as occurring with full orientation.

Mood symptoms. Of course, one classical presentation of schizophrenia is with inappropriate affect—laughter when nothing amusing has occurred, for example. However, anger, anxiety, and depression also commonly accompany psychosis, so the diagnostic criteria specify that any symptoms of depression or mania must be present for under half the total period of illness.

Absence of insight. Many patients refuse to take medicine in the mistaken belief that they are not ill, and they believe fervently in the reality of their hallucinations and delusions.

Sleep disturbance. Some patients stay up late and arise late when they are attempting to deal with the onset of hallucinations or delusions.

Substance use. Especially common is tobacco use, which affects 80% of all patients with schizophrenia.

Suicidal and violent behavior. Around 1 in 20 of patients with schizophrenia (especially newly diagnosed young men) take their own lives; many more make serious attempts. Aggressive outbursts can occur, especially in younger men, but patients with schizophrenia are far more likely to be victims than perpetrators of violence.

Lifetime risk for schizophrenia is on the order of 1 in 200 people in the general population; males and females are about equally represented. It is a disorder of younger people, beginning on average in the early 20s for men, a few years later for women. People who have a late onset (age 40 or beyond) are likely to be female; their social functioning and affect may be relatively less involved. Although there are strong genetic influences, because it is a relatively low-frequency disorder, most schizophrenia patients will not have relatives with the disorder.

Essential Features of **Schizophrenia**

All within 1 month, to a clinically important degree, the patient has at least two of: (1) delusions, (2) hallucinations, (3) speech that is incoherent or otherwise disorganized, (4) severely abnormal psychomotor behavior (catatonic symptoms), and (5) negative symptoms such as restricted affect or lack of volition. At least one of these two must be delusions, hallucinations, or disorganized speech.

The Fine Print

Don't dismiss the D's: • Duration (continuous evidence of the illness for 6+ months, with active phase symptoms for at least 1 month) • Disability (marked social, occupational, or personal impairment for a substantial amount of this time) • Differential diagnosis (**other psychotic disorders**, **mood disorder**, cognitive disorders, **physical and substance-induced psychotic disorders, schizoaffective disorder,** overvalued ideas [thoughts or beliefs—often political or religious—commonly held by a group of people]) • Demographic carve-out (if the person has a history of autism spectrum or childhood-onset communication disorder, diagnose schizophrenia *only if* there are prominent hallucinations *or* prominent delusions [plus the other requirements])

Coding Notes

Specify:

> **With catatonia** (p. 100)

If the disorder has lasted at least 1 year, specify course:

> **First episode, currently in acute episode**
> **First episode, currently in partial remission**
> **First episode, currently in full remission**
> **Multiple episodes, currently in acute episode**
> **Multiple episodes, currently in partial remission**
> **Multiple episodes, currently in full remission**
> **Continuous**
> **Unspecified**

You may specify severity, though you don't have to (p. 74).

Whereas DSM-IV (and each of its predecessors) listed several subtypes of schizophrenia, DSM-5-TR has largely done away with them. Why is this? And why were they there in the first place?

Sadly, the venerable categories of hebephrenic (disorganized), catatonic, and paranoid types, each of which had roots deep in the 19th century, simply didn't predict much—not enough, at any rate, to justify their continuing existence. Furthermore, in a given patient, they didn't necessarily hold true to type from one episode of psychosis to the next. Catatonia, encountered most often in illnesses other than schizophrenia, has now been demoted to a specifier denoting behaviors that apply not just to schizophrenia but to mood disorders and physical illnesses. And the other old categories, while interesting to discuss, have been relegated to history's dust bin, along with fever therapy and wet sheet packs.

Because schizophrenia can present in so many ways, and because it is so important (to individuals, families, society, and the history of mental disorder), I will illustrate with the stories of four patients.

Lyonel Childs

Since he was young, Lyonel Childs has been somewhat isolated, even from his two brothers and his sister. During the first few grades in school, he seemed almost suspicious if other children talked to him. He seldom appeared to feel at ease, even with those he had known since kindergarten. He never smiled or showed much emotion, so that by the time he was 10, adults said he was "nervous" and even his siblings thought he was peculiar. For a few months during his early teens, he was interested in magic and the occult; he read extensively about witchcraft and casting spells. Later he decided he would like to become a minister; he spent long hours in his room learning Bible passages by heart.

Though never much interested in sex, at age 24, still enrolled in college, he was attracted to a girl in his poetry class. Mary had blonde hair and dark blue eyes, and he noticed that his heart skipped a beat when he first saw her. She always said "Hello" and smiled when they met. He didn't want to betray too great an interest, so he waited until an evening several weeks later to ask her to a New Year's Eve party. Politely but firmly, she refused him.

Months later, Lyonel mentions to an interviewer that he thinks it strange: during the day Mary is friendly and open with him, but if he runs into her at night, she is reserved. He knows there is a message that eludes him, and it makes him feel shy and indecisive. He also notices that his thoughts have speeded up so that he can't sort them out.

"My mental energy was down," he tells the interviewer, "so I went to see the doctor. I told him I had gas forming on my intestines, and I thought it was giving me erections. And my muscles seemed all flabby. He asked me if I used drugs or was feeling depressed. I told him neither one. He gave me a prescription for some tranquilizers, but I just threw it away."

Lyonel's skin is pasty white and he looks remarkably thin, even for someone so slightly built. Casually dressed, he sits quietly without fidgeting during the interview. His speech is entirely ordinary; one thought flows logically into the next, and there are no made-up words.

By summer, he has become convinced that Mary is thinking about him. He decides that something must be keeping them apart. Whenever he has this feeling, his thoughts seem so loud that he worries other people can hear. He neglects to look for a summer job and moves back into his parents' house, where he keeps to his room, brooding. He writes long letters to Mary, most of which he destroys.

In the fall, Lyonel realizes that his relatives are trying to help him. Although they will wink an eye or tap a finger to let him know when Mary is near, it does no good. She continues to elude him, sometimes only by minutes. At times there is a ringing in his right ear, which causes him to wonder whether he is becoming deaf. His suspicion seemed confirmed by what he privately calls "a clear sign": One day while driving he notices, as if for the first time, the control button for his rear window defroster is labeled "rear def," which to him means "right-ear deafness."

When winter deepens and the holidays approach, Lyonel knows that he will have to take action. He drives off to Mary's house to confront her. As he crosses town, people nod and wink at him to signal their understanding and approval. A woman's voice, speaking clearly from just behind him in the back seat, comments "Turn right!" and "Atta boy!"

Evaluation of Lyonel Childs

Two of the five symptoms listed in DSM-5-TR's criterion A must be present for a diagnosis of schizophrenia, and at least one of them must be delusions, hallucinations, or disorganized speech. Lyonel does have two symptoms—delusions (criterion A1) and hallucinations (A2).

As with Lyonel, the hallucinations of schizophrenia are usually auditory. Visual hallucinations sometimes can indicate a substance-induced psychotic disorder or psychotic disorder due to another medical condition; they also occur in major neurocognitive disorder and delirium. Hallucinations of sense or smell are more commonly experienced by a person whose psychosis is due to some other medical condition, but their presence would not rule out schizophrenia.

As with Lyonel, auditory hallucinations are typically clear and loud; patients will often agree with an examiner who asks, "Is it as loud as my voice is right now?" Although the voices may seem to come from within the person's head, some patients will locate them elsewhere—the hallway, a household appliance, the cat.

The special messages that Lyonel received (finger tapping, eye winking) are called delusions of reference. Patients with schizophrenia may also experience other sorts of delusions, which I've listed on page 58. Delusions are often to some extent persecutory (that is, the patient feels pursued or interfered with). None of Lyonel's delusional ideas are so far from normal human experience that I'd call them bizarre. Lyonel does not have disorganized speech, catatonic behavior, or negative symptoms, but other schizophrenia patients may. His illness significantly interferes with his work (he doesn't get a summer job) and with his interpersonal relationships (he stays in his room and broods). We can infer that he is functioning much less well overall than before becoming ill (B).

Although Lyonel has heard voices for only a short time, he has been delusional for several months. The prodromal symptoms (his concerns about intestinal gas and feeling of reduced mental energy) began a year or more earlier. As a result, he easily fulfills the requirement for a total duration of at least 6 months (C).

The doctor Lyonel consults finds no evidence of another medical condition (E). Auditory hallucinations that may exactly mimic those encountered in schizophrenia can occur in alcohol-induced psychotic disorder. People who are withdrawing from amphetamines may even harm themselves as they attempt to escape terrifying persecutory delusions. We would have to rule out such a disorder had Lyonel recently used substances.

Lyonel also denies feeling depressed. Major depressive disorder with psychotic features can produce delusions or hallucinations, but often these are mood-congruent (they center around feelings of guilt or punishment that is deserved). We can exclude schizoaffective disorder because he has no prominent mood symptoms (depressive or manic, D). His symptoms have lasted longer than 6 months, so we know not to diagnose schizophreniform disorder.

Many patients with schizophrenia also have an abnormal premorbid personality. Often this takes the form of schizoid or, especially, schizotypal personality disorder. As a child, Lyonel had at least five features of schizotypal personality disorder (p. 554). These include constricted affect, no close friends, odd beliefs (interest in the occult), peculiar appearance (as judged by peers), and suspiciousness of other children. However, he has no history that should cause us to consider autism spectrum disorder (F).

With two psychotic symptoms and a duration of more than 6 months, Lyonel's illness easily matches the prototype for typical schizophrenia. I will risk monotonous repetition by asking you to note that (as with most DSM-5-TR disorders) medical and substance use causes must be ruled out, and other, more treatable mental etiologies be deemed less likely.

Throughout his current episode, Lyonel has had no reduction of symptoms that might suggest a course of illness other than continuous. He has been ill for just about 1 year. I'd peg his current GAF score at 30; his overall diagnosis would be as follows:

F20.9	Schizophrenia, first episode, currently in acute episode
F21	Schizotypal personality disorder (premorbid)
Z56.9	Unemployed

In evaluating patients who have delusions or hallucinations, be sure to consider the cognitive disorders. This is especially true in an older patient whose psychosis has developed quite rapidly. And, patients with schizophrenia who have active hallucinations or delusions should be asked about symptoms of dysphoria. They are likely to have depression or anxiety (or both) that could require additional treatment.

Bob Naples

As his sister tells it, Bob Naples was quiet when he was a kid, but not what you'd call peculiar or strange. Nothing like this had ever happened in their family before.

Bob sits in a tiny consulting room down the hall. His lips move soundlessly, and he dangles one bare leg across the arm of his chair. His sole article of clothing is a red-and-white-striped pajama top. An attendant tries to drape a green sheet across his lap, but he giggles and flings it to the floor.

His sister, Sharon, has trouble pinpointing when Bob first began to change. He has never been very sociable, she says; "You might even call him a loner." He always seemed rather distant, almost cold; he never appeared very much to enjoy anything he did. In the 5 years since he finished high school, he has lived at the home of Sharon and her husband, Dave, while working at their machine shop. But he never seemed really to live *with* them.

He's never had a romantic partner, though he sometimes used to talk with a couple of high school classmates if they dropped around. About a year and a half ago, Bob completely stopped going out and now won't even return phone calls. When Sharon asks him why, he says he has better things to do. But all he does when he isn't working is stay in his room.

Dave has remarked that, when on break at work, Bob stayed at his lathe, and talked even less than he used to. "Sometimes Dave heard Bob giggling to himself," Sharon says. "If he'd ask what's funny, Bob would kind of shrug and just turn away, back to his work."

About 2 months ago, after a year like this, Bob started staying up at night. The family would hear him thumping around in his room, banging drawers, occasionally throwing things. "Sometimes it sounds like he is talking to someone," says Sharon, "but his bedroom is on the second floor, and he has no phone."

Then, Bob stopped working. "Of course, Dave'd never fire him," Sharon continues. "But he was sleepy from being up all night, and he kept nodding off at the lathe. Sometimes he'd just leave it spinning and wander over to stare out the window. Dave was relieved when he stopped coming in."

In the last several weeks, all Bob will say is "Gilgamesh." Once Sharon asked him what it means and he answered, "It's no red shoe on the backspace." This astonished her so much that she wrote it down. After that, she gave up asking for explanations.

Sharon can only speculate how Bob came to be in the hospital. When she arrived home from the grocery store a few hours ago, he was gone. Then the phone rang, and it was the police, saying that they had him in custody: A security guard down at the mall had found him babbling something about Gilgamesh and wearing nothing but the pajama top.

Sharon blots the corner of her eye with her sleeve. "They aren't even his pajamas—they belong to my daughter."

Evaluation of Bob Naples

Do take a few moments to review Bob's history for the elements of the typical schizophrenia prototype. This is a picture to carry around in your head, against which you'll match future patients.

With several psychotic symptoms, Bob fully meets the basic criteria for schizophrenia. Besides his badly disorganized speech (criterion A3) and unfathomable behavior (leaving home undressed, A4), he has the negative symptoms of not speaking and lack of volition (he stopped going to work—A5). Although he has had active symptoms for perhaps only a few months, his reduced (even for him) sociability began well over a year ago, extending the total duration of his illness (C) well beyond the required 6-month threshold. The vignette makes clear the devastating effect of symptoms on his work and social life (B). However, even with these typical features, there are still several exclusions to be ruled out.

Bob will say only one word, so on admission we cannot determine whether he has a cognitive deficit, as would be the case in a delirium or in an amphetamine- or phencyclidine-induced psychotic disorder. Only after effective treatment could we be sure about his cognitive status. Other evidence of gross brain disease (E) could be sought with skull X-rays, MRI, and blood tests as appropriate.

Patients in a manic episode of bipolar I disorder can show a gross defect of judgment by refusing to remain clothed, but Bob does not have any of the other typical features of mania, such as euphoric mood or hyperactivity—certainly not pressured speech. The absence of prominent mood symptoms rules out major depressive episode and schizoaffective disorder (D). With manifestations of his illness present far longer than the 6-month minimum for schizophrenia, we can dismiss the possibility of schizophreniform disorder.

Several of Bob's symptoms are typical for what used to be called disorganized schizophrenia. His affect is inappropriate (he giggled at his lathe, laughed without apparent cause). Reduced lability (termed *flat* or *blunted affect*) would qualify as a negative symptom. By the time of this evaluation, his speech was reduced to a single word, but earlier it had been incoherent and peculiar enough that his sister even recorded a sample. Finally, there is loss of volition (the will to do things): He has stopped going to work and spends most of his time in his room, accomplishing, as best we can tell, nothing.

From Sharon's information, a premorbid diagnosis of some form of personality disorder would also seem warranted. Bob's specific symptoms include the following: no close friends, not desiring relationships, choosing solitary activities, lack of pleasure in activities, and no sexual experiences. This pattern, called schizoid personality disorder (p. 551), is often noted in the early histories of patients with schizophrenia.

Although Bob's ultimate diagnosis seems evident, we should await the results of lab testing to rule out causes of psychosis other than schizophrenia. Therefore, we'll add the qualifier *provisional* to his diagnosis. I'd give him a GAF score of just 15.

F20.9	Schizophrenia, first episode, currently in acute episode (provisional)
F60.1	Schizoid personality disorder (premorbid)

Disorganized schizophrenia was first recognized nearly 150 years ago. It was originally termed *hebephrenia* because it began early in life (*hebe* is Greek for *youth*). Patients with disorganized schizophrenia can appear the most obviously psychotic of all. They often deteriorate rapidly, talk gibberish, and neglect hygiene and appearance. More recent research, however, has determined that the pattern of symptoms doesn't predict enough to make disorganized schizophrenia a useful diagnostic subcategory—other than as a description of current symptoms.

Natasha Oblamov

"She's nowhere near as bad as Ivan." Mr. Oblamov is talking about his two grown children. At 30 years of age, Ivan has such severe disorganized schizophrenia (as it was once known) that, despite antipsychotic medications and a trial of electroconvulsive therapy, he could not put 10 words together so they made sense. Now Natasha, 3 years younger than her brother, has been brought to the outpatient clinic with similar complaints.

Natasha is an artist. She specializes in oil-on-canvas copies of the photographs she takes of the countryside near her home. Although she had a one-woman exhibition in a local art gallery 2 years ago, she has never earned a dollar from her artwork. She has a bedroom in her father's apartment; they are supported by his retirement income. Her brother lives on a locked ward of the state mental hospital.

"I suppose it's been going on for quite a while now," remarks Mr. Oblamov. "I should have done something earlier, but I didn't want to believe it was happening to her, too."

The signs first appeared about 10 months ago, when Natasha stopped attending class at the art institute and gave up her two or three drawing pupils. Mostly she stays in her room, even at mealtimes; she spends much of her time sketching.

Her father finally brings Natasha for evaluation because she keeps opening the door. Perhaps 6 weeks earlier, she began emerging from her room several times each evening. She will stand uncertainly for several moments, then open the front door. After peering up and down the hallway, she retreats to her bedroom. In the past week, she has reenacted this ritual a dozen times each evening. Once or twice, her father thought he heard her mutter something about "Jason." When he asked her who Jason is, she only stared past him and turned away.

Natasha is a slender woman with a round face and watery blue eyes that never seem to focus. Although she volunteers almost nothing, she answers every question clearly and logically, if briefly. She is fully oriented and denies having suicidal ideas or other problems with impulse control. Her affect is as flat as one of her canvases: She describes her most frightening experiences with no more emotion than for making a bed.

With gentle probing, the interviewer extracts more information. Jason is an instructor at the art institute. Some months earlier, when her father was out for the afternoon, Jason came to the apartment "to help me with some special stroking techniques." (She is evidently referring to her brushwork.) Although they ended up naked together on the kitchen floor, she spent most of those moments explaining why she felt she should put her clothes back on. He departed unrequited, and she never returned to the art institute.

Not long afterward, Natasha realized that Jason is hanging about, trying to see her again. She senses his presence just outside her door, but each time she opens it, he has vanished. This puzzles her, but she cannot say that she feels depressed, angry, or anxious. Now she has started hearing a voice quite a bit like Jason's, which seems to be speaking to her from the photographic enlarger she has set up in the tiny second bathroom.

"It normally just says the 'C word,'" she explains in response to a question.

"The 'C word'?"

"You know, the place on a woman's body where you do the 'F word.'" Unblinking and calm, Natasha sits with her hands folded in her lap and tells this story:

Several times in the past week or two, at night while she sleeps, Jason has slipped through her window and climbed into her bed. She awakens to feel the pressure of his body on hers; it is especially intense in her groin. After a few moments, she fully awakens, only to find him gone. And yesterday, when she went in to use the toilet, the head of an eel—or perhaps it was a large snake—emerged from the bowl and lunged at her. She slammed the lid on the animal's neck, and it disappeared. Since then, she has only used the toilet in the bathroom with the enlarger.

Evaluation of Natasha Oblamov

Natasha's variety of psychotic symptoms include visual hallucinations (the eel in the toilet—criterion A2) and a rather elaborate delusion about Jason (A1). She also has the negative symptom of flat affect (she talks about eels and her private anatomy without a hint of emotion—A5). Although her active symptoms have been evident for only a few months, the prodromal symptom of staying in her room started perhaps 10 months ago (C). I can't identify anything in the vignette I'd call lack of volition, but her disorder obviously interferes with her activities (teaching and attending art classes—B).

Nothing in Natasha's history suggests another medical condition (E) that could explain her symptoms. However, a certain amount of routine lab testing might be ordered initially: complete blood count, blood chemistries, urinalysis. No evidence is given in the vignette to suggest that she has a substance-induced psychotic disorder, and her affect, though flat, is composed—nothing like the severely depressed mood of a major depressive disorder with psychotic features (D). Furthermore, she has never had suicidal ideas, and nothing suggests a manic episode. Duration of illness longer than 6 months rules out schizophreniform disorder and brief psychotic disorder. Finally, her brother has schizophrenia. About 10% of the first-degree relatives (parents, siblings, and children) of patients with schizophrenia also have this condition. Of course, this is not a criterion for diagnosis, but it sometimes points the way.

Natasha fulfills all elements of the prototype: psychotic symptoms, duration, and absence of other causes (especially medical and substance use disorders). Age of onset isn't included in the DSM-5-TR criteria, but anyone who becomes psychotic after, say, age 35 needs to be evaluated even more carefully than usual for other causes that might possibly be treatable by other means.

In an earlier time (DSM-IV), Natasha's symptoms would have earned her a diagnostic subtype of *undifferentiated;* now everyone's diagnosis is undifferentiated. Because she's been ill less than a year (though well over the 6-month minimum), there will be no course specifier. I'd assign her a GAF score of 30. Her diagnosis would be simply this:

F20.9   Schizophrenia, first episode, acute

DSM-5-TR encourages us to rate each patient's psychotic symptoms on a 5-point scale. For the past 7 days, each of the five "A" criterion symptoms is rated as 0 = absent, 1 = equivocal (not strong or long enough to be considered psychotic), 2 = mild, 3 = moderate, or 4 = severe. In addition, the manual notes that a similar rating scheme should be used for impaired cognition, depression, and mania, because each of these features is important in the differential diagnosis of patients with psychosis. These ratings can be attached to several of the different psychotic disorders discussed in this chapter. This scheme might prove valuable for those doing research that requires meticulously scored degrees of severity, but for the rest of us, use of this enormously complicated rating system is—happily, in my judgment—optional.

Ramona Kelt

When she was 20 and had been married only a few months, Ramona Kelt was hospitalized for the first time with what was then described as "hebephrenic schizophrenia." According to records, her mood had been silly and inappropriate, her speech disjointed and hard to follow. She had been taken for evaluation after liberally sprinkling her head with coffee grounds and orange peels. She told the staff about television cameras in her closet that spied upon her whenever she had sex.

Since then, widely scattered across 25 years, she has had several subsequent episodes. Whenever she falls ill, her symptoms are the same. Each time she recovers sufficiently to return home to her husband.

Every morning Ramona's husband must prepare a list spelling out her day's activities, even including meal planning and cooking. Without it, he might arrive home to find that she has accomplished nothing that day. They have no children and few friends. Ramona's most recent evaluation is prompted by a change in medical care insurance plans.

Her new clinician notes that she still takes antipsychotics; each morning her husband carefully counts them out onto her plate and watches as she swallows them down with her orange juice. During the interview, she winks and smiles when it does not seem appropriate. She says that television cameras haven't bothered her for several years, but she does wonder whether her closet "might be haunted."

Evaluation of Ramona Kelt

Ramona has been ill for many years with symptoms that include disorganized behavior (criterion A4) and a delusion about television cameras (A1). The diagnosis of disorganized (hebephrenic) schizophrenia would at one time have been warranted, based on her inappropriate affect and bizarre speech (A3) and behavior. When acutely ill, she meets DSM-5-TR criteria for schizophrenia.

At this evaluation she is between acute episodes but shows peculiarities of affect (winking) and ideation (the closet might be haunted) that suggest attenuated psychotic symptoms. She does have the serious, ongoing negative symptom of avolition (A5): If her husband doesn't plan her day for her, she accomplishes close to nothing (this earns her a GAF score of 51). However, with only one current psychotic symptom, she appears to be partly recovered from her latest episode.

Of course, to receive a diagnosis of schizophrenia, Ramona would have to have none of the exclusions (general medical conditions, substance-induced psychotic disorder, mood disorders, schizoaffective disorder). I think we are safe in assuming that this is still the case, so her current diagnosis will be as given below. Note, too, that even the sketchy information in the vignette nicely fulfills our typical schizophrenia prototype. The course specifier equates essentially to the old diagnosis of schizophrenia, residual type.

F20.9   Schizophrenia, multiple episodes, currently in partial remission

F20.81 Schizophreniform Disorder

Its name sounds as if it must be related to schizophrenia, but the diagnosis of schizophreniform disorder (SphD) was devised in the late 1930s to deal with patients who may have something quite different. The cross-sectional appearance of these people is that of typical schizophrenia, but some of them later recover completely with no residual effects. The SphD diagnosis is valuable because it prevents closure: It alerts all clinicians that the underlying nature of the patient's psychosis has not yet been proven. (The -*form* suffix means this: The symptoms look like schizophrenia, which it may turn out to be. But with limited information, the careful clinician feels uncomfortable rushing into a diagnosis that often implies lifelong treatment and disability.)

The symptoms and exclusions required for SphD are identical to those of basic schizophrenia; where the two diagnoses differ is in terms of duration and dysfunction. As with brief psychotic disorder, DSM-5-TR doesn't require evidence that SphD has interfered with the patient's life. However, when you think about it, most people who have had delusions and hallucinations for a month or more have probably suffered some inconvenience socially or in the workplace.

The real distinguishing point is the length of time—1 to 6 months—the patient has been symptomatic. The practical importance of the interval is this: Numerous studies have shown that psychotic patients who have been briefly ill have a much better chance of full recovery than do those who have been ill for 6 months or longer. Still, over half of those who are initially diagnosed as having SphD are eventually found to have schizophrenia or schizoaffective disorder.

SphD isn't really a discrete disease at all; it's a place filler reminding us that we aren't sure what's going on but assuring us that time will yield clarity. It is used about equally for males and females, who tend to be around the same age as patients with schizophrenia when they are first diagnosed. The diagnosis is made only one-fifth as often as schizophrenia, especially in the United States and other Western countries.

In the late 1930s, the Norwegian psychiatrist Gabriel Langfeldt coined the term *schizophreniform psychosis*. In the United States it was perhaps more relevant at that time, when the diagnosis of schizophrenia was so often made for patients who had psychotic symptoms but not the longitudinal course typical of schizophrenia. As Langfeldt made clear in a 1982 letter in the *American Journal of Psychiatry,* when he devised the concept, he meant to include not only psychoses that look exactly like schizophrenia except for the duration of symptoms, but other presentations as well. These include what we would today call brief psychosis, schizoaffective disorders, and even some bipolar disorders. Time and custom have narrowed the meaning of his term, to the point where it is hardly ever used. I consider that to be a great pity; it's a useful device that helps keep clinicians on their toes and patients off chronic treatment.

Essential Features of **Schizophreniform Disorder**

All within 1 month, to a clinically important degree, the patient has at least two of: (1) delusions, (2) hallucinations, (3) speech that is incoherent or otherwise disorganized, (4) severely abnormal psychomotor behavior (catatonic symptoms), and (5) negative symptoms such as restricted affect or lack of volition. At least one of these two must be delusions, hallucinations, or disorganized speech. Note that the patient must recover fully within 6 months.

The Fine Print

The D's: • Duration (30 days to 6 months) • Disability (none required, though there may be social or other impairment) • Differential diagnosis (**physical** and **substance-induced psychotic disorders,** schizophrenia, **schizoaffective disorder, mood disorders,** cognitive disorders)

Coding Notes

Specify:

> **{With}{Without} good prognostic features,** which include: (1) psychotic symptoms begin early (in first month of illness); (2) confusion or perplexity at peak of psychosis; (3) good premorbid functioning; (4) affect not blunted. Two or more of these = with good prognostic features; none or one = without.
> **With catatonia** (p. 100)

If it's within 6 months and the patient is still ill, use the specifier *(provisional)*. Once the patient has fully recovered, within the 6 months, remove the specifier.

If the patient is still ill after 6 months, SphD can no longer apply. Change the diagnosis to schizophrenia or some other disorder.

You may specify severity, though you don't have to (p. 74).

Arnold Wilson

When he was 3, Arnold Wilson's family entered a witness protection program. At least, that's what he tells the mental health intake interviewer.

Arnold is slim, of medium height, and clean-shaven. He wears a name tag identifying him as a medical student. His gaze is direct and steady, and he sits quietly as he describes his experiences. "It was on account of my dad," he explains. "When we lived back East, he was in the Mob."

Arnold's father, the principal informant, later remarks, "OK, I'm an investment banker. You might think that's bad enough, but it isn't the Mob. Well, it's not *that* mob."

Arnold's ideas had come to him as a revelation 2 months ago. He was at his desk, studying for a physiology test, when he heard a voice just behind him. "I jumped up, thinking I must have left my door open, but there was no one in the room but me. I checked the radio and my iPhone—everything was turned off. Then I heard it again." The voice was one he recognized. "But I can't tell you whose. She told me not to."

The woman's voice speaks to him with clarity, and she moves around a lot. "Sometimes she seems to be right behind me. Other times, she stands outside whatever room I'm in." He agrees that she speaks in complete sentences. "Sometimes full paragraphs. What a gabby person!" he remarks with a laugh.

At first, the voice told him he "needed to cover my tracks, whatever *that* meant." When he tries to ignore her, "she becomes really angry, tells me to believe her, or . . ." Arnold doesn't finish the sentence. The voice points out that his last name, before he was 3, was Italian. "You know, she's really beginning to make sense."

"The name change part's true," his father explains. "When I married his mother, Arnold was part of the deal. His biological father had died—cancer of the kidney. We both thought it would be best if I adopted him." That was 20 years ago.

Arnold had difficulty in middle school. His attention wandered, and so did he. As a result, he spent a lot of time in the principal's office. Although several teachers despaired of him, in high school he hit his stride. There, he made excellent grades, got into a good college, and then he was accepted at an even better medical school. That autumn, just before starting his first year, his physical exam (and a panel of blood tests) had been completely unremarkable. He says his roommate will testify that he hasn't used any drugs or alcohol.

"It was pretty confusing, at first—the voice, I mean. I wondered if I was losing my mind. But then we talked it over, she and I. Now it seems clear."

When Arnold talks about the voice, he becomes quite animated, using appropriate hand gestures and vocal inflections. Throughout, he gives full attention to the interviewer, except once when he turns his head, as though listening to something. Or someone.

Evaluation of Arnold Wilson

Arnold's two psychotic symptoms—delusions and auditory hallucinations—are enough to get us past the criterion A requirements, which are the same for SphD as for schizophrenia. The vignette doesn't describe the extent to which his social or school functioning has been compromised, but the SphD criteria set doesn't require this information.

The clinical features of Arnold's psychosis closely resemble those of schizophrenia. Of course, that's the whole point of SphD: At the time you make the diagnosis, you don't know whether the outcome will be full recovery or long-term illness. Arnold's symptoms have been present too long for brief psychotic disorder, which lasts less than 1 month, and too briefly for schizophrenia. He doesn't misuse alcohol, and on his roommate's evidence (OK, by proxy), he doesn't use drugs at all; so we'll rule out a substance-induced psychotic disorder. The usual general medical causes of psychosis will have to be investigated, but his recent physical exam was normal. With no symptoms of mania or depression, bipolar I disorder seems vanishingly unlikely.

Whenever possible, we should make a statement of prognosis for SphD. In Arnold's case, the treating clinician notes the following evidence of good prognosis: (1) As far as anyone can tell, his illness began abruptly with prominent psychotic symptoms (auditory hallucinations). (2) His premorbid functioning (both work and social life) has been good. (3) With no flattening or inappropriateness, his affect is intact during this evaluation. The fourth good-prognosis feature DSM-5-TR specifies is perplexity or confusion. Arnold does say that he was confused at first, but by the time of his evaluation, at the height of his illness, his cognitive processes seem intact. At minimum, he has three of the features that favor a good prognosis; only two are required.

We need to add the qualifier (*provisional*) if, as with Arnold, SphD is diagnosed before the patient recovers. If he recovers completely within the 6-month time frame, we can then remove the qualifier. However, if the illness lasts longer than 6 months and it interferes with Arnold's work or social life, we will need to change the diagnosis—probably to schizophrenia.

Right now, Arnold's diagnosis should read as given below. And I'd give him a GAF score of 60: Though his psychotic symptoms are serious, his behavior hasn't been markedly affected. Yet.

F20.81   Schizophreniform disorder (provisional), with good prognostic features

---

Do you need a diagnostic place to park your patient while you collect more evidence? Even in DSM-5-TR, there persist a couple of "diagnostic sidings" that you can use to indicate that something is wrong but that you are waiting for more information before committing to a diagnosis. Of course, there's always "other specified _____" or "unspecified _____," but even beyond those useful (and vague, and sometimes indiscriminately used) locutions, some other terms carry much the same advantage.

SphD is one—it can go either way, to chronicity or to recovery. And brief psychotic disorder was manufactured to cover the month of psychosis before you can diagnose SphD. In Chapter 6, we'll see that acute stress disorder was cobbled together to cover the month before posttraumatic stress disorder kicks in. But that's about the extent of free parking. The problem is, we mental health clinicians are still dependent on our patients' appearance to inform how we view them. Other medical disciplines use lab tests, which help avoid diagnostic way stations.

F23 Brief Psychotic Disorder

Patients with brief psychotic disorder (BPsD) are psychotic for at least 1 day and return to baseline within 1 month. It doesn't matter how many symptoms they have had or whether they have had trouble functioning socially or at work. (Similar to schizophreniform disorder, any patient who remains symptomatic longer than 1 month must be given a different diagnosis.)

BPsD isn't an especially stable diagnosis: Half or more will relapse and many patients will eventually be rediagnosed with another psychotic disorder—hardly surprising for a diagnosis you can have for only 30 days. Around 5% of first-time psychotic disorder patients will have this as the initial diagnosis. It may be appropriate for some patients who experience a psychosis around the time of giving birth. Even then, it is a rare condition: The incidence of peripartum psychosis is only about 1 or 2 per 1,000 women who give birth. Indeed, BPsD is overall twice as common among women as men.

European clinicians are more likely to diagnose BPsD. (This doesn't mean that the condition occurs more frequently in Europe, just that European clinicians are apparently more alert to it—or perhaps they overdiagnose it.) BPsD may be more common among young patients (teenagers and young adults) and among patients who come from lower socioeconomic strata or who have preexisting personality disorders. Patients with certain personality disorders (such as borderline) who have very brief psychotic symptoms precipitated by stress do not require a separate diagnosis of BPsD.

Decades ago, in DSM-III-R this category was called *brief reactive psychosis*. That name and its criteria reflected the once-popular notion that it may occur in response to some overwhelmingly stressful event, such as death of a relative or financial collapse. In the DSM-5-TR criteria, this concept is retained only in the form of specifiers.

And the decisions we face about specifiers can be fraught. We must determine whether a stressor could have caused the psychosis. Of course, anything could precede the onset, and to learn what that might be and whether it was stressful could require interviewing a spouse, relative, or friend. We'd want to learn about possible traumatic events, but also about the patient's premorbid adjustment, history of similar reactions to stress, and the chronological relationship between stressor and the onset of symptoms. Even with all this, we're still stuck with a decision: Is this event a likely cause of psychosis?

The only guidance DSM-5-TR gives us is that the event(s) must be severe enough that they would stress anyone in the patient's situation and culture. But it doesn't help us at all to decide whether this psychosis is in response to that stress. My solution: Ignore the words *in response;* if there's evidence of marked stress, say so, and move on.

Essential Features of **Brief Psychotic Disorder**

All within the course of a single month, the patient develops, then recovers from an episode of psychosis that includes at least one of these symptom types: delusions, hallucinations, disorganized speech, or disorganized behavior (such as catatonia). The patient eventually returns to full premorbid functioning.

The Fine Print

The D's: • Duration (1 day to 1 month) • Disability (none required, though there may be social or other impairment) • Differential diagnosis (**mood disorders,** cognitive disorders, **psychoses caused by medical conditions or substance use, schizophrenia, catatonia,** schizophreniform disorder, personality disorders)

Coding Notes

If you make the diagnosis without waiting for recovery, you'll have to append the term *provisional.*

You can specify:

> **With peripartum onset.** Symptoms begin within 4 weeks of giving birth.
> **{With}{Without} marked stressors.** The stressors must appear to cause the symptoms, must occur shortly before symptom onset, and must be severe enough that nearly anyone would feel markedly stressed.
> **With catatonia** (p. 100)

You may specify severity, though you don't have to (p. 74).

Melanie Grayson

This was Melanie Grayson's first pregnancy, and she had been quite apprehensive about it. She'd gained 30 pounds, and her blood pressure had risen a little. But she needed only a spinal block for anesthesia, and her husband was in the room with her when she delivered a healthy baby girl.

That night she slept fitfully; the following day she was irritable. But she breastfed her gorgeous daughter and seemed to listen attentively when the nurse practitioner came to instruct her on bathing and other peripartum care.

This morning, while Melanie is having breakfast, her husband arrives to take his family home. When she orders him to turn off the radio, he looks around the room and says he doesn't hear one. "You know very well what radio," she yells, and throws a tea bag at him.

The mental health consultant notes that Melanie is alert, fully oriented, and cognitively intact. She is irritable but not depressed. She keeps insisting that she hears a radio playing: "I think it's hidden in my pillow." She unzips the pillowcase and feels around inside. "It's some sort of a news report. They're talking about what's happening in the hospital. I think I just heard my name."

Melanie's flow of speech is coherent and relevant. Apart from throwing the tea bag and looking for the radio, her behavior is unremarkable. She denies hallucinations involving any of the other senses. She insists that the voices she hears cannot be imaginary, and she doesn't think someone is trying to play a trick on her. She has never used drugs or alcohol, and her obstetrician vouches for her excellent general health. After much discussion, she agrees to remain in the hospital a day or two longer to plumb the depths of the mystery.

Evaluation of Melanie Grayson

Despite her obvious psychosis (hallucinations and delusions), the brevity of her symptoms keeps Melanie from meeting the criterion A requirements for schizophrenia, schizophreniform disorder, or schizoaffective disorder. What's left?

Although Melanie is alert and cognitively intact, any patient with abrupt onset of psychotic symptoms should be carefully evaluated for a possible delirium. (Delirious patients will often be confused, but that's also often true of people who have BPsD. Be meticulous with evaluations for psychotic thinking.) Many general medical conditions can produce psychotic symptoms. Anyone who becomes psychotic soon after entering the hospital should be evaluated for a substance-induced psychotic disorder with onset during withdrawal. Melanie has no prominent mood symptoms; if she did have any, a diagnosis of a mood disorder with psychotic features might be entertained.

It is worth noting that patients who develop psychosis after delivery may have mixtures of symptoms that include euphoria, psychosis, and cognitive changes. Many of these patients have some form of mood disorder (often bipolar I disorder). Diagnosis should be made with extreme care in all cases of peripartum psychosis; as ever, the diagnosis of schizophrenia should be made only in the most obvious, well-documented, and certain of circumstances.

With her very brief duration of psychosis and none of the exclusions, Melanie fulfills the somewhat undemanding criteria for BPsD. Until she recovers, the diagnosis will have to be provisional. I'd put her GAF score at 40. Her full diagnosis at this time would be as follows:

F23	Brief psychotic disorder, with peripartum onset (provisional)
O80	Normal delivery

F22 Delusional Disorder

Persistent delusions are the chief characteristic of delusional disorder. Often, they can seem entirely believable; however, it is not necessary that they be nonbizarre, as DSM-IV required. Still, patients tend to appear unremarkable, as long as you don't touch on one of their delusions. There are half a dozen possible themes, which I've outlined in the Coding Notes.

Although the symptoms can resemble those of schizophrenia, there are several reasons to list delusional disorder separately:

- The age of onset is often later in life (mid- to late-30s) than for schizophrenia.
- Family histories of the two illnesses are dissimilar.
- At follow-up, these patients are rarely rediagnosed as having schizophrenia.
- The infrequent hallucinations take a back seat to the delusions and are understandable in the context of those delusions.

Most importantly, compared to that of schizophrenia, the course of delusional disorder is less fraught with intellectual and work-related deterioration. In fact, behavior won't be much altered, outside of responding to the delusions: for instance, phoning the police for protection, or letter-writing campaigns to complain of sundry imagined insults or infractions. As you might suppose, resulting domestic problems are frequent—and, depending on their subtype, these patients may be swept up in litigation or endless medical tests.

Delusional disorder is uncommon (fewer than 2 per thousand in a study of a Finnish general population). Chronically reduced sensory input (being deaf or blind) may contribute to its development, as may social isolation (such as being a stranger in a foreign land). Delusional disorder may also be associated with family traits that include suspiciousness, jealousy, and secretiveness. The persecutory type is by far the most common of the subtypes; jealous type ranks a distant second.

One problem that crops up frequently is the presence of mood symptoms in patients with delusional disorder. These may be quite unsurprisingly gloomy responses to the perception that others do not agree with closely held beliefs. Depressive mood can create difficult questions of differential diagnosis: Most notably, does the patient have a primary mood disorder? The DSM-5-TR criteria do not provide a clear demarcation between primary mood disorder and psychosis from primary psychosis with depression, but the time course of two sets of symptoms—mood and psychotic—may help in the differentiation. Of course, in the case of serious question, I'd consider first the more conservative (by virtue of having a better prognosis) mood disorder. However, delusional disorder may begin to seem more likely as time passes.

Note, too, that a patient with body dysmorphic disorder whose perceptions are so fixed as to be delusional should be diagnosed not with delusional disorder, but with body dysmorphic disorder.

Shared Delusions

A situation in which others develop delusions because of close association with another delusional person is extremely rare, but also dramatic and inherently interesting. DSM-IV called this condition *shared psychotic disorder;* as long ago as 150 years it was known as *folie à deux,* which means "madness for two" (see sidebar, p. 57). Usually, two people are involved, but three, four, or more can become caught up in the delusion. Shared delusions affect women more often than men, and they typically occur within families. Social isolation may play a role in the development of this strange condition.

One of the persons affected is independently psychotic; through a close (and often dependent) association, the other comes to believe in the delusions and related experiences of the first. Though occasionally bizarre, the content of the delusion is typically believable, if unconvincing. Isolating the independently psychotic patient may cure the other(s), but this remedy doesn't always work: The parties involved, often closely related, may persist in reinforcing their mutual psychopathology.

Some patients whose delusions mirror those of people with whom they are intimately associated will, for one reason or another, not fully qualify for a diagnosis of delusional disorder. For them, you'll have to use the category of other specified (or unspecified) schizophrenia spectrum and other psychotic disorder, as described at the end of this chapter.

Essential Features of **Delusional Disorder**

For at least a month, the patient has had delusions but no other psychotic symptoms, and any mood symptoms have been relatively brief. Other than consequences of the delusions, behavior isn't much affected.

The Fine Print

OK, there might be some hallucinations, perhaps touch or smell, but only as they relate to the delusions. And they won't be prominent.

The D's: • Duration (1+ months) • Distress and disability (none, except as related to the delusional content) • Differential diagnosis (**physical** and **substance-induced psychotic disorders,** mood or cognitive disorders, schizophrenia, **obsessive-compulsive disorder with absent insight, body dysmorphic disorder,** factitious disorder, malingering)

Coding Notes

You can specify type of delusion: erotomanic, grandiose, jealous, persecutory, somatic, mixed, or unspecified (p. 58).

Specify if:

> **With bizarre content.** This denotes obviously improbable delusions (see sidebar, p. 62).

Specify course if the delusional disorder has lasted at least 1 year:

> **First episode, currently in acute episode**
> **First episode, currently in partial remission**
> **First episode, currently in full remission**
> **Multiple episodes, currently in acute episode**
> **Multiple episodes, currently in partial remission**
> **Multiple episodes, currently in full remission**
> **Continuous**
> **Unspecified**

You may specify severity, though you don't have to (p. 74).

Molly McConegal

Molly McConegal, a tiny sparrow of a woman, sits perched on the front of the waiting room chair. On her lap she tightly clutches a scuffed black handbag; her gray hair is caught up in a fierce little bun. Through spectacles as thick as highball glasses, she darts myopic, suspicious glances about the room. She has already spent 45 minutes with the consultant behind closed doors. Now she waits while her husband, Michael, has a turn.

He confirms much of what Molly has already said. They've been married for over 40 years, have two children, and have lived in the same neighborhood (the same house, in fact) nearly all their married life. Both are retired from the telephone company, and they share an interest in gardening.

"That's where it all started, in the garden," says Michael. "It was last summer, when I was out trimming the rose bushes in the front yard. Molly said she caught me looking at the house across the street. The widow woman who lives there is younger than we are, maybe 50. We nod and say 'Hi,' but in 10 years, I've never even been inside her front door. But Molly said I was taking too long on those rose bushes, that I was waiting for our neighbor—her name is Mrs. Jessup—to come out of the house. Of course, I denied it, but she insisted. Talked about it for days."

In the following months, Molly pursued the idea of Michael's supposed extramarital relationship. At first, she only suggested that he had been trying to lure Mrs. Jessup out for a meeting. Within a few weeks, she "knew" that they had been together. Soon, this had become a sex orgy.

Now Molly talks of little else and has begun to incorporate many commonplace observations into her suspicions. A button undone on Michael's shirt means that he has just returned from a visit with "the woman." The angle of the living room Venetian blinds tip her off that he was trying to semaphore messages the night before. A private detective Molly hired for surveillance only stopped by to chat with Michael, submitted an invoice for $500, and resigned.

Molly continues to do the cooking and washing for herself, but Michael now must see to his own meals and laundry. She sleeps well, eats well, and—when he isn't around—seems to be in good spirits.

Michael, on the other hand, is becoming a nervous wreck. Molly listens in on his telephone calls and steams open his mail. She told him once that she'd file for divorce, but she "wouldn't want the children to find out." Twice he has awakened at night to find her wrapped tightly in her bathrobe, standing beside his bed, glowering down at him, "Waiting for me to make my move, she tells me." Last week, she strewed thumbtacks along the hallway outside his room, so that he would cry out and awaken her when he tried to sneak away for his late-night tryst.

Michael's smile is a little wistful. "You know, I haven't had sex with anybody for nearly 15 years. Since my prostate operation, I just haven't had the ability."

Evaluation of Molly McConegal

If you compare the features of delusional disorder with those of schizophrenia, you will note many differences.

First, consider symptoms. Delusions are the only psychotic symptom found to any important degree in delusional disorder. The delusion could be any of the types listed in the Coding Notes. Molly has the jealous type, but the persecutory and grandiose types are also common. Note that apart from occasional olfactory or tactile hallucinations that support the content of delusions, patients with delusional disorder will never fulfill criterion A for schizophrenia (this nonfulfillment constitutes delusional disorder's criterion B).

The delusions need last only 1 month (A); however, by the time they come to professional attention, most patients, like Molly, have been ill much longer. The average age of patients may be around 55. The consequences are usually relatively mild for delusional disorder. Indeed, aside from the direct effects of the delusion (in Molly's case, marital harmony), work and social life may not be affected much at all (C).

However, the exclusions are pretty much the same as for schizophrenia. Always rule out another medical condition or cognitive disorder, especially a neurocognitive disorder with delusions, when evaluating delusional patients (E). This is especially important in older patients, who can be quite crafty at disguising the fact that they are cognitively impaired. Substance-induced psychotic disorders can closely mimic delusional disorder. This is especially true for amphetamine-induced psychotic disorder with onset during withdrawal, in which fully oriented patients may describe how they are being attacked by gangs of pursuers (E).

Although Molly McConegal has neither history nor symptoms to support any of the aforementioned disorders, laboratory and toxicology studies may be needed for many patients. Other than irritability when in the company of her husband, she has no symptoms of a mood disorder. Even then, her affect is quite appropriate to her content of thought. However, many patients with delusional disorder can develop mood syndromes secondary to the delusions. Then the diagnosis depends on the chronology and severity of mood symptoms. Information from relatives or other third parties is often required to determine which came first. Also, the mood symptoms must be relatively mild and brief not to derail a diagnosis of delusional disorder.

Molly has been ill a bit less than a full year, so no course of illness can be specified. Her GAF score would be 55 (highest level in the past year). Her diagnosis would be as follows:

F22   Delusional disorder, jealous type

Miriam Phillips

Miriam Phillips has lived nearly all her 23 years in the Ozarks, where she sometimes attended class in a three-room school. Although she is bright enough, she had little interest in her studies and often volunteered to stay home to care for her mother, who is unwell. She dropped out of 12th grade to keep house full time.

It is lonely living in the hills. Miriam's father, a long-distance trucker, is away most of the time. Miriam never learned to drive, and there are no close neighbors. Their television set receives mostly snow; there is little in the way of mail; and there have been no visitors at all. So she is surprised late on a Monday afternoon when two men pay a call.

After identifying themselves as FBI agents, they ask if she is the Miriam Phillips who 3 weeks ago wrote a letter to the president. When she asks how they know, they show her a faxed copy of her own letter:

> Dear Mr. President, what do you plan to do about the Cubans? They have been working on mother. Their up to no good. Ive seen the police, but they say Cubans are your job, and I guess their right. You have to do your job or Ill have a dirty job to do. Miriam Phillips.

When Miriam finally figures out that the FBI agents think she has threatened the president, she relaxes. She says she didn't mean that at all. But if no one else takes action, she'll have to crawl under the house to get the gravity machines.

"Gravity machines?" The two agents look at each other.

She explains. The machines were installed under the house by Cuban agents of Fidel Castro after the Bay of Pigs invasion in the 1960s. The machines pull your body fluids down toward your feet. They haven't affected her yet, but for years "they have bothered Mama something fierce." Miriam has seen the hideous swelling in her mother's ankles. Some days it extends almost to her knees.

The two agents listen to her politely, then depart. As they pass through town on their way to the airport, they call at the local community mental health clinic. Within a few days, a mental health worker comes to interview Miriam, who agrees to enter the hospital for a "checkup."

On admission, Miriam appears remarkably intact. She shows a full range of appropriate affect with intact cognitive capability and orientation. Her reasoning seems good, aside from the story about the gravity machines.

As far back as her teens, her mother has told her how the machines came to be installed in the crawlspace under the house. Mother had been a nurse, and Miriam always takes her word in medical matters. In the past few months, she has begun to think more about gravity machines. By some unspoken agreement, the two had never discussed the matter with Miriam's father.

After 3 days on the ward, Miriam's clinician asks whether she thought any other explanation for her mother's edema was possible. Miriam considers. She's never felt the gravity effects herself. She believes that her mother tells her the truth, but she now supposes that even Mother could have been mistaken.

Though given no medication, after a week Miriam has stopped talking about gravity machines and asks to be discharged. At the end of their shift that afternoon, two young attendants give her a lift home. As they walk her to the front door, it is opened by a short woman, quite stout, with salt-and-pepper hair. Her lower legs are neatly wrapped in elastic bandages. Through the partly opened door she darts a glance at the two men.

"Hmmm!" she says. "You look like Cubans."

Evaluation of Miriam Phillips

Though we don't know the exact duration, Miriam has had delusions far longer than a month (criterion A) without hallucinations, negative symptoms, or disordered behavior or affect. Therefore, just based on insufficient variety of symptoms (B) we can rule out schizophrenia. We can also easily discard schizophreniform and schizoaffective disorders. She isn't depressed and certainly not manic (D), and there is no history or other evidence to support substance-induced psychotic disorder or psychotic disorder due to another medical condition (E). Her delusions haven't caused any occupational or social dysfunction; her own isolation appears to have begun at least 5 years earlier, before the onset of her shared delusion (C).

After just a few days of separation from her mother, Miriam's delusions have faded. In working further with her, a therapist would also want to consider the possibility of a personality disorder, such as dependent personality disorder. Her delusion, and that of her mother, is certainly bizarre, but I'm not confident she has been ill longer than a year, so I won't give her any other specifiers. I'd give her an admission GAF score of 40.

So, what's not to like about a diagnosis of delusional disorder? Well, nothing at all, except . . .

Except that most people with delusional disorder are not in close contact with another person who has identical delusions, and most do not recover without other treatment after being separated from the other person. Indeed, that combination sounds very much like what we used to call *folie à deux*, later termed *shared psychotic disorder*. For a time, we were encouraged to diagnose such patients as having delusional disorder, which is how I formerly handled her diagnosis. Now, she still meets criteria for delusional disorder, but she also fits nicely into something that makes its home in a category called "other specified schizophrenia spectrum and other psychotic disorders." (Whew!) Which to use?

On the whole, I think I now prefer the latter because it gives us information as to probable cause and likely treatment—separating her from her mother. And no, I haven't been given explicit permission to specify the bizarre content in this context. So sue me.

F28   Delusional symptoms in the context of relationship with an
           individual with prominent delusions, with bizarre content

But I really think we should have kept the name *folie à deux*—or shared delusional disorder.

Schizoaffective Disorder

Schizoaffective disorder (SaD) is just plain confusing. Over the years, it has had many meanings for different clinicians. Partly because task force members could not agree, in 1980 DSM-III included no criteria at all. In 1987, DSM-III-R first attempted to specify criteria. These endured for 7 years, until they were substantially rewritten for DSM-IV. Showing admirable restraint, DSM-5 made relatively few changes to those criteria. Even so, in my opinion the value of this fraught diagnosis remains in question.

Most interpretations (and its name) suggest that SaD is some sort of hybrid between a mood disorder and schizophrenia. Some writers regard it as a form of bipolar disorder (certain patients seem to respond well to lithium); others believe it is more closely related to schizophrenia. Still others believe it is an entirely separate type of psychosis. And some, unfortunately, use SaD as a parking space for patients with any mixture of mood and psychotic symptoms, regardless of number or timing.

SaD can unfold in a variety of ways: mania (or depression) first, psychosis first, or both beginning together. Of course, there are the usual exclusions for substance use and general medical conditions. If we scrutinize the various time requirements, we can determine that the entire illness must last a bit longer than 1 month at minimum, though many patients will remain ill much longer.

The demographic profile of SaD remains uncertain, estimated at perhaps a third the frequency of schizophrenia, with the depressive type more common than the bipolar type. It's overall greater frequency among women reflects the fact that women are about twice as likely as men to have depressive type, with bipolar type about equally represented. Prognosis lies somewhere between that of schizophrenia and the mood disorders; bipolar type may have the better outcome.

I find it a bit easier to think of the requirements for SaD with these reminders:

- The mood symptoms must be present for over half the total duration of illness.
- The psychosis symptoms (delusions or hallucinations) must be present *by themselves* for at least 2 weeks and overall for at least 1 month.

The diagram below shows the psychosis symptoms appearing without the mood episode at the beginning of the illness, but in fact this period of "solo" psychosis can occur anywhere in its course. However, the total duration of psychotic symptoms must be at least one month. Mood symptoms can occur in the absence of psychosis symptoms—but they don't have to. Unfortunately, DSM-5-TR is silent as to whether, during the psychosis period, there can be mood symptoms that do not fully qualify as an episode of mania or depression. (DSM-IV was more forthright; it said, "in the absence of prominent mood symptoms.") Start saving for DSM-6.

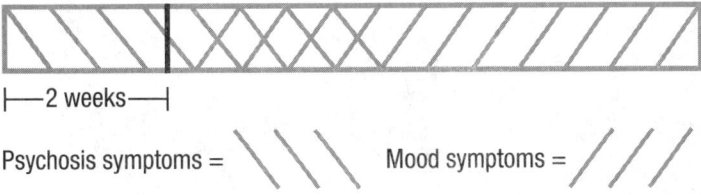

├—2 weeks—┤

Psychosis symptoms = ＼＼＼   Mood symptoms = ／／／

Essential Features of **Schizoaffective Disorder**

During a continuous period of illness the person has principal symptoms of schizo-phrenia (defined below) that coexist with those of a major depressive or manic episode. For at least 2 weeks during this illness, delusions and/or hallucinations exist *without* a mood episode. The mood episode is present for over half of the total duration of the illness, including both active and residual manifestations. Neither substance use nor a different medical illness can account for these symptoms.

The Fine Print

Schizophrenia symptoms: For at least 1 month, delusions or hallucinations plus 1+ symptoms from among hallucinations, delusions, negative symptoms, disordered speech, and disordered behavior.

Manic episode: Markedly high or irritable mood with heightened activity or energy most of the time *and* 3+ (4+ if mood is only irritable) symptoms from among grandios-ity or heightened self esteem, reduced need for sleep, markedly talkative or pressured speech, flight of ideas or racing thoughts, ready distractibility, agitation or increased goal-directed activity, and poor judgment.

Major depressive episode: Depressed mood most of day *and* 4+ symptoms from among reduced pleasure or interest in usual activities, loss or gain of appetite or weight, increased or decreased sleep most days, a sense of worthlessness or unrea-sonable guilt feelings, trouble thinking or concentrating, and repeated ideas of death or suicide.

The D's: • Duration (a total of 1+ months) • Distress and disability (none is stated, but hard to imagine without) • Differential diagnosis (psychotic mood disorders, schizo-phrenia and other psychoses, **substance use,** and **physical disorders**)

Coding Notes

Specify:

> **F25.0 Bipolar type** (if during a manic episode)
> **F25.1 Depressive type**

Specify:

> **With catatonia** (p. 100)

If the disorder has lasted at least 1 year, specify course:

> **First episode, currently in acute episode**
> **First episode, currently in partial remission**

> **First episode, currently in full remission**
> **Multiple episodes, currently in acute episode**
> **Multiple episodes, currently in partial remission**
> **Multiple episodes, currently in full remission**
> **Continuous**
> **Unspecified**
>
> You may specify severity, though you don't have to (p. 74).

Velma Dean

Velma Dean's lips curl upward, but the smile doesn't touch her eyes. "I'm really sorry about this," she tells her therapist, "but I guess—well, I don't know what." She reaches into her large shopping bag and pulls out a 6-inch kitchen knife. First, she grasps it in her hand, with her thumb along the blade. Then she tries clutching it in her fist, the tip pointed down. The clinician reaches for the alarm button under the desktop, ruefully aware of yet another course change in this patient's multifaceted history.

A month before her 18th birthday, Velma Dean joined the Army. Her father, a colonel of artillery, had wanted a son, but Velma is his only child. Over the feeble protests of her mother, Velma's upbringing was strict and militaristic. After working 3 years in the motor pool, Velma had just been promoted to sergeant when she became ill.

Her illness started with 2 days in the infirmary for what seemed like bronchitis. As the penicillin took effect and her fever resolved, the voices began. At first, they seemed to be located toward the back of her head. Within a few days they had moved to her bedside water glass. As nearly as she could tell, their pitch depended on the contents of her glass: If the glass was nearly empty, the voices were female; if it was full to the top, they spoke in a rich baritone. They were always quiet and mannerly. Often, they gave her advice on how to behave, but at times they commented on what she was doing. "They nearly drove me crazy," she complained.

A psychiatrist diagnosed Velma's condition as schizophrenia and prescribed antipsychotic drugs. Over the next several weeks, the voices improved, but never quite disappeared. She "figured out" that her illness had been caused by her first sergeant, who she believed had tried unsuccessfully to get into her bed. (When confronted later, he had laughed and said, "Hey, I'm gay.") The Army initiated discharge as medically unfit, 100% disabled. The disappointment she feels ("Another failure!") fed into the depression that grew over the next several months. Three months after her first psychotic symptoms appeared, she was well enough to travel, and her father drove her the 600 miles back home.

For treatment, Velma enrolls at her local Department of Veterans Affairs outpatient clinic. There, her new therapist verifies (1) the continuing presence (now for nearly 4 months) of her barely audible hallucinations, and (2) her deepening symptoms of depression. These include profoundly low mood (much worse in the morning than in the evening), poor self-esteem, and hopelessness. She also has experienced loss of appetite, a 10-pound weight loss over the past 2 months, insomnia that causes her to awaken early most mornings, and the guilty conviction that she has disappointed her father by "deserting" the Army before her hitch was up. She denies thoughts of injuring herself or other people. She withholds the fact that, over the 3 weeks she's been back, she has consumed nearly a pint of Southern Comfort daily.

Velma's VA clinician initially defers making a diagnosis, noting that she has been ill too long for schizophreniform disorder and that her long-standing depressive symptoms seem to argue against schizophrenia. Physical exam and laboratory testing rule out general medical conditions. Although a VA support group has helped her stop drinking, her depressive and psychotic symptoms continue.

Because Velma's psychosis may be only partly treated, her dose of antipsychotic medication is increased. This eliminates the hallucinations and delusions, but the depressive symptoms continue virtually unabated. The antidepressant imipramine at 200 mg/day produces only side effects; after 4 weeks, lithium is added. Once a therapeutic blood level is reached, her depressive symptoms melt completely away. For 6 months she remains in a good mood and free of psychosis, though she never obtains a job or does very much with her time that is constructive.

Now her clinician wonders whether Velma might be suffering from a major depressive disorder with psychotic features. And, could the antipsychotics produce side effects such as tardive dyskinesia? So with Velma's consent, they gradually reduce the antipsychotic drug by about 20% per week. For the next 3 weeks her mood remains good; except for some difficulty getting to sleep at night, she develops none of the vegetative symptoms she had formerly experienced with depression. Then she once again begins to hear voices; they direct her to run away from home. Her full former dose of antipsychotic medication is rapidly restored.

After several months of renewed stability, Velma and her therapist decide to try again. This time they began cautiously to reduce the imipramine, by 25 mg each week. Every Monday afternoon they meet to evaluate her mood and check for symptoms of psychosis. By December she has been free of the antidepressant for 2 months and has remained symptom-free (except for her habitual bland, smiling affect). Now her therapist takes a deep breath and decreases her lithium by one tablet per day. The following Monday, Velma returns to the office, depressed and hallucinating and wondering whether to hold the kitchen knife in her hand or in her fist.

Evaluation of Velma Dean

Here's how Velma's story fits into the current thinking about SaD. Her condition seems to be a mixture of mood and psychotic symptoms that constitute a single period of illness. Her only "well" periods are when she takes medication; even then, she has residual lack of initiative. She has psychotic symptoms (auditory hallucinations and a delusion that the sergeant had caused her illness) plus a major depressive episode (schizoaffective disorder criterion A). During this illness, mood symptoms, which occur both with and without psychosis, last for more than half the duration of her total illness—or disappear only with treatment (C). Because her alcohol abuse began after the onset of both psychotic and depressive symptoms, it must be a consequence of her illness, not the cause (D). The psychosis, which began first, was present at least 2 weeks before and 2 weeks after the onset of mood symptoms for a total of at least 1 month (B).

Although we can rattle off these criteria with relative ease (and, to be honest, a crib sheet), Velma's history illustrates how difficult it can be to apply them. The therapist, whose thinking has already been described in the vignette, wisely deferred diagnosis at first. This should remind us all to keep thinking about what's wrong and to reject any label that might close our minds to further diagnostic possibilities. She cannot be diagnosed as having schizophrenia because it excludes prominent, lasting mood episodes. A mood disorder with psychosis can be eliminated because she has psychotic symptoms even when not depressed. After many months of observation, she shows no evidence of another medical condition.

The relative duration of psychosis and mood symptoms is critical in SaD. DSM-5-TR states that the mood symptoms must be present for the majority of the overall duration of illness. Velma's depressive symptoms lasted for at least 2 months; there is every reason to suspect they would have continued much longer had she not received effective treatment. Her criterion A symptoms for schizophrenia were present for 2 weeks without mood symptoms. However carefully the manual tries to operationalize the duration of various symptoms, it remains to some degree a clinician's judgment call. DSM-5-TR is silent on the issue of treated depression and SaD; I'm claiming clinician's prerogative and declaring that because antidepressant treatment seems to have made all the difference, SaD should be her diagnosis.

Eventually, many patients with both mood and psychotic symptoms will comfortably fit the criteria for either schizophrenia or a mood disorder. If they are followed long enough, perhaps most patients with SaD can be rediagnosed. Given the highly restrictive nature of the current definition, it seems likely that this diagnosis should be used infrequently. Before you make the diagnosis, ask yourself first, "Have I overlooked anything?" SaD is a diagnosis best saved for patients who have a long-standing history of both sets of symptoms. Other specified (or unspecified) schizophrenia spectrum and other psychotic disorder may prove to be much more useful to most clinicians. Velma's mood symptoms were depressive, which defines her subtype diagnosis. At the time she was wielding her knife, I would place her GAF score down around 20.

F25.1   Schizoaffective disorder, depressive type

Substance/Medication-Induced Psychotic Disorder

This category includes all psychoses caused by mind-altering substances. The predominant symptoms are typically hallucinations or delusions, which, depending on the substance, can occur during withdrawal or acute intoxication. (Do not make this diagnosis if the person retains reality testing. Then, diagnose instead a substance intoxication or withdrawal.) The course is typically brief, though the symptoms can persist long enough to cause confusion with endogenous psychoses—that is, those that have no evident external cause.

Although most of these psychoses are self-limiting, early recognition is crucial. Patients have died while experiencing a substance-induced psychotic disorder, several of which can closely mimic schizophrenia. Many diagnoses are possible, if we include all the possible combinations of different substances with the type and duration of psychosis and the relation to intoxication, withdrawal, or use of medications. The incidence is unknown, though a substantial minority of first-episode psychoses may belong to this class—certainly enough that we need to remain alert for them. See the "Classes (or Names) of Medications . . ." table on page 665 for a list of medications associated with psychosis.

Essential Features of **Substance/Medication-Induced Psychotic Disorder**

After using a substance that can produce psychotic symptoms, the person develops hallucinations or delusions (or both).

For tips on identifying substance-related causation, see sidebar, page 95.

The Fine Print

The D's: • Distress or disability (work/academic, social, or personal impairment) • Differential diagnosis (**schizophrenia and its cousins,** delusional disorder, **ordinary substance intoxication** or **withdrawal, delirium,** neurocognitive disorder)

Use this diagnosis instead of substance intoxication or withdrawal only when psychotic symptoms are predominant and require clinical care.

Coding Notes

When writing down the diagnosis, use the name of the exact substance in the title: for example, methamphetamine-induced psychotic disorder.

Coding in ICD-10 depends on the substance used and whether symptoms are met for an actual substance use disorder—and how severe the use disorder is. Refer to Table 15.2 (p. 475).

Specify if:

With onset during {intoxication}{withdrawal}. This gets tacked on at the end of your string of words. It also affects the ICD-10 number.

With onset after medication use. You could alternatively use this if symptoms develop when medication is started, changed, or stopped.

You may specify severity, though you don't have to (p. 74).

Danny Finch

After enduring the ear problem for 3 days, Danny Finch finally calls for an appointment. The doctor pokes around and worries a little over Danny's tremor.

"You don't drink, do you?"

"A little. But what about my ear?"

"It's perfectly normal."

"But I hear something. It's like someone chanting. I can almost make out what they're saying. You're sure no one's put something in there, a hearing aid?" He digs at the ear with his little finger.

"Nope, clean as a whistle. Here, don't do that!" The doctor scribbles a referral to the mental health clinic down the hall. It's late on a Friday, so the clinic is closed.

On Monday afternoon, when he finally gets to his appointment, Danny can once again write his name legibly and eat solid food. But the voices are in full throat. As he talks with the interviewer, he can hardly concentrate for the shouting: "Don't tell about the drinking!" and "Why don't you just kill yourself?" Terrified, he accepts with relief a voluntary admission to the mental health ward, where his admitting diagnosis is schizophrenia. Twice a day, he tucks the potent antipsychotic medication they give him under his tongue and discards it in the tissue when he pretends to blow his nose.

He sleeps soundly at night and cleans his plate at every meal, while the voices bellow on. At the end of the week, he is visited by a consultant who learns that the voices originate about 2 feet behind him and talk in sentences. Reluctantly, Danny admits that they tell him not to talk about his drinking.

A rapid review of Danny's chart reveals no mention of alcohol use, but a little coaxing soon pries loose the whole story. Since his early 20s, he's experienced heavy drinking, loss of two jobs (with a shaky hold on his current one), and a divorce, all related to his fondness for bourbon. Most recently he has been drinking more than a pint each evening, often a fifth on the weekends. On past occasions when he's quit, he's managed to taper off; this time, a few days before he consulted the doctor about his hearing, he had stopped suddenly after a bout of what he calls "the stomach flu."

DSM-5-TR repeatedly refers to symptoms that appear caused by use of a substance. It is up to you to evaluate your patient for evidence for or against such a causation. Here are several factors, mostly based on chronology, that might constitute such evidence.

Favoring a substance-use etiology:

1. The symptoms begin during or soon after the use of a substance or soon after it is withdrawn.
2. The symptoms start after a patient has begun using a medication.
3. The drug/medication is known to have caused the symptoms in other people.
4. Of course, if your patient has had a prior episode of the same symptoms that followed use of the same substance, that's perhaps the best evidence of all.

And here are some of the reasons to resist a substance-use causation:

1. Rather obviously, a disorder with onset even marginally before substance use begins wouldn't be caused by the substance.
2. Your patient had a prior episode of the same, or very similar, symptoms that did *not* occur in the context of substance use.
3. The disorder continues long after the use of (or withdrawal from) the substance has stopped.
4. The symptoms are worse than you'd expect, considering the amount and duration of the substance misuse.

None of these is exactly iron-clad. For example, a prior history of major depressive disorder doesn't confer immunity to a subsequent depression that originates in a bottle of scotch. Still, the cues are there for your thoughtful consideration.

Evaluation of Danny Finch

Danny's auditory hallucinations (criterion A) have been present far too briefly for schizophrenia, though he describes them in similar terms. A brief psychotic disorder might seem possible, except for the requirement that a substance-induced psychotic disorder does not better explain the symptoms (C). He was recently seen by a physician who pronounced him fit; there is no evidence of any other physical condition. The fact that he seems fully oriented and can focus his attention would rule out delirium and other cognitive disorders (D). Though he appears (appropriately) frightened by his experiences (E), he presents no evidence of mood disorder (C again).

His psychosis—in the distant past it was called alcoholic auditory hallucinosis—is a disorder of withdrawal that typically occurs only after weeks or months of heavy drinking (B). By about a 4:1 ratio, it occurs much more commonly in men than in women. Auditory hallucinosis is sometimes misidentified as alcohol withdrawal delirium, though the problems with orientation and attention in the latter should make the differences clear (p. 493).

Withdrawal from other drugs can also produce psychosis. Barbiturates, which have many of the same effects as alcohol, are the most notorious of these. Some patients who use phencyclidine or other hallucinogens such as LSD experience prolonged psychosis, the risk for which may be greater in people who have personality disorders.

Danny's symptoms were clearly more serious than we'd expect in alcohol withdrawal with perceptual disturbances (which would be diagnosed had he retained insight that his experiences weren't "real"). His GAF score was only 35 on admission; his diagnosis (from Table 15.2) would be as follows:

F10.259   Severe alcohol use disorder with alcohol-induced psychotic disorder, with onset during withdrawal

Psychotic Disorder Due to Another Medical Condition

A psychosis arising in a patient who has another medical condition shouldn't be especially rare. Many diseases can produce psychosis, and some of them are relatively common. But few, if any, studies bear on questions of epidemiology. When such patients do appear, they are too often misdiagnosed as having schizophrenia or some other endogenous psychosis. This can lead to real tragedy: A patient who is not appropriately treated early enough may go on to experience (or cause) serious harm. Prevalence rates are not known exactly, but they're probably low; as you might imagine, frequency increases with age.

A person who retains insight into the unreality of hallucinations would not be given this diagnosis. Also note that a patient with mainly disorganized behavior would instead be diagnosed as having catatonic disorder due to another medical condition.

It's often a struggle to determine whether a physical illness or medical condition has caused any mental disorder. Here are a few straws in the wind that can help.

- Timing: Mental or behavioral symptoms that begin shortly after the start of the physical illness offer a pretty obvious etiological clue. And, remission follows effective treatment for the physical issue.
- Proportionality of symptoms: As the physical disorder worsens, so do the behavioral or emotional symptoms.
- Typicality of symptoms: Are the symptoms atypical for an independent psychosis? For example, you wouldn't expect first onset of psychosis in an elderly person.
- Above all, there must be a known physiological connection between the physical condition and the symptom in question. That is, we must know that the physical disorder can produce the symptom (for example, through production of chemicals, by impinging on brain structures). It cannot simply be that the prospect of having a serious illness evokes psychosis, depression, anxiety, and so forth.

OK, so these pointers aren't exactly iron-clad. Remember, they're straws, not steel.

Essential Features of Psychotic Disorder Due to Another Medical Condition

Through physiological means, a medical condition appears to have caused an illness that features obvious hallucinations or delusions.

The Fine Print

For pointers on deciding when a physical condition may have caused a mental disorder, see the sidebar above.

The D's: • Distress or disability (work/academic, social, or personal impairment) • Differential diagnosis (**delirium, another mental disorder,** substance-induced psychotic disorder, schizophrenia and its cousins, delusional disorder)

Coding Notes

In recording the diagnosis, use the name of the responsible medical condition, and list *first* the medical condition, with its code number.

Code, based on the predominant symptoms:

    F06.2 With delusions
    F06.0 With hallucinations

You may specify severity, though you don't have to (p. 74).

Rodrigo Chavez

Since retiring from teaching at age 65, Rodrigo Chavez spends most of his time sitting alone in his room. Sometimes he plays the acoustic guitar; once or twice he's shot targets at the rifle range. True to his lifelong custom, he never drinks. Other than his immediate family, he has few social contacts. "My cigarettes are my best friends," he says during the forensic examination.

When Rodrigo is nearly 70, an inoperable carcinoma of the lung is diagnosed. After a course of palliative radiotherapy, he declines further treatment and settles down in his apartment to die. Four months later, he notices right-sided headaches that will sometimes awaken him in the middle of the night. Because the doctors have told him he is terminally ill, he doesn't seek further medical attention.

Then, he begins to associate the headaches with natural gas, which he can smell coming out of the ventilator duct in his bathroom. When he calls to report the problem to Mrs. Riordan, his landlady, she sends around the building's handyman, who can find nothing wrong. But both the odors and his headaches have increased; Rodrigo recalls that, weeks earlier, Mrs. Riordan went out several times to watch while repairmen from the power company dug up the street outside the apartment building. The conclusion fairly bursts upon him: His landlady is trying to poison him.

As the odor worsens, his anger mounts. It's begun to affect his voice, which has become raspy and high-pitched. He has several shouted arguments with Mrs. Riordan. One of these they carry on through her apartment door at 2 A.M., several weeks after he first noticed the gas. He says he'll report her to the housing authority; she calls him "a crazy old coot." After he threatens her ("If I'm not safe, your life isn't worth 15 cents!"), they make simultaneous 911 calls. The police, finding nothing to charge anyone with, admonish them both to behave.

The night he is arrested, Rodrigo sits just inside his open doorway, yelling insults at Mrs. Riordan. When she lumbers to the top of the stairs to investigate, he shoots her once, just behind her left ear. The arresting officers note that he seems "strangely detached" from the murder of his landlady. One of them writes down this quotation: "It wouldn't matter, just for me. But I couldn't stand her gassing all those other people in the house."

The forensic examiner notes that Rodrigo Chavez is an elderly, slightly built man who is clean-shaven and neatly groomed. He appears gaunt; he may have lost considerable weight. Though his speech is clear, coherent, relevant, and spontaneous, his voice is high-pitched and scratchy.

At first he appears calm and describes his mood as "medium," but he becomes angry when recounting his landlady's attempts to poison him. He is oriented to person, place, and time, and he earns a perfect score on the MMSE. He is fully aware that he has lung cancer, but insight for the fact of his psychosis is nil; from recent history, his judgment has been extremely poor.

An X-ray of his chest reveals a right lung full of tumor; skull films suggest a metastatic lesion located in his right frontal lobe.

Evaluation of Rodrigo Chavez

Rodrigo Chavez is clearly psychotic: For several months he has had prominent olfactory hallucinations and an elaborate delusion about being poisoned, fulfilling criterion A. (If insight is retained that the hallucinations and delusions are a product of the patient's own mind, one would generally not diagnose a psychotic disorder.) Also note that, though Rodrigo's symptoms clearly meet the criterion A inclusion requirements for schizophrenia, they don't have to: Either hallucinations or delusions can qualify a person for psychotic disorder due to another medical condition.

Aside from his psychosis, Rodrigo's thinking is clear. He is oriented and he scores well on the MMSE, so there's no evidence of a delirium or neurocognitive disorder (D). He has no history of drinking or taking drugs, ruling out a substance-induced psychotic disorder. His mood has been angry at times, but appropriate to the content of his delusions and hallucinations, so a mood disorder with psychotic features would also seem unlikely. There is no previous history of behavior or personality change that would qualify him for a diagnosis of schizophrenia (C). Other features atypical for schizophrenia include the late age of onset and relatively brief duration. We can rule out schizophreniform disorder because another diagnosis is more likely. Mrs. Riordan's unhappy demise provides mute testimony to the seriousness of his illness (E).

Rodrigo has a cancer that is known to metastasize to the brain; his headaches suggest that it had already done so. The findings on chest X-ray and MRI confirm the diagnosis (B). His gravelly, high-pitched voice may be caused by extension of the growth or by a metastasis within his chest or neck. (Other medical conditions that can cause psychosis include temporal lobe epilepsy, primary [that is, not metastatic] brain tumors, endocrine disorders such as thyroid and adrenal disease, vitamin deficiency states, central nervous system syphilis, multiple sclerosis, systemic lupus erythematosus, Wilson's disease, and head trauma.)

Although Rodrigo has *both* hallucinations and delusions, the olfactory hallucinations appeared first and seem to predominate, resulting in the diagnosis as recorded. My assessment of his GAF score is 15.

C79.31	Cancer of the lung, metastatic to the brain
F06.0	Psychotic disorder due to metastatic carcinoma, with hallucinations
Z65.3	Arrested for murder

F06.1 Catatonia Associated with Another Mental Disorder (Catatonia Specifier)

Catatonia, which for over a century has been thought of as a classic schizophrenia subtype, was first described by Karl Kahlbaum in 1874; in 1896, Emil Kraepelin included it with the disorganized (back then it was called hebephrenic) and paranoid types as a major subgroup of what he termed *dementia praecox*. During the early part of the 20th century, each of these subtypes constituted about a third of all U.S. hospital admissions for schizophrenia. Since that time, the prevalence of the catatonic type has declined, so that it is now less usual to encounter such a patient on an acute care inpatient service. When it does occur, we would now call it catatonia associated with schizophrenia.

The catatonic features usually associated with mania include hyperactivity, impulsivity, and combativeness. These patients may also refuse to keep their clothes on. Depressed patients may show markedly reduced mobility (even to the point of stupor), mutism, negativism, mannerisms, and stereotypies.

I've omitted definitions of catatonic symptoms from various locations and gathered them all into one convenient place: right here. Each of these behaviors tends to be repeated (or ongoing) rather than a one-off occurrence.

Agitation. Excessive motor activity that appears to have neither a purpose nor an external cause.

Stupor would be more or less the polar opposite of agitation.

Catalepsy. Maintaining an uncomfortable posture, even when told it is not necessary to do so.

Echolalia. Verbatim repetition of someone else's words when a different response is indicated.

Echopraxia. Imitating another person's physical behavior, even when asked not to do so.

Exaggerated compliance. At the slightest touch, moving in the direction indicated by another person (the old German term is *mitgehen*). DSM-5-TR leaves this one out; I'm including it because it belongs.

Grimace. A facial contortion not made in response to a noxious stimulus.

Mannerisms. Repeated movements that seem to have a goal but are excessive for the purpose.

Mutism. Absence (or paucity) of speech despite evident physical ability to speak.

Negativism. Without apparent motive, the patient resists passive movement or repeatedly turns away from the examiner.

Posturing. Voluntarily assuming an unnatural or uncomfortable pose.

Stereotypy. Repeated movement that is a nonessential part of goal-directed behavior.

Waxy flexibility. Active resistance when an examiner tries to change the patient's position—similar to bending a rubber or soft wax rod.

Essential Features of Catatonia Associated with Another Mental Disorder (Catatonia Specifier)

The patient has at least three prominent symptoms of catatonia, such as catalepsy, negativism, posturing, stupor, stereotypy, grimacing, echolalia, and others (see the accompanying sidebar for definitions).

The Fine Print

Relax, it's only a specifier. No Fine Print.

Coding Notes

You can apply the catatonia specifier to manic, hypomanic, or major depressive episodes; to schizophrenia; and to schizophreniform, schizoaffective, brief psychotic, and substance-induced psychotic disorders. It can even be used for autism spectrum disorder.

List first the other mental disorder, then F06.1, then catatonia associated with [the other mental disorder].

Edward Clapham

A 43-year-old single man, Edward Clapham, is admitted to the university hospital's mental health service. He gives no chief complaint. In fact, he says nothing at all: He's entirely mute. He has been transferred from the state psychiatric hospital, where his diagnosis is listed as schizophrenia, catatonic type. For the past 8 years, he has communicated by neither speech nor writing.

According to the transfer note, throughout his hospitalization, Edward has been treated intensively with a variety of antipsychotic medications; none of them has relieved his basic symptoms. He reportedly spends the entire day every day lying on his back, toes pointing toward the foot of his bed, fists clenched and turned inward. From years of maintaining this position, he has developed severe muscle contractures at both ankles and both wrists. Most of the time he could be spoon-fed, but occasionally he refused to swallow and had to be fed by nasogastric tube. This has often been the case during the past 6 months; despite the tube feedings, he has lost about 30 pounds.

Ten days ago, Edward developed a high fever (104.6°F) and was transferred to the medical service, where the staff treated a *Klebsiella* pneumonia with tetracycline. Subsequently he was moved to the mental health service. Very little is known about Edward's background. He grew up in the Midwest, the second child of a rural family. He may have attended some college, and he worked for approximately 10 years as a tractor salesman. His admission mental status examination reads as follows:

> Mr. Clapham lies flat on his back in bed. He is totally mute, so nothing can be learned of his thought content or flow of thought. Similarly, his cognitive processes, insight, and judgment cannot be assessed. His toes point down and his fists are rotated inward. There is a noticeable tremor of his feet and his hands; he contracts the muscles of his arms and legs so strongly that they tremble.
>
> Besides being mute, he shows other signs of catatonia. *Negativism:* When he is approached from one side, he gradually turns his head so that he gazes in the opposite direction. *Catalepsy:* When a limb is placed in any position (for instance, raised high above his head), he will maintain that position for several minutes, even if told that he can relax. *Waxy flexibility:* Any attempt to bend his arm at the elbow, where there are no contractures, is met with resistance that eventually yields to pressure. It is evident that the biceps and triceps muscles are contracting together, causing motion at the joint to feel as if one were bending a rod made of wax or some other stiff substance. *Grimacing:* Every four or five minutes, he wrinkles his nose and purses his lips. This expression lasts for 10 or 15 seconds, then softens. There is no apparent purpose to these motor behaviors, and they are not accompanied by any motions of the tongue or other indications of tardive dyskinesia.

Evaluation of Edward Clapham

Counting his negative symptoms (lack of speech and affect) and his grossly abnormal motor behavior, Edward fulfills the criterion A requirements for schizophrenia. His illness has lasted far longer than the minimum 6 months (schizophrenia criterion C); it is hard to imagine how it could have had a greater effect on every aspect of his life (B). Nonetheless, his admission diagnosis is "unspecified schizophrenia spectrum and other psychotic disorder." This provisional diagnosis is given because the clinician cannot be sure from the initial presentation whether the symptoms are effects of his dehydration and loss of weight (another medical condition), schizophrenia, or another cause such as a mood disorder, which is perhaps the most frequent cause of catatonic symptoms.

The list of medical conditions that can produce catatonic behavior includes liver disease, strokes, epilepsy, and uncommon disorders such as Wilson's disease and tuberous sclerosis, an autosomal dominant genetic disorder. These possibilities should be vigorously pursued with neurological and medical consultation and with the appropriate laboratory and X-ray studies. Urine or blood screens for toxic substances or drugs of abuse should be considered a part of every such patient's workup. Any patient who presents with a first episode of catatonia should probably have an MRI. When Edward Clapham was diagnosed, MRI did not exist; we'll have to take criterion E on faith.

Many patients who have been diagnosed as having schizophrenia, catatonic type, are actually in a manic phase of bipolar I disorder (D). On the other hand, a patient with severe psychomotor slowing should be considered for major depressive disorder with melancholic features. Although patients with somatic symptom disorder are occasionally mute or have abnormal motor activity, such episodes are usually short-lived, lasting only a few hours or days, not years. Edward has been ill for years; a chronic, psychotic, catatonic mood disorder seems unlikely in the extreme.

Edward's symptoms are classic for catatonia associated with schizophrenia. He demonstrates grimacing (catatonia specifier criterion A10), muteness (A4), waxy flexibility (A3), and catalepsy (A2). He cannot be called stuporous because he is alert enough to turn away from an approaching stimulus (negativism—A5). His behavior range is insufficient to demonstrate other typical catatonic behaviors.

Because he has already been extensively (and unsuccessfully) treated with antipsychotics, Edward is given a course of electroconvulsive therapy. Although the first three bilateral treatments produce no noticeable effect, after the fourth he asks for a glass of water. After a total of 10 treatments, he converses with others on the ward, feeds himself, and walks—always on tiptoe because of the severe contractures at his ankles. Although he continues to show residual symptoms of his disease, his catatonic symptoms disappear. He eventually leaves the hospital and is lost to follow-up.

Edward's 8-year course of illness has been continuous; I'll score his GAF at discharge as 60 (on admission, it would have been pretty close to 1). After appropriate medical investigations and additional history rule out other possible causes of his abnormal behavior, his revised diagnosis is as given below.

By the way, without reference to the official DSM-5-TR severity criteria for psychosis, on admission I'd give Edward a rating of severe. I anticipate no backlash from outraged coding mavens, though I still feel that the overall global evaluation of the GAF does a better job. At discharge:

F20.9	Schizophrenia, first episode, currently in partial remission
F06.1	Catatonia associated with schizophrenia
M24.573	Contractures of ankles
M24.539	Contractures of wrists

F06.1 Catatonic Disorder Due to Another Medical Condition

In recent decades, we've come to realize that catatonia is most often found in association with various medical disorders. Each published account tends to describe only a handful of patients, but the responsible illnesses are broad, including viral encephalitis, subarachnoid hemorrhage, ruptured berry aneurysm in the brain, subdural hematoma, hyperparathyroidism, arteriovenous malformation, temporal lobe tumors, akinetic mutism, and penetrating head wounds. There has even been a description of one patient who had a reaction to fluorides. A neurologist or mental health clinician who does a lot of consulting in a busy medical center may occasionally encounter catatonic symptoms.

Whether they occur in someone with a mood disorder, with schizophrenia, or with a physical disorder, catatonic symptoms are essentially the same (see accompanying sidebar). A patient with another medical condition is more likely to have the characteristic symptoms of what has been termed *retarded* catatonia. These include posturing, catalepsy, and waxy flexibility. Such patients may also drool, stop eating, or become mute.

Essential Features of Catatonic Disorder Due to Another Medical Condition

Through physiological means, a medical condition appears to have caused an illness that features symptoms of catatonia (at least three), such as catalepsy, negativism, posturing, stupor, stereotypy, grimacing, echolalia, and others; for definitions see sidebar page 100.

The Fine Print

For pointers on deciding when a physical condition may have caused a mental disorder, see sidebar, page 97.

The D's: • Distress or disability (work/educational, social, or personal impairment) • Differential diagnosis (**delirium** or other cognitive disorder, schizophrenia and its cousins, psychotic mood disorder, obsessive–compulsive disorder)

Coding Notes

List first the actual medical condition, then F06.1, then catatonia due to [the responsible medical condition].

Marion Wright

Since graduating from high school 12 years ago, Marion Wright has worked as a sign painter. In school he had shown some aptitude for art, though he never saw himself as the next Pablo Picasso. Nor did he like school enough to study for a career in commercial art. But painting signs on buildings and billboards was undemanding, well-paying, immediately available, and largely open-air. Within a few years he was married, had two kids and a small house in a decent subdivision, and was still painting signs. He thought he was set for life.

One afternoon not long after his 30th birthday, his foreman drives by to inspect the billboard Marion has just finished. "You've painted the logo in script. The blueprint calls for block letters," the foreman points out. Marion says he thinks the script looks better, but without too much grumbling he changes it.

A week later, he completes an ad for a local premium beer; the female model holding the bottle is naked from the waist up. The following day, Marion is out of work.

Marion makes a few efforts to find a new job, but within a week he is staying at home and watching daytime TV. In the second week, his wife notes that he seems to be talking less and less, but he ignores her suggestion to seek clinical evaluation. Although he eats and sleeps as usual, his interest in sex has vanished. By week four, he has no spontaneous speech at all and will only answer a question that is put to him directly. With the added persuasion of Marion's brother, they finally get him to the clinic. Of course, he is immediately hospitalized.

On admission Marion answers questions appropriately, if briefly. Fully oriented, he denies feeling depressed or suicidal. He admits to no delusions, hallucinations, obsessions, or compulsions. He earns a perfect score on the MMSE, though the examiner notes that he is slow to carry out instructions.

The following morning, he deliberately turns away from the nurse who approaches his bedside. Although he willingly accompanies the nurse to a table in the dining room, he refuses to eat and is now completely mute. The clinician who examines him later that morning finds that Marion will readily move in any direction at the slightest touch of an examiner's hand. In the evening he seems improved, even speaks a few words.

But the next day, he lies on his back in bed, again silently refusing to cooperate. When his pillow is removed, his head remains elevated a couple of inches above the mattress. This position appears to cause him no discomfort; he seems willing to maintain it all day. Later, an examiner notes that when Marion's arm is moved to an awkward position (elevated at an angle over the bed), he maintains that position even when he is told that he can put it down.

Marion's clinicians consider the diagnosis of schizophrenia, but they note that he has been only briefly ill and has no family history of psychosis. His wife assures them that he has never abused drugs or alcohol. Despite a neurological exam that remains within normal limits, someone orders an MRI of his head. It reveals a tumor the size of a golf ball sitting on the convexity of his right frontal lobe. Once this is surgically removed, he quickly regains full consciousness. Two months later he is back on his ladder painting billboards, following instructions to the letter.

Evaluation of Marion Wright

Marion has several symptoms (three are required) that are classical for catatonia (criterion A). These include negativism (turning away from the nurse) and muteness (A5, A4), exaggerated compliance (though this is not one of the criteria DSM-5-TR mentions), a "psychological pillow" (a form of posturing in which he held his head unsupported above the mattress—A6), and catalepsy (A2).

Marion's attention doesn't wander, excluding delirium (D). Catatonic behavior can be found in schizophrenia, which his clinicians correctly reject—in part because he has been ill so briefly (C). Too few symptoms (and better choices) rule out schizophreniform disorder. Muteness and marked motor slowing, even to the point of immobility, can be encountered in a major depressive episode, but Marion specifically denies mood symptoms. Muteness may occasionally be encountered in somatic symptom disorder, malingering, and factitious disorder, but it would be unusual to encounter a full, persisting catatonic syndrome in one of these conditions.

Note that catatonic behavior can include excessive or even frenzied motor activity, which could suggest a manic episode or substance use intoxication. Of course, neither of these applies to Marion's disorder.

On laboratory examination of the surgical specimen, Marion was found to have a (benign) brain tumor, which can directly result in catatonic symptoms (B) and which caused manifest impairment (E). On admission, I'd put his GAF score at 21; his GAF score was 90 on discharge.

D32.9	Cerebral meningioma, benign
F06.1	Catatonic disorder due to cerebral meningioma

F28 Other Specified Schizophrenia Spectrum and Other Psychotic Disorder

Use this category when you want to write down the specific reason your patient cannot receive a more definite psychotic disorder diagnosis. Here's how you would record it: "Other specified schizophrenia spectrum and other psychotic disorder, attenuated psychosis syndrome."

Charles Bonnet syndrome. In this disorder (not specifically mentioned in DSM-5-TR, but first described in 1790!), people with impaired vision, many of them elderly, report complex visual hallucinations (scenes, people) but no other hallucinations or delusions. They also have insight that what they "see" is unreal. As such, they aren't truly psychotic, but one can argue that the condition belongs somewhere along the spectrum of psychotic disorders.

Attenuated psychosis syndrome. A patient has psychotic symptoms that do not meet the full criteria for any psychotic disorder (symptoms tend to be brief and less disabling, with relatively good insight).

Persistent auditory hallucinations. The patient experiences repeated auditory hallucinations without other symptoms.

Delusional symptoms in the context of relationship with an individual with prominent delusions. Most people who develop delusions in response to close association with someone who is independently psychotic can be diagnosed as having a delusional disorder. However, those who don't fulfill criteria for delusional disorder can be classified here.

Other. The patient appears to have a psychotic disorder, but the information is conflicting or too inadequate to permit a more specific diagnosis.

F29 Unspecified Schizophrenia Spectrum and Other Psychotic Disorder

This category is for symptoms or syndromes that don't meet guidelines for any of the disorders described earlier, and you do not wish to specify a reason.

Unspecified Catatonia

DSM-5-TR mentions unspecified catatonia as a possibility when the context is unclear or there is insufficient detail for a more precise diagnosis. But the coding itself is clear. First:

R29.818   Other symptoms involving nervous and musculoskeletal systems

Then:

F06.1   Unspecified catatonia

CHAPTER 3

Mood Disorders

Issues related to genetics and symptoms locate bipolar disorders as a sort of bridge between mood disorders and schizophrenia. That's why DSM-5-TR separates the deeply intertwined chapters on bipolar and depressive disorders. However, to explain mood disorders as clearly and concisely as possible, I've reunited them.

Quick Guide to the Mood Disorders

DSM-5-TR uses three groups of criteria sets to diagnose mental problems related to mood: (1) mood episodes, (2) mood disorders, and (3) specifiers describing most recent episode and recurrent course. I'll cover each of them in this Quick Guide—the longest in the book.

Mood Episodes

Simply expressed, a *mood episode* refers to any time when a patient feels unusually happy or sad. Mood episodes are the building blocks from which many of the codable mood disorders are constructed. Most patients with mood disorders will have one or more of these three episodes: major depressive, manic, and hypomanic. Without additional information, none of these mood episodes is a codable diagnosis.

Major depressive episode. For at least 2 weeks, the patient feels depressed (or cannot enjoy life) and has problems with eating and sleeping, guilt feelings, low energy, trouble concentrating, and thoughts about death (p. 112).

Manic episode. For at least 1 week, the patient feels elated (sometimes, only irritable) and may be grandiose, talkative, hyperactive, and distractible. Bad judgment leads to marked social or work impairment; often such patients require hospitalization (p. 123).

Hypomanic episode. This is much like a manic episode, but it is briefer and less severe. These patients do not need hospitalization (p. 132).

Mood Disorders

A mood disorder is a pattern of illness due to an abnormal mood. Nearly every patient with a mood disorder experiences depression at some time, but some also have highs of mood. Many, but not all, mood disorders are diagnosed on the basis of mood episodes. Most patients with mood disorders will fit into one of the codable categories listed below.

DEPRESSIVE DISORDERS

Major depressive disorder. These patients have had no manic or hypomanic episodes but have had one or more major depressive episodes. Major depressive disorder will be either recurrent or single episode (p. 116).

Persistent depressive disorder. There are no high phases, and it lasts much longer than typical major depressive disorder. This type of depression is not typically severe enough to be called an episode of major depression (though chronic major depression is now included here) (p. 139).

Disruptive mood dysregulation disorder. A child's mood is persistently negative between frequent, severe explosions of temper (p. 149).

Premenstrual dysphoric disorder. A few days before her menses begin, a woman experiences symptoms of depression and anxiety (p. 146).

Depressive disorder due to another medical condition. A variety of medical and neurological conditions can produce depressive symptoms; these need not fulfill any of the criteria sets mentioned above (p. 153).

Substance/medication-induced depressive disorder. Alcohol or other substances (intoxication or withdrawal) can cause depressive symptoms; these need not fulfill any of the criteria sets mentioned above (p. 151).

Other specified, or unspecified, depressive disorder. Use one of these categories when a patient has depressive symptoms that do not meet the criteria for the depressive diagnoses above or for any other diagnosis in which depression is a feature (p. 168).

BIPOLAR AND RELATED DISORDERS

Approximately 25% of patients with mood disorders experience manic or hypomanic episodes. Nearly all of these patients will also have episodes of depression. The severity and duration of the highs and lows determine the specific bipolar disorder.

Bipolar I disorder. There must be at least one manic episode; most patients with bipolar I have also had a major depressive episode (p. 126).

Bipolar II disorder. This diagnosis requires at least one hypomanic episode plus at least one major depressive episode (p. 135).

Cyclothymic disorder. These patients have had repeated mood swings, but none severe enough to be called major depressive episodes or manic episodes (p. 143).

Substance/medication-induced bipolar disorder. Alcohol or other substances (intoxication or withdrawal) can cause manic or hypomanic symptoms; these need not meet criteria for any of the conditions above (p. 151).

Bipolar disorder due to another medical condition. A variety of medical and neurological conditions can produce manic or hypomanic symptoms; these need not fulfill criteria for any of the conditions above (p. 153).

Other specified, or unspecified, bipolar disorder. Use one of these categories when a patient has bipolar symptoms that do not meet the criteria for the bipolar diagnoses above (pp. 165, 169).

OTHER CAUSES OF DEPRESSIVE AND MANIC SYMPTOMS

Schizoaffective disorder. In these patients, symptoms suggestive of schizophrenia coexist with a major depressive or a manic episode (p. 88).

Major and mild neurocognitive disorders with behavioral disturbance. The qualifier *with behavioral disturbance* can be coded into the diagnosis of major or mild neurocognitive disorder (p. 503). OK, so mood symptoms don't sound all that behavioral, but that's how DSM-5-TR elects to indicate the cognitive disorders with depression.

Adjustment disorder with depressed mood. This term codes one way of responding to a life stress (p. 227).

Personality disorders. Dysphoric mood is specifically mentioned in the criteria for borderline personality disorder (p. 561), but depressed mood commonly accompanies avoidant, dependent, and histrionic personality disorders.

Uncomplicated bereavement. Sadness at the death of a relative or friend is a common experience. Because *uncomplicated* bereavement is an expected reaction to a particular type of stressor, it is recorded not as a disorder, but as a Z-code (p. 607).

Prolonged grief disorder. A person of any age suffers the death of a loved one; the resulting symptoms of grief are drawn-out and disabling (p. 230).

Other disorders. Depression can accompany many other mental disorders, including schizophrenia, the eating disorders, somatic symptom disorder, sexual dysfunctions, and gender dysphoria. Mood symptoms are likely in patients with an anxiety disorder (especially panic disorder and the phobic disorders), obsessive–compulsive disorder, and posttraumatic stress disorder.

Specifiers

Two special sets of descriptors can be applied to mood episodes and mood disorders.

1. SPECIFIERS DESCRIBING CURRENT OR MOST RECENT EPISODE

These specifiers help characterize the most recent major depressive episode; all but the first two can also apply to a manic episode. Note that the specifiers for severity and remission are described on page 157.

With atypical features. These depressed patients eat a lot and gain weight, sleep excessively, and have a feeling of being sluggish or paralyzed. They are often excessively sensitive to rejection (p. 159).

With melancholic features. This term applies to major depressive episodes characterized by some of the "classic" symptoms of severe depression. These patients awaken early, feeling worse than they do later in the day. They lose appetite and weight, feel guilty, are either slowed down or agitated, and do not feel better when something happens that they would ordinarily like (p. 160).

With anxious distress. A patient has symptoms of anxiety, tension, restlessness, worry, or fear that accompanies a mood episode (p. 158).

With catatonic features. There are features of either motor hyperactivity or inactivity. Catatonic features can apply to major depressive episodes and to manic episodes (p. 100).

With mixed features. Manic, hypomanic, and major depressive episodes may have mixtures of manic and depressive symptoms (p. 161).

With peripartum onset. A manic, hypomanic, or major depressive episode (or a brief psychotic disorder) can occur in a woman during pregnancy or within a month of giving birth (p. 162).

With psychotic features. Manic and major depressive episodes can be accompanied by delusions, which can be mood-congruent or mood-incongruent (p. 163).

2. SPECIFIERS THAT DESCRIBE THE COURSE OF RECURRING MOOD EPISODES

These specifiers describe the overall course of a mood disorder, not just the form of an individual episode.

With rapid cycling. Within 1 year, the patient has had at least four mood episodes (in any combination) fulfilling criteria for major depressive, manic, or hypomanic episodes (p. 164).

With seasonal pattern. These patients regularly become ill at a certain time of the year, such as fall or winter (p. 164).

Introduction to Mood Episodes and Mood Disorders

Mood refers to the sustained emotions that color the way we view life. Recognizing when mood is disordered is extremely important, because as many as 20% of adult women and 10% of adult men may have the experience at some time during their lives. The prevalence of mood disorders seems to be increasing, accounting for half or more of a mental health practice. Mood disorders can occur in people of any race or socioeconomic status, but they are more common among those who are single and who have no mate or partner—a "significant other" who can share the joys and tribulations of their lives. A mood disorder is also more likely in someone who has biological relatives with similar problems.

Many mood disorders are built on the backs of three mood episodes: major depressive, manic, and hypomanic. I will illustrate the mood episodes with vignettes that describe patients whose illnesses depend for diagnosis on the presence of that particular episode.

Years ago, the mood disorders were called *affective disorders;* many clinicians still use the older term, which is also entrenched in the name *seasonal affective disorder.* Note, by the way, that the term *affect* covers more than just a patient's statement of emotion. It also encompasses how the patient appears to be feeling, as shown by physical clues such as facial expression, posture, eye contact, and tearfulness. Emphasis on the actual mood experience of the patient dictates the current use of mood.

Major Depressive Episode

A major depressive episode comprises five principal requirements. There must be (1) a quality of depressed mood (or loss of interest or pleasure) that (2) has existed for a minimum time period, (3) is accompanied by a required number of symptoms, (4) has resulted in distress or disability, and (5) violates none of the exclusions (listed in the Essential Features).

Major depressive episode is one of the building blocks of the mood disorders, but it's not by itself a codable diagnosis. You will use it often—it is one of the most common problems for which patients seek help. Apply it carefully after considering a patient's full history and mental status exam. (Of course, we should be careful in using every label and every diagnosis.) I mention this caution here because some clinicians tend to use the major depressive episode label almost as a reflex, without adequately considering the evidence. Once the label gets applied, too often there is a reflexive reaching for the prescription pad.

Essential Features of **Major Depressive Episode**

These people are miserable. Most feel sad, down, depressed, or some equivalent; however, some few will instead insist that they've only lost interest or pleasure in nearly all their once-loved activities. All will experience four or more additional symptoms (each of which must be a change from prior functioning) such as fatigue, inability to concentrate, feeling worthless or guilty, and a wish for death or thoughts of suicide. In three areas, symptoms may be experienced as either an increase or a decrease from normal: sleep, appetite/weight, and psychomotor activity. (For each of these, the classic picture is a decrease from what's usual—in appetite, for example—but some atypical patients will report an increase.)

The Fine Print

Children and adolescents may feel or appear only irritable, not depressed.

And, we are put on notice not to count any symptoms that are obviously caused by a different medical disorder.

Don't disregard the D's: • Duration (most of nearly every day, 2+ weeks) • Distress or disability (work/educational, social, or personal impairment) • Differential diagnosis (substance use, physical disorders)

Coding Notes

No code alert: Major depressive episode is not a diagnosable illness; it is a building block of major depressive, bipolar I, and bipolar II disorders. It may also be found in persistent depressive disorder. However, certain specifier codes apply to major depressive episodes—though you tack them on only after you've decided on the actual mood disorder diagnosis. Relax; this will all become clear as we proceed.

Quality of Mood

Depression is usually experienced as a mood lower than normal; patients may describe it as feeling "unhappy," "downhearted," "bummed," "blue," or many other terms expressing sadness. Several issues can interfere with the recognition of depression:

- Not all patients can recognize or accurately describe how they feel.
- Clinicians and patients who come from different cultural backgrounds may have difficulty agreeing that the problem is depression.
- The presenting symptoms of depression can vary greatly from one patient to another. One patient may be slowed down and crying; another will smile and

deny that anything is wrong. Some sleep and eat too much; others complain of insomnia and loss of appetite.

- Some patients don't really feel depressed; rather, they experience depression as a loss of pleasure or reduced interest in their usual activities, including sex.
- Crucial to diagnosis is that the episode must represent a noticeable change from the patient's usual functioning. Even if the patient does not notice it (some are too ill to pay attention or too apathetic to care), family or friends may report that there has been such a change.

Duration

The patient feels bad most of the day, almost every day, for at least 2 weeks. This requirement is included to ensure that major depressive episodes are differentiated from the transient "down" spells that most of us sometimes feel.

Symptoms

During the 2 weeks just mentioned, the patient must have at least five of the **bold** symptoms below. Those five must include either depressed mood or loss of pleasure, and the symptoms must overall indicate that the person is performing at a lower level than before. **Depressed mood** is self-explanatory; **loss of pleasure** is nearly universal among depressed patients. These symptoms can be counted either if the patient reports them or if others observe that they occur.

Many patients lose **appetite and weight.** More than three-fourths report trouble with **sleep.** Typically, they awaken early in the morning, long before it is time to arise. However, some people eat and sleep more than normal; many of them will qualify for the atypical features specifier (p. 159).

Depressed patients will often complain of **fatigue,** which they may express as tiredness or low energy. Their speech or physical movements may be slowed; sometimes there is a marked pause before answering a question or initiating an action. This is called **psychomotor retardation.** Speech may be very quiet, sometimes inaudible. Some patients simply stop talking completely, except in response to a direct question. At the extreme, complete muteness may occur.

At the other extreme, some depressed patients feel so anxious that they become **agitated.** Agitation may be expressed as hand wringing, pacing, or an inability to sit still. The ability of depressed patients to evaluate themselves objectively plummets; this shows up as **low self-esteem or guilt.** Some patients develop trouble with **concentration** (real or perceived) so severe that sometimes a misdiagnosis of neurocognitive disorder may be made. Thoughts of death, **death wishes,** and **suicidal ideas** are the most serious depressive symptoms of all, because there is a real risk that the patient will successfully act upon them.

To count as a DSM-5-TR symptom for major depressive episode, the behaviors listed above must occur nearly every day. However, thoughts about death or suicide need only be "recurrent." A single suicide attempt or a specific suicide plan will also qualify.

In general, the more closely a patient resembles this outline, the more reliable will be the diagnosis of major depressive episode. We should note, however, that depressed patients can have many symptoms besides those listed in the DSM-5-TR criteria. They can include crying spells, phobias, obsessions, and compulsions. Patients may admit to feeling hopeless, helpless, or worthless. Anxiety symptoms, especially panic attacks (p. 172), can be so prominent that they blind clinicians to the underlying depression. Many patients drink more (occasionally, less) alcohol when they become depressed. This can lead to difficulty in sorting out the approach to treatment: Which should be addressed first, the depression or the drinking? (Ideally, both at once.)

A small minority of patients lose contact with reality and develop delusions or hallucinations. These psychotic features can be either *mood-congruent* (for example, a depressed man feels so guilty that he imagines he has committed some awful sin) or *mood-incongruent* (imagined persecution by the FBI is not a typical theme of depression). Psychotic symptoms are indicated in the severity indicator (its verbiage you add to the diagnosis, *and* the final number in the ICD-10 code, as discussed later in this chapter). The case vignette of Brian Murphy (p. 118) includes an example.

There are three situations in which you should not count a symptom toward a diagnosis of major depressive episode:

A symptom is fully explained by another medical condition. For example, you wouldn't count fatigue in a patient who is recovering from major surgery; in that situation, you expect fatigue.

A symptom results from mood-incongruent delusions or hallucinations. For example, don't count insomnia that is a response to hallucinated voices that keep the patient awake throughout the night.

Feelings of guilt or worthlessness that occur because the patient is too depressed to fulfill responsibilities. Such feelings are too common in depression to carry any diagnostic weight. Rather, look for guilt feelings that are way outside the boundaries of what's reasonable. An extreme example: A woman believes that her wickedness caused the tragedies of 9/11.

Impairment

The episode must be serious enough to cause material distress or to impair the patient's work or school performance, social life (withdrawal or discord), or some other area of functioning, including sex. Of the various consequences of mental illness, the effect on work may the hardest to detect. Perhaps this is because earning a livelihood is so important that most people will go to great lengths to hide symptoms that could threaten their employment.

Exclusions

Regardless of the severity or duration of symptoms, major depressive episode usually should not be diagnosed in the face of clinically important substance use or a general medical disorder that could cause the symptoms.

The bereavement exclusion that was used through DSM-IV is not to be found in DSM-5-TR, because recent research has determined that depressions closely preceded by the death or loss of a loved one do not differ substantially from depressions preceded by other stressors (or possibly by none at all). There's been a lot of breast-beating over this move, or rather removal. Some claim that it places patients at risk for diagnosis of a mood disorder when context renders symptoms understandable; a substantial expansion in the number of people we regard as mentally ill could result.

I see the situation a little differently: We have now removed an artificial barrier to diagnosis and treatment. However, as with any other freedom, we must use it responsibly. Evaluate the whole situation, especially the severity of symptoms, any previous history of mood disorder, the timing and severity of putative precipitant (bereavement plus other forms of loss), and the trajectory of the syndrome (is it getting worse or better?), and reevaluate frequently; a table that parses the symptoms is included on page 607. And don't forget to consider the new diagnosis, prolonged grief disorder (p. 230).

I've included examples of major depressive episode in the following vignettes: Brian Murphy (p. 118), Aileen Parmeter (p. 121), Elisabeth Jacks (p. 129), Winona Fisk (p. 131), Iris McMaster (p. 136), Noah Sanders (p. 141), and Sal Camozzi (p. 310). In addition, there may be examples in Chapter 20, "Patients and Diagnoses"—but you'll have to find them for yourself.

Major Depressive Disorder

We'll give the diagnosis of major depressive disorder (MDD) to any patient who has one or more major depressive episodes, and no manic or hypomanic symptoms. MDD is a common condition, affecting about 7% of the general population, with a female preponderance of roughly 2:1. It typically begins in the middle to late 20s, but it can occur for the first time at any stage of life, from childhood to old age. The onset may be sudden or gradual. Although episodes last on average from 6 to 9 months, the range is enormous, from a few weeks to many years. Recovery usually begins within a few months of onset, though that, too, is greatly variable. A full recovery is less likely for a person who has a personality disorder or symptoms that are more severe (especially psychotic features).

MDD is strongly hereditary; first-degree relatives have a risk several times that of the general population.

Some patients have only a single episode during an entire lifetime; then they are diagnosed with (no surprise) MDD, single episode. However, roughly half of those who have one major depressive episode will experience another. At the point they develop a second episode (to count, it must be separated from the first by at least 2 months), we must change the diagnosis to MDD, recurrent type.

For any given patient, symptoms of depression remain pretty much the same from one episode to the next. Those with multiple recurrent episodes can expect one roughly every 4 years; there is some evidence that the frequency of episodes increases with age. Unsurprisingly, patients with recurrent episodes are also much more likely than those with a single episode to be impaired by their symptoms. One of the most severe consequences is suicide, which is the fate of about 4% of patients with MDD. Multiple episodes of depression greatly increase the likelihood of suicide attempts and completed suicide.

Perhaps 25% of patients who appear at first to have "only" major depression will eventually experience a manic or hypomanic episode, thereby requiring a change in diagnosis to some form of bipolar disorder. Several features can help predict this switch: (1) onset of depression when the person is quite young—say, during the teen years; (2) family history of a bipolar disorder (no surprise there); (3) the presence of psychosis; (4) many previous episodes; (5) poor response to antidepressant medication; (6) treatment for depression provokes switch to mania.

Essential Features of **Major Depressive Disorder, {Single Episode}{Recurrent}**

The patient has {one}{multiple} major depressive episodes and no spontaneous episodes of mania or hypomania.

The Fine Print

Two months or more without symptoms must intervene for episodes to be counted as separate.

Decide on the D's: • Duration (2+ weeks) • Differential diagnosis (**substance use** and **physical disorders,** other mood disorders, ordinary grief and sadness, schizoaffective disorder)

Coding Notes

From type of episode and severity, find code numbers in Table 3.2 (p. 166). If applicable, choose specifiers from Table 3.3 (p. 167).

Brian Murphy

When Brian Murphy was 55, his mood, which had always been "pretty medium," slid into depression. Farm chores seemed increasingly to be a burden; his tractor sat idle in its shed.

As his mood blackened, Brian's body functioning seemed to deteriorate. Although he was constantly fatigued, often falling into bed by 9 P.M., he would invariably awaken at 2 or 3 A.M. Then obsessive worrying kept him awake until sunrise. Mornings were worst for him. The prospect of "another damn day to get through" seemed overwhelming. In the evenings he usually felt somewhat better, though he'd sit around working out sums on a magazine cover to see how much money they'd have if he "couldn't work the farm" and they had to live on their savings. His appetite deserted him. Although he never weighed himself, he buckled his belt two notches smaller than he had several months before.

"Brian's just lost interest," his wife, Rachel, reports on the day he is admitted to the hospital. "He doesn't enjoy anything anymore. He spends all his time sitting around and worrying about being in debt. We owe a few hundred dollars on our credit card, but we pay it off every month. The farm's free and clear."

During the previous week or two, Brian has begun to ruminate about his health. "At first it was his blood pressure," Rachel says. "He'd ask me to take it several times a day. I still work part time as a nurse. Several times he thought he was having a stroke. Then yesterday he became convinced that his heart was going to stop. He'd get up, feel his pulse, pace around the room, lie down, put his feet above his head, do anything he could think of to 'keep it going.' That's when I decided to bring him here."

"We'll have to sell the farm." That's the first thing Brian says to his clinician when they meet. Brian is casually dressed and rather rumpled. He has prominent worry lines on his forehead, and he keeps feeling for his pulse. Several times during the interview, he seems unable to sit still; he gets up and paces over to the window. His speech is slow, but it's coherent. He talks mostly about how poor they are, how he fears that the farm will have to "go on the block." He denies hallucinating, but admits he feels tired and "all washed up—not good for anything anymore." He is fully oriented, has a full fund of information, and scores a perfect 30 on the MMSE. He admits that he feels depressed, but he denies having thoughts about death. Somewhat reluctantly, he agrees that he might need treatment.

Rachel points out that with his generous disability policy, his investments, and his pension from his former company, they have more money coming in now than when he was healthy.

"But still, we'll have to sell the farm," Brian replies.

Unfortunately, clinicians (including some mental health specialists) commonly make two sorts of mistake when evaluating patients with depression.

First, we sometimes focus too intently on a patient's anxiety, alcohol use, or psy-

chotic symptoms and ignore underlying depressive symptoms. Here's my lifelong rule, formulated from bitter experience (not all mine) as far back as when I was a resident: Always
look for a mood disorder in any new patient, even if the chief complaint is something else.

Second, the presenting depressive or manic symptoms can be quite noticeable, even
dramatic—to the point that clinicians may fail to notice, lurking underneath, the presence
of alcohol use disorder or another disorder (good examples are neurocognitive and somatic
symptom disorders). And that suggests another, equally important rule, almost the mirror
image of the first rule: Never assume that a mood disorder is your patient's only problem.

Evaluation of Brian Murphy

First, let's try to identify the current (and any previous) mood episodes. Brian Murphy
has been ill much longer than 2 weeks (criterion A). Of the major depressive episode
symptoms listed (five are required by DSM-5-TR), he has at least seven: low mood (A1),
loss of interest (A2), fatigue (A6), sleeplessness (A4), low self-esteem (A7), loss of appetite (A3), and agitation (A5). Note that either low mood or loss of interest is required
for diagnosis; Brian has both. He is so seriously impaired (B) that he requires hospitalization. Although we do not have the results of his physical exam and laboratory
testing, the vignette provides no history that would suggest another medical condition
(for example, pancreatic carcinoma) or substance use (C). However, his clinician would
need to ask both Brian and his wife about this—depressed people often increase their
drinking. He was clearly severely depressed and different from his usual self. He easily
fulfills the criteria for major depressive episode.

Next, what type of mood disorder does Brian have? He's had no manic or hypomanic episodes (E), ruling out bipolar I and II disorder. His delusions of poverty could
suggest a psychotic disorder (such as schizoaffective disorder), but he has too few psychotic symptoms, and the timing of mood symptoms versus delusions is wrong (D). He
is deluded but has no additional A criteria for schizophrenia. His mood symptoms rule
out brief psychotic disorder and delusional disorder. He therefore fulfills the requirements for MDD.

There are just two subtypes of MDD: single episode and recurrent. Although
Brian Murphy might subsequently have other episodes of depression, this is the only
one so far.

For the further description and coding of Brian's depression, let's turn ahead to
Table 3.2 (p. 166). His single episode indicates the column to highlight under MDD.
And he was delusional, so we'd code him as *with psychotic features*.

But wait: Suppose he hadn't been psychotic? What severity would we assign him
then? Even though he isn't suicidal (he doesn't want to die—he fears it), he does have
most of the required depressive symptoms, which seriously impair him. That's why
I'd rate him as severely depressed. Without psychosis, the code number changes, just
slightly.

Now we'll turn to the panoply of other specifiers, which I'll discuss toward the end of this chapter (p. 158). Brian has no manic symptoms; that rules out *with mixed features*. His delusion that he is poor and must sell the farm is *mood-congruent*—that is, in keeping with the usual cognitive themes of depression. (However, his pulse checking and worrying that his heart might stop, to me, are not delusional. I'd regard them rather as signifying the overwhelming anxiety he feels about the state of his health.) The words we'd attach to his diagnosis (so far) would be MDD, single episode, severe with mood-congruent psychotic features.

But wait; there's more. There are no abnormalities of movement suggestive of catatonic features, nor does his depression have any atypical features (for example, he doesn't eat or sleep more than normal—far from it). Of course, he would not qualify for peripartum onset. But his wife complains that he "doesn't enjoy anything anymore," suggesting that he might qualify for melancholic features. He was agitated when interviewed (marked psychomotor slowing would have also qualified for this criterion), and he has lost considerable weight. He reports awakening early on many mornings (terminal insomnia). The interviewer did not ask him whether this episode of depression differs qualitatively from how he felt when his parents died, but I'd bet that it does. So, we'll add *with melancholic features* to the mix.

I wrote this vignette before a new specifier, *with anxious distress,* was a gleam in anyone's eye, but I think Brian Murphy qualifies for it as well. He appears edgy and tense, and he is markedly restless. Furthermore, he seems to be expressing the fear that something horrible—possibly a catastrophic health event—will occur. Even though nothing was said about poor concentration, he has at least three of the symptoms required for the *with anxious distress* specifier, at a moderate severity rating. This specifier may have real prognostic importance, suggesting, in the absence of treatment, the possibility of a poor outcome—even suicide.

Some patients with severe depression also report many of the symptoms typical of panic disorder, generalized anxiety disorder, or some other anxiety disorder. In such a case, two diagnoses could be made. Usually, the mood disorder is listed first as the primary diagnosis. Anxiety symptoms that do not fulfill criteria for one of the disorders described in Chapter 4 may be further evaluated as evidence for the *with anxious distress* specifier.

Of course, Brian cannot qualify for rapid cycling or seasonal pattern; with only one episode, there can be no pattern. I'd give him a GAF score of 51, and his final diagnosis would be as given below.

Let me just say that the prospect of using so many different criteria sets to diagnose one patient may seem daunting, but a "one step at a time" approach reveals a process that is quite logical; and once you get the hang of it, it's fairly quick. The same basic methods should be applied to all examples of depression. (Of course, you could argue—*I* certainly would—that using the prototypical descriptions of depression and mania and their respective disorders simplifies things still further. But again, remember always to consider the possibility of substance use and physical causes of any given symptom set.)

F32.3   Major depressive disorder, single episode, severe with mood-congruent psychotic features, with melancholic features, with moderate anxious distress

---

There's a situation in which I like to be extra careful about diagnosing MDD. That's when a patient also has somatic symptom disorder (p. 254). The problem is that many patients who seem to have too many physical symptoms can also have mood symptoms that closely resemble major depressive episodes (and sometimes manic episodes). Over the years, I've found that these patients tend to get treatment with medication, electroconvulsive therapy (ECT), and other physical therapies that don't seem to help them much—certainly not for long. I'm not saying that drugs never work; but I maintain that if you encounter someone with somatic symptom disorder who is depressed, other treatments (such as cognitive-behavioral therapy, other forms of behavior modification) may be more effective and less fraught with complications.

Aileen Parmeter

"I just know it was a terrible mistake to come here." For the third time, Aileen Parmeter gets out of her chair and walks to the window. A wiry 5 feet 2 inches, this former Marine master sergeant (she once supervised a steno pool) weighs a scant 100 pounds. Through the slats of the Venetian blinds, she peers longingly at freedom in the parking lot below. "I just don't know whatever made me come."

"You came because I asked you to," her clinician explains. "Your nephew called and said you were getting depressed again. It's just like last time."

"No, I don't think so. I was just upset," she says patiently. "I had a little cold for a few days and couldn't play my tennis. I'll be fine if I just get back to my little apartment."

"Have you been hearing voices or seeing things this time?"

"Well, of course not." She seems rather offended. "You might as well ask if I've been drinking."

After her last hospitalization, Aileen remained well for about 10 months. Although she had taken her medicine for only a few weeks, she had remained active until 3 weeks ago. Then she stopped seeing her friends and wouldn't play tennis because she "just didn't enjoy it." She worried constantly about her health and couldn't sleep. Although she didn't complain of decreased appetite, she had lost about 10 pounds.

"Well, who wouldn't have trouble? I've just been too tired to get my regular exercise." She tries to smile, but it comes off crooked and forced.

"Miss Parmeter, what about the suicidal thoughts?"

"I don't know what you mean."

"I mean, each time you've been here—last year, and 2 years before that—you were admitted because you tried to kill yourself."

"I'm going to be fine now. Just let me go home."

But her clinician, whose memory is long, orders Aileen held for her own protection in a private room where she can be observed one-on-one.

Sleepless still at 3 A.M., Aileen gets up, smiles wanly at the attendant, and goes in to use the bathroom. Looping a strip she has torn from her sweat suit over the top of the door, she tries to hang herself. As the silence lengthens, the attendant calls out softly, then taps on the door, then opens it and sounds the alarm. The code team responds with no time to spare.

The following morning, the clinician is back at her bedside. "Why did you try to do that, Miss Parmeter?"

"I didn't try to do anything. I must have been confused." She gingerly touches the purple bruises that ring her neck. "This sure hurts. I know I'll feel better if you just let me go home."

Aileen remains hospitalized for 10 days. Once her sore neck will allow, she begins to take her antidepressant medication again. Soon she is sleeping and eating well, and she earns a perfect score on the MMSE. She is released to go home to her apartment and her tennis, still uncertain why everyone has made such a fuss.

Evaluation of Aileen Parmeter

Aileen never acknowledges feeling depressed, but she has lost interest in her usual activities. This change has lasted longer than 2 weeks, and—as in previous episodes—her other symptoms include fatigue, insomnia, loss of weight, and suicidal behavior (criterion A). (Although she reproaches herself for entering the hospital, these feelings refer exclusively to her being ill and would not be scored as guilt.) She was sick enough to require hospitalization, fulfilling the impairment criterion (B).

Aileen could have a mood disorder due to another medical condition, and this would have to be pursued by her clinician, but the history of recurrence makes this seem unlikely (C). Symptoms of apathy and poor memory raise the question of mild neurocognitive disorder, but her MMSE provides no evidence of memory impairment. She denies consuming alcohol, so a substance-induced mood disorder would also appear unlikely (her clinician has known her for so long that further pursuit of this possibility would be wasted effort).

There is no evidence that Aileen has ever had mania or hypomania, ruling out bipolar I or II disorder (E), and absence of any psychotic symptoms eliminates all psychotic disorders (D). She therefore fulfills the criteria for MDD. She's had more than one episode separated by substantially longer than 2 months, which satisfies the requirement for the term *recurrent.* Turning ahead to Table 3.2, we can reject the row there describing psychotic features (she emphatically denied having delusions or hallucinations) and remission.

Now we must consider the severity of her depression (p. 166). It is always a problem how best to score someone with so little insight. Even with the suicide attempt, Aileen appears barely to meet the five symptoms needed for major depressive episode.

According to the rules, she should receive a severity coding of no greater than moderate. However, for a patient who has nearly killed herself (more than once!), this would be inaccurate and possibly dangerous. As I've said before, the coding instructions are meant to be guides, not shackles, so I'll call Aileen's depression *severe*.

She won't qualify for any of the specifiers for the most recent episode—perhaps because her lack of insight prevents her from providing full information. (Longer observation might reveal criteria adequate for *with melancholic features*.)

Other disorders are sometimes found in patients with MDD. These include several of the anxiety disorders, obsessive–compulsive disorder, and the substance-related disorders (especially alcohol use disorder). However, Aileen has no evidence for any of these. I'd give her a GAF score of only 15 on admission. (Her GAF improves to 60 by the time she is released.) The suicidal behavior is coded as a subsequent encounter because it did not occur as a part of her initial presentation. Her complete diagnosis would be as follows:

F33.2	Major depressive disorder, recurrent, severe
T14.91XD	Current suicidal behavior, subsequent encounter

Manic Episode

The second "building block" of the mood disorders, manic episode, has been recognized for at least 150 years. The classic triad of manic symptoms consists of heightened self-esteem, increased motor activity, and pressured speech. These symptoms are obvious and often outrageous, so manic episode is not often overdiagnosed. However, the psychotic symptoms that sometimes attend manic episode can be so florid that clinicians instead diagnose schizophrenia. This tendency to misdiagnosis may have decreased since 1980, when the DSM-III criteria increased clinicians' awareness of bipolar illness. The introduction of lithium treatment for bipolar disorders in 1970 also helped promote the diagnosis.

Manic episode is much less common than major depressive episode, perhaps affecting 1% of all adults. Men and women are about equally likely to have mania. The features that must be present to diagnose manic episode are identical to those for major depressive episode: (1) A mood quality that (2) has existed for a required period of time, (3) is attended by a required number of symptoms, (4) has resulted in an important degree of disability, and (5) violates none of the listed exclusions.

Essential Features of **Manic Episode**

People in the throes of mania are almost unmistakable. They feel euphoric (though sometimes they're only irritable), and there's no way you can ignore their energy and frenetic activity. They are full of plans, which they often don't carry through—they are so distractible. They talk and laugh, and talk some more, often very fast, often with flight of ideas. They sleep less than usual ("a waste of time, when there's so much to do"), but feel great anyway. Grandiosity is sometimes so exaggerated that they become psychotic, believing that they are some exalted personage (a monarch or deity, a rock star) or that they have superhuman powers. With deteriorating judgment (they spend money unwisely, engage in ill-conceived sexual adventures or other dangerous behavior), functioning becomes impaired, often to the point that they must be hospitalized to force treatment for their own protection or for that of other people.

The Fine Print

The D's: • Duration (most of nearly every day, 1+ weeks; any duration if so ill they have to be hospitalized) • Distress or disability (work/educational, social, or personal impairment) • Differential diagnosis (**substance use** and **physical disorders,** schizoaffective disorder, neurocognitive disorders, hypomanic episodes, cyclothymia)

Coding Notes

Manic episode is not a diagnosable illness; it is a building block of bipolar I disorder.

Quality of Mood

Some patients with relatively mild symptoms just feel jolly; this good humor can be quite infectious and may make others feel like laughing with them. But as mania worsens, this humor becomes less cheerful as it takes on a "driven," unfunny quality that creates discomfort in patients and listeners alike. A few patients will have mood that is only irritable; euphoria and irritability sometimes occur together.

Duration

The patient must have had symptoms for a minimum of 1 week. This time requirement helps to differentiate manic episode from hypomanic episode.

Symptoms

In addition to the change in mood (euphoria or irritability), the patient must also have an increase in energy or activity level during a 1-week period. With these changes, at least three of the symptoms listed **in bold** below must also be present to an important degree during the same time period. (Note that if the patient's **abnormal mood** is only irritable—that is, without any component of euphoria—four symptoms are required in addition to the increased activity level.)

Heightened self-esteem, found in most patients, can become grandiose to the point that it is delusional. Then patients believe that they can advise presidents and solve the problem of climate change, in addition to more mundane tasks such as conducting psychotherapy and running the very medical facilities that currently house them. Because such delusions are in keeping with the euphoric mood, they are called **mood congruent.** Manic patients typically report feeling **rested on little sleep.** Time spent sleeping seems wasted; they prefer to pursue their many projects. In its milder forms, this **heightened activity** may be goal-directed and useful; patients who are only moderately ill can accomplish quite a lot in a 20-hour day. But as they become more and more active, agitation ensues and they may begin projects they never complete. At this point they have **lost judgment** for what is reasonable and attainable. They may become involved in risky business ventures, indiscreet sexual liaisons, and questionable religious or political activities.

Manic patients are eager to tell anyone who will listen about their ideas, plans, and work, and they do so in speech that is loud and difficult to interrupt. Manic **speech** is often **rapid and pressured,** as if there were too many dammed-up words trying to escape all at once. The resulting speech may exhibit what is called **flight of ideas,** in which one thought triggers another to which it bears only a marginally logical association. As a result, a patient may wander far afield from where the conversation (or monologue) started. Manic patients may also be **easily distracted** by irrelevant sounds or events that other people would ignore.

Some manic patients retain insight and seek treatment, but many will deny that anything is wrong. They rationalize that no one who feels this well or is so productive could possibly be ill. Manic behavior therefore continues until it ends spontaneously, or the patient is hospitalized or jailed. I consider any manic episode to be an emergency, and I don't expect many clinicians will argue.

Some symptoms not specifically mentioned in the DSM-5-TR criteria are also worth noting here.

1. Even during an acute manic episode, many patients have brief periods of depression. These "microdepressions" are relatively common; depending on the symptoms associated with them, they may suggest that the specifier *with mixed features* is appropriate (p. 161).

2. Patients may use substances (especially alcohol) in an attempt to relieve the uncomfortable, driven feeling that accompanies a severe manic episode. Less often, the substance use temporarily obscures the symptoms of the mood episode. When clinicians become confused about whether the substance use or the mania came first, the question can usually be sorted out with the help of informants.

3. Catatonic symptoms occasionally occur during a manic episode, sometimes causing the episode to resemble schizophrenia. But a history (obtained from informants) of acute onset and previous episodes with recovery can help clarify the diagnosis. Then the specifier *with catatonic features* may be indicated (p. 100).

What about episodes that don't start until the patient undergoes treatment for a depression? Should they count as fully as spontaneous mania or hypomania? To count as evidence for either manic or hypomanic episode, DSM-5-TR requires that the *full* criteria (not just a couple of symptoms, such as agitation or irritability) be present, and that the symptoms last longer than the expected physiological effects of the treatment. This declaration nicely rounds out the list of possibilities: DSM-IV stated flatly that manic episodes caused by treatment could not count toward a diagnosis of bipolar I disorder, whereas DSM-III-R implied that they could, and DSM-III kept silent on the whole matter.

The authors of the successive DSMs may have been influenced by Emerson's epigram: A foolish consistency is the hobgoblin of little minds.

Impairment

Manic episodes typically wreak havoc on the lives of patients and their associates. Although increasing energy and effort may at first improve productivity at work (or school), as mania worsens a patient becomes less and less able to focus attention. Friendships are strained by arguments. Sexual entanglements can result in disease, divorce, and unwanted pregnancy. Even when the episode has resolved, guilt and recriminations remain behind.

Exclusions

The exclusions for manic episode are the same as for major depressive episode. General medical conditions such as hyperthyroidism can produce hyperactive behavior; patients who misuse certain psychoactive substances (especially amphetamines) will appear speeded up and may report feeling strong, powerful, and euphoric.

Elisabeth Jacks had a manic episode; you can read her history beginning on page 129. Another example is that of Winona Fisk (p. 131). Look for other cases in the patient histories given in Chapter 20.

Bipolar I Disorder

Bipolar I disorder is shorthand for any cyclic mood disorder that includes at least one manic episode. Although this nomenclature is relatively recent, the concept has been recognized for over a century. Formerly, it was called manic–depressive illness; older clinicians may still refer to it this way.

Bipolar I disorder is strongly hereditary; monozygotic concordance is variously given at 40–70% (which leaves a lot of room for environmental factors such as childhood emotional trauma and recent life stresses that can include getting married and finishing college). Men and women are about equally affected for a disorder that affects a shade over 1% of the general adult population. Onset is typically in late teens or early 20s, and most people who have one episode of mania will have another. Note, however, that if the first episode is major depression, it can be hard to know whether this patient will eventually have a bipolar or major depressive disorder. Bipolar I patients are also strongly at risk for alcohol use disorder as well as a variety of physical conditions—including cardiovascular disease, sleep apnea, and obesity.

There are two technical points to consider in evaluating episodes of bipolar I disorder. First, for an episode to count as a new one, it must either represent a change of polarity (for example, from major depressive to manic or hypomanic episode), or it must be separated from the previous episode by a normal mood that lasts at least 2 months.

Second, a manic or hypomanic episode will occasionally seem to be precipitated by the treatment of a depression. Antidepressant drugs, ECT, or bright light (used to treat seasonal depression) may cause a patient to move rapidly from depression into a full-blown manic episode. Bipolar I disorder is defined by the occurrence of *spontaneous* depressions, manias, and hypomanias; therefore, any treatment-induced episode of mania or hypomania can only be used to make the diagnosis of a bipolar disorder if the symptoms persist beyond the physiological effect of that treatment. Even then, DSM-5-TR urges caution: Demand the full number of manic or hypomanic symptoms, not just edginess or agitation that some patients experience following treatment for depression.

In addition, note the warning that the mood episodes must not be superimposed on a psychotic disorder—specifically schizophrenia, schizophreniform disorder, delusional disorder, or unspecified psychotic disorder. Because the longitudinal course of bipolar I disorder differs strikingly from those of the psychotic disorders, this should only rarely cause diagnostic problems. But DSM-5-TR is concerned enough about this possibility that it issues a warning note in the bipolar I criteria: At least one manic episode must not be better explained by a psychotic disorder.

Usually, a manic episode will be current, and the patient will have been admitted to a hospital. You might occasionally use the category *current or most recent episode manic* for a newly diagnosed patient who is on a mood-stabilizing regimen. Most will have had at least one previous manic, major depressive, or hypomanic episode. However, a single manic episode is hardly rare, especially early in the course of a bipolar I disorder. Most of these patients will later have subsequent major depressive episodes, as well as additional manic ones. Males are more likely than females to have a manic first episode.

Current episode depressed (I'm intentionally shorthanding the long and unwieldy official phrase) will be one of the most frequently used of the bipolar I subtypes; nearly all patients with this disorder will receive this diagnosis at some point during their lives. The depressive symptoms will be very much like those in the major depressive disorders of Brian Murphy (p. 118) and Aileen Parmeter (p. 121). Elisabeth Jacks (p. 129), whose current episode was manic, had been depressed a few weeks before her current evaluation.

About a third of patients with a manic episode will have depressive features. Then, they may qualify for the specifier *with mixed features* (p. 161), which can predict a poorer prognosis as regards outcome and suicide attempts.

In a given patient, symptoms of mood disorder tend to remain the same from one episode to the next. However, it is possible that after an earlier manic episode, a subsequent mood upswing may be less severe, and therefore only hypomanic. (The first episode of a bipolar I disorder could be hypomanic only in retrospect, after a full mania was encountered subsequently.) Although I have provided no vignette for bipolar I, most recent episode hypomanic, I have described a hypomanic episode in the case of Iris McMaster, a patient with bipolar II disorder (p. 136).

Researchers who have followed patients with bipolar illness for many years report that some have only manias. The concept of unipolar mania has been debated off and on for a long time. There are probably some patients who never have a depression, but most will, given enough time. I have known of patients who had as many as seven episodes of mania over a 20-year period before finally having a first episode of depression. What's important here is to warn all patients with bipolar I (and II) disorder—and their families—to watch out for depressive symptoms. Patients with bipolar I have a high likelihood of completing suicide; some reports suggest that these patients account for up to a quarter of all suicides.

Essential Features of **Bipolar I Disorder**

The patient has had at least one manic episode, plus any number (including zero) of hypomanic and major depressive episodes.

The Fine Print

A manic or hypomanic episode that is precipitated by treatment (medication, ECT, light therapy) counts toward a diagnosis of bipolar I disorder *only* if the manic symptoms continue longer than the expected physiological treatment effects. And, there must be at least one manic episode that isn't better explained by a psychotic disorder.

The D's: • Differential diagnosis (**substance use** and **physical disorders, other mood disorders, psychotic disorders**)

Coding Notes

From type of episode and severity, find code numbers in Table 3.2 (p. 166). Finally, choose from a whole lot of specifiers in Table 3.3 (p. 167).

Older patients who develop a mania for the first time may have a comorbid neurological disorder. They may also have a higher mortality. First-episode mania in the elderly may be quite a different illness from recurrent mania in the elderly, and should perhaps be given a different diagnosis, such as unspecified bipolar disorder.

Elisabeth Jacks

Elisabeth Jacks operates a catering service with her second husband, Donald, who is the main informant for this history.

At age 38, Elisabeth already has two grown children, so Donald can understand why another pregnancy might upset her. Even so, from about her fourth month, she seemed unnaturally sad and spent much of each day in bed, not arising until afternoon, when her weariness might begin to ebb. Her appetite, voracious during her first trimester, fell off, so that by the time of delivery she was several pounds lighter than usual for a full-term pregnancy. She had to give up keeping the household and business accounts, because she couldn't focus her attention long enough to add a column of figures. Still, the only time Donald became really alarmed was one evening at the beginning of Elisabeth's ninth month, when she told him that she had been thinking for days that she wouldn't survive childbirth and he would have to rear their baby without her. "You'd both be better off without me, anyway," she told him.

After their son was born, Elisabeth's mood brightened almost at once. The crying spells and the hours of rumination disappeared; briefly, she seemed almost her usual self. Then late one Friday night, when the baby was 3 weeks old, Donald returned from catering a banquet to find Elisabeth, wearing only bra and panties, icing a cake. Two other just-iced cakes were lined up on the counter, and the kitchen was littered with dirty pots and pans.

"She said she'd made one for each of us, and she wanted to party," Donald tells the clinician. "I started to change the baby—he was howling in his basket—but she wanted to drag me off to the bedroom. She said 'Please, sweetie, it's been a long time.' I mean, even if I hadn't been dead tired, who could concentrate with the baby crying like that?"

All the next day, Elisabeth was out with girlfriends, leaving Donald home with the baby. On Sunday she spent nearly $300 for Christmas presents at an April garage sale. She seemed to have boundless energy, sleeping only 2 or 3 hours a night before arising, rested and ready to go. On Monday she decided to open a bakery; by telephone, she tried to charge over $1,600 worth of kitchen supplies to their Visa card. She'd have bought more the next day, but she talked so fast that the person taking her order couldn't keep up. In frustration, she slammed the phone down.

Elisabeth's behavior became so erratic that for the next two evenings Donald stayed off work to care for the baby, but his presence only seemed to provoke her sexual demands. Then there was the marijuana. Before Elisabeth became pregnant, she would have an occasional toke (she called it her "herbs"). During the past week, not all the smells in the house had been freshly baked cake, so Donald thought she might be at it again.

Yesterday Elisabeth shook him awake at 5 A.M. and announced, "I am becoming God." That prompted him to arrange for this evaluation.

Elisabeth can hardly sit still during the interview. In a burst of speech, she expresses her renewed energy and plans for the new bakery. "I've never felt better in my life," she volunteers. In rapid succession and without pause, she then describes her mood (ecstatic), how it makes her feel when she puts on her green silk dress (sexy), where she purchased the dress, how old she was when she bought it, and to whom she was married at the time.

Evaluation of Elisabeth Jacks

This vignette provides a fairly typical picture of manic excitement. Elisabeth Jacks's mood is definitely elevated. Aside from the issue of marijuana smoking (which appears to be a symptom, not a cause), her relatively late age of onset is the only atypical feature.

For at least a week Elisabeth's mood has been high (manic episode criterion A), accompanied by most of the other typical symptoms: reduced need for sleep (B2), talkativeness (B3), flight of ideas (a sample run is outlined in the last paragraph of the vignette, B4), and poor judgment (ordering baking equipment, buying Christmas gifts at the April garage sale—B7). Her disorder causes considerable distress, for her family if not for her (C)—typical of patients with a manic episode. The severity of the symptoms, not their number or type, and the degree of impairment differentiate her full-blown manic episode from a hypomanic episode.

The issue of another medical condition (D) is not addressed in the vignette. Medical problems such as hyperthyroidism, multiple sclerosis, and brain tumors would have to be ruled out by the admitting clinician before a definitive diagnosis could be made. Delirium must be ruled out for any postpartum patient, but she seems able to focus her attention well enough. Although Elisabeth may have smoked marijuana, misuse of this substance should never be confused with mania; neither cannabis intoxication nor withdrawal presents the combination of symptoms typical of mania. (Bipolar patients need a careful interview for symptoms of addiction to alcohol; comorbid alcohol use disorder is diagnosed in as many as 30%. Often the alcohol-related symptoms appear first.)

Although the depression that occurred early in her pregnancy would have met the criteria for major depressive episode, her current manic episode obviates MDD. Because the current episode is too severe for hypomania, she cannot have cyclothymic disorder. Therefore, the diagnosis will be bipolar I disorder (psychosis and hospitalization rule out bipolar II).

The course of her illness isn't compatible with any psychosis other than brief psychotic disorder, and that diagnosis specifically excludes a bipolar disorder (B). The bipolar I subtypes, as described earlier, are based upon the nature of the most recent episode. Elisabeth's, of course, is current episode manic.

Next, we'll score the severity of her mania (see the footnotes to Table 3.2). These severity codes are sufficiently self-explanatory, but for one problem: Whether Elisabeth was psychotic is not made clear in the vignette. If we take her words literally, she thought she was becoming God, in which case she would qualify for *severe with psychotic features*. These would be judged *mood-congruent* because her grandiosity is in keeping with her exalted mood. But we really ought to obtain a more accurate assessment by asking her directly, "Do you actually think you are becoming God, or do you mean something else?"

The only possible episode specifier (Table 3.3) is *with peripartum onset:* She developed her manic episode within a few days of delivery. With a GAF score of 25, the full diagnosis would be as follows:

F31.2   Bipolar I disorder, currently manic, severe with mood-congruent psychotic features, with peripartum onset

Winona Fisk

By the time she turned 21, Winona Fisk had already had two lengthy mental health hospitalizations, one each for mania and depression. Then she remained well for a year on maintenance lithium, which in the spring of her 3rd year in college she abruptly discontinued—because she "felt so well." When two of her brothers escort her to the hospital 10 days later, she has been suspended for repeatedly disrupting classes with her boisterous behavior.

On the ward, Winona's behavior is mostly a picture of manic excitement. She speaks nonstop and is constantly on the move, sometimes rummaging through other patients' purses and lockers. But many of the thoughts flooding her mind are so sad that she often spontaneously weeps for several minutes at a time. She says she feels depressed and guilty—not for her behavior in class, but because she's "such a burden" to her family. During these brief episodes, she claims to hear the heart of her father beating from his grave. Then, she wishes she could join him in death. She eats little and loses 15 pounds; she often awakens weeping at night, unable to resume sleeping.

Nearly a month's treatment with lithium, carbamazepine, and antipsychotics is largely futile. Her mood disorder eventually yields to six sessions of bilateral ECT.

Evaluation of Winona Fisk

Winona's two previous episodes of bipolar I disorder leave no room for diagnosis doubt. Now our task is to determine the type and severity of the most recent episode.

Winona's episode begins with feeling "too good" to be ill; so she ditches her lithium, and that breeds trouble. Her symptoms, which include poor judgment (she was suspended from class for her behavior), talkativeness, and increased psychomotor activity, fulfill criteria A and B for manic episode. Her clinician needs to make sure she has no other medical or substance use disorder—criterion D. She's ill enough to require hospitalization, which rules out hypomanic episode (hypomanic episode criterion E).

But at times throughout the day, she also experiences short periods of intense sadness, microdepressions that comprise several depressive symptoms. As we'll see, they fulfill the criterion A requirements for the manic episode specifier *with mixed features*. Prominent depressed mood during a manic (or hypomanic) episode (mixed features A1), inappropriate guilt (A5), and ruminations about death (A6). Because they are found in both manic and depressive episodes, problems with sleep and appetite/weight don't make the mixed features list. And I'm pretty sure her clinician has finally verified that she doesn't drink to excess or use drugs (D).

The severity of Winona's episode should be judged based on both the symptom count and the degree to which her illness affected her (and others). All things considered, her clinician judges her seriously ill, and codes her accordingly.

With a GAF score of 25, here's Winona's diagnosis:

F31.2	Bipolar I disorder, current episode manic, severe with mood-congruent psychotic features, with mixed features
Z55.9	Academic or educational problem (suspended from school)

Hypomanic Episode

Hypomanic episode is the final mood disorder building block. Comprising most of the same symptoms as found in manic episode, it is "manic episode writ small." Left without treatment, some patients with hypomanic episode may become fully manic later. But many, especially those who have bipolar II disorder, have repeated hypomanic episodes. Hypomanic episode isn't codable as a diagnosis; it forms the backbone of bipolar II disorder, and it can also be encountered in bipolar I disorder—but only if the patient has already experienced an episode of actual mania. Hypomanic episode requires (1) a mood quality that (2) has existed for a required period of time, (3) is attended by a required number of symptoms, (4) has resulted in a considerable degree of disability, and (5) violates none of the listed exclusions. (Sound familiar?) Table 3.1 compares the features of manic and hypomanic episodes.

Quality of Mood

The quality of mood in hypomanic episode tends to be euphoric without the driven quality present in manic episode, though mood can instead be irritable. However described, it is clearly different from the patient's normal, nondepressed mood.

TABLE 3.1. Comparing Manic and Hypomanic Episodes

	Manic episode	Hypomanic episode
Duration	1 week or more	4 days or more
Mood	Abnormally and persistently high, irritable, or expansive	
Activity/energy	Persistently increased	
Symptoms that are changes from usual behavior	Three or more[a] of grandiosity, ↓ need for sleep, ↑ talkativeness, flight of ideas or racing thoughts, distractibility (self-report or that of others), agitation or ↑ goal-directed activity, poor judgment	
Indicators of severity	Results in psychotic features, hospitalization, or impairment of work, social, or personal functioning	Clear change from usual functioning *and* Others notice this change *and* No psychosis, hospitalization, or impairment
Other	Rule out physical substance/medication-induced disorders With mixed features if appropriate[b]	

[a]Four or more if the only abnormality of mood is irritability.

[b]Both manic and hypomanic episodes can have the specifier *with mixed features*.

Duration

The patient must have had symptoms for a minimum of 4 days—a marginally shorter time requirement than that for manic episode.

Symptoms

As with manic episode, in addition to the change in mood (euphoria or irritability), the patient must also have an increase in energy or activity level—but again, only 4 days are required. At least three symptoms from the same list must be present to an important degree (and represent a noticeable change) during these 4 days. If the patient's *abnormal mood* is irritable and *not* elevated, four symptoms are required. Note that hypomanic episode precipitated by treatment can serve as evidence for, say, bipolar II disorder—if it persists longer than the expected physiological effects of the treatment.

The *sleep* of hypomanic patients may be brief, and *activity level* may be increased, sometimes to the point of agitation. Although the degree of agitation is less than in a manic episode, hypomanic patients can also feel driven and uncomfortable. *Judgment* deteriorates, which may lead to untoward consequences for finances or for work or social life. *Speech* may become rapid and pressured; *racing thoughts* or *flight of ideas* may be noticeable. *Easily becoming distracted* can be a feature of hypomanic episode. Heightened *self-esteem* is never so grandiose that it's delusional, and hypomanic patients are never psychotic.

In addition to the DSM-5-TR criteria, note that in hypomanic episode, as in manic episode, substance use is common.

Impairment

How severe can the impairment be without qualifying as a manic episode? This is to some extent a judgment call for the practitioner. Lapses of judgment, such as spending sprees and sexual indiscretions, can occur in both manic and hypomanic episodes—but, by definition, only a truly manic patient will be seriously impaired. If behavior becomes so extreme that hospitalization is needed or psychosis is evident, this person can no longer be considered hypomanic, and the label must be changed.

Exclusions

The exclusions are the same as those for manic episode. General medical conditions such as hyperthyroidism can produce hyperactive behavior; patients who misuse certain substances (especially amphetamines) will appear speeded up and may also report feeling strong and euphoric.

Essential Features of **Hypomanic Episode**

Hypomania is "mania lite"—many of the same symptoms, but never to the same extreme degree. These people feel euphoric (some only irritable) and they experience high energy or activity. They are full of plans, which, despite some distractibility, they may even implement. They talk a lot, reflecting their racing thoughts, and may have flight of ideas. Judgment (sex and spending) may be impaired, but not to the point of requiring hospitalization for their own protection or for that of others. Though the patients are sometimes grandiose and self-important, these features do not reach the point of delusion. You would notice the change when such a person swings into hypomania, but functioning isn't markedly impaired; indeed, sometimes these folks get quite a lot done!

The Fine Print

The D's: • Duration (most of nearly every day, 4+ days) • Disability (work/educational, social, and personal functioning are not especially impaired) • Differential diagnosis (**substance use** and **physical disorders,** other bipolar disorders)

Coding Notes

There is no severity code.
   Hypomanic episode is not a diagnosable illness; it is a building block of bipolar II disorder and bipolar I disorder.

F31.81 Bipolar II Disorder

The symptoms of bipolar II and bipolar I disorders bear important similarities. What distinguishes them from one another, however, is the degree of disability and discomfort attached to the high phase. Bipolar II never involves psychosis and never requires hospitalization.* Bipolar II disorder consists of recurrent major depressive episodes interspersed with hypomanic episodes.

Like bipolar I disorder, bipolar II may be diagnosed based on mood episodes that arise spontaneously or that are precipitated by antidepressants, ECT, or bright light therapy—*if* the induced symptoms endure beyond the expected duration of the physiological treatment effects. (Be sure to ask the patient and informants whether there has been another hypomanic episode that was *not* precipitated by treatment; many patients will have had one.) Bipolar II is also associated with an especially high rate of rapid cycling, which carries added risk for a difficult course of illness.

Though the sexes are about equally represented in bipolar I disorder, women may be more likely than men to develop bipolar II disorder. Overall, it affects under 1% of the general adult population, though prevalence among adolescents may be higher. The stresses of the peripartum period may precipitate an episode of hypomania.

Comorbidity is frequent for patients with bipolar II. Mostly they will have anxiety and substance use disorders, though eating disorders will also be in the mix, especially for female patients.

Although I earlier described hypomanic episode as "mania lite," we shouldn't imagine that bipolar II disorder is innocuous. Indeed, some studies suggest that patients with bipolar II are ill longer and spend more time in the depressive phase—which can be quite severe—than is the case for patients with bipolar I. They may also be especially likely to make impulsive, successful suicide attempts. Atypical depressive symptoms (hypersomnia, increased eating) may be more common in bipolar II. And not a few patients (in the 10% range) will eventually experience a full-blown manic episode, followed by a change of diagnosis.

Essential Features of **Bipolar II Disorder**

The patient has had at least one each of a major depressive episode (p. 112) *and* a hypomanic episode, but *no* manic episodes (p. 123) ever.

The Fine Print

There must be at least one hypomanic episode and one major depressive episode that aren't better explained by a psychotic disorder.

---

*I suppose a patient with bipolar II disorder could end up hospitalized without really needing it. In such a case, I'd go with the predominant symptoms and call it bipolar II.

The D's: • Distress or disability (distress or work/educational, social, or personal impairment, but only for the depressive episodes or for switches between episodes) • Differential diagnosis (**substance use** and **physical disorders,** other bipolar disorders, major depressive disorder, **schizoaffective disorder** or **other psychotic disorder**)

Coding Notes

Specify current or most recent episode as **{hypomanic}{depressed}.**

Choose any relevant specifiers, summarized in Table 3.3 (p. 167). For a current major depressive episode, you can mention severity (mild, moderate, severe).

Iris McMaster

"I'm a writer," says Iris McMaster. It's her first visit to the interviewer's office, and she wants to smoke. She fiddles with a cigarette but doesn't seem to know what to do with it. "It's what I do for a living. I should be home doing it now—it's my life. Maybe I'm the finest creative writer since Dostoevsky. But my friend Charlene says I should come in, so I've taken time away from working on my play and my comic novel—and here I am." She finally slips the cigarette back into the pack.

"Why does Charlene think you should come?" the interviewer wants to know.

"She thinks I'm high. Of *course* I'm high. I'm always high when I'm in my creative phase. Only she says I'm too nervous." Iris is slender and of average height; she wears a bright pink spring outfit. She gazes longingly at her pack of cigarettes. "God, I need one of those."

Her speech can be interrupted, but it is salted with bon mots, neat turns of phrase, and original similes. But Iris can also give a coherent history. Now 45, she is married to an engineer; their daughter is nearly 18. And she really is a writer, who over the last several years has sold (mainly to magazines) articles on a variety of subjects.

For 3 or 4 months Iris has been in one of her high phases, cranking out an enormous number of articles and essays on a wide range of topics. Her "wired" feeling is in a way uncomfortable, but that doesn't trouble her because she is so productive. Whenever she is creating, she doesn't need much sleep: A 2-hour nap will leave her rested and ready for another 10 hours at her computer. At those times, her husband fixes his own meals and kids her about having "a one-track mind."

Iris never eats much during her high phases, so she loses weight. But she's never gotten herself into trouble: no sexual indiscretions, no excessive spending ("I'm always too busy working to shop"). And she volunteers that she has never "seen visions, heard voices, or had weird ideas about people following me around. And I've never spent time in the funny farm."

As Iris pauses to gather her thoughts, her fingers clutch the cigarette package. She shakes her head almost imperceptibly. Without uttering another word, she grabs her purse, vaults from the chair, and sweeps through the doorway. It is the last the interviewer sees of her for a year and a half.

In November of the following year, a person announcing herself as Iris McMaster drops into that same office chair. She seems almost an impostor. She's gained 30 or 40 pounds, which she has stuffed into polyester slacks and a bulky knit sweater. "As I was saying," are the first words she utters. Just for a second, the corners of her mouth twitch upward. But for the rest of the hour, she soberly talks about her latest problem: writer's block.

About a year ago, she had finished her play and was well into her comic novel when the muse decamped. For months now, she arises around lunchtime and spends long afternoons sitting at her computer. "Sometimes I don't even turn it on!" she says. She cannot focus her thinking to create anything that seems worth clicking "save." Most nights she tumbles into bed at 9. She feels tired and heavy, as though her legs were made of bricks.

"It's cheesecake, actually," is how Iris describes her weight gain. "I have it delivered. For months I haven't been interested enough to cook for myself." The only time she felt much better was a few occasions when Charlene took her out to lunch. Then she made conversation—and ate—pretty much as she used to. "I've done that quite a lot recently, as anyone can see. Eaten." Once she returned home from her afternoon out, the depression flooded back. But she has never been suicidal.

Finally, Iris apologizes for walking out a year and a half earlier. "I didn't think I was the least bit sick," she says, "and all I really wanted to do was return to my computer and get your character on paper!"

Evaluation of Iris McMaster

This discussion will focus on the episode of elevated mood during Iris's first visit. There are two possibilities for such an episode: mania and hypomania. As far as the time requirement is concerned, either type is possible—a hypomanic episode requires 4 days (hypomanic episode criterion A). She admits that she felt "wired" back then, a feeling that was apparently sustained for several months. During her high phase, she had at least four symptoms (three required, B): high self-esteem, decreased need for sleep, talkativeness, and increased goal-directed activity (writing).

Mood in either a manic or hypomanic episode is excessively high or irritable, and it is accompanied by increased energy and activity. The real distinction between hypomania and mania consists in the effects of the mood elevation on patient and surroundings. The patient's functioning during a manic episode is markedly impaired, whereas in a hypomanic episode it is only this: a clear change from usual for the individual (C) that others can notice (D). During her high spells, Iris's writing productivity increases, and her social relationships (those with her husband and friends, though perhaps not with her hapless clinician) do not appear to suffer (E). Note that the collective effect of criteria C, D, and E is to allow some impairment of functioning, just not very much of it.

If Iris has no other medical conditions or substance-induced mood disorder (F), she will be in the ballpark for one of these three diagnoses: bipolar I, bipolar II, or cyclothymic disorder. Judging from her lack of psychosis and hospitalizations, Iris has never had a true mania, ruling out bipolar I disorder. Her mood swings aren't nearly numerous enough to qualify for a diagnosis of cyclothymic disorder.

That leaves bipolar II disorder. But to qualify for that, there must be at least one major depressive episode (bipolar II criterion A). On Iris's second visit to the clinician, her depressive symptoms included feeling depressed most of the time, weight gain, hypersomnia, fatigue, and poor concentration (her "writer's block"), which fulfill the criterion A requirements for major depressive episode. If her depression did not meet those criteria, her diagnosis would have to be unspecified (or other specified) bipolar disorder. That's the same conclusion you'd reach if a patient has never had a depression and only hypomanic episodes.

In coding bipolar II disorder, clinicians are asked to specify the most recent episode. Iris's is depression. Because it's by definition less severe than mania, bipolar II disorder provides no severity code for a hypomanic episode. However, we can rate her depression by the same criteria we'd use for any other major depressive episode. Although she has only the minimum number of symptoms needed for major depressive episode, her work has been seriously impaired. For that reason, moderate severity seems appropriate, and is reflected in her GAF score of 60. If further interview reveals additional (or more serious) symptoms, I'd consider changing her evaluation to severe. These specifiers allow leeway for clinical judgment.

Associated with her depression are several features of an episode specifier: *with atypical features*. That is, her mood brightened when she was having lunch with her friend; she also gained weight, slept excessively, and she had a sensation of heaviness (bricks—or cheesecake—in her limbs). With a total of four of these symptoms (only three are required), at the time of the second interview, her full diagnosis would read as follows:

F31.81   Bipolar II disorder, depressed, moderate, with atypical features

Sal Camozzi is another patient with bipolar II disorder; his history is given in Chapter 11.

Additional Mood Disorders

As we've discussed so far, many of the mood disorders seen in a mental health practice can be diagnosed by referring to manic, hypomanic, and major depressive episodes. These three mood episodes must be considered for any patient with mood symptoms. Next, we'll consider several other conditions that do *not* depend on these episodes for their definition.

F34.1 Persistent Depressive Disorder

This condition has gone by several names—*dysthymic disorder, dysthymia, chronic depression*, and now *persistent depressive disorder (PDD)*. Whatever we call it (I'll generally stick with plain vanilla PDD), these patients are indeed chronically depressed. For years at a time, they have many of the same symptoms found in major depressive episodes, including low mood, fatigue, hopelessness, trouble concentrating, and problems with appetite and sleep. But notice what's absent from this list of symptoms (and from the criteria): inappropriate guilt feelings and thoughts of death or suicidal ideas. In short, this illness is enduring, but relatively less severe than major depressive disorder.

Over a lifetime, perhaps 6% of adults have PDD, with women affected about twice as often as men. Although it can begin at any age, late onset is uncommon, and the classic case starts so quietly and so early in life that some patients may not recognize themselves as depressed and regard their habitual low mood as normal. In the distant past, clinicians labeled these patients as having *depressive personality* or *depressive neurosis*.

People with PDD suffer quietly, and their disability can be subtle: They tend to put much of their energy into work, with not much left over for social aspects of life. Because they don't appear severely disabled, such individuals may go without treatment until their symptoms worsen into the more obvious major depressive episode. This is the fate of many, probably most, such patients. In 1993 this phenomenon was recounted in a book that made *The New York Times* best-seller list: *Listening to Prozac*. (However, the astonishing response to medication that book reported is by no means limited to one drug.)

DSM-IV differentiated between dysthymic disorder and chronic major depressive disorder, but research did not validate the distinction. So what DSM-5-TR now calls persistent depressive disorder is a combination of two separate DSM-IV conditions. The current criteria supply some specifiers to indicate the difference. Here's what's clear: Patients who have depression that goes on and on tend to respond poorly to treatment, are highly likely to have relatives with either bipolar disorders or some form of depression, and continue to be ill at follow-up.

One other feature results from the lumping together of PDD and chronic major depression. Because some major depression symptoms do not occur in the PDD criteria set, it is possible (as DSM-5-TR notes) that a few patients with chronic major depression won't meet criteria for PDD: The combination of psychomotor slowing, suicidal ideas, and low mood/energy/interest would fit that picture (of those symptoms, only low energy appears among the B criteria for PDD). Improbable, perhaps, but there you are. We are advised that such patients should be given a diagnosis of major depressive disorder if their symptoms meet criteria during the current episode; if not, we'll have to retreat to other specified (or unspecified) depressive disorder.

Essential Features of **Persistent Depressive Disorder**

"Low-grade depression" is how these symptoms are often described, and they occur most of the time for 2 years—they are never absent for longer than 2 months running. Patients will acknowledge such symptoms as fatigue, problems with concentration or decision making, poor self-image, and feeling hopeless. Sleep and appetite can be either increased or decreased. They may meet full requirements for a major depressive episode, but they have never had a manic or hypomanic episode or cyclothymic disorder.

The Fine Print

The D's: • Duration (more days than not, 2+ years) • Distress or disability (work/educational, social, or personal impairment) • Differential diagnosis (**substance use** and **physical disorders,** ordinary sadness, persistent grief disorder, adjustment to a longstanding stressor, bipolar disorders, major depressive disorder, **psychotic disorders**)

For children, mood may be irritable rather than depressed, and the time requirement is 1 year rather than 2.

Coding Notes

Specify severity. Specify onset:

> **Early onset,** if it begins by age 20.
> **Late onset,** if it begins at age 21 or later.

Specify if:

> **With pure dysthymic syndrome.** Hasn't met full criteria for major depressive episode in the past 2 years.
> **With persistent major depressive episode.** Has met criteria throughout the past 2 years.
> **With intermittent major depressive episodes, with current episode.** Meets major depressive criteria now, but over past 2 years hasn't met criteria for 2 months at a time.
> **With intermittent major depressive episodes, without current episode.** Has met major depressive criteria in the past 2 years, though doesn't now.

A patient whose symptoms fulfill criteria for both PDD and major depressive disorder should be given both diagnoses. And one of the three specifiers just above should also be invoked.

Choose other specifiers from Table 3.3 (p. 167).

> **With anxious distress**
> **With atypical features**

Noah Sanders

For Noah Sanders, life has never seemed much fun. He was 18 when he first noticed that most of the time, he "just felt down." Although he is bright and he studied hard, throughout college he was often distracted by thoughts that he didn't measure up to his classmates. He landed a job with a leading electronics firm but turned down several promotions because he felt that he could not cope with added responsibility. It took dogged determination and long hours of work to compensate for this "inherent second-rateness." The effort left him chronically tired. Even his marriage and the birth of each of his two daughters relieved his gloom for only a few weeks, at best. His self-confidence was so low that, by common consent, his wife always made most of their family's decisions.

"It's the way I've always been. I am a professional pessimist," Noah told his family doctor one day when he was in his early 30s. The doctor guessed that he has a depressive personality.

For many years, that description seemed to fit. Then, when Noah is in his early 40s, his younger daughter leaves for college; after this, he begins to feel increasingly that life has passed him by. Over a period of several months, his depression deepens. Now he thinks he has never really been depressed before. Even visits from his daughters, which have always cheered him up, fail to improve his outlook.

Usually a sound sleeper, Noah has begun awakening at about 4 A.M. to ruminate about his mistakes. His appetite falls off, and he loses weight. When for the third time in a week his wife finds him weeping, he confesses that he feels so guilty about his failures that he believes they'd all be better off without him. That's when she drags him in for treatment.

Noah starts on an antidepressant medication. Within 2 weeks, his mood brightens, and he is sleeping soundly; at 1 month, he has "never felt better" in his life. Whereas he had once avoided oral presentations at work, he begins to look forward to them as "a chance to show what I can do." His chronic fatigue fades; he begins jogging to use up some of his excess energy. In his spare time, he starts his own small business to develop and promote some of his engineering innovations.

Ever since, Noah continues to operate his small business as a sideline—and to take his medication. Whenever he and his therapist try to reduce it, he finds himself returning to the thought, "Perhaps I am really a failure, after all."

Evaluation of Noah Sanders

For most of his adult life, Noah has had depressive symptoms that are chronic, rather than episodic. He was never without these symptoms for longer than a few weeks at a time (criterion C for PDD), and they were present most of the day, most days (A). They include general pessimism, poor self-image, and chronic tiredness, though only two symptoms are required by criterion B. Because of his indecisiveness, his wife assumed the role of family decision maker, which sounds to me an awful lot like social impairment (H). The way he felt was not different from his usual self; in fact, he says it's the way he has always been. (The extended duration is one of two main features that differentiate PDD from major depressive disorder. The other is that the required symptoms are neither as plentiful nor as severe as for major depression.) Noah has never had manic or psychotic symptoms, so we need not consider bipolar or psychotic disorders (E, F).

The differential diagnosis of PDD is essentially the same as that for major depressive disorder. Mood disorder due to another medical condition and substance-induced mood disorder must be ruled out (G). The remarkable chronicity and poor self-image invite speculation that Noah's difficulties could be explained by a personality disorder, such as avoidant or dependent personality disorder. The vignette does not address all the criteria that would be necessary to make those diagnoses. However, an important diagnostic principle holds that the more treatable conditions should be diagnosed (and treated) first. If, despite relief of the mood disorder, Noah had continued to be shy and awkward and to have a negative self-image, only then should we consider a personality diagnosis.

Now to the specifiers (Table 3.3). Though lacking psychotic symptoms, Noah had several depressive symptoms (including thoughts about death) that suggest he was severely ill. He first noticed his symptoms when he was just 18, so we'd say that his onset was early. Noah's recent symptoms would also qualify for a major depressive episode, which had begun recently and precipitated this evaluation; DSM-5-TR notes that such a patient can have symptoms that fulfill criteria for such an episode (D). We would therefore give him the specifier with intermittent major depressive episodes, with current episode.

By definition, the only standard depressive disorder specifiers that can apply to PDD are with atypical features and with anxious distress; neither of these fits.

Once treated, Noah seems almost to undergo a personality change. His mood lightens and his behavior changes to the point that, by contrast, he appears virtually hypomanic. However, these symptoms don't rise to the level required for a hypomanic episode; had that been the case, criterion E would exclude the diagnosis of PDD. (Also, remember that a hypomanic episode precipitated by treatment that does not extend past the physiological effects of treatment does not count toward a diagnosis of bipolar II disorder. It should not count against the diagnosis of PDD, either, though DSM-5-TR does not state this outright.) I thought his GAF score would be about 50 on first evaluation and a robust 90 at follow-up. In the summary, I'd note the possibility of avoidant personality traits.

Because he also meets criteria for MDD, he earns two diagnoses:

F34.1   Persistent depressive disorder, severe, early onset, with intermittent major depressive episode, with current episode, with melancholic features

F32.1   Major depressive disorder, moderate

F34.0 Cyclothymic Disorder

People with cyclothymic disorder (CD) are chronically either elated or depressed, but *for the first couple of years* they do not fulfill criteria for a manic, hypomanic, or major depressive episode. Note the phrase that's dripping with italics. I'll explain in the sidebar.

CD was at one time regarded as a personality disorder. Perhaps that was partly due to its gradual onset and prolonged duration. Some clinicians still refer to *cyclothymic temperament,* which may be a precursor to bipolar disorders.

The clinical appearance can be very variable. Some patients are nearly always dysphoric, occasionally shifting into hypomania for a day or so. Others can swing several times in a single day. Often the presentation is mixed.

Typically beginning gradually in adolescence or young adulthood, CD affects under 1% of the general population. However, clinicians diagnose it even less often than that. The sex distribution is about equal, though women are more likely to seek treatment. Not surprisingly, people usually come to clinical attention only when they are depressed. Once underway, CD tends toward chronicity.

What if your patient with CD later develops a manic, hypomanic, or major depressive episode? That happens with some frequency (up to 50%), in which case you'll have to change the diagnosis. Once a major mood episode rears its head, that patient can never revert to CD. If the new episode is major depressive, then you'll probably fall back on an unspecified (or other specified) bipolar disorder, inasmuch as, by definition, the *up* periods of CD will not qualify as a hypomanic episode.

Essential Features of **Cyclothymic Disorder**

The patient has had many ups and downs of mood that *don't* meet criteria for any of the mood episodes (major depressive, hypomanic, manic). Although symptoms occur half the time or more, up to 2 months of level mood can go by.

The Fine Print

The D's: • Duration (2+ years; 1+ year in children and adolescents) • Distress or disability (work/educational, social, or personal impairment) • Differential diagnosis (**substance use** and **physical disorders, other bipolar disorders** with rapid cycling, **psychotic disorders**)

Coding Notes

Specify if: **With anxious distress**

Honey Bare

"I'm a yo-yo!"

Without her feathers and sequins, Honey Bare looks anything but provocative. She began life as Melissa Schwartz, but she loves using her stage name. The stage in question is Hoofer's, one of the bump-and-grind joints that thrive near the waterfront. The billboard proclaims it as "Only a Heartthrob Away" from the Navy recruiting station. Since dropping out of college 4 years ago, Honey has been a front-liner in the four-girl show at Hoofer's. Every afternoon on her way to work she passes right by the mental health clinic, but this is her first visit inside.

"In our current gig, I play the Statue of Liberty. I receive the tired, the poor, and the huddled masses. Then I take off my robes."

"Is that a problem?" the interviewer wants to know.

Most of the time, it isn't. Honey likes her little corner of show biz. When the fleet is in, she plays to thunderous applause. "In fact, I enjoy just about everything I do. I don't drink much, and I never do drugs, but I do go to parties. I sing in our church choir, go to movies—I enjoy art films quite a bit." When she feels well, she sleeps little, talks a lot, starts a dozen projects, and even finishes some of them. "I'm really a happy person—when I'm feeling up."

But every couple of months, there'll be a week or two when Honey doesn't enjoy much of anything. She'll paste a smile on her face and go to work, but when the curtain rings down, the smile comes off with her makeup. She is never suicidal, and her sleep and appetite don't suffer; her energy and concentration are normal. But it's as though all the fizz has gone out of her ginger ale. She can see no obvious cause for her mood swings, which have gone on for years. She can count on the fingers of both hands the number of weeks she's been "just normal."

Lately, Honey has acquired a boyfriend—a chief petty officer who wants to marry her. He says he loves her because she is so vivacious and enthusiastic, but he has only seen her when she's bubbly. Always before, when she was depressed, he had been out to sea. Now he's written that he is being transferred to shore duty, and she fears it spells the end of their relationship. As she says this, two large tears trickle through the mascara and down her cheeks.

Four months and several visits later, Honey is back, wearing a smile. The lithium carbonate, she reports, seems to be working well. The peaks and valleys of her moods have smoothed out to rolling hills. And she still plays the Statue of Liberty down at Hoofer's.

"My sailor's been back for nearly 3 months," she says with a happy sigh, "and he's still carrying the torch for me."

As far back as the mid-19th century, Karl Kahlbaum—the German psychiatrist who first described catatonia—noted that some people experience frequent alterations between highs and lows so mild as not to require any treatment. His observations were confirmed and extended by his student and colleague, Ewald Hecker (who is best known for his description of hebephrenic schizophrenia).

But by the mid-20th century, the first DSM described cyclothymia as a cardinal personality type (along with schizoid, paranoid, and inadequate personalities). That first DSM description sounds pretty wonderful: "an extratensive and outgoing adjustment to life situations, an apparent personal warmth, friendliness and superficial generosity, an emotional reaching out to the environment, and a ready enthusiasm for competition." (I'll leave the looking-up of *extratensive* as an extra-credit exercise.) Anyway, thus was born cyclothymia as a temperament or personality style.

DSM-II also classified cyclothymic personality with personality disorders, but in 1980 it was moved to the mood disorders and rechristened with its current name. However, its relationship to other mood disorders is fraught; experts argue about it even today. Some hold that it can be prodromal to a more severe bipolar disorder. Some point out the similarities between cyclothymia and borderline personality disorder (labile, irritable moods leading to interpersonal conflict), even suggesting that borderline personality disorder belongs on the bipolar spectrum—a speculation extreme enough to provoke resistance.

All of this suggests that we still have work to do in determining CD's proper place in the diagnostic manuals. Though the DSM-5-TR criteria are a step along the road to differentiation of this venerable diagnosis, they may not signify much progress.

Evaluation of Honey Bare

The first and most obvious question is this: Has Honey ever fulfilled criteria for a manic, hypomanic, or major depressive episode (cyclothymic disorder criterion C)? When feeling down, she has no vegetative symptoms (problems with sleep or appetite) of major depressive episode. She has good concentration, has never been suicidal, and never complains of feeling worthless. At the other pole, she does indeed have symptoms similar to those of hypomania (talkative, sleeps less, is more active than at other times), but they aren't severe enough to qualify as a hypomanic episode. Honey's "up" moods aren't elevated (or irritable, or expansive) to an abnormal extent (hypomanic episode criterion A)—they are her usual level of functioning. Furthermore, she has experienced far more cycles than is typical for bipolar II disorder. We can therefore rule out any other bipolar or major depressive diagnosis.

Honey testifies that most of the time she is either up or down (we're back at cyclothymia—criterion B). Because she is never psychotic, she cannot qualify for a diagnosis such as schizoaffective disorder (D). She doesn't use drugs or alcohol, ruling out a substance-induced mood disorder (E). Again, we discard bipolar I, bipolar II, and major depressive disorders due to the lack of relevant episodes. (However, because they involve so many swings of mood, either bipolar I or II with rapid cycling can sometimes be confused with cyclothymic disorder.) Mood shifts, impulsivity, and interpersonal problems can of course be found aplenty in borderline personality disorder, but we should avoid diagnosing a personality disorder when symptoms of a major mental diagnosis are unresolved.

Symptoms present much of the time do qualify Honey for CD. She has had many mood swings; only infrequently is her mood neither high nor low. The only specifier allowed with CD, *with anxious distress*, doesn't seem to me relevant to Honey's symptoms. With a GAF score of 70 on admission and 90 at follow-up, her diagnosis is straightforward:

F34.0   Cyclothymic disorder

F32.81 Premenstrual Dysphoric Disorder

A long history of disagreement over the reality of premenstrual dysphoria caused it to languish in the appendices prior to DSM-5. But now, enough research has been published to bring it forth from the shadows.

Often beginning in the teenage years, premenstrual symptoms to some degree affect about 20% of women of reproductive age. Premenstrual dysphoric disorder affects a shade above 1% in the general population, though substantially fewer are functionally impaired. Throughout their reproductive years, these symptoms appear for perhaps a week out of each menstrual cycle. Then, these patients complain of varying degrees of dysphoric mood (which the dictionary defines as "very unhappy, uneasy, or dissatisfied"), fatigue, and physical symptoms that include sensitivity of breasts, weight gain, and abdominal swelling. Differentiation from major depressive episode and persistent depressive disorder relies principally on timing and duration.

The consequences of premenstrual dysphoric disorder can be serious: Such a patient could experience mood symptoms during an accumulated 8 years of her reproductive life. Some patients may be unaware how markedly their anger and other negative moods affect those around them, and many suffer from severe depression; perhaps 15% attempt suicide. Yet the typical patient doesn't receive treatment until she is 30, sometimes even later. Symptoms may be worse for older patients, though menopause offers a natural endpoint (duration is sometimes extended by hormone replacement therapy). Overall, this condition ranks high among the seriously underdiagnosed mental disorders.

Risk factors for premenstrual dysphoric disorder include excessive weight, stress, and trauma (including a history of abuse); there appears to be a robust genetic component. Comorbid are anxiety disorders and other mood disorders, including bipolar conditions.

Dating as far back as 1944—the term *premenstrual tension* dates at least to 1928—the premenstrual syndrome (PMS) has had a long and tempestuous life. It's been ridiculed by would-be comics, dismissed by many as pejorative, and disparaged even by some of those who practice gender politics. It should come as no surprise that it has been so ill received; as disorders go, PMS is remarkably vague and variously defined.

All told, PMS encompasses over a hundred possible symptoms. It's all anecdotal, with no specific symptoms and no minimum number required. Here are just a few: fluid retention (the symptom most often reported), especially in breasts and abdomen; craving for sweet or salty foods; muscle aches/pains, fatigue, irritability, tension, acne, anxiety, constipation or diarrhea, and insomnia; a change in sex drive; and feeling sad or moody or out of control. Most women will occasionally have one or two of these symptoms around the time of their periods—these symptoms are so common that, individually, they may be considered physiological rather than pathological. This fact causes some people to blame all such symptoms on PMS (it hardly ever goes by its full, nonabbreviated name). All women are in effect tarred with the same brush, whereas it is of crucial importance to note the exact symptoms, their timing, and their intensity.

Essential Features of **Premenstrual Dysphoric Disorder**

For a few days before menstruating, the patient experiences pronounced mood shifts, depression, anxiety, anger, or irritability. She will also admit to typical symptoms of depression, including trouble concentrating, loss of interest, fatigue, feeling out of control ("I just feel overwhelmed"), and changes in appetite or sleep. She may have physical symptoms such as sensitivity of breasts, muscle or joint pain, weight gain, and a sensation of abdominal distention. Shortly after menstruation begins, she snaps back to normal.

The Fine Print

The D's: • Duration (for several days around menstrual periods, for most cycles during the past year) • Distress or disability (social, occupational, or personal impairment) • Differential diagnosis (**substance use**—including hormone replacement therapy; **physical disorders; major depressive disorder** or **persistent depressive disorder; panic disorder; personality disorders;** ordinary grief/sadness)

Coding Note

DSM-5-TR says that the diagnosis can only be stated as *provisional* until you've obtained prospective ratings of two menstrual cycles. What you as a clinician decide to do with this is, of course, your business.

Amy Jernigan

"Look, I don't need you to tell me what's wrong. I *know* what's wrong. I just need you to fix it." One ankle crossed over the other, Amy Jernigan slouches in the consultation chair and gazes steadily at her clinician. "I brought a list of my symptoms, just so there won't be any confusion." She unfolds a half-sheet of embossed stationery.

"It always starts out 4 or 5 days before my period," she recites. "I begin by feeling uptight, like I'm waiting to take an exam I haven't studied for. Then, after a day or two, depression sets in and I just want to cry." She glances up and smiles. "You won't catch me doing that now—I'm always just fine after my period starts."

Still in her early 20s, Amy graduated from a college near her home in the Deep South. Now, while waiting for her novel to sell, she does research for a political blogger. With another glance at the paper, she continues. "But before, I'm depressed, cranky, lazy as a hound dog in August, and I don't really give a shit about anything."

Amy's mother, an antifeminist who'd campaigned against the Equal Rights Amendment, had refused to validate Amy's premenstrual symptoms, though she might have had them herself. Amy's problem began in her early teens, almost from the time of her first period. "I'd be so pissed off I'd drive away all my friends. Fortunately, I'm pretty outgoing, so they didn't—don't—stay lost for long. But reliably every month, my breasts get so sensitive they could read Braille. Then I know I'd better put a lock on my tongue, or the next week I'll be buying beers for everyone I know."

Amy tucks her list into her back pocket and sits up straight. "I hate being the feminist with PMS—I feel like a walking cliché."

Evaluation of Amy Jernigan

As Amy says, she doesn't need much discussion about what's wrong—though she doesn't have her terms quite right. Her symptoms—depression, irritability, and tension (criteria B3, B2, and B4) and breast tenderness, lethargy, and loss of interest (C7, C3, and C1)—exceed the requirement for a total of five or more. Amy herself indicates just how debilitating she considers the symptoms to be (D). The recurrence, the timing, and the absence of symptoms at times other than before her menses (A) lock in an airtight case. The duration of her low mood is too brief for either a major depressive episode or persistent depressive disorder (E). Of course, the usual inquiry must be made to rule out any substance use or another medical condition (G). I should note that, in the absence of a couple of months of prospective symptom recording, Amy's clinician needs to be extra careful to rule out major depressive disorder. It is awfully easy to ignore depressive symptoms that occur at other times of the month.

Amy's clinician would have to assess her mood through two subsequent periods to comply with criterion F. When she is ill, her GAF score will be about 60. Her diagnosis should be as follows:

F32.81   Premenstrual dysphoric disorder, provisional

The demand for prospective data before a definitive diagnosis can be made is unique in DSM-5-TR and has never been required prior to DSM-5. The rationale is to ensure that the diagnosis is made with the best data possible; the fact that such a step is not required for more diagnoses may be a nod to the realities of clinical practice. Even so, we may have just experienced the first breeze of a gathering storm.

F34.81 Disruptive Mood Dysregulation Disorder

Disruptive mood dysregulation disorder (DMDD) encompasses extremes of childhood. Most kids fight among themselves, but DMDD broadens the scope and intensity of battle. Minor provocations (insufficient cheese in a sandwich, a favorite shirt in the wash) can cause these patients to fly completely off the handle. In a burst of temper, they may threaten or bully siblings—and parents. Some may refuse to comply with chores, homework, or even basic hygiene. These outbursts occur every couple of days on average, and between storms the patient's mood is persistently unsettled—depressed, angry, or irritable.

Their behavior places children with DMDD at enormous social, educational, and emotional disadvantage. Low assessments of functioning reflect the trouble they have interacting with peers, teachers, and relatives. They require constant attention from parents, and if they go to school at all, they may need minders to assure their own safety and that of others. Some patients with DMDD suffer such intense rage that those about them fear for their lives. Even relatively mild symptoms may cause them to forego many childhood experiences, such as play dates and party invitations. In one sample, a third had been hospitalized.

Prevalence has been stated as high as 8% of 6-year-olds in the United States, tailing off with age (2.5% in 11-year-olds in Brazil). Perhaps as many as 80% of children with DMDD will also meet criteria for oppositional defiant disorder, in which case the rules say we should only diagnose DMDD. The diagnosis is more common in boys than in girls, placing it at odds with most other mood disorders, though right in line with most other childhood disorders. Although the official DSM-5-TR criteria remind us not to make the diagnosis prior to age 6, limited studies find that it is most common in preschool children. And it needs to be discriminated from teenage rebellion—the teens are a transitional period where mood symptoms are common.

The question has been asked: Why was DMDD not included in the same chapter with the disruptive, impulse-control, and conduct disorders? Of course, the original impetus was to give clinicians a mood-related alternative to bipolar I disorder. However, the prominent feature of persistently depressed (or irritable) behavior throughout the course of illness seems reason enough for placement with other mood disorders.

Partly because this diagnosis is intended for children, but mainly because I'm really worried about the validity of a newly concocted, insufficiently studied formulation (see the sidebar), I've not provided a vignette. At the same time, I'm really, *really* worried about all those kids who have been lumbered with a diagnosis of a bipolar disorder, with attendant (probably unnecessary) drug treatment.

How many disorders can you name that originated in an uncomfortable bulge in the number of patients being diagnosed with something else? I can think of exactly one, and here is how it came about.

Beginning in the mid-1990s, some prominent American psychiatrists sufficiently relaxed the criteria for bipolar disorder to allow that diagnosis in children whose irritability was chronic, not episodic. Subsequently, the number of childhood bipolar diagnoses ballooned. Many other experts howled at what they perceived to be a subversion of the bipolar criteria; thus were drawn the battle lines for diagnostic war.

Several features seem to set those youngsters well apart from traditional patients with bipolar disorder: (1) Limited follow-up studies find some increase in depression, not mania, in these children as they mature. (2) Family history studies find no excess of bipolar disorder in relatives of these patients. (3) The sex ratio is about 2:1 in favor of boys, which is disparate with the 1:1 ratio for bipolar disorder in older patients. (4) Studies of pathophysiology suggest that brain mechanisms may differentiate the two conditions. (5) The diagnosis of childhood bipolar disorder has been made far more often in the United States than elsewhere in the world. (6) Follow-up studies find far more manic or hypomanic episodes in children with bipolar disorder diagnosed according to traditional criteria than in those whose principal issue was with severe mood dysregulation.

The epic internecine battle among U.S. mental health professionals was chronicled in a 2008 *Frontline* program on PBS ("The Bipolar Child") and in a *New York Times Magazine* article by Jennifer Egan ("The Bipolar Puzzle," September 12, 2008). The dispute continues; meanwhile, the DMDD category was crafted to capture more accurately the pathology of these severely irritable children.

Essential Features of **Disruptive Mood Dysregulation Disorder**

Several times a week for at least a year, on minor provocation a child has severe tantrums—screaming or physically attacking something (or someone)—that are inappropriate for the situation and the patient's age and stage of development. Others notice that, between outbursts, the child seems mostly angry, grumpy, or sad. The attacks and intervening moods occur across multiple settings (home, school, with friends). These patients have no manic episodes.

The Fine Print

Delve into the D's: • Duration (1+ years, and never absent longer than 3 months) • Demographics (starting before age 10, the diagnosis can be first made only from age 6 through 17) • Distress or disability (symptoms are severe in at least one setting—home, school, with other kids—and present in other settings) • Differential diagnosis (**substance use** and **physical disorders, major depressive disorder, persistent depressive disorder, bipolar disorders, oppositional defiant disorder,** attention-deficit/hyperactivity disorder, **autism spectrum disorder, PTSD, separation anxiety disorder,** behavioral outbursts consistent with developmental age)

A patient who qualifies for both DMDD and oppositional defiant disorder should be diagnosed only with DMDD. DMDD should not be diagnosed with intermittent explosive disorder or bipolar disorder.

Induced Mood Disorders

Substance/Medication-Induced Mood Disorders

Substance use is an especially common cause of mood disorder. Intoxication with cocaine or amphetamines can precipitate manic symptoms, and depression can result from withdrawal from cocaine, amphetamines, alcohol, or barbiturates. Note that for the diagnosis to be tenable, it must develop in close proximity to an episode of intoxication or withdrawal from the substance, which must in turn be capable of causing the symptoms. Obviously, depression can occur with the misuse of alcohol and street drugs—perhaps 40% of individuals with a substance use disorder. However, even health care professionals can fail to recognize mood disorders caused by medications (see table on p. 665). That's why the case of Erin Finn below is a cautionary tale, probably encountered every working day in clinicians' offices around the world.

Essential Features of **Substance/Medication-Induced** {Depressive Disorder} {Bipolar and Related Disorder}

The use of some substance appears to have caused a patient to experience an obvious and enduring {depressed mood or loss of interest or pleasure in nearly all activities}{both an elevated (or expansive or irritable) mood and excessively increased energy or activity}.

For tips on identifying substance-related causation, see sidebar, page 95.

The Fine Print

The D's: • Distress or disability (work/educational, social, or personal impairment) • Differential diagnosis (physical disorders, other depressive or bipolar disorders, "ordinary" substance intoxication or withdrawal, delirium)

Use this diagnosis instead of substance intoxication or withdrawal only when mood symptoms are predominant and require clinical attention.

Coding Notes

Specify if:

With onset during {intoxication}{withdrawal}. This gets tacked on at the end of your string of words.
With onset after medication use. You could alternatively use this if symptoms develop when medication is started, changed, or stopped.

Code depending on whether there is evidence that supports a mild or moderate/severe substance use disorder (see Table 15.2 on p. 475).

Erin Finn

Erin Finn comes to the clinic straight from her job as media specialist for a political campaign. She's taken part in her state's screening program for hepatitis C, which targets people in her age group—reared before routine testing of the blood supply had reduced incidence of the disease. When her screening test came back positive and the RNA polymerase chain reaction test revealed a viral load, she'd agreed to a trial of interferon. "I sometimes feel tired, but I've had no other symptoms," she tells her clinician.

Though solidly middle-class and conservatively dressed, Erin has actually had a number of possible exposures to hepatitis C. The most likely one was a years-ago blood transfusion, but she can also claim "a wildish youth; I experimented with injectable drugs a few times, even got a tattoo. It's more or less discreet—the tattoo."

Within a few days of starting the medication she begins to notice feeling depressed—mild at first, but increasing day by day. "It feels worse than that day last year when we thought we'd lost in the primary election," she tells the interviewer. "It's been a horrible combination of sleeping poorly at night and never completely waking up during the day. And feeling draggy, and tired, and . . ." She gropes for words while fiddling with the two campaign buttons pinned to her coat.

Originally hired to do data entry, Erin has been promoted to write campaign materials for brochures and television. But most of the day her depression and resulting poor concentration produce a lot of mistakes. "I'm a crap worker," she says, "always making simple errors in grammar and spelling. It'll be my fault if we lose in November."

After a moment, she adds, "But I'm not suicidal, I'm not that dumb. Or desperate. But some days, I just wish I was dead!" She thinks for a moment. "Were dead! And my boyfriend tells me I'm useless in bed. Along with everything else, I just don't seem to care about that anymore, either."

After Erin stops the interferon, her mood and other symptoms gradually return to normal. "So the doctor thinks I ought to try the interferon again, as a sort of challenge. At first, I thought that was a total nonstarter! But then I got to worrying some more about cirrhosis, and now I think I'll give it another shot. So to speak."

She shrugs as she rolls up her sleeve. "I guess hepatitis treatment has a lot in common with politics—neither of them's bean-bag."

Evaluation of Erin Finn

Erin's symptoms would rate her a diagnosis of (relatively mild) major depressive episode, even leaving out the fatigue (which we won't count because it antedated her use of interferon). Even without all those depressive symptoms, the mere fact of having such a pronounced low mood would fulfill the requirement for medication-induced depressive disorder (criterion A). The timing is right (B1), and interferon is well known to produce depression in a sizeable number of patients (though more often in those who have had previous mood episodes—B2). And, although it is hardly a controlled experiment, her depressive symptoms did clear up soon after she discontinued the interferon. DSM-5-TR doesn't specify a challenge test (sometimes such a test is inadvisable), but a return of Erin's depressive symptoms after she resumed the medication would forge the final cause-and-effect link.

OK, so we should consider other possible causes of her depression (criteria C and D). I'll leave that as an exercise for the reader. As for criterion E (distress and disability), *res ipsa loquitur*. When we turn to Table 15.2 in Chapter 15 for ICD-10 coding, her substance is "Other" (F19), and she has obviously used it only as prescribed, so there is no use disorder. Cross-indexing with the mood disorder column yields F19.94. I would give her GAF score as 55 on admission, 90 at discharge.

B18.2	Chronic hepatitis C
F19.94	Interferon-induced depressive disorder, with onset after medication use

Mood Disorders Due to Another Medical Condition

Many medical conditions can cause depressive or bipolar symptoms, and it is vital always to consider physical etiologies when evaluating a mood disorder. This is not only because they are treatable; with today's therapeutic options, most mood disorders are *highly* treatable. It is also because some of the general medical conditions, if left inadequately treated too long, themselves have serious consequences—including death. And not a few can cause manic symptoms. I've mentioned some of these in the

"Physical Disorders That Affect Mental Diagnosis" (p. 661), though that table is by no means exhaustive.

Note this really important requirement: The medical condition must have been the direct, *physiological* cause of the bipolar or depressive symptoms. *Psychological* causation (for instance, the patient feels understandably terrible upon being told "it's cancer") doesn't count, except as the possible precipitant for an adjustment disorder.

The story of Lisa Voorhees below illustrates the importance of considering that medical conditions can cause mood disorders.

Essential Features of {Depressive Disorder} {Bipolar and Related Disorder} Due to Another Medical Condition

Through physiological means, a medical condition appears to have caused an illness that features obvious and enduring {depressed mood or loss of interest or pleasure in nearly all activities}{both an elevated (or expansive or irritable) mood and excessively increased energy or activity}.

The Fine Print

For pointers on deciding when a physical condition may have caused a mental disorder, see sidebar, page 97.

The D's: • Duration (none stated, though it would not be fleeting) • Distress or disability (work/educational, social, or personal impairment) • Differential diagnosis (substance use disorders, **other depressive** or **bipolar disorders,** other mental disorders, delirium)

Coding Notes

Specify for: **Depressive disorder due to another medical condition**

   F06.31 With depressive features. You cannot identify full symptomatic criteria for a major depressive episode.
   F06.32 With major depressive–like episode. You can.
   F06.34 With mixed features. Manic or hypomanic symptoms are evident but not predominant over the depressive symptoms.

Specify for: **Bipolar and related disorder due to another medical condition**

   F06.33 With manic- or hypomanic-like episode. You can identify full symptomatic criteria for mania or hypomania.
   F06.33 With manic features. Full mania or hypomania criteria are not met.
   F06.34 With mixed features. Depressive symptoms are evident but not predominant over the manic symptoms.

It was only with DSM-5 that criteria specifically differentiated medically precipitated bipolar and depressive disorders. What if you can't tell? Some mood disorders, in their early stages, may be too indistinct to call. You might then be reduced to diagnosing unspecified mood disorder (F39).

Lisa Voorhees

By the time she arrives at the mental health clinic, Lisa Voorhees has already seen three doctors, each of whom dismissed her problem as "entirely mental." She has "been 39 for several years," but she is slender and smart, and she knows she is still attractive to men.

She intends to stay that way. Her job as personal secretary to the chairman of the department of English and literature at a large Midwestern university introduces her to a lot of eligible males. And that is where Lisa first noticed the problem that makes her think she is losing her mind.

"It's this gorgeous assistant professor of Romance languages," she tells the interviewer. "He's always in and out of the office, and I'd done everything short of sexual harassment to get him to notice me. Then one day last spring, he asked me out to dinner and a show. And I turned him down! I just wasn't interested. It was as if my sex drive had gone on sabbatical!"

For weeks she continued to feel uninterested in men, and then one morning she woke up next to "this odious creep from the provost's office" she'd avoided for months. She felt disgusted with herself, but before she kicked him out, they had sex again anyway.

For the next several months, Lisa's sexual appetite suddenly changes every 2 or 3 weeks; privately, she invokes Henry James, calling it "The Turn of the Screw." During her active phase, she feels airy and light, and can pound away at her keyboard 12 hours a day. But the rest of the time, nothing pleases her. She is depressed and grouchy at the office, sleeps badly (and alone), and jokes that her keyboard and mouse are conspiring to make her feel clumsy.

Even Lisa's wrists feel weak. She buys a wrist rest to use when she is typing, and that helps for a while. But she can find neither splint nor salve for the fluctuations of her libido. One doctor tells her it is "the change" and prescribes estrogen; another diagnoses "manic–depression" and offers lithium. A third suggests pastoral counseling. Instead, she attends the clinic.

In frustration, Lisa rises from her chair and paces to the window and back. "Wait a minute—do that again," the interviewer urges.

"Do what? All I did was walk across the room."

"I know. How long have you had that limp?"

"I don't know. Not long, I guess. What with the other problems, I hardly notice. Does it matter?"

It proves to be the key. Three visits to a neurologist, some X-rays, and an MRI later,

Lisa's diagnosis is multiple sclerosis. The neurologist explains that multiple sclerosis sometimes causes mood swings. With treatment for multiple sclerosis underway, Lisa returns to the mental health clinic for psychotherapy.

Evaluation of Lisa Voorhees

On paper, the various criteria sets make reasonably clear-cut the differences between mood disorders with "emotional" causes and those caused by general medical conditions or substance use. In practice, it isn't always obvious.

Lisa's mood symptoms have alternated between periods of highs and lows. Although they last 2 weeks or longer, none of these extremes is severe enough to qualify as a manic, hypomanic, or major depressive episode. The depressed period is too brief for persistent depressive disorder; the whole episode hasn't lasted long enough for cyclothymic disorder; and there is no evidence for a substance-induced mood disorder.

Depressive (or bipolar) disorder due to another medical condition must fulfill two important criteria. The first is that symptoms must be directly produced by physiological mechanisms of the illness itself, not simply by an emotional reaction to being sick. For example, patients with cancer of the head of the pancreas are known to have a special risk of depression, which doesn't occur just as a reaction to the news or continuing stress of having a serious medical problem.

Several lines of evidence could bear on a causal relationship between a medical condition and mood symptoms. A connection may exist if the mood disorder is more severe than the general medical symptoms seem to warrant or than the psychological impact would be on most people. However, such a connection would not be presumed if the mood symptoms begin before the patient learns of the general medical condition. Similar mood symptoms developing upon the disclosure of a different medical problem would argue against a diagnosis of either bipolar or depressive disorder due to another medical condition. By contrast, arguing for a connection would be clinical features different from those typical of a primary mood disorder (such as atypical age of onset). None of these conditions obtains in the case of Lisa Voorhees.

A known pathological mechanism that can explain the development of the mood symptoms in physiological terms obviously argues strongly in favor of a causal relationship. Multiple sclerosis, affecting many areas of the brain, satisfies this criterion. A high percentage of patients with multiple sclerosis have reported mood swings. Periods of euphoria have also been reported in these patients; anxiety may be more common still.

Many other medical conditions can cause depression. Endocrine disorders are important causes: Hypothyroidism and hypoadrenocorticalism are associated with depressive symptoms, whereas hyperthyroidism and hyperadrenocorticalism are linked with manic or hypomanic symptoms. Infectious diseases can cause depressive symptoms (many otherwise normal people have noted lassitude and low mood when enduring a bout of the flu; Lyme disease has received a lot of attention for years). Space-occupying lesions of the brain (tumors and abscesses) have also been associated with depressive symptoms, as have vitamin deficiencies. Finally, about one-third of patients with Alzheimer's disease, Huntington's disease, or stroke may develop serious depressive symptoms.

The second major criterion for a mood disorder due to another medical condition is that the mood symptoms must not occur only during a delirium. Delirious patients can have difficulties with memory, concentration, lack of interest, episodes of tearfulness, and frank depression that closely resemble major depressive disorder. Lisa presents no evidence to suggested delirium.

As to the specifier, we could choose between *with manic features* and *with mixed features* (see Essential Features, above). At different times, Lisa has both extremes of mood; neither predominates, so I'd go with . . . well, see below, along with a GAF score of 70. The code and name of the general medical condition would be included, as follows, with the name of the medical condition:

G35   Multiple sclerosis
F06.34   Bipolar disorder due to multiple sclerosis, with mixed features

Modifiers of Mood Diagnoses

Table 3.3 (p. 167) shows at a glance when and how to apply each of the modifiers of mood disorders covered below.

Severity and Remission

Severity Codes

No mood episode—major depressive, manic, or hypomanic—is codable by itself (sorry, I *know* you've heard this before). Instead, we use each as the basis for other diagnoses. However, they do have severity codes attached to them, and the same approach to severity coding is used for major depressive and manic episodes. Use these codes for the current or most recent major depressive episode in major depressive, bipolar I, or bipolar II disorders, or the current or most recent manic episode in the two bipolar disorders. (Hypomanic episode is by definition relatively mild, so it gets no severity specifier.)

The basic severity codes for manic and major depressive episodes are these:

Mild. Symptoms barely fulfill the criteria. For major depressive episode, they result in only minor distress or interference with the patient's ability to work, study, or socialize.

Moderate. Intermediate between mild and severe. For manic episode, there is a marked increase in activity level or impaired judgment.

Severe. There are several symptoms more than the minimum for diagnosis, and they markedly interfere with patient's work, social, or personal functioning. For mania, nearly continual supervision is needed to prevent bodily harm to others or self.

Remission Codes

Most patients with bipolar disorders recover completely between episodes (and most of them will have subsequent episodes). Still, up to a third of patients with bipolar I disorder do not recover completely. The figures for patients with major depressive disorder are not quite so grim. Following are two specifiers for current status of either of these disorders, as well as bipolar II disorder and persistent depressive disorder.

> **In partial remission.** A patient who previously met full criteria and now either (1) has fewer than the required number of symptoms or (2) has had no symptoms at all, but for under 2 months.

> **In full remission.** For at least 2 months, the patient has had no important symptoms of the mood episode.

Specifiers That Describe the Most Recent Mood Episode

The episode specifiers describe features of the patient's current or most recent episode of illness. No additional code number is assigned for these features; you just write out the verbiage. Again, Table 3.3 (p. 167) shows when you can use each of the following special qualifiers.

With Anxious Distress

Someone with bipolar I, bipolar II, cyclothymic, major depressive, or persistent depressive disorder may experience symptoms of high anxiety. Such a patient may have a greater than average potential for suicide and for chronicity of illness.

Essential Features of **With Anxious Distress**

During a major depressive/manic/hypomanic episode or persistent depressive disorder or cyclothymic disorder, the patient feels notably edgy or tense, and may be extra restless. Typically, there is difficulty focusing attention because of worries—"I'm afraid something terrible could happen," or "I could lose control and . . . [fill in the awful consequence]."

Coding Notes

Specify severity: **mild** (2 symptoms of anxious distress), **moderate** (3 symptoms), **moderate–severe** (4–5 symptoms), **severe** (4–5 symptoms plus physical agitation)
    See Table 3.3 for application (p. 167).

There's something kind of funny here. We've been given a mood specifier that has its own severity scale, derived (as are manic and major depressive episodes) by counting symptoms. DSM-5-TR notes that high anxiety may indicate poor outcome: suicide risk, nonresponse to treatment, long duration of illness, so this is important stuff. Still, if there's any other place in DSM-5-TR where it's possible to have two separate severity ratings in the same diagnosis, I don't recall it. (Other specifiers have several symptoms to count; for example, why don't we also rate severity of *with melancholic features?*) Furthermore, it is at least theoretically possible a patient could have mild depression with severe anxious distress. Of course, you can rate each part independently, but it could be confusing, and it sounds a little silly. My approach would be to focus on the severity of the mood episode. The specifier will probably get along just fine on its own.

With Atypical Features

Not all seriously depressed patients have the classic vegetative symptoms typical of melancholia (see below). Patients who have atypical features seem almost the reverse: Instead of sleeping and eating too little, they sleep and eat too much. This pattern is especially common among younger (teenage and college-age) patients. Indeed, it is common enough that it might better be called *nonclassic depression.*

Two reasons make it important to specify *with atypical features.* First, because such patients' symptoms often include anxiety and sensitivity to rejection, they risk being mislabeled as having an anxiety disorder or a personality disorder. Second, they may respond differently to treatment than do patients with melancholic features. Patients with atypical features may respond to specific antidepressants (monoamine oxidase inhibitors) and may also show a favorable response to bright light therapy for seasonal (winter) depression.

Iris McMaster's bipolar II disorder includes atypical features (p. 136).

Essential Features of **With Atypical Features**

A patient experiencing a major depressive episode (or persistent depressive disorder) feels better when something good happens ("mood reactivity," which obtains whether the patient is depressed or well). The patient also has other atypical symptoms: an increase in appetite or weight (the classic depressed patient reports a decrease), excessive sleeping (as opposed to insomnia), a feeling of being sluggish or paralyzed, and long-existing (not just when depressed) sensitivity to rejection.

The Fine Print

The *with atypical features* specifier cannot be used along with these specifiers: *with melancholia* or *with catatonic features.* See Table 3.3 (p. 167) for application.

With Catatonia

This specifier, also mentioned in Chapter 2 in association with the psychotic disorders, can also be used when catatonic features are present during a major portion of major depressive or manic (but not hypomanic) mood episodes. You can find the definitions of the various terms in the page 100 sidebar. When you use this specifier, you must add a line of extra code after listing and coding the other mental disorder:

F06.1   Catatonia associated with [state the mental disorder]

I've given examples in the histories of Edward Clapham (p. 101) and Marion Wright (p. 105), though neither had a primary mood disorder.

With Melancholic Features

This specifier refers to a negative view of the world and the classical "vegetative" symptoms of severe depression. Patients with melancholic features awaken too early in the morning, feeling worse than they do later in the day. They also have reduced appetite and may lose weight. They take little pleasure in their usual activities (including sex) and are not cheered by the presence of people whose company they normally enjoy. This loss of pleasure is not merely relative, but total or nearly so.

Melancholic features are especially common among patients who first develop severe depression in midlife. This condition was once called *involutional melancholia*, from the observation that it seemed to occur in middle to old age (life's so-called involutional period). However, it is now recognized that melancholic features can affect people of any age; they are especially likely to occur during a psychotic depression. Depression with melancholia typically responds well to somatic treatments such as antidepressant medication and ECT.

Again, see Table 3.3 (p. 167) for details of when to apply this specifier. Brian Murphy (p. 118) is an example of such a patient; Noah Sanders (p. 141) is another.

Essential Features of **With Melancholic Features**

In the depths of a major depressive episode, the patient cannot find pleasure in accustomed activities or feels no better if something good happens (OK, could be both). Such a patient also experiences several of these: a mood that is deeply despondent and hopeless; diurnal variation of mood (more depressed in the morning); terminal insomnia (awakening at least 2 hours early); change in psychomotor activity (sometimes agitated, more often slowed down); marked loss of appetite or weight; and guilt feelings that are unwarranted or extreme. This form of depression is extremely severe and can border on psychosis. Indeed, it is more common among patients who also have psychotic features.

> **Coding Notes**
>
> You can apply this specifier to a major depressive episode wherever it occurs: major depressive disorder (single episode or recurrent), bipolar I or II disorder, or persistent depressive disorder. See Table 3.3 (p. 167).

With Mixed Features

In 1921, Emil Kraepelin described mixed forms of mania and depression. DSM-IV and its predecessors included a mixed episode among the mood disorders. But that's been retired, and DSM-5-TR offers *with mixed features* as a specifier to use with patients who, within the same time frame, have symptoms of depression *and* mania (or hypomania). The features of the two opposite poles occur more or less at the same time, though some patients experience the gradual introduction (then fading away) of, say, depression within a manic episode.

However, researchers are only just ascertaining the degree to which such a patient differs from someone with "pure" episodic mania or depression. Patients who have mixed features appear to have more total episodes and more depressive episodes, and they remain ill longer. They may tend to have more comorbid mental illness and greater suicide risk. Their work is more likely to be impaired. Patients with major depressive disorder who have mixed features are especially likely to develop a bipolar disorder in the future.

Despite this attention, we'll probably continue to use the *with mixed features* specifier less often than could be justified. Several studies suggest that a third or more of patients with a bipolar disorder have at least one episode with mixed symptoms; some reports suggest that mixed mood states are more frequent in women than in men.

You can apply this specifier to episodes of major depression, mania, and hypomania (see Table 3.3, p. 167). Because of the greater impairment and overall severity of mania symptoms, if you have a patient who meets full criteria for both mania and major depression, you should probably go with the diagnosis of bipolar I disorder with mixed features, rather than major depressive disorder with mixed features. Winona Fisk (p. 131) had bipolar I disorder with mixed features.

The criteria for with mixed features omit some of the mood symptoms found in manic and major depressive episodes. That's because they might conceivably belong on both lists, and hence not indicate a mixed presentation. These symptoms include certain problems with sleep, appetite/weight, irritability, agitation, and concentration. Note, by the way, that the patient must meet full criteria for major depressive, manic, or hypomanic episode.

The criteria are silent as to how long each day (or, actually, the majority of days) the mixed features must be present, and I don't know of any data that would help us understand this question better. Right now, even a few minutes a day, repeated day after day, would seem enough to earn this specifier. One day, additional research will help us understand whether that's a sensible time frame—or too short, or too long. Right now, that picture is decidedly, well, mixed.

Essential Features of **With Mixed Features**

Here, there are two ways to go.

On most days, a patient with a manic or hypomanic episode also has several noticeable symptoms of depression: depressed mood, low interest or pleasure in most activities, an activity level that is speeded up or slowed down, feeling tired, feeling worthless or guilty, repeated thoughts about death or suicide. (See Coding Note.)

Most days, a patient with a major depressive episode also has several noticeable symptoms of mania: heightened mood, grandiosity, increased talkativeness, flight of ideas (or racing thoughts), increased energy level, poor judgment (such as excessive spending, sexual adventures, imprudent financial speculations), reduced need for sleep.

In either case, other people can notice these symptoms, which are different from normal for the person.

Coding Note

The impairment and severity of full-blown mania suggest that patients who simultaneously meet full episode criteria for *both* manic and depressive episodes should be recorded as having manic episode, with mixed features.

With Peripartum Onset

Over half of all women have "baby blues" after giving birth: They may feel sad and anxious, cry, complain of poor attention, and have trouble sleeping. This lasts a week or two and is usually of little long-term consequence. But about 10% of new mothers have enough symptoms to be diagnosed as having a mood disorder; these patients often have a previous history of mental disorder. An episode of hypomania may be especially likely after childbirth. Recurrences are common. Only about 2 out of 1,000 new mothers actually become psychotic.

The *with peripartum onset* specifier has the briefest Essential Features in this book. Though Elisabeth Jacks had a manic episode after giving birth (p. 123), a major depressive episode would be much the more common response. *With peripartum onset* can apply to bipolar I and bipolar II disorders, to major depressive disorder, and to brief psychotic disorder (see Table 3.3, p. 167).

Essential Features of **With Peripartum Onset**

A new mother's mood disorder starts during pregnancy or within a month of delivery.

Coding Notes

See Table 3.3 (p. 167) for application.

With Psychotic Features

Irrespective of the severity rating, some patients with manic or major depressive episodes will have delusions or hallucinations. (Of course, most of these patients you will have rated as being severely ill, but it is at least theoretically possible that a patient could have just a few symptoms—including psychosis—that somehow haven't posed a huge inconvenience.) Around half of patients with bipolar I disorder will have psychotic symptoms; far fewer patients with major depressive disorder will be psychotic.

Psychotic symptoms may be mood-congruent or mood-incongruent. Specify, if possible:

> **With mood-congruent psychotic features.** The content of the patient's delusions or hallucinations is completely in accord with the typical themes of the relevant mood episode. For major depression, these include death, disease, guilt, delusions of nihilism (nothingness), personal inadequacy, or punishment that is deserved. For mania, they include exaggerated ideas of identity, knowledge, influence, self-worth, or relationship to God or someone else powerful or famous.

> **With mood-incongruent psychotic features.** The content of the patient's delusions or hallucinations is not in accord with the typical themes of the mood episode. For either mania and major depression, these might include delusions of persecution, control, thought broadcasting, and thought insertion.

Essential Features of **With Psychotic Features**

The patient has hallucinations or delusions in the course of a major depressive or manic episode.

Coding Notes

Specify, if possible:

> **With mood-congruent psychotic features.** The psychotic symptoms match what you'd expect from the basic manic or depressive mood (see above).
> **With mood-incongruent psychotic features.** They don't match.

Specifiers That Describe Episode Patterns

Two specifiers describe the frequency or timing of mood episodes. Their appropriate uses are summarized in Table 3.3 (p. 167), as are those for the other types of specifiers.

With Rapid Cycling

A patient who does *not* cycle rapidly will typically experience months (perhaps 3–9) of depression, followed by a somewhat shorter period of mania or hypomania. With advancing years, the entire cycle tends to speed up, but most patients have no more than one up-and-down cycle per year, even after five or more complete cycles.

Some patients, however, especially women, experience these mood swings much more rapidly: Within a few weeks they may go from mania to depression to mania again. Their symptoms meet full mood episode requirements—that's how they differ from cyclothymic disorder. Other than frequency, the individual episodes meet full criteria for major depressive, manic, or hypomanic episodes.

Recent research suggests that patients who cycle rapidly are more likely to originate from higher socioeconomic classes; in addition, a history of rapid cycling predicts that this pattern will continue in the future. Rapid cyclers may be more difficult than other patients to manage with standard maintenance regimens, and they may have a poorer overall prognosis. *With rapid cycling* can apply to bipolar I and bipolar II disorders.

Essential Features of **With Rapid Cycling**

A bipolar patient has four or more episodes per year of major depression, mania, or hypomania.

Coding Notes

To count as a separate episode, an episode must be marked by remission (part or full) for 2+ months or by a change in polarity (such as from manic or hypomanic to major depressive episode). Episodes precipitated by medical illness or substance use don't count.

With Seasonal Pattern

Here is yet another mood disorder specifier that has only been recognized in the last few decades. In the usual pattern, depressive symptoms (these are often also atypical) appear during fall or winter months and remit in the spring and summer. Patients with winter depression may report other difficulties, such as pain disorder symptoms or a craving for carbohydrates, during their depressed phase. Winter depressions occur more commonly in polar climates, especially in the far North, and younger people may be more susceptible. *With seasonal pattern* can apply to bipolar I and bipolar II disorders and to major depressive disorder, recurrent type. There may also be seasonality to manic symptoms, although this is far less well established. (Bipolar I patients may experience the seasonal pattern with one type of episode, not with the other.)

Sal Camozzi's (p. 310) bipolar II disorder included a seasonal pattern.

Essential Features of **With Seasonal Pattern**

The patient's mood episodes repeatedly begin (and end) at about the same times of year. For at least the past 2 years, *only* seasonal episodes have occurred. Lifelong, seasonal episodes markedly outnumber nonseasonal ones.

The Fine Print

Disregard examples where there is a clear external cause, such as a worker who is laid off every summer.

Putting It All Together: Coding and Labeling the Mood Disorders

Coding and labeling the mood disorders, especially major depressive disorder and bipolar I disorder, have always been complex undertakings—and DSM-5-TR and ICD-10 have further complicated them. (And wait 'til you clap eyes on ICD-11!) Table 3.2 lays out the possible codes for bipolar I and major depressive disorders. A footnote to this table gives examples of how to label presentations of these disorders.

In addition to the three bipolar types listed in Table 3.2, there is also the possibility of bipolar I, unspecified type. That's mainly intended for the folks who work on coding when we neglect to indicate the polarity of the most recent episode. We clinicians should ordinarily have little occasion to use this code. Because the episode type is unknown, no episode specifiers can apply.

Table 3.3 (p. 167) summarizes all the descriptors and specifiers that can apply to mood disorders and indicates with which disorders each modifier can be used.

Other Specified and Unspecified Mood Disorders

F31.89 Other Specified Bipolar and Related Disorder

Use other specified bipolar and related disorder when you want to write down the specific reason you cannot give your patient a more definite bipolar diagnosis. To prevent

TABLE 3.2. Coding for Bipolar I and Major Depressive Disorders

Severity	Bipolar I, current or most recent episode			Major depressive, current or most recent episode	
	Manic[a]	Hypomanic	Depressed[b]	Single	Recurrent
Mild	F31.11	F31.0 (no severity, no psychotic symptoms for hypomanic episodes)	F31.31	F32.0	F33.0
Moderate	F31.12		F31.32	F32.1	F33.1
Severe	F31.13		F31.4	F32.2	F33.2
With psychotic features[c]	F31.2	—	F31.5	F32.3	F33.3
In partial remission[d]	F31.73	F31.71	F31.75	F32.4	F33.41
In full remission[e]	F31.74	F31.72	F31.76	F32.5	F33.42
Unspecified	F31.9	F31.9	F31.9	F32.9	F33.9

Note. The order is name → episode type → severity/psychotic/remission → other specifiers. And here are two examples of how you put it together: (1) bipolar I disorder, manic, severe with mood-congruent psychotic features, with peripartum onset, with mixed features; (2) major depressive disorder, recurrent, in partial remission, with seasonal pattern. Severity for mood episodes is judged on number and severity of symptoms and degree of impaired functioning.

[a]Manic episode: *mild* = minimum (3 or slightly more) manic symptoms that are distressing but interfere minimally with functionality; *moderate* = markedly increased activity or impaired judgment; *severe* = nearly constant supervision needed to safeguard patient or others.

[b]Major depressive episode: *mild* = minimum symptoms with manageable distress and impairment; *moderate* = intermediate symptoms, distress, and impairment; *severe* = markedly more symptoms than the minimum required, distress is serious and unmanageable, and there is much interference with functioning.

[c]If psychotic features are present, use these code numbers regardless of severity (it will almost always be severe, anyway). Record psychotic features as mood-congruent or mood-incongruent (p. 163).

[d]Partial remission. Symptoms are still present, but no longer meet criteria.

[e]Full remission. For 2 months or more, the patient has been essentially free of symptoms.

overuse and "medicalization" of the typical ebb and flow of mood, the patient must have symptoms that don't qualify for a more specific bipolar disorder diagnosis *and* that cause distress or interfere with normal functioning. DSM-5-TR gives several examples:

Short-duration hypomanic episodes (2–3 days) and major depressive episodes. Such a patient will have had at least one fully qualified major depressive episode, plus at least one episode of hypomania too brief (2–3 days) to justify a diagnosis of bipolar II disorder. Because the depression and hypomania don't occur together, a *with mixed features* designation wouldn't be appropriate.

Hypomanic episodes with insufficient symptoms and major depressive episodes. Such a patient will have had least one major depressive episode but no actual manic or hypomanic episodes, though there will have been at least one episode of *subthreshold hypomania*. That is, the high phase is long enough (4 days or more) but is a symptom or two shy of the number required for a hypomanic episode (elevated mood plus one or two of the other symptoms of a hypomanic episode, or irritable mood plus two or three of the other symptoms of hypomania). The hypomanic

TABLE 3.3. Descriptors and Specifiers That Can Apply to Mood Disorders

Disorder	Severity (p. 157)	Remission (p. 158)	With mixed features (p. 161)	With anxious distress (p. 158)	With catatonia[a] (p. 160)	With atypical features (p. 159)	With melancholic features (p. 160)	With peripartum onset (p. 162)	With psychotic features (p. 163)	With rapid cycling (p. 164)	With seasonal pattern (p. 164)
Major depression											
Single episode	X		X	X	X	X	X	X	X		
Recurrent	X		X	X	X	X	X	X	X		X
Bipolar I											
Most recent manic	X	X	X	X	X			X	X	X	X
Most recent depressed	X	X	X	X	X	X	X	X	X	X	X
Most recent hypomanic		X	X	X				X		X	X
Most recent unspecified											
Bipolar II											
Most recent hypomanic		X	X	X				X		X	X
Most recent depressed	X	X	X	X	X	X	X	X	X	X	X
Cyclothymia				X		X					
Persistent depressive[b]	X	X	X	X							

Note. This table can help you to choose the sometimes lengthy string of names, codes, and modifiers for the mood disorders. Start reading from left to right in the table, putting in any modifiers that apply in the order you come to them.

[a]The catatonia specifier requires its own line of code and description (p. 160).
[b]Also with intermittent major depressive episodes, {with}{without} current episode; with pure dysthymic syndrome; with persistent major depressive episode (p. 139).

and major depressive symptoms don't overlap, so you can't call it major depressive episode with mixed features.

Hypomanic episode without prior major depressive episode. Here you'd classify (no surprise) someone with an episode of hypomania who hasn't ever fully met criteria for a major depressive episode or a manic episode.

Short-duration cyclothymia. In a period less than 2 years (less than 1 year for a child or adolescent), such a patient will have had multiple episodes of both hypomanic symptoms and depressive symptoms, all of which will have been either too brief or have too few symptoms to qualify for a major depressive or hypomanic episode. Of course, there will be no manias and no symptoms of psychosis. Patients with short-duration cyclothymia will have symptoms for most days and will have no symptom-free periods longer than 2 months.

Manic episode superimposed on schizophrenia (or another psychotic disorder). Use this when the patient has a manic episode and a psychotic disorder that lacks defined mood episodes.

Note that DSM-5-TR cautions us not to use bare-bones "other specified bipolar disorder" or "other specified depressive disorder" as the actual diagnosis. Rather, we are also supposed to state, in full, one of the (often cumbersome) titles given in the bipolar list just above and the depressive list below. One thing we can rely on: Regardless of which of the several discrete terms we choose, there is just one code number for bipolar disorders, one for depressive.

F32.89 Other Specified Depressive Disorder

Use other specified depressive disorder in the same way as described above for other specified bipolar and related disorder. DSM-5-TR provides the following examples of other specified depressive disorder:

Recurrent brief depression. Every month for 12+ months, lasting from 2 to 13 days at a time, these patients have low mood plus at least four other symptoms of depression that aren't associated with menstruation. The patients have never fulfilled criteria for another mood disorder, and they've not been psychotic.

Short-duration depressive episode. These patients would meet criteria for major depressive episode except for duration—their episodes last 4–13 days. Here's the full run-down: depressed mood; at least four other major depressive symptoms; clinically significant distress or impairment; has never met criteria for other mood disorders; not currently psychotic; and doesn't meet criteria for other conditions.

Depressive episode with insufficient symptoms. These patients would meet criteria (duration, distress) for major depression, except that they have too few symptoms. They don't have another psychotic or mood disorder. I've used just this descriptor for Enoch Dimond in Chapter 11 (p. 343).

Major depressive episode superimposed on schizophrenia (or another psychotic disorder). Use this when the patient has a major depressive episode and a psychotic disorder that lacks defined mood episodes. However, oftentimes when a psychotic patient becomes depressed, the depressive symptoms can be regarded as features associated with the principal diagnosis—no additional coding required.

F31.9 Unspecified Bipolar and Related Disorder

And here you'd include patients for whom you don't care to indicate the reason you aren't diagnosing a well-defined bipolar condition.

F32.A Unspecified Depressive Disorder

As for unspecified bipolar and related disorder, when you don't care to indicate the reason for a well-defined diagnosis, you can use the unspecified depressive disorder category.

F06.30 Mood Disorder Due to Known Physiological Condition, Unspecified

OK, it's not in DSM-5-TR. But ICD-10 claims it for its own.

F39 Unspecified Mood Disorder

DSM-5-TR has finally fixed a problem introduced by DSM-5: the lack of a parking spot for a patient who has a mood disorder, but you don't (yet) even know whether it will turn out to be bipolar or depressive. Unspecified mood disorder resurrects the concept held in mood disorder not otherwise specified, from DSM-IV. It will surely be received gratefully by clinicians who have been forced into unwise choices by the chapter structure of DSM-5.

CHAPTER 4

Anxiety Disorders

Quick Guide to the Anxiety Disorders

One or more of the following conditions may be diagnosed in patients who present with prominent anxiety symptoms; a single patient may have more than one anxiety disorder.

Primary Anxiety Disorders

Panic disorder. These patients experience repeated panic attacks—brief episodes of intense dread accompanied by a variety of physical and other symptoms, together with other related mental and behavioral changes and worry about having additional attacks (p. 172).

Agoraphobia. These people fear situations or places, such as entering a store, where they might have trouble obtaining help if they became anxious (p. 178).

Specific phobia. These patients fear specific objects or situations. Examples include animals, storms, heights, blood, airplanes, being closed in, or any situation that may lead to vomiting, choking, or developing an illness (p. 181).

Social anxiety disorder. These patients imagine themselves embarrassed when they speak, write, or eat in public or use a public urinal (p. 184).

Selective mutism. A child chooses not to talk, except when alone or with select intimates (p. 186).

Generalized anxiety disorder. Although they experience no episodes of acute panic, these patients feel tense or anxious much of the time and worry about many different issues (p. 190).

Separation anxiety disorder. The individual becomes anxious when separated from a parent or other attachment figure (p. 187).

Anxiety disorder due to another medical condition. Panic attacks and generalized anxiety symptoms can be caused by numerous medical conditions (p. 195).

Substance/medication-induced anxiety disorder. Use of a substance or medication has caused panic attacks or other anxiety symptoms (p. 192).

Other specified, or unspecified, anxiety disorder. Use these categories for disorders with prominent anxiety symptoms that don't fit neatly into any of the groups above (p. 197).

Other Causes of Anxiety and Related Symptoms

Obsessive–compulsive disorder. These patients are bothered by repeated thoughts or behaviors that can appear senseless, even to them (p. 199).

Posttraumatic stress disorder. A severely traumatic event, such as combat or a natural disaster, is relived over and over with accompanying anxiety (p. 218).

Acute stress disorder. This condition is much like posttraumatic stress disorder, except that it begins during or immediately after the stressful event and lasts a month or less (p. 223).

Avoidant personality disorder. These timid people are so easily wounded by criticism that they hesitate to become involved with others (p. 569).

With anxious distress specifier for major depressive disorder. Some patients with major depressive disorder have much accompanying tension and anxiety (p. 158).

Somatic symptom disorder and **illness anxiety disorder.** Panic and other anxiety symptoms are often part of various somatic symptom disorders (pp. 254 and 263).

Introduction

The conditions discussed in this chapter are characterized by anxiety, fear, and the behaviors people use to combat them. Panic disorder, the various phobias, and generalized anxiety disorder are collectively among the most frequently encountered of all mental disorders listed in DSM-5-TR. Yet, in discussing them, we must also keep in mind three other facts about anxiety.

The first of these is that a certain amount of anxiety isn't just normal, but is adaptive and perhaps vital for our well-being and functioning. For example, when we are about to take an examination or speak in public (or write a book), the fear of failure spurs us on to adequate, perhaps extraordinary, preparation. Similarly, normal fear lies behind our healthy regard for excessive debt, violent criminals, and poison oak.

Anxiety is also a symptom—one that's encountered in many mental disorders. Because it is so dramatic, we sometimes focus our attention on the anxiety to the exclusion of historical data and other symptoms (depression, substance use, and problems with memory, to name just a few) that are crucial to diagnosis. I've interviewed countless patients whose anxiety symptoms have masked mood, somatic symptom, or other disorders—conditions that are often not only highly treatable when they are recognized, but sometimes deadly when they are not. Indeed, anxious people are especially at risk for suicidal behavior; moving from suicidal thoughts to attempts may be more likely in a person who has panic disorder, specific phobia, or generalized anxiety disorder.

The third issue I want to emphasize is that anxiety symptoms can sometimes indicate the presence of a substance use problem, another medical condition, or even a different mental disorder altogether (such as a mood, somatic symptom, or cognitive disorder). These conditions should be considered for any patient who presents with anxiety or avoidance behavior.

Once again, I've eschewed DSM-5-TR's organization, which seems to rely on the typical age of onset (most anxiety disorders begin when the patient is relatively young). Rather, I've started with panic attacks, because they are pervasive throughout the anxiety (and many other) disorders.

Panic Attack

Someone in the throes of a panic attack feels foreboding—a sense of disaster that is typically accompanied by cardiac symptoms (such as irregular or rapid heartbeat) and trouble breathing (shortness of breath, chest pain). The attack begins abruptly and builds rapidly to a peak; the whole, miserable experience usually lasts less than half an hour.

Here are some important facts about panic attacks:

- They are common (perhaps 30% of all adults have experienced at least one). In a 12-month period, over 10% of Americans will have one (though they are far less common among Europeans).
- Women are more often affected than men.
- DSM-5-TR notes that smoking may be a risk factor.
- They can occur as isolated experiences in most adults; then, there is no diagnosis at all.
- Panic attacks may occur within a broad spectrum of frequency, from just a few episodes in the lifetime of some individuals to many times per week in others. Some people even awaken at night with *nocturnal* attacks, which may indicate a more severe form of panic disorder.
- Untreated, they can be severely debilitating. Many patients change their behavior in reaction to the fear that the attacks mean they are psychotic or physically ill.
- Treatment is sometimes easy, perhaps just by providing a little reassurance or a paper bag to breathe into.

- Sometimes panic attacks mask other illnesses that range from mood disorders to heart attacks.

- Some panic attacks are triggered by specific situations, such as crossing a bridge or roaming a crowded supermarket. Such attacks are said to be *cued* or *situationally bound*. Others have no relationship to a specific stimulus but arise spontaneously, as in panic disorder. These are termed unexpected or *uncued*. A third type, *situationally predisposed* attacks, consists of attacks in which the patient often (but not always) becomes panic-stricken when confronted by the stimulus.

- The person can be calm or anxious when the panic attack begins.

- By themselves, panic attacks are not codable. I've described them here so they can be identified and applied as a specifier to whatever disorder may be appropriate. Of course, they always occur in panic disorder, but then you don't have to specify them—they go with the territory.

Pathological panic attacks usually begin in a person's 20s. Panic attacks may occur without other symptoms (when they may qualify for a diagnosis of panic disorder) or in connection with a variety of other disorders, which may include agoraphobia, social anxiety disorder, specific phobia, posttraumatic stress disorder (PTSD), mood disorders, and psychotic disorders. They can also feature in anxiety disorder due to another medical condition and in substance-induced anxiety disorder.

Essential Features of **Panic Attack**

A panic attack is fear (sometimes stark terror!) that begins suddenly and is accompanied by a variety of classic "fight-or-flight" symptoms, plus a few others—chest pain, chills (sometimes feeling too hot), choking, shortness of breath, rapid or irregular heartbeat, tingling or numbness, heavy sweating, nausea or abdominal discomfort, dizziness or feeling faint, and tremor. As a result, these people may feel "unreal" or afraid that they are losing their minds or dying. There must be at least four of the described physical and emotional sensations.

Coding Notes

Panic attack is not a codable disorder. It provides the basic information for panic disorder and it can be attached as a specifier to other diagnoses. These include PTSD, all other anxiety disorders, and other mental disorders (including eating, mood, psychotic, personality, and substance use disorders). Panic attacks are even found in medical conditions affecting the heart, lungs, and gastrointestinal tract.

Shorty Rheinbold

Seated in the clinician's waiting room, Shorty Rheinbold should feel relaxed. The lighting is soft, the music soothing; the sofa on which he sits is comfortably upholstered. Angel fish swim lazily in their sparkling glass tank. But Shorty feels anything but calm. Perhaps it's the receptionist—he wonders whether she's competent to handle an emergency with his sort of problem. Barricaded behind her computer, she looks something like a badger.

For several minutes he has felt worse with every heartbeat. His heart is the key; when Shorty first sat down, he hadn't even noticed it, quietly ticking away inside his chest, just doing its job. But now, with no warning, it has begun to demand attention. At first, it only skips a beat or two, but soon it begins a ferocious assault on his rib cage. Every beat has become a painful, bruising thump that causes him to clutch at his chest. He tries to keep his hands under his jacket so as not to attract too much attention.

Then, right on schedule, the shortness of breath begins. It seems to arise from his left chest area, where his heart is doing all the damage. It claws its way up through his lungs and into his throat, gripping him around the neck so he can breathe only in the briefest of gasps.

The pounding heart and chest pain can mean only one thing—after 2 months of an attack every few days, Shorty gets the message. He is dying! Of course, the cardiologist he consulted last week claimed that his heart was sound as a brass bell, but this time he knows it's about to fail. He cannot fathom why he hasn't died before; with every attack, he's feared it more. Now it seems impossible that he could survive this one. Does he even want to? The thought nearly makes him retch.

Shorty leans forward so he can grip both his chest and his abdomen as unobtrusively as possible. But he can hardly hold anything at all: The familiar tingling and numbness has started up in his fingers, and he can sense the shaking of his hands as they try to contain the various miseries that have taken over his body.

He glances across the room to see whether Miss Badger has noticed. No help from that quarter: She is still pounding away at her keyboard, oblivious to his wretchedness. Perhaps all the patients behave this way? Perhaps—but suddenly, there *is* an observer. Shorty is watching himself! Some part of him has floated free to hang suspended, halfway up the wall. From this vantage point, he can look down and view with pity and scorn the quivering flesh that is, or had been, Shorty Rheinbold.

Now the Spirit Shorty can see how fiery red Shorty's face has become. Hot air has filled his head, which seems to expand with every gasp. He floats farther up the wall and the ceiling melts away; he soars out into the brilliant sunshine. He squeezes his eyes shut but cannot keep out the blinding light.

Depression is so often found in patients who complain of recurrent panic attacks that the association cannot be overemphasized. Some studies suggest that over half the patients with panic disorder also have major depressive disorder. Clearly, we must carefully evaluate for symptoms of a mood disorder everyone who presents with panic symptoms.

Evaluation of Shorty Rheinbold

Shorty has experienced a typical panic attack: It began suddenly, developed rapidly, and included a generous helping of the required symptoms. His shortness of breath (criterion A4) and heart palpitations (A1) are classic panic attack symptoms; he also had chest pain (A6), lightheadedness (A8), and numbness in his fingers (A10). Shorty's fear that he will die (A13) is typical of the concerns patients have during an attack. The sensation of watching himself (depersonalization—A11) is a less common symptom of panic. He needs only four of these symptoms to substantiate the fact of panic attack.

Shorty's panic attack is uncued, which means one that seems to happen spontaneously; he is unaware of any event, object, or thought that might have triggered it. Uncued attacks are typical of **panic disorder,** which can also involve a cued (or situationally bound) attack. The panic attacks that develop in **social anxiety disorder** and **specific phobia** are cued to the stimuli that repeatedly and predictably pull the trigger.

Panic attacks can occur in several **medical conditions.** One of these is acute myocardial infarction, the very condition many panic patients fear. Of course, whenever indicated, patients with symptoms like Shorty's should be evaluated for myocardial infarction and other medical disorders. These include low blood sugar, irregular heartbeat, mitral valve prolapse, temporal lobe epilepsy, and a rare adrenal gland tumor called a pheochromocytoma. Panic attacks also occur during intoxication with several **psychoactive substances,** including **amphetamines, marijuana,** and **caffeine.** (Note that in addition, some patients misuse alcohol or sedative drugs in an effort to reduce the severity of their panic attacks.)

There is no code number associated with panic attack. We'll get to Shorty's complete diagnosis later.

F41.0 Panic Disorder

Panic disorder is a common anxiety condition in which the patient experiences *unexpected* panic attacks (usually many, but always more than one) and worries about having another. Though the panic attacks are usually uncued, situationally predisposed attacks and cued/situationally bound attacks also can occur (see definitions above). A strong minority of patients will have nocturnal panic attacks as well as those that occur while awake; these patients may have a more severe form of the panic disorder. Perhaps half of patients with panic disorder also have symptoms of agoraphobia (p. 178).

Panic disorder typically begins during the patient's early 20s. It is one of the most common anxiety disorders, found in 2–3% of the general adult population. Children have panic attacks, but panic disorder is infrequent, rising gradually through the teen years. It is especially common among women. Frequency declines in older populations, a rare benefit of the aging process.

Essential Features of **Panic Disorder**

As a result of repeated surprise panic attacks (see the Essential Features on p. 173), the patient fears that they will happen again or tries to avert further attacks by taking inadvisable, often ineffective action, such as abandoning once-favored activities or avoiding places where attacks have occurred.

The Fine Print

Don't forget the D's: • Duration (1+ months) • Distress or disability (as above) • Differential diagnosis (**substance use** and **physical disorders, other anxiety disorders,** mood and psychotic disorders, **OCD, PTSD,** actual danger)

Shorty Rheinbold Again

Shorty opens his eyes to discover that he is lying on his back on the waiting room floor. Two people bend over him—the receptionist, and another person he doesn't recognize. He guesses this must be the mental health clinician he is supposed to see.

"I feel like you saved my life," Shorty says.

"Not really," the clinician replies. "You're just fine. Does this happen often?"

"Every 2 or 3 days now." Shorty warily sits up. After a moment or two, he lets them help him to his feet and into the interview room.

Just when his problem began wasn't quite clear at first. Shorty is 24 and had spent 4 years in the Coast Guard. Since his discharge, he'd knocked around a bit, and then moved in with his folks while he worked in construction. Six months ago, he got a job as cashier in a service station and repair shop.

He likes this gig just fine. He sits in a glassed-in booth all day making change, running credit cards through the scanner, selling snacks. The wages aren't exciting, but he doesn't have to pay rent. Even with eating out almost every evening, Shorty still has enough at the end of the week to take his girl out on Saturday nights. Neither one of them drinks or uses drugs, so dating doesn't set him too far back.

The problem began when Shorty had been working for a couple of months. The boss told him to go out on the wrecker with Bruce, one of the mechanics. They had stopped along the eastbound interstate to pick up an old Buick Skylark with a blown head gasket. For some reason, they had trouble getting it into the sling. Shorty was on the traffic side of the truck, trying to manipulate the hoist in response to Bruce's shouted directions. Suddenly, a caravan of tractor-trailer trucks roared past. The noise and the blast of wind caught Shorty off guard. He spun around into the side of the wrecker, fell, and rolled to a stop, inches from huge, screaming tires.

Now, with Shorty's color and heart rate returned to normal, he can tell the remainder of his story. He continues to go out on the wrecker, even though he feels near panic every time he does so. He'll only go when Bruce is along, and he carefully avoids the traffic side of the vehicles.

That isn't the worst of the problem—he could always quit and get another job. But lately, Shorty has been having these attacks at other times, when he least expects them. Now the attacks are triggered by nothing at all; they just happen, though not when he is at home or in his glass cage at work. When shopping last week, he had to abandon the cart full of groceries he was buying for his mother. He doesn't even want to go to the movies with his girlfriend. For the last few weeks he has suggested that they spend Saturday night at her place watching TV instead. She hasn't complained yet, but he thinks it's only a matter of time.

"I have just about enough strength to tough it out through the workday," Shorty says. "But I've got to get a handle on this thing. I'm too young to spend the rest of my life like a hermit in a cave."

Further Evaluation of Shorty Rheinbold

The fact that Shorty experiences panic attacks has already been established. They were originally associated with the specific situation of working around the wrecker. But for months now, they have occurred every few days, usually catching him unaware (panic disorder criterion A). Undeniably worried and concerned (B1), he has altered his activities with his girlfriend (B2). Although several medical conditions can cause panic attacks, a cardiologist recently pronounced Shorty medically fit. Substance-induced anxiety disorder (C) is also eliminated by the history: Shorty doesn't use drugs or alcohol. (But watch out for patients who medicate their panic attacks with drugs or alcohol.) With no other mental disorder more likely (D), his symptoms fully support a diagnosis of panic disorder.

But wait, as they say, there's more, for which we'll have to consider the symptoms of agoraphobia. Recently, Shorty has feared all sorts of other situations that involve being away from the safety of home—driving, shopping, even going to the movies (agoraphobia criterion A)—which nearly always provoke panic (C). As a result, he either avoids the situations or has to be accompanied by Bruce or by his girlfriend (D). As a result of his fears, Shorty's life space has already begun to contract. Without treatment, it seems only a matter of time before he will have to quit his job and remain at home (G). These symptoms are typical; we won't quibble about the exact duration because they are so severe (F). They'll fulfill the requirements for agoraphobia, assuming we can rule out other etiologies for his symptoms (H, I). Sure, we should inquire further to determine that he's driven by the fear that help would be unavailable or that escape would be difficult (B), but knowing Shorty, I'm pretty sure of the answer.

The diagnosis of specific phobia or social anxiety disorder would seem unlikely because the focus of Shorty's anxiety is not a single issue (such as enclosed places) or a social situation. Patients with somatic symptom disorder also complain of anxiety symptoms, but this is an unlikely diagnosis for a physically healthy man.

Although the vignette doesn't address this possibility, about half the time, major depressive disorder is comorbid with panic disorder. Often-dramatic anxiety symptoms may overshadow the more subtle depressive symptoms, so there is danger that a clinician could overlook them completely. Shorty's mood is anxious, neither depressed nor irritable. Nonetheless, in those cases where the criteria for both an anxiety and a mood disorder are fulfilled, both disorders should be listed. Other anxiety disorders can be comorbid in panic disorder patients; these include generalized anxiety disorder and specific phobia.

I'd give Shorty a GAF score of 61 and list his diagnosis as follows:

F41.0	Panic disorder
F40.00	Agoraphobia

It can be really hard to differentiate panic disorder and agoraphobia from other anxiety disorders that involve avoidance (especially specific phobia and social anxiety disorder). The final decision often comes down to clinical judgment, though the following sorts of information can help:

- How many panic attacks does the patient have, and what type are they (cued, uncued, situationally predisposed)? Uncued attacks suggest panic disorder; cued attacks suggest specific phobia or social anxiety disorder. But they can be inter-mixed.
- In how many situations do they occur? Limited situations suggest specific phobia or social anxiety disorder; attacks that occur in a variety of situations suggest panic disorder and agoraphobia.
- Does the patient awaken at night with panic attacks? This is more typical of panic disorder.
- What is the focus of the fear? If it is having a subsequent panic attack, panic disorder may be the correct diagnosis—unless the panic attacks occur only when the patient is, say, riding in an airplane, in which case you might correctly diagnose specific phobia, situational type.
- Does the patient constantly worry about having panic attacks, even when in no danger of facing a feared situation (such as riding in an elevator)? This would suggest panic disorder and agoraphobia.

F40.00 Agoraphobia

The *agora* was the marketplace to ancient Greeks. In contemporary usage, *agorapho-bia* refers to the fear some people have of being in any situation or place where escape seems difficult or embarrassing, or where help might be unavailable should anxiety symptoms occur. Open or public places such as theaters and crowded supermarkets qualify; so does any travel from home. People with agoraphobia either avoid the feared place or situation entirely, or, if they must confront it, require the presence of a companion or tough it out with intense anxiety. In any event, *agoraphobia* is a concept the Greeks didn't have a word for; its first recorded use was in 1873.

Agoraphobia usually involves such situations as being away from home, standing in a crowd, staying home alone, crossing a bridge, and traveling by bus, car, or train. Agoraphobia can develop rapidly, within just a few weeks, in the wake of a series of panic attacks, when fear of recurrent attacks causes the patient to avoid leaving home or participating in other activities. Some people develop agoraphobia without any preceding panic attacks.

In recent years, estimates of the prevalence of agoraphobia have risen to the neighborhood of 1–2%. As with panic disorder, women are more susceptible than men; the disorder usually begins in the teens or 20s, though some patients have their first symptoms after the age of 40. Often, panic attacks precede the onset of the agoraphobia. It is strongly heritable.

Essential Features of **Agoraphobia**

People with agoraphobia almost invariably experience inordinate anxiety or dread when they must face specific feared situations: riding a bus or airplane (or any other mass transit); shopping, attending a theatrical entertainment, or any activity that occurs indoors. For some, it's something as ordinary as walking in an open space (flea market, playground), being part of a crowd, or waiting in a queue. What they fear can be as simple as standing alone outside where they live. When you explore their thinking, these folks are afraid that, should they have panic symptoms (p. 172) or another medical emergency (a fall, sudden diarrhea), escape could be impossible or help unavailable. So they avoid these situations or brave them only when accompanied by a trusted friend; if all else fails, they endure them with lots of suffering.

The Fine Print

Symptoms of fear/avoidance obviously exceed the threat they face from any actual medical condition they might have—DSM-5-TR gives as examples inflammatory bowel disease and Parkinson's.

Don't duck the D's: • Duration (6+ months) • Distress or disability (distress, work/ educational, social, or personal impairment) • Differential diagnosis (other anxiety disorders, mood and psychotic disorders, **OCD, PTSD, social** and **separation anxiety disorders, situational phobias,** panic disorder, **body dysmorphic disorder**)

Lucy Gould

"I'd rather have her with me, if that's all right." Lucy Gould is responding to the clinician's suggestion that her mother wait outside the office. "By now, I don't have any secrets from her."

Since age 18, Lucy hasn't gone anywhere without her mother. In fact, in those 6 years she's hardly been anywhere at all. "There's no way I could go out by myself—it's like entering a war zone. If someone's not with me, I can barely stand even to go to doctor appointments and stuff like that. But I still feel awfully nervous."

By nervousness, Lucy doesn't mean actual panic attacks; she's never felt that she can't breathe or is about to die. What she experiences is a motor agitation so intense that it has caused her to flee from shopping malls, supermarkets, and movie theaters. Nor can she ride on public transportation; buses and trains both terrify her. She has the feeling, vague but always present, that something awful will happen there. Perhaps she will become so anxious that she will pass out or wet herself, with no one who can help her. She hasn't been alone in public since the week before her high school commencement. Then, she could climb the steps to receive her diploma because she was with her best friend, who knew what to do if she needed help.

Lucy has always been a timid, rather sensitive girl. The first week of kindergarten, she cried each time her mother left her by herself at school. But her father insisted that she "toughen up," and within a few weeks she had nearly forgotten her terror. She subsequently maintained a nearly perfect attendance record at school. Then, shortly after her 17th birthday, her father died of leukemia. Her terror of being away from home began within a few weeks of his funeral.

Only partly to make ends meet, her mother sold their house, and they moved into a condominium across the street from the high school. "It's the only way I got through my last year," Lucy explains.

For several years, Lucy has kept house while her mother assembles circuit boards at an electronics firm outside town. Lucy feels perfectly comfortable in that role, even though her mother is away for hours at a time. Her physical health is good; she has never used drugs or alcohol; and she has never had depression, suicidal ideas, delusions, or hallucinations. But a year ago Lucy developed insulin-dependent diabetes, which requires frequent trips to the doctor. She tried to take the bus by herself, but after several failures—once, in the middle of traffic, she forced open the rear door and sprinted for home—she has given up. Now her mother is applying for disability assistance so she can remain at home to provide the aid and attendance Lucy requires.

Evaluation of Lucy Gould

Because of her fears, which are inordinate and out of proportion to the actual danger (criterion E), Lucy avoids a variety of situations and places, including supermarkets, malls, buses, and trains (A). If she does go, she requires a companion (D). She can't state exactly what might happen—only that it would be awful and embarrassing (she might even lose bladder control), and that help might not be available (B). Although her symptoms only came to light when another problem (type 2 diabetes) forced her to leave the house, her agoraphobic fears are clearly not related to the diabetes (H). OK, you'll have to read between the lines of the vignette to verify criteria C (the situations almost always provoke anxiety) and G (the patient experiences clinically important distress or impairment).

Lucy's symptoms are too varied for specific phobia or social anxiety disorder. (Note also that in agoraphobia, the perceived danger comes from the environment; in social anxiety disorder, it lies in the relationship with other people.) Her problem isn't that she fears being left alone, as would be the case with separation anxiety disorder—although when she was 5, she clearly had had elements of that disorder. She hasn't had a major trauma, as would be the case in PTSD; the death of her father was traumatic, but her own symptoms don't focus on reliving this experience. There is no indication that she has OCD. And so (finally!) we can dispose of criterion I.

Agoraphobia can accompany a variety of diagnoses, the most important of which are mood disorders that involve major depressive episodes. However, Lucy denies having symptoms of depression, psychosis, and substance use. Although she has diabetes, it developed years after her agoraphobia symptoms became apparent. Besides, it's hard to imagine a physiological connection between agoraphobia and diabetes, and her anxiety symptoms are far more extensive than the realistic concerns you'd expect from the typical individual with diabetes. (You'd need to apply the same reasoning to any other medical condition an agoraphobic patient might have.)

Because Lucy has never experienced a discrete panic attack, she won't meet the criteria for panic disorder in addition to her agoraphobia. By the way, the fact that she is housebound nets her a low GAF score of 31.

F40.00	Agoraphobia
E10.9	Insulin-dependent diabetes mellitus

Specific Phobia

People with specific phobias have unwarranted fears of specific objects or situations. Those recognized best are phobias of animals, blood, heights, travel by airplane, being closed in, and thunderstorms. The anxiety produced by exposure to one of these stimuli may take the form of a panic attack or of a more generalized sensation of anxiety, but it is always directed at something specific. (However, these patients can also worry about what they might do—faint, panic, lose control—if they must confront whatever it is they are afraid of.) Generally, the closer they are to the feared stimulus and the more difficult it would be to escape, the worse they feel.

Patients usually have more than one specific phobia (the median is three). A person who is about to face one of these feared activities or objects will immediately begin to feel nervous or panicky—a condition known as *anticipatory anxiety.* The degree of discomfort is often mild, however, so most people do not seek professional help. When it causes a patient to avoid feared situations, anticipatory anxiety becomes a major inconvenience; it can even interfere with working. Patients with specific phobias involving blood, injury, or injection may experience what is called a *vasovagal response;* this means that reduced heart rate and blood pressure cause the patients to faint.

In the general population, specific phobia is one of the most frequently reported anxiety disorders. Perhaps 10% of U.S. adults have suffered to some degree from one of the specific phobias, though clinical significance is hard to judge.

Onset is usually in childhood or adolescence; animal phobias especially tend to begin early. Some begin after a traumatic event, such as being bitten by an animal. A situational fear (for example, being closed in or traveling by air) is more likely than other types of specific phobia to have a comorbid disorder such as depression and substance misuse, though comorbidity with a wide range of mental disorders is the rule. Females outnumber males perhaps 2:1.

Essential Features of **Specific Phobia**

A specific situation or thing habitually causes such immediate, inordinate (and unreasonable) dread or anxiety that the person avoids it or endures it with much anxiety.

The Fine Print

The D's: • Duration (6+ months) • Distress or disability (work/educational, social, or personal impairment) • Differential diagnosis (substance use and physical disorders, **agoraphobia, social anxiety disorder, panic disorder, separation anxiety disorder,** mood and psychotic disorders, anorexia nervosa, **OCD, PTSD**)

Coding Notes

Specify all types that apply with individual ICD-10 codes:

> **F40.218 Animal type** (snakes, spiders)
> **F40.228 Natural environment type** (thunderstorms, heights)
> **Blood–injection–injury type** (syringes, operations):
>> **F40.230 Blood**
>> **F40.231 Injections and transfusions**
>> **F40.232 Other medical care**
>> **F40.233 Injury**
> **F40.248 Situational type** (traveling by air, being closed in)
> **F40.298 Other type** (situations where the person could vomit or choke; for children, loud noises or people wearing costumes)

Esther Dugoni

A slightly built woman of nearly 70, Esther Dugoni is healthy and fit, though in the last year or two she has developed a tremor: She has early Parkinson's disease. For the several years since she retired from her job teaching horticulture in junior college, she has worked hard on her own garden. At the flower show a year ago, her rhododendrons won first prize.

But 10 days ago, her mother died, and she and her sister have been appointed co-executors. The estate is large; to probate the will and dispose of the house, she will have to make several trips to Detroit, over halfway across the country. That means flying, which is why she has sought help at the mental health clinic.

"I can't fly!" she tells the clinician. "I haven't flown anywhere in 20 years."

As a child, Esther never had an opportunity to fly. With five children of her own to care for on her husband's schoolteacher pay, she didn't travel much as an adult, either. She made a couple of short hops years ago, when two of her children were getting married "in different cities, of course." On one of those trips, her plane circled the field in Omaha for nearly an hour, trying to land between thunderstorms. The ride was wretchedly bumpy; the plane was full; and many of the passengers were airsick, including the men seated on either side of her. There was no one to help—the flight attendants remained strapped in their seats. She kept her eyes closed and breathed through her handkerchief to try to filter out the odors that filled the cabin.

They finally landed safely, but it was the last time Esther ever flew anywhere. "I don't even like to go to the airport to meet someone," she says. "Even that makes me feel short of breath and kind of sick to my stomach. Then I get this sort of dull pain in my chest, and I start to shake—I feel like I'm about to die, or something else awful will happen. It all seems so silly."

Esther really has no alternatives to flying. She can't remain in Detroit until all the business has been taken care of; it will take months. The train doesn't connect, and the bus is impossible. So of course, she's panicking.

Evaluation of Esther Dugoni

Esther's anxiety symptoms are cued by the prospect of airplane travel (criterion A); even going to the airport invariably produces anxiety (B), and she has avoided plane travel for years (C, E). She recognizes that this fear is unreasonable ("silly"), and it embarrasses her (D), but it's about to interfere with the conduct of her personal business (F).

Specific phobia is not usually associated with any general medical condition or substance-induced disorder. In response to delusions, patients with schizophrenia will sometimes avoid objects or situations (a telephone that is "bugged," food that is "poisoned"), but such patients lack the required insight that their fears are unfounded. Of course, specific phobias must be differentiated from fears associated with other disorders (such as agoraphobia, OCD, PTSD, social anxiety disorder—G). And Esther's clinician should ask about possible comorbid diagnoses. Pending that, and with a GAF score of 75, her diagnosis will be as given below. (Esther has only one phobia, a situational one; the median is three, each of which would be listed on a separate line with its own number.)

F40.248	Specific phobia, situational (fear of flying)
G20	Parkinson's disease
Z63.4	Uncomplicated bereavement

Fears involving animals of one sort or another are remarkably common. Children are especially susceptible to animal phobias, and many adults don't much care for spiders, snakes, or cockroaches. But a diagnosis of specific phobia, animal type, should not be made unless a patient is truly impaired by the symptoms. For example, you wouldn't diagnose a snake phobia in a prisoner serving a life sentence—under which circumstances confrontation with snakes and activity restriction as a result would be unlikely.

F40.10 Social Anxiety Disorder

Social anxiety disorder (SAD) is a fear of appearing clumsy, silly, or shameful. Patients dread social gaffes such as trembling when writing or being unable to perform competently when speaking or playing a musical instrument. Using a public urinal will cause anxiety for some men. Fear of blushing affects especially women, who may not be able to put into words what's so terrible about turning red. Fear of further eating in public is sometimes acquired after an episode of choking on food; it can occur any time from childhood to old age. Some patients fear (and avoid) multiple such public situations.

Many people, men and women, have noticeable physical symptoms with SAD: blushing, hoarseness, tremor, and perspiration. Such patients may have actual panic attacks. Children may express their anxiety by clinging, crying, freezing, shrinking back, throwing tantrums, or refusing to speak.

Studies of general populations report a lifetime occurrence of SAD of about 7%, though it's lower in Europe. Whatever the actual figure, these findings contradict previous impressions that SAD is rare—perhaps interviewers tend to overlook a common condition that patients silently endure. Women predominate in general population samples, though males and females are roughly equal in treatment settings.

Onset is typically in the early to middle teens. The symptoms of SAD overlap with those of avoidant personality disorder; the latter disorder is more severe, but both begin early, tend to last for years, and have some commonalities in family history. Indeed, SAD is reported to have a strong genetic basis.

Essential Features of Social Anxiety Disorder

Inordinate anxiety is attached to circumstances where others could closely observe the patient—public speaking or performing, eating or having a drink, writing, perhaps just speaking with another person. Because these activities almost always provoke disproportionate fear of embarrassment or social rejection, the patient avoids the situations or endures them with much anxiety.

The Fine Print

For children, the "others" who could closely observe the patient must include peers, not just adults.

The D's: • Duration (6+ months) • Distress or disability (work/educational, social, or personal impairment) • Differential diagnosis (**substance use** or **physical disorders,** mood and psychotic disorders, **panic disorder, body dysmorphic disorder, autism spectrum disorder,** anorexia nervosa, OCD, avoidant personality disorder, ordinary shyness, other anxiety disorders—especially agoraphobia)

Coding Notes

Specify if:

> **Performance only.** The patient fears public speaking or performing, but not other situations.

Valerie Tubbs

"It starts right here, and then it spreads like wildfire. I mean, like real fire!" Valerie Tubbs points to the right side of her neck, which she keeps carefully concealed with a blue silk scarf. "It" has been happening for almost 10 years, any time she is with people; it is worse if she's with a lot of people. Then she's sure everybody notices.

Although she has never tried, Valerie doesn't think that her reaction is something she can control. She just blushes whenever she thinks people are watching her. It started when she had to give a talk during a high school speech class. She had become confused about the difference between a polyp and a medusa, and one of the boys noticed that a red spot had appeared on her neck. "He said it looked like a bull's-eye," she says. To the general amusement of the class, she quickly flushed all over and had to sit down.

Since then, Valerie has tried to avoid the potential embarrassment of saying anything to more than a handful of people. She gave up her dream of becoming a fashion buyer for a department store because she couldn't tolerate the scrutiny the job would entail. Instead, she has spent the last 5 years dressing mannequins for the same store—behind closed curtains.

Valerie knows it's "stupid" to be so afraid. It isn't just that she turns red; she turns *beet*-red. "I can feel prickly little fingers of heat crawling out across my neck and up my cheek. My face feels like it's on fire, and my skin is being scraped with a rusty razor." Whenever she blushes, she doesn't feel exactly panicky. It's a sense of anxiety and restlessness that makes her wish her body belonged to someone else. "Even the thought of meeting new people makes me feel irritable and keyed up."

Evaluation of Valerie Tubbs

For years, Valerie has feared being embarrassed by the blushing that occurs whenever she speaks with other people (in one sentence, criteria A, B, C, and F). Though
insight isn't required for the diagnosis, her fear is excessive (E) and she knows it. Her
reluctance to speak publicly and her scarf help her avoid exposure to scrutiny (D). Her
anxiety also prevents her from working at the job she would prefer (G).

With no actual panic attacks, and in the absence of anxiety disorder due to another
medical condition and substance-induced anxiety disorder (H), determining her diagnosis comes down to the differential diagnosis of phobias (I). In the absence of a typical history, we can quickly dismiss specific phobia. People who have agoraphobia may
avoid dining out because they fear the embarrassment of having a panic attack in a
public restaurant. Then you would only diagnose SAD present prior to the onset of the
agoraphobia and unrelated to it. (Sometimes even clinicians who specialize in evaluating and treating the anxiety disorders can have trouble deciding between those two
diagnoses.) Patients with anorexia nervosa avoid eating, but the focus is on their weight,
not on the embarrassment that might result from gagging or leaving crumbs on their
lips.

It is important to differentiate SAD from the ordinary shyness that is so common
among children and other young people; this shows the value of insisting that symptoms must be present for at least half a year, required by DSM-5-TR for adults as well
as for children. Also keep in mind that many people worry about or feel uncomfortable
with social activities such as speaking in public (stage fright or microphone fright). They
should not receive this diagnosis unless in some important way it affects their work,
social, or personal functioning.

SAD is often associated with suicide attempts and mood disorders. Anyone with
SAD may be at risk for self-treatment with drugs or alcohol; Valerie's clinician should
ask carefully about these conditions. SAD has elements in common with avoidant personality disorder, which, often comorbid in these patients, may be a warranted diagnosis in a patient who is generally inhibited socially, is overly sensitive to criticism, and
feels inadequate. Other mental disorders you might sometimes need to rule out—not
at issue for Valerie—would include panic disorder, separation anxiety disorder, body
dysmorphic disorder, and autism spectrum disorder.

Valerie's fears involved far more than performances, so the performance specifier
won't apply. With a GAF score of 61, her diagnosis would be as follows:

F40.10   Social anxiety disorder

F94.0 Selective Mutism

Selective mutism denotes children who remain silent except when alone or with a small
group of intimates. The disorder typically begins during preschool years (ages 2–4),
after speech has developed. Such a child, who speaks appropriately at home among

family members but becomes relatively silent when among strangers, may not attract clinical attention until formal schooling begins. Although often shy, most such children have normal intelligence and hearing. When they do speak, they tend to use ordinary articulation, sentence structure, and vocabulary. The condition often improves spontaneously within weeks or months, though no one can predict which patient will improve.

Selective mutism is uncommon, with a prevalence of under 1 in 1,000. It usually begins by age 5 and probably affects girls and boys about equally. Family history is often positive for social anxiety disorder or selective mutism. Comorbid conditions include other anxiety disorders (especially separation anxiety disorder and social anxiety disorder). Patients with selective mutism tend not to have externalizing disorders such as oppositional defiant or conduct disorder.

Essential Features of **Selective Mutism**

Despite speaking normally at other times, the patient consistently does not speak in certain situations where it is expected, such as in class.

The Fine Print

The first month of a child's first year in school is often fraught with anxiety; exclude behaviors that occur during this time.

The D's: • Duration (1+ months after first month of school) • Distress or disability (social or work/academic impairment) • Differential diagnosis (unfamiliarity with the language to be used; a **communication disorder** such as **stuttering; psychotic disorders, autism spectrum disorder,** intellectual developmental disorder, social anxiety disorder)

F93.0 Separation Anxiety Disorder

For years, separation anxiety disorder (SepAD) was diagnosed in childhood—and stayed there. More recently, however, evidence has accumulated that the condition also affects adults. This can happen in two ways. Perhaps a third of children with SepAD continue to have symptoms of the disorder well into their adult years. However, some patients, perhaps precipitated by loss due to divorce or death of a loved one, develop symptoms de novo in their late teens or even later—sometimes even beginning in old age. SepAD is more common in females than in males, though boys may be more likely to be referred for treatment. Its prevalence in children is probably in the 2–4% range.

In children, SepAD may begin with a precipitant such as moving to a new home or school, a medical procedure or serious physical diagnosis, or the loss of an important friend or pet (or a parent). Symptoms often show up as school refusal, but younger children may even show reluctance at being left with a sitter or at day care. Children may enlist physical complaints, imagined or otherwise, as justification for remaining home with parents.

Adults, too, may fear that something horrible will happen to an important attachment figure—perhaps a spouse, or even a child. As a result, they are reluctant to leave home (or any other safe place); they may fear even sleeping alone, and they experience nightmares about separation. When apart from the principal attachment figure, they may need to telephone or otherwise touch base several times a day. Some may try to ensure safety by setting up a routine of closely shadowing the other person.

When the onset is early in childhood, this condition is likely to remit; with later onset, symptoms are more likely to continue into adulthood and to confer more severe disability (though the intensity may wax and wane). Children with SepAD tend to drift into subclinical forms or nonclinical status. Most adults and children with SepAD also have other disorders (especially mood, anxiety, and substance use disorders), though SepAD is often the condition present the longest.

Children with SepAD often have parents with an adult form of the same disorder. As with most anxiety disorders, there is a strong genetic component.

Essential Features of **Separation Anxiety Disorder**

Because they fear what might happen to a parent or someone else important in their lives, these patients resist being alone. They imagine that the parent will die or become ill or lost (or that *they* will); even the thought of separation can cause anxiety, nightmares, or perhaps vomiting spells, headaches, or other physical complaints. They are therefore reluctant to attend school, go out to work, or sleep away from home—or perhaps even in their own beds.

The Fine Print

The D's: • Duration (6+ months in adults, though extreme symptoms such as total school refusal could justify diagnosis after a shorter duration; 4+ weeks in children) • Distress or disability (work/educational [notably, school refusal], social, or personal impairment) • Differential diagnosis (mood disorders, other anxiety disorders [e.g., **agoraphobia, generalized anxiety disorder, psychotic disorders, autism spectrum disorder, illness anxiety disorder,** PTSD])

Nadine Mortimer

She is 24 years old, but Nadine Mortimer still lives at home. The only reason for her evaluation, she tells the clinician, is that her mother and stepfather have just signed on to join the Peace Corps; she, Nadine, will be left behind. "I just know I won't be able to stand it." She sobs into her Kleenex.

Being alone has frightened Nadine from the time she was very small. She thinks she can trace it back to her father's death: He was a mechanic who drove a racing car for fun—until the weekend he encountered a wall at the far turn of their hometown track. Her mother's response was strangely stoic. "I think I took on the job of grieving for both of us," Nadine comments. Within the year, her mother had remarried.

Her first day of first grade, Nadine had been so fearful that her mother remained in the classroom. "I was afraid something terrible would happen to her, too, and I wanted to be with her, for safety." After several weeks, Natalie could tolerate being left at school, but the following year, she threw up when Labor Day rolled around. After a few miserable weeks in second grade, she was withdrawn and home-schooled.

In 10th grade, she was reading and doing math at 12th-grade level. "But my socialization skills were near nil. I'd never even been to a sleepover at another girl's house," she says. So, her parents bribed her with a cell phone and the promise that she could call any time; with it, she could endure short absences from them. By the time Nadine started junior college—hardly farther away than her high school—she'd negotiated for smart phones with a "Find my phone" app. Now she could track her mother's whereabouts to within a few feet. With that, she reports, she could "roam comfortably, stores and whatnot, as long as I can check Mom's location whenever I want." Once, when her battery died, she suffered a panic attack.

Nonetheless, she still didn't graduate from junior college, and after a semester she just stayed home to feel close to her mother. "I know it seems weird," she tells the interviewer, "but I always imagine that someday she won't come home to me. Just like Daddy."

Evaluation of Nadine Mortimer

From the time she started school (criterion B), Nadine had clear symptoms of SepAD. She worried that harm might befall her mother, and she became severely distressed when they were separated; she'd vomited at the mere prospect of a new school year (A). As a result, she had almost no friends and had never slept away from home (C). There was no sign of other disorders to exclude (D).

Modified by her adult status, many of these same symptoms persist—panic symptoms when she can't keep close tabs on her mother, from whom she refuses to live apart. She even retains the same fear of harm befalling her mother should they ever separate. The prospect of her parents' leaving for a new career deeply troubles her. Even if Nadine hadn't had symptoms as a child, her adult disorder is troubling enough to qualify for the diagnosis of SepAD.

A significant problem remains in the differential diagnosis of SepAD: How does one distinguish it from agoraphobia? There is some overlap, but patients with SepAD fear being away from a parent or other significant person, whereas a person with agoraphobia fears places from which escape would be difficult or help unavailable. The symbolic testimony of her smart phone suggests that Nadine's anxiety is of the former type, not the latter. I would put her current GAF score at 45.

F93.0   Separation anxiety disorder

The DSM-IV criteria for SepAD employed several behaviors only appropriate to children; perhaps this explains why it wasn't recognized in adults earlier. Even now, panic symptoms may sometimes draw clinicians off the scent of adult SepAD.

F41.1 Generalized Anxiety Disorder

Generalized anxiety disorder (GAD) can be hard to diagnose. The symptoms are relatively unfocused; the nervousness is low-key and chronic; panic attacks are not required. It is, after all, just worry, and that's something that touches all of us. But there are differences. Ordinary worry is somehow less serious; we are able (well, most of the time) to put it aside and concentrate on other, more immediate issues. The worry of GAD often starts of its own accord, seemingly without cause. And GAD worry is at times hard to control. It carries with it a collection of physical symptoms that pile onto the sense of agitated restlessness in a cascade of misery.

Although some patients with GAD may be able to state what it is that makes them nervous, others cannot. GAD worry is typically about far more issues ("everything") than objective facts can justify. The disorder typically begins at about 30 years of age; many patients with GAD have been symptomatic for years without coming to the attention of a clinician. Perhaps this is because the degree of impairment in GAD is often not all that severe. Genetic factors play an important role in the development of GAD. It is found in up to 3% of the general adult population and 1% of adolescents (12-month prevalence), and, as with nearly every other anxiety disorder, females predominate.

Essential Features of Generalized Anxiety Disorder

Hard-to-control, excessive worrying about a variety of issues—health, family problems, money, school, work—results in physical and mental complaints: muscle tension, restlessness, becoming tired easily, irritability, poor concentration, and trouble with sleep.

The Fine Print

Three symptoms are required for adults, only one for children.

The D's: • Duration (on most days for 6+ months) • Distress or disability (work/educational, social, or personal impairment) • Differential diagnosis (**substance use** and **physical disorders,** mood disorders, **panic disorder, social anxiety disorder, somatic symptom disorder, anorexia nervosa, body dysmorphic disorder, illness anxiety disorder, separation anxiety disorder, schizophrenia, delusional disorder, OCD, PTSD,** realistic worries)

Bert Parmalee

Bert's been a worrywart for most of his adult life—at age 35, he sometimes still dreams that he is failing all his college electrical engineering courses. For the past year he has been the administrative assistant to the chief executive officer of a Fortune 500 company, where he had previously worked in product engineering. Now he feels that he is walking a tightrope.

"I took the job because it seemed a great way to move up the corporate ladder," he said, "but almost every day I have the feeling my foot's about to slip off the rung."

Each of his company's six ambitious vice-presidents sees Bert as a personal pipeline to the CEO. His boss is a hard-driving workaholic who constantly sparks ideas that he wants implemented yesterday. Several times he has told Bert that he is pleased with his performance; in fact, Bert's doing the best job of any administrative assistant he's ever had. But that doesn't seem to reassure Bert.

"I've felt uptight just about every day since I started this job," Bert says with a sigh. "My boss expects action and results. He has zero patience for thinking about how it should all fit together. Our vice-presidents all want to have their own way. Several of them hint pretty broadly that if I don't help them, they'll put in a bad word with the boss. I'm always looking over my shoulder."

Now Bert has trouble concentrating at work; at night, though exhausted, he has trouble getting to sleep. Once he does, he sleeps fitfully. He has become chronically irritable at home; he yells at his children for no reason. But he's never had a panic attack, and he doesn't think he's depressed. In fact, he still takes pleasure in his two favorite activities: Sunday afternoon football on TV and Saturday night lovemaking with his wife. Recently, she offered to take the kids to her mother's for a few weeks, to relieve some of the pressure. This has only resurrected some of his old insecurities—that he isn't good enough for her, that she might leave him for someone else.

Bert is carefully dressed, slightly overweight, and balding. He appears apprehensive, fidgeting just a bit; his speech is clear, coherent, relevant, and spontaneous. He denies having obsessions, compulsions, phobias, delusions, or hallucinations. On the MMSE, he scores a perfect 30. He says that his main problem—his only problem—is "this nagging uneasiness."

Valium makes him drowsy. He's tried meditating, but that seems only to help him focus on his problems. For a few weeks he has tried having a glass of wine before dinner, which both relaxes him and prompts worries about alcoholism. Once or twice he even went with his brother-in-law to an Alcoholics Anonymous meeting. "The only good that did is, now I've decided to try dreading one day at a time."

Evaluation of Bert Parmalee

Bert worries about multiple aspects of his life (his job, being an alcoholic, losing his wife); each of these worries seems excessive for the facts (criterion A). The excessiveness of his worries would differentiate them from the usual sort of anxiety that is not pathological. Despite repeated efforts (meditation, medication, reassurance), he has been unable to control these fears (B). In addition, he has at least four physical or mental symptoms (only three are required): trouble concentrating (C3), fatigue (C2), irritability (C4), and sleep disturbance (C6). He has been having difficulty nearly every day for longer than the required 6 months (A). And his symptoms cause him considerable distress, perhaps even more than is usual for patients with GAD (D).

One of the difficulties in diagnosing GAD is that so many other conditions must be excluded (E). A number of physical illnesses can cause anxiety symptoms; a complete workup of Bert's anxiety would have to consider these possibilities. From the information contained in the vignette, a substance-induced anxiety disorder would appear unlikely.

Anxiety symptoms can be found in nearly every category of mental disorder, including psychotic, mood (depressed or manic), eating, somatic symptom, and cognitive disorders. From Bert's history, none of these seem remotely likely (F). For example, we can eliminate an adjustment disorder with anxiety because Bert's symptoms meet the criteria for another mental disorder.

We need to make sure that Bert's worry and anxiety aren't focused solely on the features of another mental disorder, especially another anxiety disorder. For example, it shouldn't be "merely" worry about weight gain in anorexia nervosa, about contamination (OCD), separation from attachment figures (separation anxiety disorder), public embarrassment (social anxiety disorder), or having physical symptoms (somatic symptom disorder). Nevertheless, note that a patient can have GAD in the presence of another mental disorder—most often, mood and other anxiety disorders—provided the symptoms of GAD are serious enough to merit clinical intervention.

The only specifier possible for GAD is the optional *with panic attacks*. Bert's diagnosis, other than a GAF score of 70, would be an unvarnished:

F41.1   Generalized anxiety disorder

It is reasonable to ask this question: Does diagnosing GAD in a patient who has depression help with your evaluation? After all, the anxiety symptoms may disappear once the depression has been sufficiently treated. The value is that flagging the anxiety symptoms gives a more complete picture of the patient's pathology. And, it warns of the potential for suicide.

Substance/Medication-Induced Anxiety Disorder

When the symptoms of anxiety or panic can be attributed to the use of a chemical substance, make the diagnosis of substance/medication-induced anxiety disorder. It can occur during acute intoxication (or heavy use, as with caffeine) or during withdrawal (as with alcohol or sedatives), but the symptoms must be more severe than you'd expect for ordinary intoxication or withdrawal, and serious enough to warrant clinical attention.

Many substances can produce anxiety symptoms, but those most associated are marijuana, amphetamines, and caffeine. See Table 15.1 (p. 412) for a summary of the substances for which intoxication or withdrawal can be expected to create anxiety. If more than one substance is involved, you'd code each separately. Quite frankly, in the general population these disorders are probably rare.

Essential Features of **Substance/Medication-Induced Anxiety Disorder**

The use of some substance appears to have caused the patient to experience prominent and severe anxiety symptoms or panic attacks.

For tips on identifying substance-related causation, see sidebar, page 95.

The Fine Print

The D's: • Distress or disability (work/educational, social, or personal impairment) • Differential diagnosis (ordinary substance intoxication or withdrawal, **delirium,** physical disorders, mood disorders, other anxiety disorders)

Use this diagnosis instead of substance intoxication or withdrawal only when anxiety symptoms are predominant and require clinical care.

Coding Notes

Specify:

With onset during {intoxication}{withdrawal}. This gets tacked on at the end of your string of words.

With onset after medication use. You could alternatively use this if symptoms develop when medication is started, changed, or stopped.

For specific coding procedures, see Table 15.2 (p. 475).

Bonita Ramirez

Bonita Ramirez, a 19-year-old first-year college student, is accompanied to the emergency room by two friends. Alert, intelligent, and well informed, she cooperates fully in providing the intake information.

Bonita's parents both hold graduate degrees and are well established in their professions. They live in a well-to-do suburb of San Diego. Bonita is their oldest child and only daughter. Strictly reared in the Catholic faith, she wasn't allowed to date until a year ago. Until sorority rush week, the only alcohol she ever tasted was Communion wine. By her account and that of her companions, she had been happy, healthy, and vivacious when she arrived on campus a fortnight ago.

Two weeks has made a remarkable difference. Bonita now sits huddled on the examination table, feet drawn up and her arms wrapped around her knees. She trembles noticeably; although it is only September, she wears a sweater and complains of feeling cold. She keeps reaching for the emesis basin beside her, as though she might need it again.

Her voice quavers as she says that nothing like this has ever happened to her before. "I had some beer last week. It didn't bother me at all, except for the headache the next morning."

This evening, during a "big sister, little sister" party at the sorority Bonita has pledged, she drank some beer. That emboldened her to take a few hits from the marijuana joint they were passing around. The beer must have numbed her throat, because she found she could draw the smoke deep into her lungs and hold it, the way her friends showed her. For about 10 minutes afterward, Bonita hadn't noticed anything at all. Then her head began to feel tight, "as though my hair were a wig that didn't fit right." Suddenly, when she tried to take a deep breath, her chest "screamed in pain"; unable to breathe, she became instantly aware that she was about to die. She vomited, then she tried to run, but her rubbery legs refused to obey.

Her new sorority sisters hadn't had much experience with drug reactions, so they called to the fraternity house next door, and one of the fellows came over and tried to talk Bonita down. After an hour, she still felt the panicked certainty that she would die or go mad; her shortness of breath and nausea hadn't abated. That was when they decided to bring her to the emergency room.

At length she says, "They told me it would relax me and expand my consciousness. I just want to contract it again."

Evaluation of Bonita Ramirez

Bonita's history—she was healthy until the ingestion of a substance that is known to produce anxiety symptoms, especially in a naïve user—is a dead giveaway for the diagnosis (criteria A, B). Other drugs that commonly produce anxiety symptoms include amphetamines, which can also produce panic attack symptoms, and caffeine when used heavily. However, because anxiety symptoms can be encountered at some point during the use of most substances, you can code an anxiety disorder secondary to the use of nearly any of them, provided that the anxiety symptoms are worse than you would expect for ordinary substance withdrawal or intoxication. Because she required emergency evaluation and treatment, and because she had symptoms atypical of cannabis intoxication (nausea, shortness of breath, chest pain, feeling doomed to die), we would judge this to be the case for Bonita (E). Despite the proximity of the development of her symptoms to substance use (C), her clinician would want to be sure that she did not have another medical condition (or treatment with medication for a medical condition) that could provide an alternative explanation for her anxiety symptoms.

Although she arrived at the emergency room in a severe panic state, I would score Bonita's GAF as a relatively high 80, because her symptoms have caused her no actual disability (plenty of distress) and should be transient; other clinicians might disagree. She hasn't used cannabis before, so of course she has no use disorder; the code we'll use comes from the "none" row for cannabis in Table 15.2 (p. 475).

F12.980   Cannabis-induced anxiety disorder, with onset during intoxication

F06.4 Anxiety Disorder Due to Another Medical Condition

Many medical disorders can produce anxiety symptoms, which will often resemble those of panic disorder or generalized anxiety disorder. Occasionally, they may take the form of obsessions or compulsions. Most anxiety symptoms won't be caused by a medical disorder, but it is supremely important to identify those that are. The symptoms of an untreated medical disorder can evolve from anxiety to permanent disability or worse—consider the dangers of a growing brain tumor.

Essential Features of Anxiety Disorder Due to Another Medical Condition

Through physiological means, a medical condition appears to have caused an illness that features panic attacks or marked anxiety.

The Fine Print

For pointers on deciding when a physical condition may have caused a disorder, see sidebar, page 97.

The D's: • Distress or disability (work/educational, social, or personal impairment) • Differential diagnosis (substance use disorders, **delirium, other mental disorders** such as mood disorders, illness anxiety disorder, adjustment disorder)

Coding Notes

In recording the diagnosis, use the name of the responsible medical condition, and list first the medical condition, with its code number.

Millicent Worthy

"I wonder if we could just leave the door open." Millicent Worthy gets up from the chair and opens the examining room door. She has fidgeted throughout the first part of the interview. Part of that time, she has hardly seemed to be paying attention at all.

"I feel better not being so closed in," she offers. Once she finally settles down, she tells this story.

Millicent is 24 and divorced. She has never touched drugs or alcohol. In fact, until about 4 months ago, she's been well all her life. She visited a mental health clinic only once before, when she was 12: Her parents were having marital problems, and everyone had gone for family counseling.

Her first hint of nervousness occurred while tending the checkout counter at the video rental outlet where she works. She felt cramped, hemmed in, as if she needed to walk around. One afternoon, when she was the only employee in the store and she had to stay behind the counter, her heart began to pound, and she perspired and became short of breath. She thought she was about to die.

Over the next several weeks, Millicent gradually became aware of other symptoms. Her hand had begun to shake; she noticed it one day at the end of her shift when she was adding up her cash register receipts. Now, her appetite is voracious, yet in the past 6 weeks her weight has dropped nearly 10 pounds. She still loves watching movies, but lately she feels so tired at night that she can barely stay awake in front of the TV. Her mood, she confesses, has been somewhat irritable.

"As I thought about it, I realized that all this started about the time my boyfriend and I decided to get married. We've been living together for a year, and I really love him. But I've been burned before, in my first marriage. I thought that might be what was bothering me, so I gave back his ring and moved out. If anything, I feel even worse now than I did then."

Several times during the interview Millicent shifts restlessly in her chair. Her speech is rapid, though she can be interrupted. Her eyes seemed to protrude slightly, and although she has lost weight, there is a fullness in her neck that suggests a goiter—an enlargement of the thyroid gland. She agrees that she has been having trouble tolerating heat. "There's no air conditioner in our store. Last summer it was no problem because we kept the door open. But now it's terrible! And if I wear any less clothing to work, they'll have to give me a desk in the adult video section."

Millicent's thyroid function studies prove markedly abnormal. Within 2 months an endocrinologist brings her hyperactive thyroid under control, and her anxiety symptoms disappear completely. Six months later, she and her fiancé tie the knot.

Evaluation of Millicent Worthy

Millicent has had at least one panic attack (criterion A); her distress is palpable (E). The only remaining requirement involves ruling out other causes of her problem.

If she'd had repeated panic attacks and if the symptoms of her goiter had been overlooked, she could have been misdiagnosed as having panic disorder. Her restlessness could have been misinterpreted as generalized anxiety disorder; her feelings of being closed in sound like a specific phobia. (Even Millicent interpreted her own symptoms as psychological, C.) Such scenarios reinforce the wisdom of placing physical conditions at the top of our lists of differential diagnoses.

Irritability, restless hyperactivity, and weight loss also suggest a manic episode, but that is usually accompanied by a subjective feeling of high energy, not fatigue. Millicent's rapid speech could be interrupted; in bipolar mania, often it cannot. Her lack of previous depressions or manias also argues, if softly, against any mood disorders. Her history rules out a substance/medication-induced anxiety disorder. And her attention span and orientation are good, so we can discard delirium (D). Finally, and importantly, we know that the physiological effects of hyperthyroidism can cause anxiety symptoms of the sort Millicent experienced (B).

The broken engagement is noteworthy, not as a cause of her anxiety symptoms, but as a relationship problem that needs attention in the overall treatment plan. I'd put her GAF score at an almost-healthy, but still-needs-to-be-addressed 85. Before treatment, her diagnosis would be:

E05.00	Hyperthyroidism with goiter without thyroid storm
F06.4	Anxiety disorder due to hyperthyroidism
Z63.0	Breakup with fiancé

F41.8 Other Specified Anxiety Disorder

Patients who have prominent symptoms of anxiety, fear, or phobic avoidance that don't meet criteria for any specific anxiety disorder can be coded as having other specified anxiety disorder—and the reason for not including them in a better-defined category should be stated. DSM-5-TR suggests several different possibilities:

Limited-symptom attacks. This would include panic attacks or GAD with too few symptoms.

The presentation is atypical. DSM-5-TR gives the example of GAD that occurs less often than "more days than not."

Cultural syndromes. DSM-5-TR mentions two on page 261.

F41.9 Unspecified Anxiety Disorder

CHAPTER 5

Obsessive–Compulsive and Related Disorders

Quick Guide to the Obsessive–Compulsive and Related Disorders

People who are preoccupied with obsessional ideas or certain repetitive behaviors may qualify for the disorders listed here.

Obsessive–compulsive disorder. These people are bothered by repeated thoughts or behaviors that appear senseless, even to them (p. 199).

Body dysmorphic disorder. In this disorder, physically normal people believe that parts of their bodies are misshapen or ugly (p. 203).

Hoarding disorder. An individual accumulates so many objects (perhaps of no value) that they interfere with life and living (p. 206).

Trichotillomania (hair-pulling disorder). Pulling hair from various parts of the body is often accompanied by feelings of "tension and release" (p. 209).

Excoriation (skin-picking) disorder. Patients so persistently pick at their skin that they traumatize it (p. 211).

Obsessive–compulsive and related disorder due to another medical condition. Obsessions and compulsions can be caused by various medical conditions (p. 214).

Substance/medication-induced obsessive–compulsive and related disorder. Various substances can lead to obsessive–compulsive symptoms that don't fulfill criteria for any of the above-mentioned disorders (p. 213).

Other specified, or unspecified, obsessive–compulsive and related disorder. Use one of these categories to code disorders with prominent obsessive–compulsive symptoms that do not fit neatly into any of the groups above (p. 215).

Introduction

This chapter—which was new in DSM-5—pulls together disorders that have in common intrusive thoughts and time-consuming, repetitive behaviors: skin picking, hoarding, checking for body defects, and of course the classic component symptoms of obsessive–compulsive disorder (OCD). These behaviors aren't all unwanted—at least not at first, as with the pursuit of physical perfection (body dysmorphic disorder) or an accumulation of goods (hoarding). However they begin, the behaviors eventually become symptoms that are burdensome to those whose once-voluntary acts have morphed into duties that are performed—or resisted—at the cost of anxiety and distress.

Other features bind together this seemingly disparate collection of conditions: onset when young, similar comorbidities, a family history of OCD, response to similar treatments, and hints of dysfunction in the frontostriatal brain circuitry (caudate hyperactivity).

F42.2 Obsessive–Compulsive Disorder

Obsessions are recurring thoughts, beliefs, or ideas that dominate a person's mental content. They persist even though the person may believe they are unrealistic and tries to resist them. *Compulsions* are acts (either physical or mental) performed repeatedly in a way that the person may realize is neither appropriate nor useful. So why do them? For the most part, the aim is to neutralize the obsessional thinking. Note, then, that repeated thoughts can themselves sometimes be compulsions, if their purpose is to reduce the obsessional anxiety.

Compulsions can be comparatively simple, such as uttering or thinking a word or phrase of protection against an obsessive thought. But some are almost unbelievably complex. For instance, an elaborate dressing, bedtime, or washing ritual, if not performed exactly as specified by intricate rules, must be repeated until the person gets it right. Of course, that sort of behavior can soak up hours every day.

Although obsessions without compulsions do occur, most patients have both, and they are usually accompanied by anxiety and dread. And most patients recognize them as being irrational and want to resist. OCD comprises four major symptom patterns, whose features sometimes overlap.

- The most common is a fear of *contamination* that leads to excessive handwashing or cleaning.
- *Harm* that might be done intentionally or by dint of failure to perform some action ("Did I turn off the cooktop?") lead to excessive checking: The patient returns repeatedly to be sure that the cooktop is well and truly cold.
- *Symmetry* (putting things into a specific order, counting things).
- Ideas that are unacceptable on grounds of morality or taste (*taboos*): These include sexual aggression and sacrilegious ideas and actions.

Obsessions and compulsions consume huge blocks of time; they affect some people to the point that it can take hours just to finish breakfast or other daily routines. And by the way, in an effort to "help," relatives will sometimes become so involved in these maladaptive rituals that it encourages the person to continue with behaviors they would rather abandon.

One feature that helps classify patients with OCD is their degree of insight. Most patients are pretty well aware that their behavior is odd or peculiar; in fact, they often feel embarrassed and try to hide it. But others—perhaps 10–25% of all patients with OCD—either have never recognized the irrationality of their behavior or have now to some degree lost that insight. Poor insight often indicates a worse prognosis. A few patients have so little of it that they are actually delusional; however, their OCD can be distinguished from delusional disorder by the presence of their obsessions, so you don't need to give them an additional diagnosis of a psychosis. Children often don't have the experience to judge the reasonableness of their own behavior, so insight specifiers may not apply to them.

OCD is clinically important because it is often chronic and debilitating. Though symptoms may wax and wane, it puts people at risk for celibacy or marital discord and interferes with performance at school and work. Comorbidity is the rule, with two-thirds of patients experiencing major depression. Perhaps 15% attempt suicide.

OCD typically begins in adolescence (males) or young adult life (females), but it may take a decade or more before patients come to clinical attention. When it begins before puberty, compulsions may start first, often accompanied by tics and comorbid disorders.

Men and women are about equally likely to be affected by OCD. Its prevalence, which hovers just above 1% on the general population, is reported to be greater in individuals of high intelligence and higher socioeconomic classes. OCD is strongly familial (risk for first-degree relatives is 12%) and probably at least in part inherited. However, it is still unclear how genetics and environmental influences interact.

Tic Specifier

DSM-5 added a specifier concerning a patient's experience with a tic disorder. These patients, usually male, tend to have a very early onset of OCD—often before the age of 11. They are especially likely to obsess over issues of precision and symmetry; their compulsions concern ordering and arranging things. Some studies seem to suggest that a chronic tic disorder may reduce patients' response to antidepressant medications (though not to cognitive-behavioral therapy), and that antipsychotic drugs may help. However, it isn't clear that the history of tics denotes a patient who is more seriously ill. The tic specifier will apply to about 30% of patients with OCD.

The December 2008 issue of *The Atlantic* reported asking for a term that would describe the irresistible impulse to rearrange the contents of a dishwasher. Numerous readers suggested "obsessive compulsive dishorder."

Essential Features of **Obsessive–Compulsive Disorder**

The patient has distressing obsessions or compulsions (or both) that occupy so much time they interfere with accustomed routines.

The Fine Print

Obsessions are recurring, unwanted ideas that intrude into awareness; the patient tries to suppress, disregard, or neutralize them—perhaps by performing a compulsive ritual. *Compulsions* are repeated physical (sometimes mental) behaviors that follow strict rules (or respond to obsessions) in an attempt to prevent something awful from happening or to alleviate distress; the patient may try to resist them. The behaviors are unreasonable, meaning that they have no realistic chance of helping the distress.

The D's: • Distress or disability (typically, the obsessions and/or compulsions occupy an hour a day or more or cause work/educational, social, or personal impairment) • Differential diagnosis (**substance use** and **physical disorders,** "normal" superstitions and rituals that don't cause actual distress or disability, **major depressive** and **psychotic disorders,** anxiety and **impulse-control disorders, conduct disorders, eating disorders,** Tourette's disorder, obsessive–compulsive personality disorder, **illness anxiety disorder, hoarding disorder, generalized anxiety disorder, body dysmorphic disorder, trichotillomania, excoriation disorder, autism spectrum disorder, stereotypic movement disorder, gambling disorder, paraphilic disorders**)

Coding Notes

Specify degree of insight:

> **With good or fair insight.** The patient realizes that the OCD thoughts and behaviors are not (or probably not) true.
> **With poor insight.** The patient thinks that the OCD concerns are probably true.
> **With absent insight/delusional beliefs.** The patient strongly believes that the OCD concerns are true.

Specify if:

> **Tic-related.** The patient has a history (current or past) of a tic disorder.

Leighton Prescott

Pausing for a moment, Leighton Prescott leans forward to straighten a stack of journals on the interviewer's desk. The chapped skin on the backs of his hands is the color of dusty bricks. Apparently satisfied, he resumes his narrative.

"I get this feeling that semen could be on my hands and that it might be transferred to a woman and get her pregnant, even if I only shook hands with her. So, I started washing extra carefully each time I masturbated."

Leighton is 23 and a graduate student in plant physiology. Though he is enormously bright and dedicated to science, his performance has slipped badly over the past few months. He attributes this to the handwashing rituals. Whenever he has the thought that he might have contaminated his hands with semen, he feels compelled to scrub them vigorously.

A year earlier, this had only meant 3 or 4 minutes with a bar of soap and water as hot as he could stand it. Soon he required a nail brush; still later he was brushing his hands and wrists as well. Now he has evolved an elaborate ritual. First, he scrapes under his nails with a blade; then he uses the brush on them. He then lathers surgical soap up to his elbows and scrubs with a different brush, 15 minutes per arm. Then he must start over with his nails, which might be harboring semen he has scrubbed off his arms. If he has the thought that he hasn't performed one of the steps exactly, he will have to start all over again. In recent weeks, starting over has become the norm.

"I know it seems crazy," he says with a glance at his hands. "I'm a biologist. That part of me knows that spermatozoa can't live longer than a few minutes on the skin. But if I don't wash, the pressure just builds up and up, until I *have* to wash—washing is the only thing that relieves the anxiety."

Leighton doesn't think he is depressed, though he certainly is appropriately concerned about his symptoms. His sleep and appetite haven't changed; he has never felt guilty or suicidal.

"Just stupid, especially when my girl stopped seeing me. I used the bathroom in a restaurant I took her to. After 45 minutes, she had to send the manager in for me." He laughs without much humor. "She says she might see me again, if I'd clean up my act."

Evaluation of Leighton Prescott

Leighton's obsessions and compulsions (criterion A) both easily fulfill the requirements for OCD. He tries to suppress the recurrent thoughts about contamination, which he recognizes as the unreasonable products of his own mind (good insight). He feels compelled to ward off these ideas by repetitive handwashing, which he acknowledges to be grossly excessive—and worthless. By the time he seeks help, his symptoms occupy several hours each day, interfere with his schooling and social life, *and* cause him severe distress (B). He has no other identifiable mental disorder that might account for his symptoms (D).

An important step in evaluating anyone for OCD is to determine whether the patient's focus of concern is pathological. For example, for someone who lives in a ghetto or a war zone it might be prudent to triple-lock the doors and frequently check security. Had Leighton been excessively concerned about numerous real-life problems (such as passing his exams or succeeding with his girlfriend), he might instead warrant a diagnosis of generalized anxiety disorder.

Though repetitive behavior is also characteristic of Tourette's disorder and temporal lobe epilepsy, patients with other medical conditions rarely present with obsessions or compulsions (C). However, occasionally a person will develop obsessions or compulsions because of substance use. Inquire carefully about past or present tics, reported in about one-quarter of all OCD patients. Not only is there a relationship between OCD and Tourette's disorder, but an outsized percentage of patients with OCD (though not Leighton) report a history of chronic tics.

Obsessional thinking or compulsive behavior can be found in a variety of other mental disorders. People may obsessively pursue any number of activities, such as gambling, drinking, and sex. The differential diagnosis also includes body dysmorphic disorder (the patient obsesses about body shape) and illness anxiety disorder (the focus is health). Patients with psychotic disorders sometimes maintain their obsessional ideas to a delusional degree. And of course, there is something a bit obsessive in the eating behaviors of patients with anorexia nervosa and bulimia nervosa.

Perhaps 20% of patients with OCD have premorbid obsessional traits. Because of its name, obsessive–compulsive personality disorder can be confused with OCD. Patients with only the personality disorder may not have obsessions or compulsions at all. They are perfectionistic and become preoccupied with rules, lists, and details. These people may accomplish a task slowly because they keep checking to be sure it is being performed exactly right, but they do not have the desire to resist this behavior. OCD and obsessive–compulsive personality disorder can coexist, in which case the OCD is often extra severe. Some clinicians believe that the border zone between OCD and schizotypal personality disorder is also a common problem in differential diagnosis.

Leighton's clinician needs to ensure that he doesn't have one of the (numerous) other conditions that often accompany OCD. Besides the two personality disorders just mentioned, I'd especially check for mood disorders (both depressive and bipolar) and anxiety disorders (generalized anxiety disorder, social anxiety disorder, and panic disorder). Indeed, earlier DSMs classified OCD itself as an anxiety disorder.

Although most patients with OCD recognize that their obsessions and compulsions are unreasonable or excessive, some lose insight as the illness wears on. Leighton recognizes that he is being unreasonable; we'll classify him accordingly. With a GAF score of 60, his diagnosis will be the following:

F42.2   Obsessive–compulsive disorder, with good insight

F45.22 Body Dysmorphic Disorder

Patients with body dysmorphic disorder (BDD) worry that there is something wrong with the shape or appearance of a body part—most often breasts, genitalia, hair, or some facial feature such as the nose. The ideas these patients have about their bodies are not delusional; as in illness anxiety disorder, they are overvalued ideas. At one time the disorder was called *dysmorphophobia;* although some clinicians may still call it that, it isn't a phobia at all (irrational fear doesn't really enter into it).

This disorder can be devastating. Although they frequently request medical procedures (such as dermabrasion) or plastic surgery to correct their imagined defects, patients are often dissatisfied with the results. For that reason, surgery is usually con-traindicated. They may also seek reassurance (which helps only briefly), try to hide their perceived deformities with clothing or makeup, or avoid social situations; some even become housebound. The preoccupation causes clinically important distress of other sorts—depressed mood, for example, even suicide ideas and attempts. Insight varies, though it's mostly poor.

In the general population, the rate of BDD is probably about 2%. It may account for as many as 10% of patients who consult a dermatologist and a third of patients seeking rhinoplasty. Though patients with BDD are relatively young (it tends to begin during the teen years), incidence may peak again after the age of menopause. Although the question is not settled, men and women are probably about equally affected. However, males are more often concerned about genitals and hair.

DSM-5-TR mentions BDD by proxy, in which a patient becomes concerned with imagined defects in the appearance of another person—usually a spouse or close relative. It's been little studied, and though likely pretty rare, prevalence isn't known.

Essential Features of Body Dysmorphic Disorder

In response to a miniscule, sometimes invisible physical flaw, the patient repeatedly checks in a mirror, asks for reassurance, or picks at patches of skin—or makes mental comparisons with other people.

The Fine Print

The D's: • Distress or disability (work/educational, social, or personal impairment) • Differential diagnosis (substance use and physical disorders, mood and psychotic disorders, **eating disorders** such as anorexia nervosa, OCD, generalized anxiety disorder, social anxiety disorder, illness anxiety disorder, ordinary dissatisfaction with personal appearance, gender dysphoria)

Coding Notes

Specify if:

> **With muscle dysmorphia.** These patients believe that their bodies are too small or lack adequate musculature.

Specify degree of insight:

> **With good or fair insight.** The patient realizes that the BDD thoughts and behaviors are definitely (or probably) not true.
> **With poor insight.** The patient thinks that the BDD concerns are probably true.
> **With absent insight/delusional beliefs.** The patient strongly believes that the BDD concerns are true.

Muscle Dysmorphia Specifier

The muscle dysmorphia specifier for BDD is found almost exclusively in men, who typically believe (with little insight) that they are too small or slightly built. As a result, they will often take dieting or weightlifting to extremes, and may misuse anabolic steroids or other drugs. (These patients may also be concerned about other body features—skin, hair, or whatever.)

Cecil Crane

Cecil Crane is only 24 when referred. "He came in here last week asking for a rhinoplasty," says the plastic surgeon on the telephone, "but his nose looks perfect to me. I told him that, but he insisted there was something wrong with it. I've seen this kind of patient before—if I operate, they're never satisfied. It's a lawsuit waiting to happen."

When Cecil appears a few days later, he has the most beautiful nose the clinician has ever seen, apart from one or two Greek statues. "What seems to be wrong with it?"

"I was afraid you'd say that," says Cecil. "Everybody says that."

"But you don't believe it?"

"Well, they look at me funny. Even at work—I sell suits at Macy's—I sometimes feel that the customers notice. I think it's this bump here."

Viewed from a certain angle, the area Cecil pointed out bore the barest suggestion of a convexity. He complains that it cost him his girlfriend, who always claimed it looked fine to her. Weary of Cecil's trying to inspect his profile in every mirror he passed and banging on about plastic surgery all the time, she'd finally sought greener pastures.

Cecil feels unhappy, though not depressed. He admits that he is making a mess of his life, but he has nevertheless maintained his interests in reading and going to the movies. He thinks his sex interest is good, though it's been untested since his girlfriend decamped. His appetite is good, his weight about average for his height. His flow of thought is unremarkable; its content, aside from concern about his nose, seems quite ordinary. He even admits that it is possible that his nose is less ugly than he fears, though he thinks that unlikely.

Cecil cannot say exactly when his worry about his nose began. It may have been about the time he started shaving. He recalls frequently gazing at a silhouette of his profile that had been cut from black paper during a seashore vacation with his family. Although numerous relatives and friends remarked that it was a good likeness, something about the nose had bothered him. One day he removed the silhouette from its frame and, with a pair of scissors, tried to put it to rights. Within moments the nose lay in snippets on the kitchen table and Cecil was grounded for a month.

"I sure hope the plastic surgeon is a better artist than I am," he comments.

Evaluation of Cecil Crane

The criteria for BDD are straightforward. Cecil is preoccupied with his flawless nose (criterion A), which causes him enough distress to seek surgery—and lose his girlfriend (C). More than one person has tried to assure him that his nose is normal, even gorgeous, so his distress evidently exceeds usual concerns regarding appearance. And his constant checking in the mirror satisfies the requirement for behaviors that address his concern (B). Despite this full checklist of symptoms, there are several disorders in the differential diagnosis we should consider.

In illness anxiety disorder, it isn't appearance that preoccupies the patient; rather, it is fear of having a disease. In anorexia nervosa, people have distorted self-image, but only in the context of concern about overweight. In the somatic type of delusional disorder, patients lack insight that their complaints might be unreasonable, whereas Cecil will entertain the notion that others might see his nose differently. (However, some patients with BDD completely lack insight; then the differentiation turns on the content of the delusion, which in delusional disorder will involve not the appearance of body parts but their function or sensations.) Complaints from patients with schizophrenia about appearance are sometimes bizarre (one woman reported that when she looked into the mirror, she noticed that her head had been replaced by a mushroom). In gender dysphoria, patients' distress is limited to their gender identity being different from their sex assigned at birth.

None of these was the focus of Cecil's concern. However, his clinician would do well to look carefully for social anxiety disorder, obsessive–compulsive disorder, and major depressive disorder, all of which can be comorbid with body dysmorphic disorder. Pending investigation for these conditions, Cecil's full diagnosis would be as given below, with a GAF score of 70:

F45.22   Body dysmorphic disorder, with fair insight

F42.3 Hoarding Disorder

First written down over a thousand years ago, the Beowulf legend referred to a *hoard* as a mass of something valuable (especially money or other treasure) laid by for the future. Nowadays, we stand this definition on its head to mean worthless stuff that's kept beyond all practical use.

The motivations behind hoarding can be varied. Some people believe their things are valuable when they're not. Others may be imitating behavior they've encountered in family members (a genetic component is also suspected). Still others apparently feel comforted by the presence of possessions they've grown used to having, or that they think they might need later. Whatever the impetus, a hoarder's living space becomes cluttered, perhaps eventually filling up completely; if living areas remain habitable, it's probably because someone else tidies up the mess. One social consequence of hoarding is that children dread having visitors to the home; they sure don't learn the basics of housekeeping there! There are now online support groups for hoarders' children, who are otherwise left with their own hopeless attempts at coping with the unsightly, the unsanitary, and the unsafe.

A condition that's said to affect perhaps 2% of the general population, hoarding disorder was new in DSM-5. It was once considered a variant of OCD; however, not even 20% of hoarders meet OCD criteria—partly because they don't regard their behavior as intrusive, unpleasant, or distressing. Indeed, distress often develops only when they are forced to get rid of the stuff they've so persistently carried home.

Hoarding disorder comprises several special types: people who hoard books, or animals (think a houseful of cats), or food that is—ugh!—way past its pull date. Animal hoarders also save other items, some of which may at least have the advantage of decent sanitation. The disorder begins young and worsens with time, so that it is more often found among older adults; males may outnumber females. It appears to be strongly hereditary.

Essential Features of **Hoarding Disorder**

These people are in the grip of something powerful: the overwhelming urge to accumulate stuff. They experience trouble—indeed, distress—when trying to part with or discard their possessions, even those that appear to have little value, sentimental or otherwise. As a result, unless someone else intervenes, things quite literally pile up, cluttering living areas to render them unusable, even dangerous.

The Fine Print

The D's: • Duration (not stated, other than "persistent") • Distress or disability (work/ educational, social, or personal impairment) • Differential diagnosis (substance use and **physical disorders** [especially involving brain damage], **mood** and **psychotic disorders, neurocognitive disorder, OCD, autism spectrum disorder,** normal collecting)

Coding Notes

Specify if:

> **With excessive acquisition.** If symptoms are accompanied by excessive collecting, buying, or stealing of items that are not needed or for which there is no space available.

Specify degree of insight:

> **With good or fair insight.** The patient realizes that these thoughts and behaviors cause problems.
> **With poor insight.** The patient mostly believes that hoarding isn't a problem.
> **With absent insight/delusional beliefs.** The patient strongly believes that hoarding is not a problem.

Langley Collyer

More than half a century on, the Collyer case remains celebrated in the annals of hoarding.

Though well educated (Columbia University) and a talented pianist, Langley Collyer probably never held gainful employment. He and his older brother, Homer, lived in the Harlem house left them by their parents, an obstetrician and his wife who were first cousins. Trained as a lawyer, Homer worked for a time, but his vision deteriorated, and he suffered from arthritis. So, as they grew older, the brothers lived on their inherited money. They didn't require much: They had no gas, electricity, or telephone service. Even the water was eventually turned off. For decades, they essentially camped out indoors.

Langley would walk miles to the store for supplies that he'd pull along home in a wagon. On these journeys, he also collected much of the debris that ultimately invaded their living space. Although he wore clothes long out of fashion, Langley was not completely asocial. As reported from accounts of those who knew him, he was pleasant, at times grateful for company. He even admitted that he was too reclusive.

In 1947, at age 61, Langley died, crushed under the weight of the booby traps he'd designed and installed over a period of years to prevent criminals from stealing the brothers' possessions. Encountering doorways stuffed with 10-foot-high walls of bailed newspaper and other debris, police had to chop their way in. It took them over 2 weeks to find Langley's body, which lay just 10 feet from where Homer had subsequently died of starvation.

After the bodies were removed, workers cleared the house of its holdings. They found dressmaker's dummies, sheets of Braille, a doll carriage, bicycles, a photograph of Mickey Rooney, old advertisements, firearms and ammunition, parts for old radios, chunks of concrete, and shoelaces. The brothers had stored portions of their body waste in jars. There was a two-headed baby preserved in formaldehyde (probably an artifact from their father's medical practice), a canoe, a disassembled Model T automobile, two pipe organs, thousands of empty tin cans, and 14 pianos. There were also tons of newspapers, saved so that Homer could catch up on the news, once he regained his sight. In all, the house eventually yielded 180 tons of junk, with everything covered in the dust of decades.

Evaluation of Langley Collyer

The analysis of Langley's condition requires a little forgiveness. That's because, candidly, we must infer one criterion important for hoarding disorder: that no other medical disorder can better explain the symptoms (criterion E). Langley and Homer famously refused to seek medical attention, hence Homer's crippling arthritis and, perhaps, his blindness. But Langley eschewed alcohol and drugs, and he appeared well enough for decades until the very end of his life—when everything came, quite literally, crashing down.

Hoarding can occur as a symptom of OCD, but as with most patients who hoard, Langley displayed no evidence of actual obsessions or (other) compulsions (F). Although there is no evidence for another mental disorder, neither have we evidence that Langley did not suffer from, say, major depressive disorder (it and OCD are often comorbid with hoarding disorder).

As for the other requirements of the syndrome, Langley was undeniably a collector whose accumulated tonnage didn't just impinge upon but engulfed the living space of the two hermit brothers (A, B, C). It imperiled their own health and that of any public service personnel who might need to give assistance; failing to maintain a safe environment satisfies the stress or impairment requirement (D).

In the absence of direct testimony from Langley, we cannot know how deeply he understood his condition, so we must ignore the insight specifiers. However, we can probably agree that his collecting habits qualify for the specifier *with excessive acquisition*—as is the case in most hoarders. Although we are no longer able to code something on the order of "personality disorder, diagnosis deferred," if Langley were a living patient I'd make some sort of note in my summary to that effect—to alert me or another clinician down the road that more diagnostic work remained to be done. I'd give him a GAF score of 60.

F42.3   Hoarding disorder, with excessive acquisition

F63.3 Trichotillomania (Hair-Pulling Disorder)

Trichotillomania comes from the Greek, meaning "passion for pulling hair." As with pyromania and kleptomania, many such patients (but not all) feel a mounting tension until they succumb to the urge. Then, when they pull a strand, they experience release. With onset ordinarily in childhood, people with trichotillomania repeatedly extract their own hair, beards, eyebrows, or eyelashes. Less often, they will pull hair from armpits, the pubic area, or other body locations. They usually don't report pain associated with this behavior, although they may note a tingling sensation.

Some people put the hair into their mouths; about 30% swallow it. Long hair can accumulate in the stomach or intestines as a bezoar (hairball) that may require surgical removal. Some patients are referred for mental health care by dermatologists, who note patchy hair loss.

Trichotillomania is embarrassing to patients, who tend to be secretive, so it's unclear just how common it is. Some hair pulling can be found in up to 3% of the adult population, especially women, though far fewer (probably under 1%) meet full criteria for the disorder. It is far more common in females than in males, and it is especially common in people with intellectual developmental disorder. Many such patients also repetitively attack their bodies in other ways: They crack their knuckles, bite their nails, or pick at their skin.

Though it is not a requirement for diagnosis, the feeling of tension before hair pulling, and release or relief of stress afterward, characterizes many sufferers. These patients may be in for a more severe course of the illness than those who don't report this feature.

Trichotillomania usually arises in childhood or adolescence; when it begins in an adult, it may be associated with psychosis. The condition tends to wax and wane but is often chronic. In an overall population prevalence of 1–2%, females far outnumber males.

Essential Features of **Trichotillomania**

These patients repeatedly pull out of their own hair, resulting in bald patches and multiple attempts to control the behavior.

The Fine Print

The D's: • Duration ("recurrent") • Distress or disability (work/educational, social, or personal impairment) • Differential diagnosis (substance-related disorders, **physical disorders,** mood and psychotic disorders, **body dysmorphic disorder,** OCD, ordinary grooming)

Rosalind Brewer

"I don't know why I do it, I just do it." Rosalind Brewer comes to the mental health clinic on referral from her dermatologist. "I get to feeling sort of uptight, and if I just pop one little strand loose, somehow it relieves the tension." She selects a single strand of her long blonde hair, twines it neatly twice around her forefinger, and tweaks it out. She gazes at it a moment before dropping it onto the freshly vacuumed carpet.

Rosalind has been pulling out her hair for nearly half her 30 years. She thinks it started during her second or third year in high school, when she was studying for final exams. Perhaps the tingling sensation on her scalp helped her stay awake, though she doesn't really remember. "Now it's a habit. I've always only pulled hairs from the very top of my head."

The top of Rosalind's head bears a round, almost bald spot about the size of a poker chip. Only a few broken hairs and a sparse growth of new hair sprout there. It resembles a tiny tonsure.

"It used to make my mom really angry. She said I'd end up looking like Dad. She'd order me to stop, but you know kids. I used to think I had her by the short hairs." She laughs a little. "Now that I want to stop, I can't."

Rosalind sucked her thumb until the age of 8, but her childhood was otherwise unremarkable. Her physical health is good; she has no other compulsive behaviors or obsessive thinking. She denies using drugs or alcohol. She has no significant symptoms of depression, and she admits that her hair pulling is a serious problem. She can wear a hairpiece to hide her bald spot, but knowing it's there has kept her from forming any close relationship with a man.

"It's bad enough looking like a monk," Rosalind says. "But this has got me living like one, too."

Evaluation of Rosalind Brewer

Rosalind's symptoms of repeated hair pulling (criterion A) include the classic "tension and release" that used to be required for a diagnosis of trichotillomania, but now is only a frequent feature. She has no evidence of a dermatological disorder or other general medical condition (D) that might explain the condition. The mental conditions that might be confused with trichotillomania include OCD, in which compulsions are performed not as an end to themselves, but as a means of preventing anxiety. Hair pulling is sometimes found in body dysmorphic disorder, but all will agree that Rosalind has an actual cosmetic issue. Factitious disorder, another possibility, would be ruled out because Rosalind gives no indication that she wants to be a patient. She has no psychosis or other evident mental disorder (especially mood disorder, E), except for the distress (C) at her inability to stop (B).

With a GAF score of 70, her complete diagnosis is straightforward:

F63.3   Trichotillomania

F42.4 Excoriation (Skin-Picking) Disorder

Excoriation (skin-picking) disorder usually begins by adolescence, though sometimes later. These patients spend much time—perhaps hours each day—digging at their skin. Most will focus on head or face; fingernails tend to be the instruments of choice, though some patients use tweezers. As with other disorders of impulse such as pyromania, tension prior to the act is a frequent finding in these patients. Then the act of picking may yield gratification; subsequent embarrassment or shame can delay treatment. Infections are common, sometimes producing ulceration. Patients may use cosmetics to conceal the scratches and scarring.

Patients may avoid social events, but for others, consequences can be dire. One patient picked so persistently at his neck and scalp that he dug right through his skull and developed an epidural abscess. The resultant quadriplegia resolved only partially; confined to a wheelchair, he ultimately resumed picking. This is an extreme; however, scarring and less harmful infections are common. Many patients will spend an hour or more each day engaged in picking behavior or dealing with its consequences.

A third of people with excoriation disorder currently have some other mental disorder, most notably trichotillomania, a mood disorder, or OCD; some bite their nails. Nearly half of those with body dysmorphic disorder also pick at themselves. Excoriation is found in people with developmental disabilities, especially in those with Prader–Willi syndrome (see sidebar, p. 214).

Described as far back as 1889, excoriation disorder is relatively common; its prevalence is probably 2% or so. It tends to begin in adolescence and runs a chronic course. Most patients are female; many have relatives similarly afflicted.

Essential Features of **Excoriation (Skin-Picking) Disorder**

The patient frequently tries to stop the repeated digging, scratching, or picking of skin that has caused lesions.

The Fine Print

The D's: • Duration ("recurrent") • Distress or disability (work/educational, social, or personal impairment) • Differential diagnosis (**substance use** [cocaine] and **physical disorders** [such as scabies or acne], **psychotic disorders**, OCD, **body dysmorphic disorder, stereotypic movement disorder, nonsuicidal self-injury**)

Brittany Fitch

The evidence is stark: Brittany Fitch's face is replete with pitting and scars. A few of the lesions are still inflamed, and one on her forehead has scabbed over. She has covered her fingernails with tape.

When she was 11, Brittany had acne, which her mother would "relieve" by squeezing the pustules and blackheads. Brittany endured long minutes standing with her head wedged into a corner, her mother's muscular fingers digging away "as if for gold," Brittany recalls years later. Released at last, she'd run to the bathroom and dab cool water on her smarting, spotted face. She'd hated her mother.

Now in college, Brittany has taken over the squeezing and picking job, though she knows it only leads to more skin damage. Several times a week she will attack herself, perhaps for just a few minutes at a time, but longer if she's alone in the bathroom. She feels drawn to mirrors to inspect, to criticize her complexion; those inspections, inevitably, usher in further episodes of destruction. Because she feels ashamed of the damage she's wreaked, she avoids dating. It's been 6 months since she's attended a play or a concert, even by herself.

"I hope you can help me," she says with a wry smile. "More than anything, I want to stop being my mother."

Evaluation of Brittany Fitch

Brittany's condition isn't hard to diagnose. The spots and scars (criterion A) and the taped fingernails (B) tell much of the story, and her clinic visit testifies to the distress her symptoms cause (C). The most important question at this point would be this: Could another mental (or medical) disorder explain her symptoms? For that, her clinician will have to dig a little deeper, so to speak, into her history to make sure she doesn't have OCD (E). Of course, she doesn't have body dysmorphic disorder: Her skin condition is perfectly evident to anyone who looks.

If her clinician can find no evidence of a medical condition (perhaps scabies or some other dermatological disease) or a substance use disorder (such as use of cocaine or methamphetamines, in which the sensation of bugs crawling on or under the skin can precipitate picking, D), Brittany's diagnosis seems secure. I would base her GAF score of 60 on the degree of social disability she experiences.

F42.4   Excoriation disorder

Substance/Medication-Induced Obsessive–Compulsive and Related Disorder

Reports link obsessive–compulsive symptoms to use of codeine, cocaine, ecstasy, and methamphetamine. If these criteria look an awful lot like those for substance-induced anxiety disorders, it's because, back in DSM-IV, the two sections were combined. That's one reason I've elected not to include an additional vignette here. The other is that these conditions are probably vanishingly rare.

A principal example is the foraging behavior noted in users of crack cocaine. For a few hours at most, heavy users will inspect the carpet or bare floor looking for bits of the drug they might have dropped. It always occurs as a withdrawal phenomenon, and though they realize it is in vain, they feel helpless to resist.

Essential Features of **Substance/Medication-Induced Obsessive–Compulsive and Related Disorder**

The use of some substance appears to have caused obsessions, compulsions, hoarding, hair pulling, excoriation, or other recurring symptoms involving the patient's own body.
    For tips on identifying substance-related causation, see sidebar, page 95.

The Fine Print

The D's: • Distress or disability (work/educational, social, or personal impairment) • Differential diagnosis (ordinary substance intoxication or withdrawal, **delirium,** physical disorders, OCD, anxiety disorders)
    Use this diagnosis instead of substance intoxication or withdrawal only when obsessive–compulsive symptoms are predominant and require clinical care.

Coding Notes

Specify:

> **With onset during {intoxication}{withdrawal}.** This gets tacked on at the end of your string of words.

With onset after medication use. You could alternatively use this if symptoms develop when medication is started, changed, or stopped.

For specific coding procedures, see Table 15.2 (p. 475).

F06.8 Obsessive–Compulsive and Related Disorder Due to Another Medical Condition

Occasionally you'll encounter obsessive–compulsive symptoms that are associated with another medical condition. Of course, association doesn't prove causation, but an etiological relationship has been claimed for Japanese B encephalitis and arachnoid cyst, among others.

Obsessive–compulsive symptoms are also found with Sydenham's chorea, which can accompany streptococcal infection in children. Much has been written about the pediatric autoimmune neuropsychiatric disorders associated with streptococcal infection (PANDAS), in which young children develop obsessions and compulsions as well as tics and other symptoms, but without the motor disorder of chorea. After years of study, a lot still isn't known—including whether PANDAS is an actual entity, and whether the alleged association is even genuine. (In 2013, a young man was arrested for planning to bomb his own high school near Portland, Oregon. In his defense, he cited OCD due to PANDAS.)

Prader–Willi syndrome is a rare (about 1 in 50,000) disorder associated with a portion of DNA missing from chromosome 15. The condition may be identified at birth by genetic testing of markedly hypotonic babies. Though some individuals with this syndrome have borderline normal intelligence, mild to moderate intellectual developmental disorder is common. Patients typically have short stature and hypogonadism; insatiable appetite often results in severe obesity. Some have mood symptoms and problems with impulse control; others can also have hoarding behavior, foraging for food, skin picking, and obsessions with cleanliness—almost a clean sweep of the disorders this chapter comprises.

Essential Features of Obsessive–Compulsive and Related Disorder Due to Another Medical Condition

Through a physiological mechanism, a medical condition appears to have caused an illness that features obsessions, compulsions, hoarding, hair pulling, excoriation, or other recurrent symptoms concerning the patient's own body.

The Fine Print

For pointers on deciding when a physical condition may have caused a mental disorder, see sidebar, page 97.

The D's: • Distress or disability (work/educational, social, or personal impairment) • Differential diagnosis (substance use disorders, **delirium, other mental disorders such as mood and anxiety disorders, OCD**)

Coding Notes

Depending on presentation, specify:

> **With appearance preoccupations.** For symptoms similar to body dysmorphic disorder.
> **With obsessive–compulsive disorder-like symptoms**
> **With hair-pulling symptoms**
> **With hoarding symptoms**
> **With skin-picking symptoms**

F42.8 Other Specified Obsessive–Compulsive and Related Disorder

This category (which you use, remember, when a patient has obsessive–compulsive features but doesn't fully qualify for a diagnosis, and you want to say *why*) might be appropriate in several situations, including these:

> **Symptoms similar to body dysmorphic disorder, but with actual flaws.** The flaws are there, all right, but the concern seems excessive.
>
> **Obsessional jealousy.** Without qualifying for any other mental disorder, the patient is distressed (or impaired) by a partner's alleged infidelity; as a result, repetitive behavior or thoughts occur.
>
> **Olfactory reference disorder (aka syndrome).** The belief that one has an offensive body odor (when none is appreciable by others) leads to repetitive showering, checking for body odor, or masking with scents. Japanese mental health professionals know it as *jikoshu-kyofu.*
>
> **Symptoms similar to body dysmorphic disorder, but without repetitive behaviors.**

F42.9 Unspecified Obsessive–Compulsive and Related Disorder

The patient has obsessions or compulsions or other behaviors that belong in this chapter, and you *don't* care to explain your thinking.

CHAPTER 6

Trauma- and Stressor-Related Disorders

Quick Guide to Trauma- and Stressor-Related Disorders

Various types of stress and trauma are responsible for the disorders we'll consider in this chapter.

Primary Trauma- and Stressor-Related Disorders

Reactive attachment disorder. There is evidence of pathogenic care in a child who habitually doesn't seek comfort from parents or surrogates (p. 235).

Disinhibited social engagement disorder. There is evidence of pathogenic care in a child who fails to show expected reticence in the company of strangers (p. 235).

Posttraumatic stress disorder. These adolescents or adults repeatedly relive a severely traumatic event, such as combat or a natural disaster (p. 218).

Posttraumatic stress disorder in preschool children. Children repeatedly relive a severely traumatic event, such as car accidents, natural disasters, or war (p. 222).

Acute stress disorder. This condition is much like posttraumatic stress disorder, except that it begins during or immediately after the stressful event and lasts a month or less (p. 223).

Prolonged grief disorder. Someone of any age suffers the death of a loved one; the resulting symptoms of grief are drawn-out and disabling (p. 230).

Adjustment disorder. Following a stressor, an individual develops symptoms that disappear once the cause of stress has subsided (p. 227).

Other specified, or unspecified, trauma- and stressor-related disorder. Patients in whom stress or trauma causes presentations different from those above may be classified in one of these categories (p. 237).

Other Problems Related to Trauma or Stress

Problems related to abuse or neglect. An astonishing number of Z-codes cover the categories of difficulties that arise from neglect or from physical or sexual abuse of children or adults (p. 613).

Separation anxiety disorder. The patient becomes anxious when separated from parent, other attachment figure, or home (p. 187).

Introduction

This chapter incorporates certain diagnoses formerly listed as anxiety, developmental, or adjustment disorders. The unifying factor here is that something traumatic or stressful in the patient's history appears to be at least partly responsible for the symptoms that develop. It is part of a trend toward grouping together patients of any age who have the right mix of symptoms, rather than separating patients by developmental stage.

Many diagnoses include statements about what is not causative, but other than substance-related disorders, here is the only full DSM-5-TR section that presumes to identify any etiology at all, let alone something that's rooted in the psychology of a pathological developmental process.

In the instances of reactive attachment and disinhibited social engagement disorders, there must be evidence of pathogenic care; for posttraumatic stress disorder (PTSD) and its cousins, a horrific event; for adjustment disorder a stressful—well, stressor. The respective criteria sets permit us to check off the fulfilled criteria and go on our way, perhaps thinking that we've solved the puzzle.

While we rejoice that we've successfully determined a cause–effect relationship, nagging at the back of our minds must be a sense that there is more to the story. Otherwise, why do some people become symptomatic while others, exposed to (as best we can determine) the exact same stimuli, go untrammeled on their way? Furthermore, studies have demonstrated that, sooner or later, significant stressors will visit the majority of us. Shouldn't we conclude that the stimulus in question is necessary, but not sufficient, for the outcome observed?

At least this DSM-5-TR chapter has herded most of these etiology-specific diagnoses into one corral, where we can keep a watchful eye on them.

F43.10 Posttraumatic Stress Disorder

Many people who survive severely traumatic events will develop PTSD. Survivors of combat are the most frequently affected, but it is also encountered in those who have experienced other disasters, both natural and contrived. These include rape, floods, abductions, and airplane crashes, as well as the threats that may be posed by a kidnapping or hostage situation. Children can have PTSD from inappropriate sexual experience, even without actual physical injury. PTSD can be diagnosed even in those who have only learned about severe trauma (or its threat) suffered by someone to whom they are close—children, spouses, other close relatives. One or two in every 1,000 patients who have undergone general anesthesia have later reported awareness of pain, anxiety, helplessness, and the fear of impending death during the procedure; up to half of them may subsequently develop PTSD symptoms. Implicitly excluded from the definition are stressful experiences of ordinary life, such as bereavement, divorce, and serious illness. Awakening from anesthesia while your surgery is still in progress, however, would qualify as a traumatic event, as would learning about a spouse's sudden, accidental death or a child's life-threatening illness. Watching TV images of a calamity is not a sufficient stressor (except if the viewing is related to the person's job).

After a delay (symptoms usually don't develop immediately after the trauma), the person in some way relives the traumatic event and tries to avoid thinking about it. There are also symptoms of physiological hyperarousal, such as an exaggerated startle response. Patients with PTSD also express negative feelings such as guilt or a sense of personal responsibility ("I should have prevented it").

Aside from the traumatic event itself, other factors may play a role in the development of PTSD. Individual factors include the person's innate character structure and genetic inheritance. Relatively low intelligence and low educational attainment are positively associated with PTSD. Environmental influences include relatively low socioeconomic status and membership in a minority racial or ethnic group.

In general, the more horrific and enduring the trauma, the more likely PTSD is to develop. The risk runs to one-quarter of the survivors of heavy combat and two-thirds of former prisoners of war. Those who have experienced natural disasters such as fires or floods are generally less likely to develop symptoms. (Overall lifetime prevalence of PTSD is on the order of 7%, though European researchers report substantially lower rates.) Older adults are less likely to develop symptoms than are younger ones, and women tend to have somewhat higher rates than do men. About half the patients recover within a few months; others can experience years of incapacity.

In children, the general outline is pretty much the same as the five general points given in the list of typical symptoms, though the emphasis on symptom numbers differs, as you can note in Table 6.1 (p. 224).

Mood, anxiety, and substance use disorders are frequently comorbid. A recent specifier reflects findings that in perhaps 12–14% of patients, dissociation is important in the development and maintenance of PTSD symptoms.

Essential Features of **Posttraumatic Stress Disorder**

Something truly awful has happened. One person has been gravely injured or perhaps sexually abused; another has viewed death, injury, or sexual trauma occurring to someone else; a third has only learned that a close associate has experienced an accident or other form of violence. Emergency workers (police, firefighters) may be traumatized through repeated exposure during their work.

As a result, for many weeks or months these people repeatedly relive their event, perhaps through upsetting nightmares or dreams, through intrusive mental images, or through dissociative flashbacks. Some respond to reminders of the event with physiological sensations (racing heartbeat, shortness of breath) or marked emotional distress.

In addition, the person in some way creates distance from the event—perhaps by suppressing associated memories or emotions or by avoiding locations, people, or activities that could serve as reminders.

And, there must be two or more expressions of cognitive disturbance. These might include negative moods (anger, fear, guilt, shame); or gloomy thoughts ("I'm useless," "The world's a mess," or "I can't believe anyone"). Or, distorted thinking causes patients to cast inappropriate blame on themselves or others. They may lose interest in important activities or come to feel detached from other people. Some will experience amnesia for aspects of the trauma; others become unable to experience positive emotions—to love or to experience joy.

Finally, there must be at least a couple of expressions of reactivity and hyperarousal: These include irritability, reckless or self-harmful behavior, excessive vigilance, trouble concentrating, trouble sleeping, and an intense startle response.

The Fine Print

See Table 6.1 (p. 224) for diagnostic differences relevant to children under age 7.

The D's: • Duration (1+ months) • Distress or disability (work/educational, social, or personal impairment) • Differential diagnosis (**substance use** and **physical disorders** [especially traumatic brain injury], mood and anxiety disorders, dissociative and psychotic disorders, adjustment disorder, normal reactions to stressful events)

Coding Notes

Specify if:

With delayed expression. Symptoms sufficient for diagnosis didn't fully accumulate until at least 6 months after the event.
With dissociative symptoms:
Depersonalization. This indicates feelings of detachment, as though dreaming, from the patient's own mind or body.
Derealization. To the patient, the surroundings seem distant, distorted, dreamlike, or otherwise unreal.

Barney Gorse

"Those rats! They're shooting! They're g—"

Someone behind Barney Gorse has dropped a book onto the tile floor of the mental health clinic waiting room. The sudden noise has set him off. Now, backed into a corner, he swallows his words and cocks his fist for action. His pupils are widely dilated; perspiration stands out on his forehead. He pants heavily and points a shaky finger at a student standing petrified across the room. "Get this goddam rat out of here!" He lumbers toward the hapless student.

"Hang on, Barney. It's OK." Barney's new therapist takes him firmly by the elbow and leads him to a private office. They sit there in silence for a few minutes, while Barney's breathing gradually slows, and the clinician reviews his chart.

Barney Gorse is 39 now, but he was barely 20 when his draft number came up and he joined the Ninth Infantry Division in Vietnam. At that time President Nixon was "winding down the war," which made it seem all the more painful when Barney's squad was hit by mortar fire from North Vietnamese regulars.

He has never talked about it, even during "anger displacement" group therapy with other veterans. Whenever they ask him to tell his story, he flies into a rage. But something truly devastating must have happened to Barney that day. The reports mention a wound in the upper thigh; he was the only member of his squad to survive the attack. He had been awarded a Purple Heart and a full pension.

There are several hours of the attack Barney can't remember at all. And he has always been careful to avoid films and television programs about war. He says he's had enough of it to last everybody's lifetime; in fact, he has gone to some lengths to avoid thinking about it. He celebrated his discharge from the Army by getting drunk, and he remained that way for 6 years. When he finally sobered up, he turned to drugs. Even they couldn't obliterate the nightmares that still haunt him; several times a week, he awakens screaming. Sudden noises startle him into a panic attack.

Thanks to disulfiram and a chaplain in the county jail where he was once held as a persistent public nuisance, Barney has been clean and sober for 6 months. On the condition that he would seek treatment for his substance use, he was released. The specialists in substance misuse treatment quickly recognized that other problems have led him here.

Now the therapist reminds him again that he needs to dig into his feelings about the past. Barney responds that he doesn't have any feelings; they've dried up on him. For that matter, the future doesn't look so good, either: "Got no job, no wife, no kids. I just wasn't meant to have a life." He gets up and puts his hand on the doorknob to leave. "It's no use. I just can't talk about it."

Evaluation of Barney Gorse

Let's summarize and restate the criteria that must be fulfilled to diagnose PTSD.

1. There must be *severe trauma* (criterion A). Barney's occurred in the context of combat, but a variety of civilian stressors can also culminate in death, serious

injury, or sexual abuse. Two features must be present for a stressor to be considered sufficiently traumatic: (a) It must involve the fact or threat of death, severe wounds or injuries, or sexual violation; and (b) it must be personally experienced by the patient in some way—through direct observation (not viewed on TV), through personal involvement, or through information obtained later that it involves a relative or close friend. A first responder (police officer, fire fighter, emergency medical technician on an ambulance) could also qualify through repeated exposure to consequences of the horrific event (think workers at Ground Zero shortly after 9/11). Divorce, or death of a spouse from cancer, though undeniably stressful, are relatively commonplace and expected; they don't qualify.

2. Through some intrusive mechanism, the patient *relives the stress*. Barney has flashbacks (B3), during which he imagines himself back in Vietnam. He also experiences intense responses to an external cue (seeing a staff member who, to him, resembles a Viet Cong soldier). Less dramatic forms of recollection could include recurrent memories, dreams, and any other reminder of the event that results in distress or physiological symptoms.

3. The patient attempts (wittingly or not) to achieve *emotional distance* from the stressful event by avoiding reminders of the trauma. The reminders can be either internal (feelings, thoughts) or external (people, places, activities). Barney refuses to watch movies and TV programs or to talk about Vietnam (C).

4. The patient also has two or more expressions of *negative mood and thoughts* related to the trauma. Barney's include amnesia for much of his time in combat (D1), a persistently negative frame of mind ("I wasn't meant to have a life"—D4), and the lack of positive mood states (his feelings have "dried up," D7).

5. Finally, PTSD patients must have at least two symptoms of *heightened arousal and reactivity* associated with the traumatic event. Barney suffers from insomnia (E6) and a severe startle response (E4); others may experience general irritability, poor concentration, reckless or self-harmful behavior, or excessive vigilance. As with all symptoms, the clinician must determine that these symptoms of arousal had not been apparent before Barney's Vietnam trauma.

Barney's symptoms have persisted far longer than the required minimum of 1 month (F); are obviously stressful and impair his functioning in several areas (G); and cannot be attributed to the direct physiological effects of substance use—now that he's been clean and sober for half a year (H).

The experience of severe trauma in combat and the typical symptoms would render any other explanation for Barney's symptoms unlikely. A patient with intermittent explosive disorder might become aggressive and lose control but wouldn't have the history of trauma. Still, clinicians must always be alert to the possibility of another medical condition (H) that might produce anxiety symptoms and could be diagnosed instead of or in addition to PTSD. For example, head injuries are relatively common among veterans of combat or other violent trauma; we'd have to mention and code any accompanying brain injury. Situational adjustment disorder shouldn't be confused with PTSD: The severity of the trauma would be far less, and the effects would be transient and less dramatic.

In PTSD, comorbidity is the rule rather than the exception. Barney has used drugs and alcohol; his clinician would have gathered additional information about using other substances and mentioned them in Barney's diagnostic summary. Of combat veterans who have PTSD, half or more also have a problem with a substance use disorder, and use of multiple substances is common. Anxiety disorders (phobic disorders, generalized anxiety disorder) and mood disorders (major depressive disorder and persistent depressive disorder) are likewise common in this population. Dissociative amnesia may also occur. Any coexisting personality disorder would be explored, but it is hard to make a definitive diagnosis when a patient is acutely ill with PTSD. Malingering is also a diagnosis to consider whenever there appears to be a possibility of material gain (insurance, disability, relief from legal problems) resulting from an accident or physical attack.

Although the vignette is imprecise on this point, Barney's symptoms had probably begun by the time he was discharged from the military, so he would not rate the specifier *with delayed expression*. The vignette doesn't provide encouragement to add *with prominent dissociation*. I'd give him a GAF score of 35. Pending further information on substance use, Barney's diagnosis would read as follows:

F43.10	Posttraumatic stress disorder
F10.20	Alcohol use disorder, moderate, in early remission
Z60.2	Lives alone
Z56.9	Unemployed

There is still considerable controversy over the specifier *with delayed expression*. Some experts deny that symptoms of PTSD can begin many months or years after the trauma. Nonetheless, it is there to use, should you ever find it appropriate.

Posttraumatic Stress Disorder in Preschool Children

When preschool children are exposed to traumatic events, it is mostly by way of car accidents, natural disasters, abuse, and war—in short, all the benefits contemporary life has to offer. The question is, do very young children respond with typical PTSD symptoms? The best evidence would seem to indicate that they do, but with a likelihood much lower (0–12%) than for older children.

Table 6.1 compares the DSM-5-TR criteria for PTSD in young children, PTSD in adults, and acute stress disorder. The revamped criteria for PTSD in young children are, as we would hope, more sensitive to symptoms relevant to in this age group. Based on interviews with parents, they yield rates in children who have survived severe burns of 25% and 10% at 1 month and 6 months, respectively.

F43 Acute Stress Disorder

Based on the observation that some people develop symptoms immediately after a traumatic stress, acute stress disorder (ASD) was devised several decades ago. Even then, this wasn't exactly new information; something similar was noted as far back as 1865, just after the U.S. Civil War. For many years it was termed "shell shock." Like PTSD, ASD can also be found among civilians. Overall rates of ASD, depending on the nature of the trauma and personal characteristics of the individual, center on 20%, with women outnumbering men.

Though different in number and distribution of symptoms, the criteria embody the same elements required for PTSD:

- Exposure to an event that threatens body integrity
- Reexperiencing the event
- Avoidance of stimuli associated with the event
- Negative changes in mood and thought
- Increased arousal and reactivity
- Distress or impairment

The symptoms usually begin as soon as the patient is exposed to the event (or learns about it), but they must be experienced farther along than 3 days after the stressful event to fulfill the criterion for duration. This gets us past the stressful event itself and to its immediate aftermath. Should symptoms last longer than 1 month, they are no longer acute and no longer constitute ASD. Then, the diagnosis of many patients will roll over into PTSD—the case for as many as 80% of ASD patients. However, patients with PTSD often don't enter through the ASD doorway; half are identified farther along the road than the first month.

Essential Features of **Acute Stress Disorder**

Something truly awful has happened. One person has been gravely injured or perhaps sexually abused; another has viewed death, injury, or sexual trauma occurring to someone else; a third has learned that a close associate has experienced an accident or other form of violence. Emergency workers (police, firefighters) may be traumatized through repeated exposure during their work.

As a result, for up to a month the patient experiences many symptoms such as intrusive, distressing memories concerning the event; related bad dreams; dissociative

TABLE 6.1. Features of PTSD in Preschool Children, PTSD in Adults, and Acute Stress Disorder

Child PTSD (<7 years)	Adult PTSD	Acute stress disorder
	Trauma	
Direct experience	Direct experience	Direct experience
Witness	Witness	Witness
Learn of	Learn of	Learn of
	Repeat exposure (not just TV)	Repeat exposure (not just TV)
Intrusion symptoms (1/5)[a]	*Intrusion symptoms (1/5)*	*All symptoms (9/14)*
• Memories	• Memories	• Memories
• Dreams	• Dreams	• Dreams
• Dissociative reactions	• Dissociative reactions	• Dissociative reactions
• Psychological distress	• Psychological distress	• Psychological distress *or* physiological reactions
• Physiological reactions	• Physiological reactions	
Avoidance/negative emotions (1/6)	*Avoidance (1/2)*	
• Avoids memories	• Avoids memories	• Avoids memories
• Avoids external reminders	• Avoids external reminders	• Avoids external reminders
	Negative emotions (2/7)	• Altered sense of reality of self or surroundings
	• Amnesia	• Amnesia
	• Negative beliefs	
	• Distortion → self-blame	
• Negative emotional state	• Negative emotional state	
• Decreased interest	• Decreased interest	
• Social withdrawal	• Detached from others	
• Decreased positive emotions	• No positive emotions	• No positive emotions
Physiological (2/5)	*Physiological (2/6)*	
• Irritable, angry	• Irritable, angry	• Irritable, angry
	• Reckless, self-destructive	
• Hypervigilance	• Hypervigilance	• Hypervigilance
• Exaggerated startle	• Exaggerated startle	• Exaggerated startle
• Poor concentration	• Poor concentration	• Poor concentration
• Sleep disturbance	• Sleep disturbance	• Sleep disturbance
	Duration	
>1 month	>1 month	3 days–1 month

[a]Fractions indicate the number of symptoms required of the number possible in the following list.

experiences such as flashbacks or feeling unreal; or amnesia for parts of the event. There may be severe mental distress precipitated by internal or external reminders, or the inability to experience joy or love. Patients will attempt to avoid reminders (refusing to watch films or television or to read accounts of the event), pushing thoughts or memories out of consciousness. Also included are symptoms of hyperarousal: irritability, hypervigilance, trouble concentrating, insomnia, or an intense startle response.

The Fine Print

The D's: • Duration (3 days to 1 month) • Distress or disability (work/educational, social, or personal impairment) • Differential diagnosis (**substance use** and **physical disorders** (especially **traumatic brain injury**), **brief psychotic disorder,** panic disorder, mood disorders, dissociative disorders, PTSD, adjustment disorders)

Marie Trudeau

Marie Trudeau and her husband, André, sit in the intake interviewer's office. Although André does most of the talking, Marie is the patient. She spends most of the time rubbing the knuckles of one hand and gazing vacantly into the room.

"I just can't believe the change in her," he says. "A week ago, she was completely normal. Never had anything like this in her life. Heck, she's never had anything wrong with her, period. Then, all of a sudden, boom! She's a mess."

At André's exclamation, Marie jerks around to face him and rises half out of her chair. For a few seconds she stands there, frozen except for her gaze, which darts about the room.

"Aw, geez, I'm sorry, honey. I forgot." He puts his arm around her. Grasping her shoulders firmly but gently, he eases her back into the chair. He holds her there until she relaxes her grip on his arm.

He continues the story. A week earlier, Marie had just finished her gardening and was sitting in the backyard with a lemonade, reading a book. When she heard airplane engines, she looked up and saw two small planes flying high overhead, directly above her. "My God," she thought, "they're going to collide!" As she watched in horror, they did collide.

She could see perfectly. The sun was low, brilliantly highlighting the two aircraft against the deep blue of the late afternoon sky. Something seemed to have been torn off one of them—the news media later reported that the right wing of one plane had ripped right through the cockpit of the other. Thinking to call 911, Marie picked up her phone, but she didn't dial. She could only watch as two tiny objects suddenly appeared beside the stricken airplanes and tumbled toward her in leisurely arcs.

"They weren't objects, they were people." It's the first time she has spoken during the interview. Marie's chin trembles, and a lock of hair falls across her eye. She doesn't try to brush it back.

As she continued to watch, one of the bodies hurtled into her yard 15 feet from where she was sitting. It burrowed 6 inches deep into the soft earth behind her rose bushes.

What happened next, Marie seems to have blanked out completely. The other body landed in the street a block away. Half an hour later, when the police knocked on her door, they found her in the kitchen peeling carrots for supper and crying into the sink. When André arrived home an hour after that, she seemed dazed. All she would say was "I'm not here."

In the 6 days since, Marie hasn't changed much. Although she might start a conversation, something will appear to distract her, and she tends to trail off midsentence. She can't focus much better on her work at home. Amy, their 9-year-old daughter, seems to be taking care of her. Sleep has slipped to a restless struggle, and 3 nights running Marie has awakened from a dream, trying to cry out but managing only a terrified squeak. She keeps the kitchen blinds closed, so she won't even have to look into the backyard.

"It's like someone I saw in a World War II movie," André concludes. "You'd think she's shell-shocked."

Evaluation of Marie Trudeau

Anxiety and depressive symptoms are nearly universal following a severe stress. Usually these are relatively short-lived, however, and do not include the full spectrum of symptoms required for ASD. This diagnosis should only be considered when major symptoms last 3 days or more after personal exposure to a horrific event. Such an event is the plane crash Marie witnessed (criterion A2). She is dazed (B6) and emotionally unresponsive (B5) and cannot recall what happened during part of the incident (B7). When she can sleep at all (B10), she has nightmares (B2); she also avoids looking into the backyard (B9), startles easily (B14), and even in the interviewer's office appears hypervigilant (B12). From her inability to finish conversations, we infer poor concentration (B13), as she was distracted by intrusive recollections of the event (B1). DSM-5-TR requires 9 of the 14 symptoms listed in criterion B; as far as we are aware, prior to witnessing the accident she'd had none of them. Since the event, just a week earlier (C), she has been unable to carry on with her work at home (D).

Would any other diagnosis be possible? According to André, Marie's previous health has been good, reducing the likelihood of another medical condition (E). We aren't told whether she uses alcohol or drugs, though the fact that she was drinking lemonade at the time of the crash could suggest that she did not. (OK, I'm definitely out on a limb here; her clinician needs to rule out a substance use disorder.) Brief psychotic disorder would be ruled out by the lack of delusions, hallucinations, or disorganized behavior or speech.

Patients with ASD can have severe depressive symptoms ("survivor's guilt"), to the point that a concomitant diagnosis of major depressive disorder may sometimes be justified; Marie deserves further investigation along those lines. Until then, with a GAF score of 61, her diagnosis would be straightforward:

F43.0   Acute stress disorder

Adjustment Disorder

People with adjustment disorder (AD) may be responding to one stress or to many; the stressor may happen once or repeatedly. If the stressor goes on and on, it can even become chronic, as when a child lives with parents who fight continually. In clinical situations, the stressor has usually affected only one person, but it can affect many (think flood, fire, and famine). However, almost any relatively commonplace event could be a stressor for someone. For adults, examples most often cited are getting married or divorced, moving, and financial problems; adolescents often cite problems at school. Whatever the nature of the stressor, the patients feel overwhelmed by the demands of something in the environment.

As a result, they develop emotional symptoms such as low mood, crying spells, complaints of feeling nervous or panicky, and other depressive or anxiety symptoms— which must not, however, meet criteria for another defined mood or anxiety disorder. Some patients have mainly behavioral symptoms—especially some we might think of as conduct symptoms, such as driving dangerously, fighting, or defaulting on responsibilities.

The course tends to be brief; DSM-5-TR criteria specify that the symptoms must not persist longer than 6 months after the end of the stressor or its consequences. (Some studies report that a large minority of patients continue to have symptoms longer than the 6-month limit.) Of course, if the stressor is ongoing, such as a chronic illness, it may take a very long time for the patient to adjust.

Although AD has been reported in 10% or more of adult primary care patients, and in huge percentages of mental health patients, one study found a prevalence of only 3%; many of these patients were being inappropriately treated with psychotropic medications, and in only two cases had the AD diagnosis been made. The discrepancies probably rest on the somewhat flimsy criteria and on the (mistaken) view of AD as a residual diagnosis.

AD is found in all cultures and age groups, including children. It may be more firmly anchored in adults than in adolescents, whose early symptoms often evolve into other, more definitive mental disorders. The reliability and validity of AD tend to be quite low. In one study, fewer than two-thirds of patients receiving the clinical diagnosis of AD could be subsequently confirmed by ICD-10 criteria.

Personality disorders or cognitive disorders may make a person more vulnerable to stress, and hence to AD. Patients in whom AD is diagnosed often misuse substances as well.

Essential Features of **Adjustment Disorder**

An obvious stressor causes someone to develop depression, anxiety, or behavioral symptoms—but the response exceeds what you'd expect for most people in similar circumstances. After the stressor has ended, the symptoms might drag on a bit, but not longer than 6 additional months.

The Fine Print

The D's: • Duration (starts within 3 months of stressor's onset, stops within 6 months of stressor's end) • Distress or disability (work/educational, social, or personal impairment) • Differential diagnosis (just about everything you can name: substance use and physical disorders, **other mental disorders** such as mood and anxiety disorders, PTSD and acute stress disorder, somatic symptom disorder, psychotic disorders, conduct and other behavior disorders, milder reactions to life's stresses, **prolonged grief disorder, normal bereavement**)

Coding Notes

Specify:

F43.21 With depressed mood. The patient is mainly tearful, sad, or hopeless.

F43.22 With anxiety. The patient is mainly nervous, tense, or fearful of separation.

F43.23 With mixed anxiety and depressed mood. Symptoms combine the two above.

F43.24 With disturbance of conduct. The patient behaves inappropriately or unadvisedly, perhaps violating societal rules, norms, or the rights of others.

F43.25 With mixed disturbance of emotions and conduct. The clinical picture combines emotional and conduct symptoms.

F43.20 Unspecified. Use for other maladaptive stress-related reactions, such as physical complaints, social withdrawal, work or academic inhibition.

Specify if:

Acute. The condition has lasted less than 6 months.

Persistent (chronic). 6+ months duration of symptoms, though still not lasting more than 6 months after the stressor has ended.

Clarissa Wetherby

"I know it's temporary, and I know I'm overreacting. I sure don't want to, but I just feel upset!"

Clarissa Wetherby is referring to her husband's new work schedule. Arthur Wetherby is foreman on a road-paving crew whose current job is to widen and resurface a portion of the interstate highway just a few miles from the couple's house. Because the current section of the road involves an interchange with another major highway, the work must take place at night.

For the past 2 months, Arthur has slept days and left for work at 8:00 P.M. Clarissa works the day shift as cashier in a restaurant. Except on weekends, when he tries to sleep normal hours so they can be together, they hardly ever see one another. "I feel like I've been abandoned," she says.

The Wetherbys have been married only 3 years, and they have no children. Each is 35; each was married once before. Neither drinks or uses drugs. Clarissa's only previous encounter with the mental health system occurred 7 years ago, when her first husband left her for another man. "I respected his right not to continue living a lie," she says, "but I felt terribly alone and humiliated."

Clarissa's symptoms now are much as they were then. Most of the time when she is at work, she feels "about normal" and maintains good interest in what she is doing. But when alone at home in the evenings, waves of sadness overwhelm her. This leaves her virtually immobilized, unable even to turn on the television for company. She often cries to herself (and feels guilty for giving in to her emotions). "It's not as if someone died, after all," she says. Although she has some difficulty getting to sleep at night, she sleeps soundly in the morning. Her appetite is good, her weight has been constant, and she has had no suicidal ideas or death wishes. She does not report any problems with her concentration. She denies ever having symptoms of mania.

When she sought help before, she remained depressed and upset until a few weeks after the divorce was final. Then, suddenly, she seemed able to put it behind her and begin dating once again.

"I know I'll feel better, once Arthur gets off that schedule," she says. "I guess it just makes me feel worthless, playing second fiddle to an overpass."

Evaluation of Clarissa Wetherby

Clarissa herself recognizes that some might consider her reaction to the stress of her husband's work schedule to be extreme. That is one of the important features of this disorder: The patient's misery seems disproportionate to the stress that has apparently caused it (criterion B1). Her history provides a clue as to the source of her reaction: She is reminded of that awful time when her first husband abandoned her—for good, and under humiliating circumstances. It is important, however, always to consider carefully whether a patient's reaction occurs as a nonpathological response to a genuine danger. That wasn't the case with Clarissa.

The time course of Clarissa's symptoms is right for AD: They developed shortly after she first encountered Arthur's new work schedule (A). Although we cannot know how long this episode might last, her previous episode ended after a few months, when the aftermath of her divorce subsided (E). Of course, bereavement doesn't enter into her differential diagnosis (D).

Note that AD is not intended as a residual diagnosis, though it is often used that way. Nonetheless, it does come at the end of a long differential diagnosis that comprises many other DSM-5-TR conditions (C). For Clarissa, the symptoms of mood disorder are the most prominent. She has never been manic, so cannot qualify for a bipolar disorder. She has low mood, but only when alone in the evenings (not most of the day). She maintains interest in her work (rather than experiencing loss of interest in nearly all activities). Without at least one of those symptoms, there cannot be a diagnosis of major depressive disorder, regardless of her guilt feelings, low energy, and trouble getting to sleep at night. Of course, her symptoms have lasted far less than 2 years, ruling out persistent depressive disorder. Although she remains fully functional at work, she is seriously distressed, fulfilling the severity requirement.

The question of PTSD (or acute stress disorder) often arises in the differential diagnosis of AD. Each of those diagnoses requires that the stressor threaten serious harm and that the patient react with a variety of responses; Clarissa's situation does not fulfill these conditions. Similarly, she doesn't have symptoms that would suggest generalized anxiety disorder, another diagnosis prominent in the differential for AD. A personality disorder may worsen (and hence become more apparent) with stress, but there is no hint that Clarissa had any lifelong character pathology. I'd assign her a GAF score of 61.

F43.21   Adjustment disorder, with depressed mood, acute

Although some data support the utility of AD, which has been used clinically for decades, I recommend reserving it as a diagnosis of "almost last resort." There are several reasons for this warning.

For one thing, we probably too often use it when we simply have no better idea of what is going on. For another, the DSM-5-TR criteria do not tell us how we are to differentiate ordinary events from those that are stressful enough to cause depression, anxiety, or aberrant behavior. I suspect that events are often singled out on the basis that they cause an emotional or behavioral problem, and that seems to me a tad circular. But in the end, the determination of extraordinary stress rests with the patient, not with the observer.

F43.81 Prolonged Grief Disorder

When a loved one dies, we grieve. How we mourn the loss—the expressions whereby we convey our feelings—can take many forms and run a gamut of intensity from wearing somber clothing to maintaining stiff-lipped stoicism to repeated outbursts of despair and agony.

The emotions and the behaviors of our experience with grief derive from a variety of sources: our cultural norms, our connection to the one who has died, the support from others we care about, and our own innate personality factors. For a time after a death, reality typically intrudes in bursts or waves, elicited by reminders of the one we have lost. Then, though anniversary recurrences are common, within a few weeks or months the episodes gradually lessen before resolving to the point that we can focus on other issues in our lives. In a word, we move on.

But not everyone follows this trajectory. For perhaps 2–5% of bereaved individuals, especially females, and especially for those who might have been dependent on the deceased person for love or support (a child, for example, or a spouse), the experiences related to grief persist; symptoms crowd out other thoughts and behaviors long past the first-year anniversary of the death. These people have entered the realm of prolonged grief disorder (PGD).

People with this condition experience longing for or preoccupying thoughts of the departed that is accompanied by emotional pain or numbness; by cognitive issues such as rejection of the idea that the death has occurred or a view that life has become meaningless; by problems with their own identities (feeling partly dead); and by behavioral issues that include avoiding reminders of the death, and trouble rebuilding their own lives.

To a degree, this condition resembles posttraumatic stress disorder. In PTSD, however, the intrusive thoughts focus on the traumatic event itself, whereas in PGD the patient is preoccupied not with the death, but with the relationship with and yearning for the one who has died. (DSM-5-TR notes that when the traumatic event responsible for PTSD is a death, it must be "unnatural." So, a death due to a violent physical attack or automobile accident qualifies for PTSD; one caused by heart attack or cancer does not.) Of course, some of those with prolonged grief will also experience PTSD. That is, both PTSD and PGD can result from the same, violent, traumatic incident—but become evident in the differing time frames specified by these two diagnoses.

Another condition likely to be confused with PGD is severe depressive disorder. Of course, bereaved people typically express gloomy thoughts. But in prolonged grief, the morbid thoughts will be focused on the loss; in depression, they range more broadly, and may be accompanied by hopelessness. Additional symptomatic differences and similarities have been noted; for convenience, I have gathered them into a table (see Table 6.2).

As the DSM's newest disorder, much remains unclear about PGD. It affects only a small proportion of bereaved individuals—probably well under 10%, but just how far down into single digits is flat-out unknown. Rates may be higher in teenagers. Although first symptoms begin soon after learning of the death, full expression may take time. It tends to be worse if PTSD is also present. Males and females are probably about equally affected; older people may be more at risk, which is greater if the death is of a spouse or partner, or a child. And the death of a child may presage a course that is especially long or arduous.

Essential Features of **Prolonged Grief Disorder**

After the death of a close friend or relative, the person's depth of grief is demonstrated by powerful longings for or by preoccupying thoughts or memories of the dead person. (Circumstances of the death may preoccupy children or adolescents.)

Sorrow provokes three or more of the following eight symptoms: marked emotional pain; marked loneliness; emotional numbness (feelings have become less intense or absent); disbelief that the death has really happened; disrupted identity (e.g., the patient may feel partly dead); a feeling that life has become meaningless; avoidance of reminders of the death; trouble moving on with life (such as meeting with friends, making plans).

The Fine Print

The D's: • Duration (at least 12 months, 6 months in children; symptoms strongly present most days since the death, and nearly every day for the past month) • Distress or disability (work/educational, social, or personal impairment) • Differential diagnosis (normal grief, **PTSD,** major depressive disorder, **substance use disorders,** or any **other mental** or **medical disorder**) • Demographic carve-outs (accepted cultural, religious, and social customs cannot explain symptoms)

TABLE 6.2. Comparison of Major Depression with Prolonged Grief

	Major depression	Prolonged grief
Depressive thoughts	Generalized misery	Focus on the deceased
Sense of hopelessness	Often present	Not a characteristic
Main affects	Low mood, can't feel pleasure	Emptiness, loss
Intense longing for deceased	Not associated	Associated
Loss of personal worth; feels self-contempt	Associated	Not associated
Depressed mood is	Persistent	Comes in waves
Seeks smells, voice recordings of deceased	Not associated	Associated
Global guilt feelings; "I'm a burden"	Associated	Not associated
Avoidance behavior	General withdrawal	Associated with deceased
Death wishes	"I don't deserve to live"	"Wish to be with [deceased]"
Sleep disturbance	Common	Common
Appetite loss, weight loss	Common	Not common
Psychomotor retardation	Perhaps	

Note that the text describing some DSM-5-TR disorders (for example, delusional disorder, depersonalization/derealization disorder, fetishistic disorder) requests that we take into consideration cultural, age-appropriate, and religious background in determining whether the patient qualifies for the diagnosis. Other than a brief mention in the criteria for general personality disorder and in social anxiety disorder, prolonged grief disorder is the first time cultural considerations have been folded into the actual diagnostic criteria for a particular mental condition.

Maureen Kidd

On a Saturday afternoon, Maureen Kidd stands in a church vestibule, awaiting her groom. At age 27, she has never before ventured onto the bridal path. She and Jake have planned the day meticulously, right down to the choreographed first dance. She and her party (matron of honor, five bridesmaids, an adorable flower girl) wait half an hour before someone receives a text message: Jake isn't coming.

After an hour of frantic calls and texts, Maureen learns that he has met another woman with whom he is even now slinking out of town. Deeply distressed and horribly embarrassed, Maureen dissolves into tears. But as the days pass, she can rationalize, "Everything happens for a purpose; I just haven't found this one yet." Two years later, when she marries Matthew, the horticulture expert at the farm center where they both work, she realizes her purpose was just a little slow in appearing.

"Matthew is the best thing that's ever happened to me," Maureen tells everyone who will listen. Where Jake had been excitable and loud, Matthew is calm and soothing. "And he's thoughtful and generous and, let's be honest, Jake was pretty much a tightwad—he even had me buy my own ring." Months after the ceremony, she starts taking a botany class at the junior college so she can better help with new stock propagation at the nursery. She knows she sounds monotonous, but she loves to recite her new mantra: "In his work, in his person—Matt is perfect for me; our life together is perfect."

But in the early weeks of the COVID-19 pandemic, Matthew and Maureen reluctantly attend a company-sponsored party where there's a lot of hugging and back-slapping—and maybe a little coughing with not a mask in sight—and they both catch COVID-19. "I pulled through," she tells her therapist, "but after a short stint in the ICU and a boatload of heroic treatments, Matthew . . . Matthew died." She clenches her fists and bitterly weeps.

Though devastated, she assumes she'll work her way through. "That's the way it went with Mom when Dad died, more than a decade ago." Only, with Maureen, it doesn't go that way at all. "No matter how I force myself, I can't get past the feeling that the only thing left for me is to write my own obituary."

She drops her botany class and loses all interest in seeing her friends. "And that's probably fine with them—all I ever talk about is Matt. Of course, they tell me how sorry they are, but even I can see that I've become a total bore. When he died, he took so much of me with him."

She suffers the abiding desire for his embrace, his support, the deep connection they shared. "I'll awaken in the night with the loneliness, the enormity of my loss—it's like a physical weight that threatens to crush my chest. But no Advil or Tylenol can ever touch it. I've never been on a deserted island, but that's how it feels: abandoned and forever lost, even when I'm with other people."

Alone in the wee hours, she will ruminate about how needlessly he died, how stupid it was, how *criminal* that he was exposed to the virus. And her anger! For that holiday party, their boss had refused to hold the event outside. "My beloved husband—sacrificed to the god of commerce," she repeats over and over.

For a year now, she has slept in the guest room—even entering the bedroom she once shared with Matthew reduces her to acid tears. "I wake up in the night and, when he's not there beside me, I feel an emptiness I can never fill."

Evaluation of Maureen Kidd

There are three parts to the event that qualifies Maureen, or anyone, for consideration of prolonged grief disorder: (1) the death of someone dear (criterion A) leads to (2) intense grief, characterized by longing for (B1) or repetitive thinking about (B2) the dead person that (3) persists for 12 months or more and for the past month occurs every day, or nearly. Maureen's story easily ticks each of these boxes. Now we must determine that most days for the year (and nearly every day for the previous month) she has the majority of the eight possible social, emotional, and intellectual symptoms, each of which we must judge markedly intense. Let's see . . .

Sleeping in the guest bedroom would qualify as avoiding reminders of Matthew (criterion C3), and dropping her botany classes tells us that, far from moving on with her life, she's stuck on the off ramp of his death (C5). As for loneliness (C8), that's the very word she used with her therapist. And the crushing discomfort in her chest that no analgesic can ever address—that'll serve for emotional pain (C4). Would you count the statement about her obituary as one of identity disruption (C1)? I would, and so, I'm pretty sure, would Maureen.

Among the symptoms she *doesn't* have is disbelief that Matthew has died (C2)—she believes it, all right, it's right there in her face, every day. Though we could infer that she finds her life meaningless, to count it as a symptom (C7), we'd need to practice due diligence and ask. Also, far from emotional numbness (C6), she expresses stark anger at her needless loss. (Could a person experience both emotional numbness *and* intense emotional pain? Sequentially, perhaps, but at the same time? That would be a stretch.)

Then there's the fine print: duration, 12 months—*check;* distress and/or disability—*check and double check* (obvious distress *and* problematic work/social interactions, D). Demographic carve-outs (E)—we haven't explored her cultural, religious, and social background, but we do know that she hasn't followed her mom's example of grief recovery.

What about the differential diagnosis? We have no evidence of other mental or physical disorders; she doesn't drink alcohol or use drugs, and, though the death of a loved one could qualify for a diagnosis of posttraumatic stress disorder if it's violent, Matthew's death, though tragic and preventable, was from "natural causes"—a clear *no* for PTSD. But wait a minute—shouldn't we consider a mood disorder? She certainly is sad!

Here's where we can put to use Table 6.2, which shows the differences between mood disorder and the low mood associated with prolonged grief. To be brief, several of her symptoms (depressive thoughts, intense longing, avoidance behavior) fall into the prolonged grief column; none would I place in the depression column—save, perhaps, hopelessness, which we'll have to infer because we didn't think to ask. Of course, bereaved people can also have a diagnosable mood disorder, and we should be alert for one in Maureen. But at this evaluation, it isn't apparent, and puts paid to criterion F.

I'd put Maureen's GAF at somewhere below 50. Her diagnosis will be:

F43.81   Prolonged grief disorder

F94.1 Reactive Attachment Disorder

F94.2 Disinhibited Social Engagement Disorder

In two apparently rare but extremely serious disorders, children who have been mistreated (by accident or design) respond by becoming either markedly withdrawn or pathologically outgoing. For neither disorder do we have a lot of information, placing these two among the least well understood of mental disorders that affect children—or adults, for that matter.

Each disorder is conceived as a reaction to an environment in which the child experiences caregiving that is inconstant (frequent change of parent or surrogate) or pathological (neglect). One of two patterns then develops.

In reactive attachment disorder (RAD), even young infants withdraw from social contacts, appearing shy or distant. Inhibited children will resist separation by tantrums or desperate clinging. In severe cases, infants may exhibit failure-to-thrive syndrome, with length, weight, and head circumference hovering around the 3rd percentile on standard growth charts.

By contrast, a child's response in disinhibited social engagement disorder (DSED) borders on the promiscuous. Rather than showing typical wariness, small children boldly approach strangers; instead of clinging, they may appear indifferent to the departure of a parent. In both types, the abnormal responses are more obvious when the main caregiver is absent.

Factors that indicate increased risk for either RAD or DSED include being reared in an orphanage or other institution; protracted hospitalizations; multiple and frequent changes in caregivers; severe poverty; abuse (the gamut of physical, emotional, and sexual); and a family riven by death, divorce, or discord. Complications associated with these disorders include stunted physical growth, low self-esteem, delinquency, anger management issues, eating disorders, malnutrition, depression or anxiety, and later substance misuse.

In either disorder, a constant, nourishing relationship with a sensitive caregiver is required to reestablish adequate physical and emotional growth. Without such a remedy, the conditions tend to persist into adolescence. There have been almost no studies of follow-up into adult life; despite a dearth of reliable information, you will (of course) find websites. DSM-IV listed these two conditions as subcategories of one disorder. Because of differences in symptoms, course, treatment response, and other correlates, DSM-5-TR treats them as separate diagnoses—despite their supposed common etiology. However, some patients will appear withdrawn when very young, then become disinhibited later, whereas others have symptoms of both conditions simultaneously. The upshot is that some observers find the dichotomy a bit forced.

Neither disorder is encountered often, even in clinical populations, and DSM-5-TR notes that the majority of neglected children develop neither set of symptoms.

Essential Features of **Reactive Attachment Disorder**

Adverse child care (neglect, caregiving that is insufficient or changed too frequently) has apparently caused a child to withdraw emotionally; the child habitually neither seeks nor responds to soothing from an adult. Such children will show little emotional or social response to other people; far from having positive affect, they may experience periods of unprovoked irritability, fear, or sadness—even when with reassuring caregivers.

The Fine Print

The presumption of causality stems from the temporal relationship of the traumatic child care to the disturbed behavior.

The D's: • Demographics (begins before age 5; the child has a developmental age of at least 9 months) • Differential diagnosis (**autism spectrum disorder,** intellectual developmental disorder, depressive disorders)

Coding Notes

Specify if:

> **Persistent.** Symptoms are present longer than 1 year.
> **Severe.** All symptoms are present at a high level of intensity.

Essential Features of **Disinhibited Social Engagement Disorder**

Adverse child care (neglect, caregiving that is insufficient or changed too frequently) has apparently caused a child to become unreserved in approaching and interacting with unfamiliar adults. Such children, rather than showing typical first-acquaintance shyness, will little hesitate to pair off with a strange adult; they readily show excessively familiar physical or verbal behavior and don't "check in" with known caregivers—even in strange settings. Their behavior crosses usual cultural and social boundaries.

The Fine Print

The presumption of causality stems from the temporal relationship of the traumatic child care to the disturbed behavior.

The D's: • Demographics (child has developmental age of at least 9 months) • Differential diagnosis (autism spectrum disorder, intellectual developmental disorder, **ADHD**)

Coding Notes

Specify if:

> **Persistent.** Symptoms are present longer than 1 year.
> **Severe.** All symptoms are present at a high level of intensity.

F43.89 Other Specified Trauma- or Stressor-Related Disorder

This diagnosis will serve to categorize those patients for whom there is an evident stressor or trauma, but who for a specific, stated reason don't fulfill criteria for any of the standard diagnoses already mentioned above. DSM-5-TR gives several examples, including two forms of adjustment-like disorders (one form with delayed onset and another with prolonged duration relative to adjustment disorder). Others are as follows:

> **Adjustment-like disorders with onset of symptoms delayed beyond 3 months after the stressor.**

> **Adjustment-like disorders lasting beyond 6 months without prolonged stressor.**

The official titles as printed in DSM-5-TR of these are way longer than need be; I couldn't resist truncating them.

> **Persistent response to trauma with PTSD-like symptoms.** The symptoms don't fully meet PTSD criteria and last longer than 6 months.

> **Various cultural syndromes.** You'll find a number of these in an appendix in DSM-5-TR, page 874.

F43.9 Unspecified Trauma- or Stressor-Related Disorder

This diagnosis will cover those patients for whom there is an evident stressor or trauma, but who don't fulfill criteria for any of the standard diagnoses already mentioned above, and for whom you do not care to specify the reasons why the criteria are not fulfilled.

CHAPTER 7

Dissociative Disorders

Quick Guide to the Dissociative Disorders

Dissociative symptoms are principally covered in this chapter, but there are some conditions (especially involving loss or lapse of memory) that are classified elsewhere.

Primary Dissociative Disorders

Dissociative amnesia. The patient cannot remember important information that is usually of a personal nature. This amnesia tends to be stress-related (p. 243).

Dissociative identity disorder. One or more additional identities intermittently seize control of the patient's behavior (p. 240).

Depersonalization/derealization disorder. The patient has episodes of feeling detached from the patient's own self or mind or from the (unreal-seeming) environment. In this condition, there is no actual memory loss (p. 249).

Other specified, or unspecified, dissociative disorder. Patients who have symptoms suggestive of any of the disorders above, but who do not meet criteria for any one of them, may be placed in one of these two categories (p. 251).

Other Causes of Marked Memory Loss

When dissociative symptoms are encountered in the course of other mental diagnoses, a separate diagnosis of a dissociative disorder is not ordinarily given.

Panic attack. Some patients may experience depersonalization or derealization as part of an acute panic attack (p. 172).

Posttraumatic stress disorder. A month or more following a severe trauma, the patient may not remember important aspects of personal history (p. 218).

Acute stress disorder. Immediately following a severe trauma, patients may not remember important aspects of personal history (p. 223).

Somatic symptom disorder. Patients who have a history of multiple somatic symptoms that distress them or cause marked disruption to their daily lives may forget important aspects of personal history (p. 254).

Non-rapid eye movement sleep arousal disorder, sleepwalking type. Sleepwalking resembles the dissociative disorders, in that there is amnesia for purposeful behavior. But it is classified with all the other sleep disorders (p. 336).

Borderline personality disorder. When severely stressed, these people will sometimes experience episodes of dissociation, such as depersonalization (p. 561).

Malingering. Some people consciously feign symptoms of memory loss. Their object is material gain, such as avoiding punishment or obtaining money or drugs (p. 616).

Introduction

Dissociation occurs when one group of mental processes becomes separated from the rest. In essence, some of an individual's thoughts, feelings, or behaviors are removed from conscious awareness and control. An example: An otherwise healthy college student cannot recall any of the events of the previous 2 weeks.

As with so many other mental symptoms, you can have dissociation without disorder; if it's mild, it can be entirely normal. (For example, while enduring a boring lecture, did you ever daydream about your weekend plans, unaware that you'd been called on for a response?) There's also a close connection between the phenomena of dissociation and hypnosis. Indeed, over half the people interviewed in some surveys have had some experience of a dissociative nature.

Episodes of dissociation severe enough to constitute a disorder have several features in common:

- They usually begin and end suddenly.

- They are perceived as a disruption of information that is needed by the individual. They can be *positive*, in the sense of something added (for example, flashbacks) or *negative* (an event or a time period for which the person has no memory).

- Although clinicians often disagree as to etiology, many episodes appear to be precipitated by psychological conflict.

- Often, they are encountered in people who have suffered trauma of one sort or another.

- Although they are generally regarded as rare, their numbers may be increasing.

- In most disorders (except depersonalization/derealization), there is a profound disturbance of memory.

- Impaired functioning or a subjective feeling of distress is required only for dissociative amnesia and depersonalization/derealization disorder.

In its introduction to dissociative disorders, DSM-5-TR informs us that, because patients often dissociate following traumatic experiences, the dissociative disorders are placed next to the trauma-caused disorders in the book—as a physical verification of their close relationship. I can't think of any other such juxtaposition in DSM-5-TR.

F44.81 Dissociative Identity Disorder

In dissociative identity disorder (DID), which previously achieved notoriety as multiple personality disorder, the person possesses two or more distinct identities. Ranging up to 200 in number, they may not even be of the patient's own gender, these identities may have their own names. Some may be symbolic, such as "The Worker." They can vary widely in age and style: If the patient is usually shy and quiet, one identity may be outgoing or even boisterous.

The identities may to some degree be aware of one another, though only one interacts with the environment at a time. The transition from one to another is often sudden, perhaps precipitated by stress. Most patients are aware of the loss of time that occurs when another identity is in control. However, some only become aware of their peculiar state when the alterations in character with time are pointed out. Note that, even among DID patients, it is unusual to encounter full expression of identity—names, clothing, accents, handwriting, and other features of person and personality.

Of special diagnostic note are states of pathological possession, which can have characteristics similar to DID. They may be described by the patient as a spirit or other external being that has taken over the person's functioning. If this behavior is part of a recognized, accepted cultural or religious practice, it will not usually qualify for diagnosis as DID. But a person who has recurrent states of possession that cause distress and otherwise conform to DSM-5-TR criteria may well qualify for diagnosis. Of course, we would not diagnose DID in a child who has an imaginary playmate.

The onset of this perhaps too-fascinating disorder is usually in childhood, though it is not commonly recognized then. Affecting up to 1% of the general population, most of the patients are female, and many may have been sexually abused. Indeed, DSM-5-TR notes that PTSD is frequently comorbid. DID tends toward chronicity. It may run in families, but the question of genetic transmission is also unresolved.

Essential Features of **Dissociative Identity Disorder**

A patient appears to have at least two clearly individual personalities, each with unique attributes of mood, perception, recall, and control of thought and behavior. The result: memory gaps for personal information and recent experience that common forgetfulness cannot begin to explain.

The Fine Print

The D's: • Distress or disability (work/educational, social, or personal impairment) • Differential diagnosis (**substance use** and **physical disorders,** major depressive or bipolar disorder, anxiety disorders, psychotic disorders, PTSD, other dissociative disorders, religious possession states or cultural practices, childhood imaginary playmates/fantasy play), malingering, factitious disorder • Demographic carve-out (symptoms are not related to widely accepted cultural or religious practices)

DID is diagnosed much more commonly by clinicians in North America than in Europe. This fact has engendered a long-running dispute. European clinicians (naturally) claim that the disorder is rare, and that by paying so much attention to patients who dissociate, New World clinicians encourage the development of cases. At this writing, the two camps continue to argue—as if possessed.

Effie Jens

On her first visit to the mental health clinic, Effie cries and talks about her failing memory. On some days, at age 26—"way too young for Alzheimer's," she sobs—she feels senile. For several months she has noticed holes in her memory. These sometimes last 2 or 3 days. Her recall isn't just spotty; for all she knows about her activities on those days, "I might as well have been under anesthesia." However, from telltale signs—such as food that has disappeared from her refrigerator and recently arrived letters that have been opened—she knows she must have been awake and functioning during these times.

On the proceeds of the property settlement from her recent divorce, Effie lives alone in a small apartment; her relatives all dwell in a distant city. She enjoys quiet pastimes, such as reading and watching television. She is shy and has trouble meeting people; there is no one she sees often enough to help her account for the missing time.

For that matter, Effie isn't all that clear about the details of her earlier life. The second of three daughters of an itinerant preacher; her early childhood memories are a jumble of labor camps, cheap hotel rooms, and Bible-thumping sermons. By the time she reached her teens, she had attended 15 different schools.

Late in the interview, she reveals that she has virtually no memory of the entire year she was 13. Her father's preaching had been moderately successful, and they had settled in a small town in southern Oregon—the only time she had started and finished a year in the same school. But what had happened to her during the intervening months? Of that period, she recalls nothing whatsoever. Evidently puzzled, she carefully grips the arms of her chair.

The following week, she returns to the clinic. But she seems a different person. "Call me Liz," she says as she drops her shoulder bag onto the floor, sits, and crosses her legs. Without prompting, she launches into a long, detailed, and frankly dramatic recounting of the past 3 days. She went out for dinner and dancing with a man she'd met in the grocery store; afterward, they hit a couple of bars together.

"But I only had ginger ale," she says with a smile. "I never drink. It's terrible for the figure."

"Are there any parts of last week you can't remember?"

"Oh, no. *She's* the one with amnesia."

"She" is Effie Jens, whom Liz clearly regards as a person quite different from her own self. Liz is happy, carefree, and sociable; Effie is introspective and prefers solitude. "I'm not saying that she isn't a decent human being," Liz concedes, "but you've met her—don't you think she's just a tad mousy?"

Although for many years she has "shared living space" with Effie, it wasn't until after the divorce that Liz began to come out. At first, this was for only an hour or two, especially when Effie was tired or depressed and needed a break. Recently, Liz takes control for longer and longer periods of time. Once, Liz stayed out for 3 days.

"I try to be careful, it frightens her so," Liz says with a worried frown. "I've begun to think seriously about taking control for all time. I think I can do a better job. I certainly have a more interesting social life."

Besides being able to recount her activities during the blank times that drove Effie to seek care, Liz can give eyewitness account of all of Effie's conscious activities. She even knows what had happened during Effie's "lost" year when she was 13.

"It was Daddy," Liz says with a curl of her lip. "He said it was part of his religious mission to 'practice for a reenactment of the Annunciation.' But it was really just another randy male groping his own daughter, and worse. Effie told Mom. At first, Mom wouldn't believe her. And when she finally did, she made Effie promise never to tell. She said it would break up the family. All these years, I'm the only other one who's known about it. No wonder she's losing her grip—it even makes me feel nauseous."

Evaluation of Effie Jens

Effie's two personalities (criterion A) are typical of DID: One is quiet and unassuming, the other assertive. (But Effie's history is atypical: More than two personalities is the rule.) What happens when Liz is in control is unknown to Effie, who experiences these episodes as amnesia. This difficulty with recall is vastly more extensive than you'd expect from common forgetfulness (B). It is distressing enough to send Effie in search of help (C).

Several other causes of amnesia should be considered in the differential diagnosis of this condition. Of course, any possible medical condition must be ruled out, but Effie/Liz has no history suggestive of either a seizure disorder or substance use (I'm thinking of partial seizures and alcoholic blackouts). Even though Effie has a significant problem with amnesia, it isn't her main problem, as would be the case with dissociative amnesia, which is less often recurrent and does not involve multiple, distinct identities. Note, too, the absence of any information that Effie belongs to a cultural or religious group whose practices included trances or other rituals that could explain her amnesia (D).

Schizophrenia has sometimes been confused with DID, primarily by laypeople who equate "split personality" (which is how some in the general public characterize schizophrenia) with multiple personality disorder, the old name for DID. However, although bizarre behavior may be encountered in DID, the identities are not usually psychotic. As with other dissociative disorders, discrimination from malingering can be difficult; information from others about possible material gain provides the most valuable data. Effie's history is not typical for either of these diagnoses.

Some patients with DID will also have borderline personality disorder. The danger is that only the latter will be diagnosed by a clinician who mistakes alternating personae for the unstable mood and behavior typical of borderline personality disorder. Substance-related disorders sometimes occur with DID; neither Effie nor Liz drinks alcohol (E). GAF score would be 55.

| F44.81 | Dissociative identity disorder |
| Z63.5 | Divorce |

F44.0 Dissociative Amnesia

There are two main requirements for dissociative amnesia (DA): (1) The patient has forgotten something important, and (2) other disorders have been ruled out. Of course, the central feature is the inability to remember significant events. Over 100 years ago, clinicians like Pierre Janet recognized several patterns in which this forgetting can occur:

Localized (or circumscribed). The patient has recall for none of the events that occurred within a particular time frame, often during a calamity such as a wartime battle or a natural disaster. This is the most common pattern in patients with DA.

Selective. Certain periods of time, such as the birth of a child, have been forgotten. This type is less common.

The next three types are much less common, and may eventually lead to a diagnosis of dissociative identity disorder (see below):

Generalized. All the experiences during the patient's entire lifetime have been forgotten. It is classically found in combat survivors and victims of sexual assault and may be associated with fugue.

Continuous. The patient forgets all events from a given time forward to the present. This is now extremely rare.

Systematized. The patient has forgotten certain classes of information, such as those relating to family or to work—or being abused.

DA begins suddenly, usually following severe stress such as physical injury, guilt about an extramarital affair, abandonment by a spouse, or internal conflict over sexual issues. Sometimes the patient wanders aimlessly near home. Duration ranges widely, from minutes to perhaps years. The amnesia usually ends abruptly with complete recovery of memory. In some individuals, it may occur again, perhaps more than once.

DA has still received insufficient study, so too little is known about demographic patterns, family occurrence, and the like. Beginning during early adulthood, it is most commonly reported in young women; it may occur in under 1% of the general population, though recent surveys have pegged it somewhat higher—even an astonishing 1.8% in one small U.S. community. Many patients with DA have reported childhood sexual trauma, with a high percentage who cannot remember the actual abuse.

Dissociative Fugue

In the subtype of DA known as dissociative fugue, the amnesic person suddenly journeys from home. This often follows a severe stress, such as marital strife or a natural or human-made disaster. The individual may experience disorientation and a sense of perplexity. Some will assume a new identity and name, and for months may even work at a new occupation. However, in most instances the episode is a brief period of travel, lasting a few hours or days. Occasionally, there may be outbursts of violence. Recovery may be sudden, with subsequent amnesia for the episode.

Dissociative fugue is another of those extraordinarily interesting disorders—fodder for novels and motion pictures—that are reportedly common but about which there has been far too little solid research. It was demoted from an independent diagnosis in DSM-IV to a specifier for dissociative amnesia in DSM-5 and later. It is interesting that fugue also occurs with dissociative identity disorder, yet the specifier is not applied to DID.

Essential Features of **Dissociative Amnesia**

Far beyond common forgetfulness, the person cannot recall important (usually distressing or traumatic) personal information.

The Fine Print

The D's: • Distress or disability (work/educational, social, or personal impairment) • Differential diagnosis (**substance use** and **physical disorders** [especially **seizure disorders** and **traumatic brain injury**], **neurocognitive disorders, PTSD, acute distress disorder, dissociative identity disorder, somatic symptom disorder,** ordinary forgetfulness, malingering and factitious disorder)

Coding Note

If relevant, specify:

F44.1 With dissociative fugue

Holly Kahn

A mental health clinician presents the following case history to a medical center ethicist.

A 38-year-old woman has been seen several times in the outpatient clinic. She complains of depression and anxiety, both of which are relatively mild. These symptoms seem focused on the fact that she is 38 and unmarried, and her "biological clock is ticking." She has had no problems with sleep, appetite, or weight gain or loss, no thoughts about suicide.

For many months Holly Kahn had so longed for a child that she intentionally became pregnant by her then boyfriend. When he discovered what she had done, he broke off their relationship. The following week she miscarried. Stuck in her boring salesclerk job, she says she's come to the clinic for help in "finding meaning for her life."

The oldest girl in a Midwestern family, Holly spent much of her adolescence caring for younger siblings. Although she attended college for 2 years during her mid-20s, she left school with neither degree nor career to show for it. In the last decade, she has lived with three different men; her latest relationship lasted the longest and had seemed the most stable. She has no history of drug or alcohol abuse and is in good physical health.

The clinician's verbal description is of a plain, no longer young (and perhaps never youthful), heavy-set woman with a square jaw and stringy hair. "In fact, she looks quite a lot like this." The clinician produces a drawing of a woman's head and shoulders. It is somewhat indistinct and smudged, but the features closely match the verbal description. The ethicist recognizes it as a flyer that has recently received wide distribution. Below the picture, the copy reads: "Wanted by FBI on suspicion of kidnapping."

A day-old infant has been abducted from a local hospital's maternity ward. The first-time mother, barely out of her teens, had handed her baby girl to a woman wearing operating room scrubs. The woman had introduced herself as a nursing supervisor and said she needed to take the baby for a final weighing and examination before discharge. That was the last time anyone could remember seeing either the woman or the baby. The picture was drawn by a police artist from a description given by the distraught mother. A reward was being offered by the baby's grandparents.

The mental health clinician continues. "The next-to-last time I saw my patient, we were trying to work on ways she could take control over her own life. She seemed quite a bit more confident, less depressed. The following week she came in late, looking dazed. She claimed to have no memory of anything she had done for the past several days. I asked her whether she'd been ill, hit on the head, that sort of thing. She denied all of it. I started probing backward to see if I could jog her memory, but she became more and more agitated and finally rushed out. She said she'd return the next week, but I haven't seen her since. It wasn't until yesterday that I noticed her resemblance to the woman in this picture."

The therapist sits gazing at the flyer for a few seconds, then says: "Here's my dilemma. I think I know who committed this awful crime, but I have a privileged relationship with the person I suspect. Just what is my ethical duty?"

Evaluation of Holly Kahn

Whether Holly took the baby is not the point here. At issue is the cause of her evident amnesia, which is her most pressing recent problem (criterion A). She has been under stress because of her desire to have a baby, and this could have provided the stimulus for her amnesia. The episode was itself evidently stressful enough that she broke off contact with her clinician (B).

The vignette provides no information that might support other (mostly biological) causes of amnesia (D). Specifically, we know of no head trauma that might have induced a major neurocognitive disorder due to traumatic brain injury. Substance-induced neurocognitive disorder, persistent would be ruled out by Holly's history of no substance use (C). Her general health has been good and there is no history of abnormal physical movements, reducing the likelihood of epilepsy. Although she has had a miscarriage, too much time has passed for a postmiscarriage psychosis to be a possibility. Some patients with amnesia are also mute; they may be misdiagnosed as having another medical condition with catatonic symptoms. And, just to be complete, we should note that her loss of memory is far more striking and significant than ordinary forgetfulness—which we humans experience all the time.

Holly has no history of a recent, massive trauma that might indicate acute stress disorder. If she is malingering, she does it without an obvious motive (if she is trying to avoid punishment for a crime, simply staying away from the medical center would serve her better). It certainly wouldn't appear to be a case of typical daydreaming. Holly is clear about her personal identity, and she has not traveled from home, so she doesn't qualify for the dissociative fugue specifier and code change. Although we must be careful to avoid diagnosing a patient we have not personally interviewed and for whom we lack adequate collateral information, if what material we do have is borne out by subsequent investigation, her diagnosis would be as below. I'd give her GAF score as 31.

Functional neurological (conversion) symptoms are typical of the somatic symptom disorders and dissociation and tend to involve the same psychic mechanisms. Whenever you encounter a patient who dissociates, consider whether such a diagnosis is also warranted.

F44.0   Dissociative amnesia

John Doe

When he walks into the homeless shelter, he hasn't a thing to his name, including a name. He's been referred from a hospital emergency room, but he tells the clinician on duty that he's only looking for a place to stay. As far as he's aware, his physical health is good. His problem is that he doesn't remember a thing about his life prior to waking up at dawn this morning on a park bench. Later, when filling out the paperwork, the clinician pencils "John Doe" in the space for "patient's name."

If you ignore the fact that he can give a history spanning only about 8 hours, John Doe's mental status exam seems unremarkable. He appears to be in his early 40s. He is dressed casually in slacks, a pink dress shirt, and a nicely fitting corduroy sports jacket with leather patches on the elbows. His speech is clear and coherent; his affect is generally pleasant, though the loss of memory obviously troubles him. He denies having hallucinations or delusions ("as far as I know"), though he points out logically enough that "I can't vouch for what kind of crazy ideas I might have had yesterday."

John Doe appears intelligent, and his fund of information is good. He can name five recent presidents in order and discuss recent national and international events. He repeats eight digits forward and six backward without error. He scores 29 out of 30 on the MMSE, failing only to identify the county in which the shelter is located. Although he surmises that he must be married (he wears a wedding ring), after a half-hour conversation he still can remember nothing pertaining to his family, occupation, place of residence, or personal identity.

"Show me the inside of your sports coat," the clinician says.

After a moment of perplexed hesitation, John Doe unbuttons the jacket and holds it open. The label bears the name of a men's clothing store in Cincinnati 500 miles away.

"Let's try there," the clinician suggests. Several telephone calls later, the Cincinnati Police Department identifies John Doe as an attorney whose wife reported him missing 2 days ago.

The next morning John Doe is on a bus for home. Days later, the clinician learns the rest of the story. A 43-year-old specialist in wills and probate, John Doe had been accused of comingling the bank accounts of clients with his own. He protested his innocence and has hired his own attorney, but the Ohio State Bar Association stands ready to proceed against him. The pressure to straighten out his books, maintain his law practice, and defend himself in court and against his own state bar has been enormous. Two days before he disappeared, he told his wife, "I don't know if I can take much more of this without losing my mind."

Evaluation of John Doe

John Doe is classically unable to recall important autobiographical information—in fact, all of it (criterion A). It is understandable—and required for the diagnosis (B)—that this troubles him.

Neither at the time of evaluation nor at follow-up is there evidence of alternative disorders (D). John has not switched repeatedly between identities, ruling out dissociative identity disorder (you wouldn't diagnose these two together). Other than obvious amnesia, there is no evidence of a cognitive disorder. At age 43, a new case of temporal lobe epilepsy would be unlikely, but a complete evaluation should include a neurological workup. Of course, any patient who has episodes of amnesia must be evaluated for substance-related disorders (especially as concerns alcohol, C).

The conscious imitation of amnesia of malingering can be very difficult to discriminate from the amnesia involved in DA with dissociative fugue. However, although John Doe does have legal difficulties, these would not be relieved by feigned amnesia. (When malingering appears to be a possibility, collateral history from relatives or friends of previous such behavior or of antisocial personality disorder can help.) A history of lifelong multiple medical symptoms might suggest somatic symptom disorder. John has no cross-sectional features that would suggest either a manic episode or schizophrenia, in either of which wandering or bizarre behaviors can occur.

Epilepsy is prominent in the differential diagnosis of the dissociative disorders. However, epilepsy and dissociation should not be too hard to tell apart, even without the benefit of an EEG. Epileptic episodes usually last no longer than a few minutes and involve speech and motor behaviors that are repetitive and apparently purposeless. Dissociative behavior, on the other hand, may continue for days or longer, involving complex speech and motor actions that appear purposeful.

Although John Doe's case is not quite classical (he did not assume a new identity and inhabit a new life), he did travel far from home and purposefully set about seeking shelter. That sets up the specifier for his diagnosis. And along the way, I'd put his GAF at 55.

| F44.1 | Dissociative amnesia, with dissociative fugue |
| Z65.3 | Investigation by state bar association |

Note that the fugue subtype has a different code number than plain vanilla dissociative amnesia. This reflects the fact that, in ICD-10, a fugue state is a diagnosis separate and apart from dissociative amnesia. So, the number change is a feature, not a bug.

F48.1 Depersonalization/Derealization Disorder

We'll define *depersonalization* as a sense of being cut off or detached from oneself. This feeling may be experienced as viewing one's own mental processes or behavior; some people feel as though they are in a dream; others may experience lack control of their own bodies—rather like a robot. When a person is repeatedly distressed by episodes of depersonalization, and there is no other disorder that better accounts for the symptoms, you can diagnose depersonalization/derealization disorder (DDD).

DSM-5-TR offers another route to that diagnosis: through the experience of *derealization*. This is the feeling that the exterior world appears unreal or odd, as though the patient were dreaming or perhaps viewing things through a fog. Patients may notice that the appearance of objects (size, shape, color) has changed, or that other people seem robotic or even dead. Always, however, the person retains insight that it is only a change in perception—that the world itself has remained the same.

The fact that about half of all adults have had at least one such episode requires that we limit who receives this diagnosis. It should not be made unless the symptoms are persistent or recurrent, and unless they impair functioning or cause significant distress—something considerably beyond the bemused reflection, "Well, *that* was weird!" In fact, depersonalization and derealization are much more commonly encountered as symptoms than as a diagnosis. For example, derealization or depersonalization is a qualifying symptom for panic attack (p. 172).

Episodes of DDD are often precipitated by stress; they may begin and end suddenly. The disorder usually has its onset in the teens or even earlier; it may be initially precipitated by drug use such as marijuana, ketamine, or ecstasy; however, if it is only experienced with drug use, it won't be called DDD. Perhaps half the population has experienced a brief episode at some time, but general population prevalence rates for DDD in full appear to be down around 1–2%, with males and females nearly equal. Once begun, it tends to be chronic.

Essential Features of **Depersonalization/Derealization Disorder**

A patient repeatedly experiences depersonalization or derealization, during which reality testing remains intact. (For definitions, see above).

The Fine Print

The D's: • Distress or disability (work/educational, social, or personal impairment) • Differential diagnosis (**substance use** and **physical disorders, major depressive** and **panic disorders, psychotic disorders, PTSD, acute stress disorder, schizophrenia, other dissociative disorders**)

Francine Parfit

"It feels like I'm losing my mind." Francine Parfit is only 20 years old, but she has already worked as a bank teller for nearly 2 years. With several pay raises already to her credit, she believes that she is good at her job—conscientious, personable, and reliable. And healthy, though she's been increasingly troubled by what she calls her "out-of-body experiences."

"I'll be standing behind my counter and, all of a sudden, I'm also standing a couple of feet away. I seem to be looking over my own shoulder as I'm talking with my customer. And in my head, I'm commenting to myself on my own actions. It's like I'm a different person who I'm watching. Stuff like 'Now she'll have to call the assistant manager to get approval for this transfer of funds.' I came to the clinic because I saw something like this on television a few nights ago, and the person got shock treatments. That's when I began to worry something really awful was wrong."

Francine denies that she has ever had blackout spells, convulsions, blows to the head, severe headaches, or dizziness. In high school she smoked pot a time or two, but otherwise she's kept herself free of drugs and alcohol. Her physical health has been excellent; her only visits to physicians have been for immunizations, Pap smears, and a preemployment physical exam 2 years ago.

Each episode begins suddenly, without warning. First Francine will feel anxious; then she'll notice that her head seems to bob up and down; it's only a slight nodding, but it's beyond her control. Occasionally she'll feel a warm sensation on the top of her head, as if someone has cracked a parboiled egg that's now dribbling yolk through her hairline.

These episodes seldom last longer than a few minutes, but they are becoming more frequent—several times a week now. If they occur while she's at work, she can usually take a break until they pass. But several times it's happened when she is driving. She worries she might lose control of her car.

Francine has never heard voices or had hallucinations of other senses, but she acknowledges that, when she's having an episode, the world seems "a little fuzzy"; she denies ever feeling in any way talked about or plotted against. She has never had suicidal ideas and doesn't feel depressed.

"Just scared," she concludes. "It's so spooky to feel that you've sort of died."

Evaluation of Francine Parfit

The sensation of being an outside observer of yourself can indeed be quite unsettling; it is one that many people who are not patients have had a time or two. What makes Francine's experience stand out is that it returns so often (criterion A1) and so forcibly that she seeks an evaluation (C). (She is a little unusual in that her episodes didn't seem to be precipitated by stress; in many people, they are.) Notice that she describes her experience "like I'm a different person," not "I *am* a different person." This tells us that she has retained contact with reality (B).

Francine's experiences and feelings are much like those of Shorty Rheinbold (p. 174); however, his depersonalization occurred as a symptom of **panic disorder.** A variety of other conditions include depersonalization as a symptom: **posttraumatic stress disorder; anxiety, cognitive, mood, personality,** and **substance-related disorders; schizophrenia;** and **epilepsy** (D, E). However, Francine does not complain of panic attacks or have symptoms of other disorders that could account for the symptoms. Francine could also have received this diagnosis had she experienced only symptoms of derealization.

With a GAF score of 70, her diagnosis would be:

F48.1   Depersonalization/derealization disorder

F44.89 Other Specified Dissociative Disorder

This category is for patients whose symptoms represent a change in the integrative functions of identity, memory, or consciousness, but who do not meet criteria for one of the specific dissociative disorders listed above. Here are some examples; a particular condition should be stated after the other specified diagnosis is given.

Identity disturbance due to prolonged and intense coercive persuasion. People who have been brainwashed or otherwise indoctrinated may develop mixed dissociative states.

Syndromes of mixed dissociative symptoms. With no frank dissociative amnesia, such a person might experience chronic or recurrent milder symptoms that wouldn't qualify for a better-defined dissociative diagnosis.

Acute dissociative reactions to stressful events. DSM-5-TR mentions that these often last just a few hours, always less than a month, and are characterized by mixed dissociative symptoms (depersonalization, derealization, amnesia, disruptions of consciousness, stupor).

Dissociative trance. The patient experiences reduced awareness of the here and now, becoming unresponsive to stimuli. (Someone engaging in an accepted religious or cultural ritual would not qualify as an example of dissociative trance.)

F44.9 Unspecified Dissociative Disorder

Here we can categorize those patients who have evident dissociative symptoms but do not fulfill criteria for any of the standard diagnoses already mentioned above, and for whom we do not care to specify the reasons.

CHAPTER 8

Somatic Symptom and Related Disorders

Quick Guide to the Somatic Symptom and Related Disorders

When somatic (body) symptoms are a prominent reason for evaluation by a clinician, the diagnosis will often be one of the disorders (or categories) listed below.

Primary Somatic Symptom Disorders

Somatic symptom disorder. Formerly called somatization disorder, these patients have a history of multiple somatic symptoms that distress them or cause marked disruption to their daily lives (p. 254).

Somatic symptom disorder, with predominant pain. The pain in question has no apparent physical or physiological basis, or it far exceeds usual expectations, given the patient's actual physical condition (p. 260).

Functional neurological symptom disorder (formerly conversion disorder). These patients complain of isolated symptoms that seem to have no physical cause (p. 266).

Illness anxiety disorder. Formerly called hypochondriasis, this is a disorder in which physically healthy people have an unfounded fear of a serious, often life-threatening illness such as cancer or heart disease, but little in the way of somatic symptoms (p. 263).

Psychological factors affecting other medical conditions. A patient's mental or emotional issues influence the course or care of a medical disorder (p. 270).

Factitious disorder imposed on self. Patients who want to occupy the sick role (perhaps they enjoy the attention of being in a hospital) consciously fabricate symptoms to attract attention from health care professionals (p. 272).

Factitious disorder imposed on another. A person induces symptoms in someone else, often a child, possibly for the purpose of gaining attention or sympathy (p. 273).

Other specified, or unspecified, somatic symptom and related disorder. These are catch-all categories for patients whose somatic symptoms fail to meet criteria for any better-defined disorder (p. 279).

Other Causes of Somatic Complaints

Actual physical illness. Psychological causes for physical symptoms should be considered only after physical disorders have been eliminated.

Mood disorders. Pain with no apparent physical cause is characteristic of some patients with major depressive disorder (p. 116) and bipolar I disorder, current or most recent episode depressed (p. 126).

Substance use. Patients who use substances may complain of pain or other physical symptoms. These may result from the effects of substance intoxication (p. 419) or withdrawal (p. 410).

Adjustment disorder. Some patients who are experiencing a reaction to environmental circumstances will complain of pain or other somatic symptoms (p. 227).

Malingering. These people know that their somatic or psychological symptoms are fabricated, and their motive is some form of material gain, such as avoiding punishment or work, or obtaining money or drugs (p. 616).

Introduction

For centuries, clinicians have recognized that physical symptoms and concerns about health can have emotional origins. DSM-III and its successors have gathered such diagnoses under one umbrella. Collectively, these are now called the somatic symptom and related disorders because their presentations are concerned with somatic (bodily) disease. Like so many other groups of disorders discussed in this book, these conditions are not bound together by common etiologies, family histories, treatments, or other factors. This chapter is simply another convenient collection—in this case, of conditions that prominently involve physical symptoms.

Several sorts of problem can suggest somatic symptom disorder. These include the following:

- Pain that is excessive or chronic
- Functional neurological symptoms (p. 266)

- Chronic, multiple symptoms that seem to lack an adequate explanation

- Physical complaints that don't improve, despite treatment that helps most patients

- Excessive concern with health or body appearance

Patients with somatic symptom and related disorders have usually been evaluated many times for physical illness. These evaluations often lead to testing and treatments that are expensive, time consuming, ineffective, and sometimes dangerous. The result of these efforts may be only to reinforce the person's fearful belief in some nonexistent physical illness or process. At some point, health care personnel recognize that whatever is wrong has strong emotional underpinnings and refer the patient for a mental health evaluation.

It is important to acknowledge that, with the obvious exception of factitious disorder, these patients are not faking their symptoms. Rather, they often believe that they have something seriously wrong; this belief can cause them enormous anxiety and impairment. Without meaning to, they inflict great suffering on themselves and on those around them.

On the other hand, we must also remember that the mere presence of a somatic symptom disorder is no guarantee that another medical—or mental—condition will not subsequently develop.

F45.1 Somatic Symptom Disorder

DSM-5-TR criteria for somatic symptom disorder (SSD) require only a single somatic symptom and 6 months duration, but that symptom (or symptoms) must cause distress or markedly impair the person's functioning. Nonetheless, the classic patient has a pattern of multiple physical and emotional symptoms that can affect various (often many) areas of the body, with the pattern of concerns lasting far beyond the minimum 6 months. The symptom areas involved can include pain symptoms, problems with breathing or heartbeat, abdominal complaints, and menstrual disorders. Functional neurological symptoms (apparent body malfunctioning such as paralysis or blindness that has no anatomical or physiological cause) may also be encountered. Treatment that usually helps symptoms caused by actual physical disease is often ineffective for these patients.

SSD begins early in life, usually in the teens or early 20s, and can last for many years—perhaps throughout the patient's lifetime.* Often overlooked even by health care professionals, we still have far too little information about prevalence and distribution. With its more liberal criteria, SSD was found in a questionnaire study to

---

*Much of the information on SSD presented here and elsewhere in this chapter is based on studies of patients defined by DSM-IV criteria.

affect 7–17% of the general population. The DSM-IV version accounted for 7–8% of mental health clinic patients and perhaps nearly that percentage of hospitalized mental health patients. By any criteria, women outnumber men (the true ratio is uncertain), and these disorders have a strong tendency to run in families. Transmission is probably both genetic and environmental, found more frequently in patients with low socioeconomic status and limited education.

Half or more of patients with SSD have anxiety and mood symptoms. There is an ever-present danger that clinicians will diagnose an anxiety or mood disorder and ignore the underlying SSD. Then the all-too-common result is that the patient receives treatment specific for the mood or anxiety disorder, rather than an approach that might address the underlying SSD.

Essential Features of **Somatic Symptom Disorder**

Concern about one or more distressing or disruptive somatic symptoms leads the patient to express a high level of health anxiety, to invest excessive energy and time in health care, or to think excessively about the seriousness of symptoms.

The Fine Print

The D's: • Duration (a single symptom may be brief, but the overall duration must be 6+ months) • Differential diagnosis (substance use and physical disorders, illness anxiety disorder, functional neurological symptom disorder, mood disorders, panic and generalized anxiety disorders, delusional disorder, obsessive–compulsive disorder, dissociative disorders, body dysmorphic disorder, factitious disorder, malingering)

Coding Notes

Specify if:

> **With predominant pain.** For patients who complain mainly of pain. See the additional discussion on page 260.
> **Persistent.** If the course is marked by serious symptoms, lots of impairment, and a duration greater than 6 months.

Consider the following behaviors related to seriousness of patient's symptoms: excessive thoughts, persistent high anxiety, excessive energy/time expended. Then rate severity:

> **Mild.** One of the behaviors mentioned above.
> **Moderate.** 2+.
> **Severe.** 2+, along with numerous somatic complaints (or one extremely severe complaint).

Within my own professional experience, this mental disorder has borne four different names. Over 2,000 years ago the Greeks spoke of *hysteria,* in the belief that symptoms arose from a uterus (*hystera*) that wandered throughout the body, producing pain, or stopping the breath, or clogging the throat. That ancient term remained in vogue until the middle of the 20th century, when it was gradually replaced by a new label and a more complicated definition.

Briquet syndrome was coined in honor of the 19th-century French physician who first described the disorder's typical polysymptomatic presentation. Diagnosis required 25 symptoms (of a possible 60), each of which, the clinician had to determine, was unsubstantiated by objective physical or laboratory examination. Besides ordinary physical complaints, the list included pseudoneurological symptoms (such as temporary blindness and aphonia) as well as emotional symptoms such as depression, anxiety attacks, and hallucinations.

The Briquet criteria identified a group of patients who, on follow-up interview, had not developed actual physical disease and who had responded well to psychological treatment and behavioral management. But 25 symptoms were just too many for some clinicians. In 1980, the authors of DSM-III devised the term *somatization disorder,* which reduced the number of symptoms and discarded all the mental and emotional symptoms from the Briquet symptoms list.

DSM-III-R and DSM-IV further redefined and shortened the list ("dumbed it down," some would say). Even with the simpler somatization disorder symptoms, however, few patients were ever diagnosed; perhaps clinicians didn't want to take the trouble, or perhaps the symptoms were simply too restrictive for practical purposes. DSM-5-TR states that non-mental health clinicians found the criteria hard to understand, and that emphasizing a lack of medical explanation was pejorative and demeaning.

It is noteworthy that, as the names have progressively lengthened, the criteria sets have been getting shorter—with the obvious exception of hysteria itself, which was a seat-of-the-pants diagnosis that required but a single symptom, often of the pseudoneurological "conversion" type. Now, with SSD, we are back where we started: A single symptom, attended by a certain degree of concern on the part of the patient, will suffice for a DSM-5-TR diagnosis.

It remains to be seen how well the current criteria will delimit a homogeneous group of patients from those with physical illness or other mental disorders. But I fear that we may have truly come full circle, to the point where we are once again in danger of misidentifying people whose symptoms are perplexing, even mysterious, but which could well presage ultimate physical or severe mental disorder.

One other issue deserves our scrutiny: DSM-5-TR criteria do not require us to rule out other possible causes for the patient's symptoms. That places the SSD criteria in select company (intellectual developmental disorder, substance use disorders, anorexia nervosa, and the paraphilias) as requiring no consideration of a differential diagnosis.

In a previous edition of this book, I recommended against using the current diagnostic criteria. That may have been swimming against too swift a current, so here's my current suggestion for using DSM-5-TR criteria for SSD:

- Look for a long duration of symptoms, far beyond the 6 month minimum.
- Interview carefully to try to identify the patient who has multiple symptoms extending over this extended time period.
- Obtain information from other health care providers to help identify symptoms that have not responded to usual treatment interventions.
- Carefully rule out other possible causations, including mood and anxiety disorders and the use of substances.
- And follow the patient carefully: You never know what turn in the road you may both encounter.

Cynthia Fowler

Cynthia Fowler cries when she tells her story to the most recent in her series of health care professionals. At age 35, her history is long and complicated. It begins in her mid-teens with arthritis that seemed to move from one joint to another. She was told that these were "growing pains," but over the intervening 20 years, they continue to come and go. Although she has been subsequently diagnosed as having various types of arthritis, laboratory tests have substantiated none of them. A long succession of treatments has proven fruitless.

In her mid-20s, Cynthia was evaluated for left flank pain, but again no pathology was found. Later, abdominal pain and vomiting spells were worked up with gastroscopy and barium X-rays. Each of these studies proved normal. A histamine antagonist was added to her growing list of medications, which by now included various anti-inflammatory agents, as well as prescription and over-the-counter analgesics.

At one time, Cynthia thought that many of her symptoms were aggravated by her premenstrual syndrome, which she recognized after reading about it in women's magazines. She was invariably irritable with cramps before her period, which used to be so heavy that she would sometimes stay in bed for several days. When she was 26, she'd had a total hysterectomy. Six months later, persistent vomiting led to an endoscopy; other than adhesions, no abnormalities were found. Alternating diarrhea and constipation then caused her to experiment with a series of preparations to regulate her bowel movements.

When questioned about sex, Cynthia shifts uncomfortably in her chair. She doesn't care much for it and has never experienced a climax. Her lack of interest is no problem to her, though each of her three husbands complained a lot. She finally admits that, when a young teenager, something sexual might have happened to her, but that's a part of her life she really cannot recall. "It's as if someone cut a whole year out of my diary," she explains.

One way or another, each of Cynthia's previous clinicians has disappointed her.

"None of the others knew how to help me. But I just know you'll find out what's wrong. Everyone says you're the best in town." Through her tears, she manages a confident smile.

Evaluation of Cynthia Fowler

At a glance, we can affirm that Cynthia has distressing somatic symptoms (criterion A) that have for years (C) occupied a great deal of time and attention (B). There, in a nutshell, are the requirements for a DSM-5-TR diagnosis of SSD. However, I'd prefer to analyze her condition in light of the old DSM-IV somatization disorder guidelines (sidebar, p. 259).

Cynthia needs at least eight symptoms across the four symptom areas. She has *pain* (abdominal, flank, joint, and menstrual); *gastrointestinal* (diarrhea, vomiting); *sexual* (excessive menstrual bleeding, sexual indifference); and a lone *pseudoneurological* symptom (amnesia). DSM-IV criteria required that these symptoms not be explainable based on physical disease, and that they impair the patient's functioning in some way—I don't think I'll get much disagreement there, either. They started well before she turned 30, and there is nothing to suggest that she has intentionally feigned anything. Q.E.D.

Even so, as with nearly every mental disorder, another medical condition is the first possibility that I would seek to rule out. Among the medical and neurological disorders to consider are multiple sclerosis, spinal cord tumors, and diseases of the heart and lungs. Cynthia has already been worked up for a variety of medical conditions and has been prescribed multiple medications, none of which has done her much good. Judging by the last paragraph of the vignette, her previous clinicians might have been at a loss to diagnose or treat her effectively.

Setting Cynthia's experience apart from patients with organic disease are (1) the number and variety of the symptoms (though neither quantity nor diversity is required by DSM-5-TR SSD criterion A); (2) the absence of an adequate explanation for the symptoms based on history, lab findings, or physical examination (which is not required for SSD, either); and (3) inadequate relief from treatments that are ordinarily helpful for the symptoms in question (yup, not required). Note once again that although the SSD criteria allow a diagnosis based on far fewer symptoms than Cynthia has, her history is typical of a group of patients whom clinicians have been treating in vain for millennia.

Certain other somatic symptom and related disorders require discussion. In SSD with predominant pain, the patient focuses on severe, sometimes incapacitating physical pain. Although Cynthia complains of pain in a variety of locations, that is only one aspect of a much broader picture of somatic illness. Patients with illness anxiety disorder (formerly hypochondriasis) can have multiple physical symptoms, but their concern focuses on the fear of having a specific physical disease, not, as with Cynthia, particular symptoms.

Cynthia has no classical physical conversion symptoms (e.g., stocking or glove anesthesia, hemiparalysis), but many patients with SSD do. Then functional neurological symptom disorder enters the differential diagnosis. DSM-5-TR makes the point that functional neurological symptom disorder can be diagnosed along with SSD. I can see a benefit to this practice: It allows us to highlight certain symptoms for which there is no discernable physical causation. But to me, it doesn't cover any new diagnostic ground.

We should always inquire carefully about substance-related disorders, which are found in a quarter or more of patients with SSD. And when patients come to the attention of mental health providers, it is often because of a concomitant mood or anxiety disorder. Cynthia's amnesia might also qualify for the diagnosis of dissociative amnesia if it were the predominant problem.

Many patients with SSD also have one or more personality disorders. Especially prevalent is histrionic personality disorder, though borderline and antisocial personality disorders may also be found. Cynthia's words to the clinician in the last paragraph of the vignette make one wonder about a personality disorder, but with insufficient information, I'd defer that diagnosis for now. There's no way to code it out, so I would mention in my summary that further evaluation is needed.

With a GAF score of 61, Cynthia's current diagnosis would read as follows:

F45.1   Somatic symptom disorder

For the only time in this book, I am providing DSM-IV criteria. Imperfect as they may be, I hope that they will give you a couple of perspectives. First, with them you can appreciate the breadth of physical and emotional symptoms that can affect patients who present with somatic symptoms. Perhaps more importantly, it provides a tool to identify the patients most likely to benefit from a treatment approach that doesn't just futilely reprise the medication and surgical interventions used in the past.

And here is my personal guarantee: Any patient diagnosed by this standard will also qualify for a DSM-5-TR diagnosis of SSD.

Outline of the DSM-IV somatization disorder:

- From an early age, these patients have numerous physical complaints that wax and wane, with new ones often beginning as old ones resolve. With treatment typically ineffective, patients tend to switch health care providers in search of cure.
- The wide variety of possible symptoms fall into several groups.
  - Pain (several different sites are required): in the head, back, chest, abdomen, joints, arms or legs, or genitals; or related to body functions, such as urination, menstruation, or sexual intercourse
  - Gastrointestinal (other than pain): bloating, constipation, diarrhea, nausea, vomiting spells (except during pregnancy), or intolerance of several foods (nominally, three or more)
  - Sexual or reproductive systems (other than pain): difficulty with erection or ejaculation, irregular menses, excessive menstrual flow, or vomiting that persists throughout pregnancy

○ Pseudoneurological (not pain): blindness, deafness, double vision, lump in throat or trouble swallowing, inability to speak, poor balance or coordination, weak or paralyzed muscles, retention of urine, hallucinations, numbness to touch or pain, seizures, amnesia (or any other dissociative symptom), or loss of consciousness (other than fainting)

- The typical patient will have eight or more symptoms, with four (or more) from the pain group, two from the gastrointestinal group, and at least one each from the other two groups. Most patients will have far more symptoms than eight. Symptoms require treatment or impair social, personal, or occupational functioning.

- DSM-IV required an onset by age 30, but most patients have been ill from their teens or early 20s. Symptoms must be unexplained by any medical condition (including substance misuse). Patients who also have actual physical illnesses often react to them with greater anxiety than you might expect.

- Of course, actual physical illness should be first on the list of differential diagnoses, and, because SD can be difficult to treat, there are many other mental and emotional disorders that need to be ruled out. These include mood or anxiety disorders, psychotic disorders, and dissociative or stress disorders. Substance use disorders can be comorbid with SD. I would include factitious disorder and malingering on the differential list, but at the bottom.

From *DSM-IV Made Easy* (pp. 294–295) by James Morrison. Copyright © 1995 The Guilford Press. Reprinted by permission.

With Predominant Pain Specifier for Somatic Symptom Disorder

Some patients with SSD experience mainly pain, in which case the specifier *with predominant pain* is indicated. DSM-IV called it pain disorder and listed it as an independent condition with its own criteria. (From here on, I'll refer to it as SSD–Pain.) Whatever we call it, we need to keep in mind these facts:

- Pain is subjective—individuals experience it differently.
- There is no gross anatomical pathology.
- Measuring pain is hard.

So it's hard to know that a patient who complains of chronic or excruciating pain, and apparently lacks adequate objective pathology, has a mental disorder at all. (In DSM-5-TR, patients who have actual pain but show excessive concern can be diagnosed with SSD–Pain.)

The pain in question is usually chronic and often severe. It can take many forms, but especially common is pain in the lower back, head, pelvis, or temporomandibular joint. Typically, SSD–Pain doesn't wax and wane with time and doesn't diminish with distraction; it may respond only poorly to analgesics, if at all.

Chronic pain interferes with cognition, causing patients to have trouble with memory, concentration, and completing tasks. It is often associated with depression, anxiety, and low self-esteem; sleep may be disturbed. Such patients may experience slower response to stimuli; fear of worsening pain may reduce their physical activity. Of course, work suffers. Over half the time, clinicians manage chronic pain inadequately.

SSD–Pain usually begins in the 30s or 40s, often following an accident or some other physical illness. It is more often diagnosed in women than in men. As its duration lengthens, it can lead to increasing incapacity for work and social life, and sometimes to complete invalidism. Although some form of pain affects many adults in the general population—perhaps as high as 30% in the United States—no one knows for sure the prevalence of SSD–Pain.

Ruby Bissell

Ruby Bissell places a hand on each chair arm and shifts uncomfortably. She has been talking for nearly half an hour, and the dull, constant ache has worsened. Pushing up with both hands, she hoists herself to her feet. She winces as she presses a fist into the small of her back; the furrows on her face add a decade to her 45 years.

Although Ruby has had this problem for nearly 6 years, she isn't exactly sure when it began. Perhaps it was when she helped move a patient from the operating table to a gurney. The first orthopedist she consulted explained that her pulled ligament was mild, so she continued her work as an operating room nurse for nearly a year. But whether she is sitting or standing, her back hurts so much she's had to resign from her job. Now she can't maintain any physical position longer than a few minutes at a time.

"They let me do supervisory work for a while," she says, "but I had to quit that, too. My only choices were sitting or standing, and I have to spend part of each hour flat on my back."

From her blue-collar parents, Ruby inherited a solid work ethic. She's supported herself since she was 17, so her forced retirement was a blow. But she can't say she feels depressed about it. In fact, she has never been very introspective about her feelings, and she can't really explain how she feels about many things. She does deny ever having hallucinations or delusions; aside from her back pain, her physical health has been good. Although she occasionally awakens at night with back pain, she has no real insomnia; appetite and weight have been normal. When asked whether she's ever had death wishes or suicidal ideas, she seems a little offended and strongly denies them.

A variety of treatments have made little difference in Ruby's condition. Pain medication provides almost no relief at all, so she's quit them all before she could get hooked. Physical therapy made her hurt even more, and an electrical stimulation unit seemed to burn her skin.

Finding no anatomical pathology, a neurosurgeon explained to Ruby that a laminectomy and spinal fusion were unlikely to improve matters. Besides, her own husband's experience causes her to distrust any surgical intervention. He was injured in a trucking accident a year before her own difficulty began; his subsequent laminectomy left him not only disabled for work, but impotent. With no children to support, the two live in reasonable comfort on their combined disability incomes.

"Mostly we just stay at home," Ruby remarks. "We care a lot for each other. Our relationship is the one part of my life that's really good."

The interviewer asks whether they are still able to have any sort of a sex life. Ruby admits that they do not. "We used to be very active, and I enjoyed it a lot. Since his accident, he can't perform, and Gregory feels terribly guilty that he can't satisfy me. Now my back pain would keep me from having sex, regardless. It's almost a relief that he doesn't have to bear all the responsibility."

Evaluation of Ruby Bissell

For several years (far longer than the 6 months required by SSD criterion C), Ruby has complained of severe pain (A) that has markedly affected her life, especially her ability to work. She has clearly spent a great deal of time and effort (B) trying to manage her pain. And with that, we've covered the three DSM-5-TR requirements for SSD–Pain.

Although criteria don't require us to rule out other causes, we're responsible clinicians, so of course we'll do so anyway. Principally, we need to know that her pain isn't caused by another medical condition. The vignette makes clear that she has been thoroughly evaluated by her orthopedist, who reports that she doesn't have pathology adequate to account for the severity of her symptoms. (Even if she did have defined pathology, SSD–Pain might also be suspected should the distribution, timing, or description of the pain be atypical for that physical illness.)

Could Ruby be malingering? This question is especially relevant to anyone who receives compensation for a work-related injury. But her suffering seems genuine, and the vignette gives no indication that she is physically more able-bodied for leisure than for work. Her referral wasn't made within a legal context, and she cooperated fully with the examination. Furthermore, malingering would seem inconsistent with her long-held work ethic.

Pain is often a symptom of depression; indeed, many practitioners will automatically recommend a course of antidepressant medication for someone who complains of severe or chronic pain. Although Ruby denies feeling especially depressed, her pain symptoms might be a stand-in for a mood disorder. However, she has had no suicidal ideas or disturbance of sleep or appetite that would support such a diagnosis. Although patients with substance-related disorders will sometimes fabricate (or imagine) pain to obtain medications, Ruby has been careful to avoid becoming dependent on analgesics.

If present at all, physical symptoms in people with illness anxiety disorder tend to be mild; these folks are preoccupied not with symptoms but with having a specific disease, and Ruby doesn't seem all that worried. Pain is not a focus for functional neurological symptom disorder. People with adjustment disorder will sometimes have physical symptoms, but such conditions are associated with identifiable precipitants and disappear with the stressor.

DSM-5-TR doesn't require us to identify psychological factors that could underlie pain. Indeed, the presumption that there be a psychological mechanism is not a criterion for SSD. It is useful, however, to think about possible psychological factors that could contribute to the production or maintenance of a given patient's pain experience. Ruby's history includes several such possibilities. These include her perception of her husband's feeling about his impotence, her anxiety at being left as the sole breadwinner, and possibly her own resentment at having worked since she was a teenager. (For many patients, we could identify multiple psychological considerations.)

Psychological factors that might be causing or worsening Ruby's pain thus include stress resulting from relationships, work, and finances. With her GAF score of 61, her diagnosis would be as follows:

F45.1   Somatic symptom disorder, with predominant pain

Occasionally a patient, like Ruby, will be completely unable to describe the emotional component of pain. The inability to verbalize the emotions one feels has been termed *alexithymia*, Greek for "without expression of mood."

F45.21 Illness Anxiety Disorder

People with illness anxiety disorder (IAD) worry terribly that they might have a serious illness. This concern persists despite medical evidence to the contrary and reassurance from health care professionals. Common examples include fear of heart disease (which might start with an occasional heart palpitation) and of cancer (ever wonder about that mole—it seems to have darkened a bit?). Patients with IAD are not psychotic: They may agree temporarily that their symptoms could be emotional in origin, though they quickly revert to their fearful obsessing. Then, they reject any suggestion that they do not have physical disease and may even become outraged and refuse mental health consultation.

Perhaps three-quarters of the patients diagnosed in DSM-IV with hypochondriasis actually have physical symptoms that would qualify them in DSM-5-TR for somatic symptom disorder. However, the remaining quarter have all the concern about being sick, but not much in the way of actual somatic symptoms. Occasionally, a patient with demonstrable organic disease will still have hypochondriacal symptoms that are out of proportion to the seriousness of the actual medical condition. To delineate these patients more clearly, DSM-5 renamed the condition (*hypochondriasis* is considered pejorative) and wrote new criteria.

Though known for centuries, IAD still hasn't been carefully enough studied; much of what is known is extrapolated from older studies of hypochondriasis. By all accounts, however, it is fairly common (perhaps 5% of the general population), especially in the offices of non-mental health practitioners. IAD tends to begin in the 20s or 30s, with peak prevalence at about 30 or 40. It is probably about equally frequent in men and women. Any hereditary influence is likely to be modest. Although they do not have high rates of current medical illnesses, patients with IAD report a high incidence of childhood illness.

Historically, hypochondriasis has been a source of fun for cartoonists and playwrights (read Molière's *The Imaginary Invalid*), but the disorder causes genuine misery. Although it can resolve completely, it more often runs a chronic course, for years interfering with work and social life. Many patients go from doctor to doctor in the effort to find someone who will validate their concerns and relieve them of the serious disorders they feel sure they have; for a few, like Molière's poor creature, Argan, it leads to complete invalidism.

Essential Features of **Illness Anxiety Disorder**

Despite the absence of serious physical symptoms, the patient is inordinately concerned about being ill. High anxiety coupled with a low threshold for alarm yields recurring behaviors concerning health (seeking reassurance, checking over and over for physical signs). Some patients cope instead by avoiding hospitals and medical appointments.

The Fine Print

The D's: • Duration (6+ months, though the focus of concerns may move from one condition to another) • Differential diagnosis (physical disorders, mood disorders, **generalized anxiety disorder, panic disorder, obsessive–compulsive disorder, delusional disorder, body dysmorphic disorder, somatic symptom disorder,** adjustment disorder)

Coding Notes

Specify subtype:

  Care-seeking type. The patient uses medical services more than usual.
  Care-avoidant type. Due to heightened anxiety levels, the patient avoids seeking medical care.

Julian Fenster

"Wow! My chart must be 2 inches thick." Julian Fenster is checking in for his third emergency room visit in the past month. "That's just Volume 3," the nurse tells him.

At age 24, Julian lives with his mother and a teenage sister. Years ago, he enrolled at a college several hundred miles away. After only a semester, he moved back home. "I didn't want to be that far from my doctors," he explains. "When you're trying to prevent heart disease, you can't be too careful." With a practiced hand, he adjusts the blood pressure cuff around his upper arm.

When Julian was a young teenager, his dad died. "His death was self-inflicted," Julian points out. "He'd had rheumatic fever as a child, which gave him an enlarged heart. And the only thing he ever exercised was his right to eat anything fried, including Twinkies. And he smoked—he was a proud two-pack-a-day man. Look where that got him."

None of these health risks apply to Julian, who is nothing if not careful about what he puts into his body. He has spent hours searching the Internet for information on diet, and he once attended a lecture by Dean Ornish. "I've followed a plant-based diet ever since," Julian said. "I'm especially keen on tofu. And broccoli."

Julian has never complained much about having symptoms—just the odd palpitation, maybe "hot flushes" on an especially humid day. "I don't feel bad," he explains. "I just feel scared."

This time, he's heard a report on NPR about young people with heart disease. It startled him so much he dropped the dish he had been putting into the cupboard. Without even cleaning up the mess, he caught the next bus to the ER.

Julian agrees that he needs a different approach to his health care needs and thinks he might be willing to give cognitive-behavioral therapy a try. "But first," he asks, "could you check my blood pressure just once more?"

Evaluation of Julian Fenster

The requirements for IAD are not onerous; Julian handily meets them all. He has a disproportionate concern for a condition he's been assured he does not have (criterion A). He has both high anxiety and a low threshold for alarm (it took only a report on the radio to frighten him into the ER once again, C). His actual symptoms aren't just mild—they are pretty much nonexistent (B)—so we can rule out somatic symptom disorder. He's invested huge amounts of time in trolling the Internet for health information (D). Finally, he has had these symptoms far longer than the 6-month minimum required (E) for the diagnosis of IAD.

As with any condition discussed in this chapter (other than the disparaged [by me] somatic symptom disorder), the first issue to rule out on our list is another medical condition: Marked, if not inordinate, health anxiety is pretty common in medical outpatients. Physical illnesses can be easy to miss, especially if the patient has had a long history of complaints that seem without physical basis. However, Julian's symptoms have been evaluated over and again, to the point that there seems little danger anything has been missed. Still, people with hypochondriacal behavior are not immortal, so physical disorders would remain a significant rule-out that his clinicians must always keep in mind.

Anxious concern about health can occur in other mental disorders, but we can find some differences to help discriminate. Among these are OCD, body dysmorphic disorder, and anxiety disorders (for example, generalized anxiety disorder and panic disorder). Julian's symptoms suggest none of these. When somatic concerns emerge in schizophrenia, they tend to be delusional and bizarre ("My brain is turning to bread"). In major depressive disorder, they are ego-syntonic but may be influenced by melancholia (For a severely depressed patient I might understand "My bowels have turned to cement" as metaphoric, not delusional.) As keen as I am on looking for depression in almost every mental health patient, I don't see depressive symptoms here. I'd give him a GAF score of 65.

The girth of Julian's chart supports the care-seeking subtype specifier.

F45.21   Illness anxiety disorder, care-seeking type

Functional Neurological Symptom Disorder (Conversion Disorder)

Let's define a functional neurological symptom as (1) a change in how the body functions when (2) there is clinical evidence that the symptom does not reflect a medical or neurological disorder. These symptoms are sometimes termed *pseudoneurological* and used to go by the moniker of conversion symptoms; now the term *functional neurological* has seized top billing. By any name, they include both sensory and motor symptoms.

Conversion symptoms (for convenience, I'll continue using this hoary term) usually don't conform to the anatomical pattern we'd expect for a condition with a well-defined physical cause. An example would be a *stocking anesthesia,* in which the patient complains of numbness of the foot that ends abruptly in a line encircling the lower leg. The actual pattern of nerve supply to the foot and ankle is quite different; it would not cause numbness defined by such a neat boundary. Other examples of sensory conversion symptoms include blindness, deafness, double vision, and hallucinations. Examples of motor deficits that are conversion symptoms include impaired balance or staggering gait (which used to be called *astasia-abasia*), weak or paralyzed muscles, lump in throat or trouble swallowing, loss of voice, and retention of urine.

For decades, clinicians were required to judge that an emotional conflict or specific psychological stress caused the conversion symptom (for example, a man develops blindness after viewing his wife in bed with a neighbor). DSM-5-TR has abandoned this requirement, in view of the potential for disagreement as to causation: One clinician may see a causal link between two events, whereas another strenuously argues against the connection.

Note that the criteria don't require patients to undergo laboratory or imaging tests. The requirement is only that, after a careful physical and neurological evaluation, the symptom cannot be explained by a known medical or neurological disease process. The stocking anesthesia I mentioned above would fill that requirement; so would total blindness in a patient whose pupils constrict in response to a bright light. Other evidence might include a change in findings from positive to negative when a different test is used (or the patient is distracted), or impossible findings such as tunnel vision. There is a rich and entertaining literature of clinical tests for functional neurological symptoms.

Conversion symptoms occur widely, throughout various medical populations; up to one-third of adults have had at least one such symptom during their lifetime. However, functional neurological symptom disorder is rarely encountered—perhaps in only 1 of 10,000 general population. It is usually a disorder of young people and is probably far more common among women than men. It is somewhat more likely to be found in patients with less than average education and medical sophistication and who live where medical practice and diagnosis are still emerging. It may be diagnosed more often among patients seen in consultation in a general hospital and in neurology clinics.

Having a conversion symptom may not allow meaningful predictions about a patient's future course. Follow-up studies find that many people who have had a conversion symptom do not have a mental disorder. Years later, many will be well, with no physical or mental disorders. Some have somatization (or somatic symptom) disorder or another mental disorder. A few turn out to have an actual physical (sometimes neurological) illness, including brain or spinal cord tumors, multiple sclerosis, or a variety of other medical and neurological disorders. Although clinicians have undoubtedly improved in their ability to discriminate conversion symptoms from "real disease," it remains distressingly easy to make mistakes.

Essential Features of **Functional Neurological Symptom Disorder**

The patient experiences changes in sensory or voluntary motor functioning that appear clinically inconsistent with any known medical or neurological condition. The symptom causes marked distress or disability or deserves a medical evaluation.

The Fine Print

The D's: • Distress or disability (work/educational, social, or personal impairment) • Differential diagnosis (**physical disorders,** any **other mental disorder,** but especially mood disorders, panic disorder, body dysmorphic disorder, dissociative disorders, factitious disorder, malingering)

Coding Notes

Specify if:

> **Acute episode.** Symptoms have lasted under 6 months.
> **Persistent.** Symptoms have lasted 6+ months.

Specify: **{With}{Without} psychological stressor**

Specify type of symptom:

> **F44.4 With weakness or paralysis; with abnormal movement** (tremor, dystonia, myoclonus, abnormal gait)**; with swallowing symptoms;** *or* **with speech symptom** (dysphonia, slurring)

F44.5 With attacks or seizures
F44.6 With anesthesia or sensory loss; *or* **with special sensory symptom**
(hallucinations or other disturbance of vision, hearing, smell)
F44.7 With mixed symptoms

There's something missing from the DSM-5-TR criteria for functional neurological symptom disorder. In DSM-IV, we clinicians had to rule out intentional production of symptoms—specifically, malingering and factitious disorder. Although we are still asked to assure ourselves that no other diagnosis better explains the symptom, those two diagnoses aren't explicitly mentioned. In my opinion, this is a good thing, because it's hard (sometimes impossible) to determine for sure that a patient is faking. But with conversion symptoms, we should always keep the possibility in mind and do all we can to rule out factitious disorder and malingering, along with every other confounding diagnosis.

Rosalind Noonan

Rosalind Noonan comes to her university's student health service because of a stutter—remarkable because she is 18 and has been stuttering for only 2 days.

It began on Tuesday afternoon during her women's issues seminar. The class had been discussing sexual harassment, which gradually morphed into a consideration of sexual molestation. To foster discussion, the graduate student leading the seminar asked each participant to comment. When Rosalind's turn came, she stuttered so badly that she gave up trying to talk at all.

"I still ca-ca-ca-can't understand it," she tells the interviewer. "It's the first time I've ever had this pr-pr-pro-pro—difficulty."

Rosalind is a first-year student who plans to major in psychology "to help me learn more about myself." What she already knows includes the following.

When she was only a week old, Rosalind was adopted by a high school physics teacher and his wife, who have no other children. Her father is a rigid and perfectionistic man who dominates both Rosalind and her mother. She has no information about her biological parents.

As a young child, Rosalind was overly active; during her early school years she'd had difficulty focusing her attention. She would probably have qualified for a diagnosis of ADHD, but the only evaluation she ever had was from their family physician, who thought it was "just a phase" she would soon outgrow. Despite that lack of diagnostic rigor, when she was 12, she did begin to grow out of it. By the time she entered high school, she was doing nearly straight-A work.

Although she had many friends in high school and has dated extensively, she's never had a serious boyfriend. Her physical health is excellent, with visits to doctors only for immunizations. Her mood is almost always bright and cheerful; she has no history of delusions or hallucinations, and she has never used drugs or alcohol. "I g-g-grew up healthy and happy," she protests. "That's why I d-d-d-don't understand this!"

"Hardly anyone reaches adulthood without having some problems." The pause for a response yields nothing, so the interviewer continues: "For example, when you were a child, did anyone ever approach you for sex?" Rosalind's gaze seems to lose focus as tears trickle down her cheeks. Haltingly at first, then in a rush, the following story emerges.

When she was 9 or 10, her parents had become friendly with a married couple, both of whom taught English at her father's school. When Rosalind was 14, the woman suddenly died; subsequently, the man was invited for dinner on several occasions. One evening he consumed too much wine and was put to bed on their living room sofa. Rosalind awakened to find him lying on top of her in her bed, his hand covering her mouth. She was never certain whether he penetrated her, but her struggles apparently caused him to ejaculate. After that, he left her room. He never again returned to their home.

The following day she confided her story to her mother, who at first assured Rosalind that she must have been dreaming. When confronted with the evidence of the stained sheets, her mother urged her to say nothing about the matter to her father. It was the last time the subject had ever been discussed in their house.

"I'm not sure what we thought Daddy would do if he found out," Rosalind comments, with notable fluency, "but we were both afraid of him. I felt I'd done something to be punished for, and I suppose Mom must have worried he'd attack the other teacher."

Evaluation of Rosalind Noonan

Rosalind's stuttering is a classic conversion (OK, functional neurological) symptom: It suggests or mimics a medical condition, and its sudden appearance at college age isn't what we'd expect for the stuttering of speech fluency disorder (criteria A, B). Many clinicians would agree that it was precipitated by the stress of discussing long-buried sexual abuse. This aspect of the disorder—the putative psychological factors related to the symptoms—is one criterion for diagnosis that DSM-5-TR no longer carries. However, it is still something to note when you encounter it.

The most serious mistake a clinician can make in this context is to diagnose functional neurological symptom disorder when the symptom is caused by another medical condition (C): Sometimes, very peculiar symptoms eventually turn out to have a medical basis. However, the abrupt onset of stuttering in an adult is almost certain to have no identifiable organic cause. The fact that Rosalind's difficulty disappeared during the evaluation would be additional evidence that this was a conversion symptom.

Rosalind says that her health has always been good, but her clinician should nonetheless ask about other symptoms that could indicate somatic symptom disorder (somatization disorder in DSM-IV), in which conversion symptoms are so commonly encountered. Her focus on the symptom, rather than on a fear of having some serious disease, eliminates illness anxiety disorder (hypochondriasis) from our consideration. Although the criteria don't exclude pain, by convention conversion symptoms don't usually include pain; when pain occurs as a symptom that is caused or increased by psychological factors, the diagnosis is likely to be somatic symptom disorder, with predominant pain. Another condition in which conversion symptoms are sometimes encountered is schizophrenia, but there is no evidence that Rosalind has ever been, or is now, psychotic. Neither is there evidence that she has consciously feigned her symptom, ruling out factitious disorder and malingering.

Rosalind is concerned about her stuttering (D), which is quite the opposite from the unconcerned indifference (sometimes referred to as *la belle indifférence*) often associated with conversion symptoms. Although many patients with functional neurological symptom disorder will also have a diagnosis of histrionic, dependent, borderline, or antisocial personality disorder, in Rosalind we don't see any of these. As in somatic symptom disorder, mood, anxiety, and dissociative disorders are often associated.

Although Rosalind is still stressed by the sexual molestation, her overall functioning is good; I'd peg her GAF score at 75. The type of symptom and presumed psychological stressor are detailed in the final diagnosis:

F44.4   Functional neurological symptom disorder, with speech symptom (stuttering), acute episode, with psychological stressor (concerns about molestation)

F54 Psychological Factors Affecting Other Medical Conditions

Mental health professionals deal with all sorts of problems that can influence the course or care of a medical condition. Indeed, you might find a psychological factor (or two) at play in most any patient. The diagnosis of psychological factors affecting other medical conditions can be used to identify such patients. Although it is coded as a mental disorder and with mental disorders, it does not actually constitute one, so I've not provided a full vignette—just a few snippets to illustrate how the diagnosis might be applied.

Some Examples

DSM-IV included six specific categories of factors that could change the course of a medical condition. Partly because they were hardly ever used, DSM-5-TR has ditched these categories, though it does offer some suggestions. I've melded the lists below. If more than one psychological factor is present, choose the most prominent one.

Mental disorder. For 15 years Philip's compliance with treatment for schizophrenia has been spotty. Now the voices warn him to refuse dialysis for kidney failure.

Symptoms of psychological distress (insufficient for a DSM-5-TR diagnosis). With few other symptoms, Alice's mood has been so low that she hasn't bothered filling prescriptions for her type 2 diabetes.

Personality traits or coping style. Gordon's lifelong hatred of authority figures has led him to reject his doctor's recommendation for a stent.

Maladaptive health behaviors. Weighing in at nearly 400 pounds, Tim knows he should avoid sweetened drinks, but nearly every day his love of Big Gulps wins out.

Stress-related physiological response. April's job as the Governor's spokesperson is so demanding that she's had to double up on her antihypertensive drugs.

Other or unspecified psychological factors. Harold's religion prohibits him from accepting a blood transfusion. In Nanja's culture, a woman mustn't allow any man not her husband to see her unclothed; her new internist is Derek.

And finally, a nonexample, courtesy of DSM-5-TR: If a patient seeks care through alternative healing, the intent is to access health care. This should not be recorded as an issue in this section.

Essential Features of **Psychological Factors Affecting Other Medical Conditions**

A patient's physical symptom or illness is negatively affected by a psychological or behavioral issue in one or more of these ways: the issue interferes with treatment, creates additional health risks for the patient, or, by adversely affecting underlying pathology, brings forth more symptoms or need for medical care. Or, timing shows a causal relationship between the psychological/behavioral issue and negative effect on the medical condition.

The Fine Print

The D's: • Differential diagnosis (other mental disorders, such as panic disorder, mood disorders, somatic symptom disorder and illness anxiety disorder, posttraumatic stress disorder, adjustment disorders, mental disorders due to another medical condition)

Coding Notes

Specify current severity:

   Mild. The factor increases medical risk.
   Moderate. The factor worsens the medical condition.
   Severe. It causes an ER visit or hospitalization.
   Extreme. It results in severe, life-endangering risk.

Code the name of the relevant medical condition first.

Psychological factors is the only condition in DSM-5-TR that is neither an actual disorder nor a specifier for one. In truth, it should have been given a Z-code and stuck in the back of the book with other such issues, but that wasn't an option: ICD-10 makes the rules. But I think it's confusing to have it up in the front seat.

F68.X Factitious Disorder

Factitious means something that is artificial. In the context of mental health patients, it refers to a disorder that looks like *bona fide* disease but isn't. Such patients accomplish this by simulating symptoms (for example, complaining of pain) or physical signs (such as warming a thermometer in coffee or submitting a urine specimen that's been supplemented with sugar). Sometimes they will complain of psychological symptoms, including depression, hallucinations, delusions, anxiety, suicidal ideas, and disorganized behavior. Because they are subjective, manufactured mental symptoms can be very hard to detect.

DSM-5-TR includes two subtypes of factitious disorder: in one, behaviors affect the patient; in the other, behaviors affect another person.

F68.10 Factitious Disorder Imposed on Self

People affected by factitious disorder imposed on self (FDIS) can have remarkably dramatic symptoms, accompanied by outright lying about the severity of the distress. We become suspicious when the overall pattern of signs and symptoms is atypical for the alleged illness or when the story varies with repetition. Other patients with FDIS, however, know a lot about the symptoms and terminology of disease; then the diagnosis can be extremely difficult to determine. Some people willingly undergo many procedures (some of them painful or dangerous) to continue in the patient role. With treatment that is ordinarily adequate to address their supposed disease, their symptoms either do not remit or they evolve new complications.

Once hospitalized, patients with FDIS often tend to complain bitterly and to argue with staff members. They characteristically remain hospitalized for a few days, have few if any visitors, and leave against medical advice once their tests prove negative. Many travel from city to city in the quest for medical care. The most persistent travelers and confabulators among these are sometimes said to have Münchausen syndrome, named for the fabled 18th-century German baron who told outrageous lies about his adventures.

DSM-5-TR doesn't require speculation as to possible motives for FDIS (or its sibling, FDIA, discussed below)—a blessing for those of us who reject the implication that clinicians can read minds. It is enough to detect the pattern in a patient whose behavior involves no other person.

Patients with FDIS differ profoundly from malingerers, who may show some of the same behaviors—silting a urine specimen, embellishing the subjective reports of their suffering. However, malingerers do these things to qualify for financial compensation (such as insurance payments), to obtain drugs, or to avoid work, punishment, or, in days gone by, military service. The motivation in FDIS appears more complex: These patients may need the security of being cared for, the satisfaction of duping medical personnel, or the pleasure of receiving a whole lot of attention from important people. For whatever reason, they manufacture physical or psychological symptoms in a manner that they may claim they cannot control.

The diagnosis of FDIS is made by excluding physical disease and other disorders. It is conceivable that a patient might manufacture a personality disorder, but I know of no such cases. Indeed, many probably have a genuine personality disorder.

FDIS begins early in life; often it starts with a hospitalization for genuine physical problems. No one knows how rare it is, though it appears to be more common in males than in females. It results in severe impairment: People with FDIS are often unemployed and do not maintain close ties with family or friends. Their lives are complicated (and sometimes put at risk) by tests, medications, and unnecessary surgical procedures.

F68.A Factitious Disorder Imposed on Another

A condition that has been recognized for only a few years, in DSM-IV factitious disorder imposed on another (FDIA) emerged from an appendix to enter the body of the DSM (there's an unsettling image!). It used to be called factitious disorder (or Münchausen) *by proxy*, because it isn't the patient who has symptoms. Rather, the caregiver both causes factitious symptoms in another person and bears the diagnosis. That "other" is almost always a child, though my Medline search revealed the occasional elderly person and at least one dog.

Three-quarters, sometimes more, of the perpetrators are female—usually the mother of a symptomatic child. Because many people with FDIA have a background in health care, it can be hard to catch them out. When apprehended, they often turn out to have a mood or personality disorder, or both; actual psychosis is rare. Some also have a history of FDIS. And note that a parent or other caregiver who fakes illness in another person to avoid legal proceedings would not be given this diagnosis, which is specifically excluded when the behavior is pursued to achieve material benefit.

Some parents with FDIA appear to believe that their children are ill; they tend to behave as "doctor addicts" who need the attention that comes with having a desperately ill child. Individuals with FDIA typically limit themselves to the false reporting of signs and symptoms of disease, such as seizures or apnea. Others, however, will induce symptoms—most commonly by suffocation or poisoning, but also by falsifying urine or stool samples or other lab specimens. Perhaps half the victims have an actual physical illness, in addition.

Medical personnel may be persuaded to prescribe treatment that the child doesn't need—and is perhaps harmful. Indeed, the person most taken in may be the physician: One will occasionally become angry at staff members who have accumulated evidence of the caregiver's perfidy. Some experts recommend against informing the doctor when covert surveillance is planned, to lessen the risk that the perpetrator will be tipped off.

The suspicions of medical personnel may be alerted by a parent who seems insufficiently concerned about a sick child, by symptoms that seem to make no sense, or by a child whose symptoms continue despite treatment that should be adequate. In some cases, however, the parent perpetrator appears so distraught that the clinician remains in steadfast ignorance of the potential for foul play. Then, the injuries will continue until the perpetrator is apprehended, the child dies, or with the march of time, the perpetrator moves on to involve another, probably younger child. In one survey, over 70% of victims sustained disfigurement or permanent disability.

Overall, FDIA is probably uncommon, though the true prevalence is unknown—health care providers are often loath to write down the correct diagnosis. However, one study of general hospital patients found close to 1% may have this diagnosis.

Victims are about equally male and female. Though most are under age 5, some are older. Most perpetrators are female and not single parents; often they are described as exemplary parents, though they may react inappropriately (for example, excitement) upon receiving bad health news. As you would expect, when a teen is involved, there is often a degree of collusion with the perpetrator. The overall mortality rate among victims is an appalling 10%; death occurs most often when poisoning or suffocation is involved.

Patients with factitious disorder sometimes take on symptoms of new (and often poorly investigated) illnesses—the "disorder *du jour*" phenomenon. The criteria for such a diagnosis may be nonspecific, so the patients can be difficult to manage. Often, they are disagreeable. It is far too easy to dismiss them with a diagnosis of factitious disorder without taking steps to ensure that we have first ruled out every other possible causative mental (and physical) condition.

I'd also point out that here in the differential diagnosis, I've used the term *malingering*—a rare occurrence in this book. Why is that? Surely people malinger other symptoms and disorders. Of course they can, and sometimes do. But I strongly believe it incumbent on clinicians to be extremely chary of malingering as a diagnostic formulation.

Essential Features of **Factitious Disorder**

To present a picture of someone who is ill, injured, or impaired, {the patient}{another person acting for the patient} feigns physical or mental symptoms or signs of illness or induces an illness or injury. This behavior occurs without evident benefit (such as financial gain, revenge, or avoiding legal responsibility).

The Fine Print

Note that, in the case of factitious disorder imposed on another, it is the perpetrator who receives the diagnosis. The victim may be given a different diagnosis to reflect the abuse: T74.12X (p. 613).

The D's: • Differential diagnosis (substance use and physical disorders, psychotic disorders, somatic symptom disorders, personality disorders, malingering)

Coding Notes

Diagnose:

> **Factitious disorder imposed on self.** The perpetrator is also the recipient.
> **Factitious disorder imposed on another.** The perpetrator and victim are separate individuals. (The perpetrator receives the factitious disorder code; the victim receives a Z-code reflecting the abuse.)

For either type, specify:

> **Single episode**
> **Recurrent episodes**

Jason Bird

Jason Bird carries no health care card—he claims he lost his billfold to a mugger hours before coming to the emergency room of a Midwestern hospital late one Saturday night. He complains of crushing substernal chest pain. Although his electrocardiogram (EKG) is markedly abnormal, it does not show the changes typical of an acute myocardial infarction. The cardiologist on call, noting his ashen pallor and obvious distress, orders him admitted to the cardiac ICU, then waits for the cardiac enzyme results.

The following day, Jason's EKG is unchanged, and the serum enzymes show no evidence of heart muscle damage. But his chest pain continues, and he loudly complains of being ignored. The cardiologist requests an urgent mental health consultation.

At age 47, Jason is a slightly built man with a bright, shifting gaze and a 4-day growth of beard. He speaks with a nasal Boston accent. His right shoulder bears the tattoo of a boot and the legend "Born To Kick Ass." Throughout the interview he frequently complains of chest pain, but he breathes and talks without evident effort and displays no anxiety about his physical condition.

He says he grew up in Quincy, Massachusetts, the son of a physician. After high school he attended college for several years, but discovered he is "too creative" to stick with a profession or a conventional job. Instead, he turned to inventing medical devices, and numbers among his successes the positive-pressure respirator that bears his name. Although he made several fortunes, he has lost nearly everything to his penchant for playing the stock market. He was visiting in the area, relaxing, when the chest pain struck.

"And you've never had it before?" asks the interviewer, looking through the chart.

Jason denies that he's had any previous heart trouble. "Not even a twinge. I've always been blessed with good health."

"Ever been hospitalized?"

"Nope. Well, just a tonsillectomy when I was a kid."

Further questioning is similarly unrevealing. As the interviewer departs, Jason is demanding extra meal service.

Playing a hunch, the interviewer begins telephoning emergency room physicians in the Boston area to ask about a patient who has Jason's name or peculiar tattoo. The third try strikes pay dirt.

"Jason Bird? I wondered when we'd hear from him again." The voice on the other end of the line chuckles. "He's been in and out of half the facilities in the state. His funny-looking EKG—probably an old MI—looks pretty bad, so he always gets admitted, but there's never any evidence of anything acute going on. But I don't think he's addicted to pain meds. A couple of years ago, he was admitted for a genuine pneumonia and got through a week without analgesia—and with no withdrawal symptoms. He'll stay in the ICU a couple of days and rag on the staff about—whatever. Then he'll split. He seems to enjoy needling medical people."

"He told me that he was the son of a physician and that he was a wealthy inventor."

The Boston informant sighs. "The old respirator story. I checked into that one the third time he was admitted here. That was a different Bird altogether. I don't know that Jason's ever invented anything in his life—other than his medical history. As for his father, he might have been a chiropractor."

Returning to the ward to add a note to the chart, the interviewer discovers that Jason has discharged himself against advice, leaving for the hospital administrator a letter of complaint.

Evaluation of Jason Bird

Jason's story illustrates the principal difficulty of diagnosing factitious disorder: The criteria depend heavily on the clinician's ability to determine that the signs and symptoms presented are intentionally falsified (criterion A). Sometimes that's easy, as when you catch the patient scratching open a wound or parking a thermometer on the radiator. But often the intent to deceive must be deduced, as in Jason's case, from a string of visits to diverse health care facilities for the same fanciful complaint. Jason's EKG did not evolve, and his cardiac enzymes weren't elevated, so his interviewer inferred that Jason was feigning or markedly exaggerating his chest pain. That assumption may have been correct, but it was supported not by proof, only by reports from the emergency room.

Jason presented himself as ill (B), even in the absence of external motivation such as monetary gain or escape from punishment (C). That is important, for such behavior is the principal ingredient that differentiates factitious disorder from malingering—which of course we must consider, if only to refute it. Malingering carries with it no criteria, but we commonly agree that it occurs when a person consciously pretends to have a disorder to gain something of value: money (from insurance, a lawsuit, compensation); drugs (from a sympathetic physician); avoidance of a conviction for a crime; or release from, for example, military service. (I suppose that's a criterion of sorts.) For Jason, no such material gain is apparent.

The list of other differential diagnoses is predictable. Most important, of course, FDIS must be differentiated from physical illnesses. This was soon accomplished in Jason's case. Then other mental disorders must be ruled out. Patients with somatic symptom disorder may also complain of symptoms that have no apparent organic basis. Those with antisocial personality disorder may lie about symptoms, but they usually have some material gain in mind (to avoid punishment, to obtain money). Some patients with schizophrenia have a bizarre lifestyle that could be confused with the wanderings of classic Münchausen syndrome, but their content of thought will usually include clear delusions and hallucinations. Patients who feign psychological symptoms may look as though they have neurocognitive disorder or brief psychotic disorder. None of these disorders could be supported by Jason's history or current presentation.

Several other disorders may accompany FDIS. These include substance-related disorders (involving sedatives and analgesics) and dependent, histrionic, and borderline personality disorders. Of course, we have far too little information for any of these in Jason's case; when we do have an inkling, we should mention the possibility in the summary we dictate. With a GAF score of 41, here is how I'd diagnose Jason Bird:

F68.A   Factitious disorder imposed on self

Claudia Frankel

Police reports are typically pretty dull; they don't often moisten the eye. The Frankel case proves the exception to that rule.

When Rose Frankel was only 2 years old, she began having intestinal and other complaints that would define the next 6 years of her life. It started with spells of vomiting that seemed intractable to treatment. In all, she was carried back and forth to the pediatrician's office and to the hospital some 200 times. Each visit led to new tests and more attempts at treatment that led nowhere. She underwent nearly two dozen operative procedures, and swallowed numerous medications for diarrhea, infections, seizures, and spells of vomiting.

Then—finally!—nurses on the pediatric intensive care unit noticed that Rose would appear to be on the mend until her mother, Claudia, arrived and would take her into a private room. They'd hear Rose crying, and her health would take another turn for the worse—sometimes, just when she seemed ready for discharge.

In all, Rose suffered nearly a dozen serious infections; one of them, a life-threatening sepsis, involved multiple organisms. Through it all, Claudia worked closely with their family doctor. They would speak in person or on the phone several times a day, and Dr. Bhend often spoke of Claudia as his "good right arm" in trying to get to the bottom of the calamity that was engulfing their patient.

Throughout her medical ordeal, the only time that Rose remained healthy longer than a month was when Claudia left town to nurse her own mother through what proved to be the old lady's final illness. For the last few weeks of her kindergarten year, Rose bloomed. But she sickened again, shortly after Grandma died and Claudia returned home.

Several on the hospital nursing staff were beyond suspicious. Once, they'd found a bottle of Ipecac discarded in the room Rose had occupied. On another occasion, a monitoring device that three staff members had checked within the hour had been found turned off. As they told the investigating officers, most staff members concluded that Claudia was responsible for her daughter's illness, so they hid a camera in the private room Claudia always used during Rose's many admissions. When he found out, Dr. Bhend, concerned about the loss of trust, warned Claudia of the "impending sting." That afternoon, she checked Rose out of the hospital, and they were lost to follow-up. The staff revealed the full details to the police, who opened a file but were never able to pull together adequate solid information.

Evaluation of Claudia Frankel

Two of the criteria required for a diagnosis of factitious disorder are easily satisfied. There is nothing to suggest an external reward for Claudia's behavior such as financial gain (criterion C), and she certainly did present Rose as being impaired (D). Two other criteria we must take on faith: Although the circumstantial evidence was strong that Rose's symptoms were fabricated, the staff just missed nailing down proof (A). And we cannot be sure that Claudia had no other mental disorder such as a delusional disorder that could better explain her behavior (D). Therefore, our current diagnosis should be treated as provisional. I would make a note in her chart to the effect that further investigation would be needed regarding a personality disorder; in ICD-10, we cannot code "diagnosis deferred" in that category.

Assigning Claudia's GAF score requires some thought. Should we base our judgment on the fact that she was able to function well in most areas of her life, or on the effect of her behavior on Rose and on their relationship? In my opinion, the determining factor would be the disastrous consequences of her impaired judgment (not to mention the potential for future damage); hence the low GAF score of 30. However, others might see her situation differently and choose to argue.

Note that Rose herself would be given the code T74.12 to reflect the fact that she has suffered from physical abuse by a parent.

F68.A   Factitious disorder imposed on another (provisional)

F45.8 Other Specified Somatic Symptom and Related Disorder

This category is for patients whose somatic symptoms do not fulfill criteria for any of the somatic symptom and related disorders discussed above, but about which we have some information. Any diagnosis suggested here has not yet been studied enough for formal inclusion in DSM-5-TR and should be considered tentative. Keep in mind that with more information, such a patient may qualify for a diagnosis in a different chapter or for another diagnosis in this one.

> **Pseudocyesis.** The word *pseudocyesis* means "false pregnancy," and it refers to patients' incorrect belief that they are pregnant. They develop signs of pregnancy such as protruding abdomen, nausea, amenorrhea, and breast engorgement—and even such sensations as fetal movement and labor pains.

> **Illness anxiety disorders without excessive health-related behaviors or maladaptive avoidance.**

> **Brief illness anxiety disorder.**

> **Brief somatic symptom disorder.** I'll leave these last two definitions as homework—for extra credit, of course.

F45.9 Unspecified Somatic Symptom Disorder

Use this category when full criteria for any of the disorders discussed in this chapter are not met, and you do not wish to specify a reason or a possible presentation.

CHAPTER 9

Feeding and Eating Disorders

Quick Guide to the Feeding and Eating Disorders

Primary Feeding and Eating Disorders

Each of the primary feeding and eating disorders involves abnormal behaviors concerning the act of consumption. Anorexia nervosa is less common than bulimia nervosa, and both are less common than the newbie, binge-eating disorder. The overall prevalence of these three disorders may be increasing. The three remaining specific disorders were transplanted from the old childhood/adolescence section of DSM-IV.

Anorexia nervosa. Even though they are severely underweight, these patients perceive themselves as fat (p. 281).

Bulimia nervosa. These patients eat in binges, then prevent weight gain by self-induced vomiting, purging, and exercise. Although appearance is important to their self-evaluations, they do not have the body image distortion characteristic of anorexia nervosa (p. 285).

Binge-eating disorder. These patients eat in binges, but do not try to compensate by vomiting, exercising, or using laxatives (p. 289).

Pica. The patient eats material that is not food (p. 293).

Rumination disorder. The patient persistently regurgitates and re-chews food already eaten (p. 294).

Avoidant/restrictive food intake disorder. The patient's failure to eat enough leads to weight loss or a failure to gain weight (p. 296).

Other specified, or unspecified, feeding or eating disorder. Use one of these categories for a disorder of feeding or eating that does not meet the criteria for any of those mentioned above (p. 297).

Other Causes of Abnormal Appetite and Weight

Mood disorders. Patients with a major depressive episode (or persistent depressive disorder) can experience either anorexia with weight loss or increased appetite with weight gain (pp. 116 and 139).

Schizophrenia and other psychotic disorders. Bizarre eating habits are occasionally encountered in psychotic patients (p. 63).

Somatic symptom disorder. Complaints of marked weight fluctuation and appetite disturbance may be encountered in these patients (p. 254).

Kleine–Levin syndrome. This rare disorder causes people to eat voraciously and sleep profoundly (sidebar, p. 318).

Simple obesity. This is not a DSM-5-TR diagnosis (there's no evidence that it is associated with any defined mental or emotional pathology). But emotional problems that contribute to the development or maintenance of obesity can be coded as psychological factors affecting other medical conditions (p. 270). There is now also a separate medical code for overweight or obesity (E66.9).

Introduction

Eating too little and eating too much have probably caused problems as long as there have been eaters. Nearly everyone has pursued one of these behaviors at one time or another. But like so many behaviors, when carried to extremes, they can be dangerous; sometimes they turn deadly. Although the criteria crisply distinguish one from another, patients can move between the disorders and subclinical presentations.

Anorexia Nervosa

Recognized for nearly 200 years, anorexia nervosa (AN) has three main components. The patient (1) restricts food intake to the point of markedly reduced body weight, yet (2) remains inordinately concerned about obesity or weight gain, and (3) has the distorted self-perception of being overweight. Even if patients recognize their overall thinness, they may focus hypercritical attention on certain body parts—("My butt's just gross").

Other symptoms are elaborations of maladaptive eating behaviors—food restriction, excessive exercise, and vomiting or other methods of purging. Although many female patients stop menstruating, the absence of menses didn't provide a meaningful distinction, so it's no longer used as a criterion. Patients with AN may have abnormal vital signs (slow heart rate, low blood pressure); abnormal lab values and other tests can also occur (anemia, loss of bone density, EKG changes).

Let's note two additional features of the presentation. One has to do with the duration of symptoms, which DSM-5-TR doesn't specify in the diagnostic criteria. Therefore, we'll have to deduce from the statement that for subtype diagnosis, a patient must have symptoms for at least 3 months. The other is insight, which is pretty much absent in patients with AN. Despite severe weight loss (some can look downright skeletal), they do not seem to recognize just how underweight they are.

AN carries with it serious health consequences. Although two-thirds of community sample patients have remitted at 5 years, mortality (due to substance use, suicide, and malnutrition) is about six times that of the general population. Clinical populations may (no surprise) fare worse. Those who binge and then purge to maintain low weight tend to be older and sicker, and to have worse outcomes than those who only restrict their intake. Crossover between subtypes occurs—more often from the restrictor type than to it—limiting predictive accuracy. Depression and anxiety are frequently concomitants.

Around 1.5% of the female population is affected by AN (lifetime prevalence); the rate for males is perhaps a fifth of that. Adolescents and young adults are most at risk for first episode; it's especially common among those who are figure skaters or gymnasts (women) or jockeys or long-distance runners (men). The restricting type is the more usual. The concordance rate is higher in identical than in fraternal twins, indicating a degree of genetic underpinning. The value Western cultures place on being thin is also a likely contributing factor.

Essential Features of **Anorexia Nervosa**

People with AN (1) eat so little that they lose too much weight for their height and body frame (many look gaunt), yet (2) remain fearful of obesity or weight gain (or continue to undereat) and (3) have the distorted self-perception that they are fat.

The Fine Print

Some patients may not admit to fear of overweight but take steps to avert (needed) weight gain anyway.

The D's: • Duration (3+ months) • Differential diagnosis (substance use and physical disorders, mood or anxiety disorders, schizophrenia, obsessive–compulsive disorder, social anxiety disorder, body dysmorphic disorder, avoidant/restrictive food intake disorder, bulimia nervosa)

Coding Notes

Specify type that applies to the previous 3 months:

F50.02 Binge-eating/purging type. The patient has repeatedly purged (vomited; misused enemas, laxatives, or diuretics) or eaten in binges.

F50.01 Restricting type. The patient has not recently binged or purged, but loses weight by dieting, exercise, or fasting.

Based on body mass index (BMI; kg/(height in meters)^2), specify severity (level may be increased, depending on symptoms and degree of functional impairment). For adults, levels are as follows:

Mild. BMI of 17 or more.
Moderate. BMI of 16–17.
Severe. BMI of 15–16.
Extreme. BMI under 15.

Specify if:

In partial remission. For a substantial period, the patient no longer is seriously underweight, but remains overly concerned about weight or misperceives own body weight/shape.
In full remission. For a substantial period, the patient has met no AN criteria.

Marlene Richmond

A statuesque blonde at 5 feet 7 inches tall, on the day she is admitted Marlene Richmond weighs just over 80 pounds. Dressed in a jogging suit and leg warmers, she spends part of the initial interview doing deep knee bends. Information for her history is also provided by her older sister, who accompanies her to the hospital.

Marlene grew up in a small town in southern Illinois. Her father, who drills wells for a living, has a drinking problem. Her mother, severely overweight, starts numerous fad diets but never has much success with any of them. One of Marlene's earliest memories is her own resolve that she will grow up to be like neither of her parents.

Back in 10th grade, the concerns of her social circle revolved around appearance, clothing, and diet. That year alone, Marlene dropped 15 pounds from her highest weight ever, which was 125 pounds; even then she complained to her friends that she was too fat. Throughout her high school career, she remained fascinated by food. She took both introductory and advanced family and consumer sciences, and she spent much of her time in computer science class devising a database that could total up the calories in any recipe.

Whenever allowed to do so, Marlene ate in her bedroom while watching television. If forced to eat with the family, she mostly just rearranged the food on her plate or mashed it with a fork. Those bites she did take were the smallest that wouldn't fall through the tines.

"It's not as if I'm not hungry," she says during her admission interview. "I think about food most of the time. But I look so bloated and disgusting—I can't stand to see myself in the mirror. If I eat even a little bit too much, I feel so stuffed and guilty that I have to bring it back up."

Two years ago, Marlene started vomiting whenever she thought she had overeaten. At first, she would stick her finger or the blunt end of a pencil down her throat; once she tried some Ipecac she found in the medicine cabinet at a friend's house. She soon learned simply to vomit at will, without any chemical or mechanical aids. She also reduced her weight by using diuretics and laxatives. The diuretics helped her shave off a pound or two, but they left her so thirsty that she would soon gain it back. Once or twice a week, she now binges on high-carbohydrate food (she prefers corn chips and cola), then vomits up what she has eaten.

Other than her remarkable thinness—and her pallor, which is subsequently attributed to anemia—Marlene looks like a typical 20-year-old woman. She stops exercising when the interviewer requests it, but later she asks to use a stair-step exerciser. Her mood is cheerful, her flow of thought logical. She has no delusions or hallucinations, though she admits that she is terrified of gaining weight. However, she denies having any other phobias, obsessions, or compulsions; she has never had a panic attack. Most of her spontaneous comments concern meal planning and cooking, and she volunteers that she might like to become a dietitian. She appears bright and attentive and earns a perfect score on the MMSE.

Marlene's only health concern is that she hasn't had a menstrual period for 5 or 6 months. She knows she isn't pregnant—she hasn't had so much as a date for a year. "I think I'd be more attractive if I could just lose another couple of pounds," she says.

Evaluation of Marlene Richmond

Even though she is markedly underweight for her height (criterion A), Marlene continues to express concerns about gaining weight (B). Her disgust at her own image in the mirror suggests the distorted view patients with AN have of themselves (C). Her loss of weight is so profound that she hasn't had a menstrual period for several months. Although not all patients take active steps to avoid weight gain (some only restrict intake), Marlene's vomiting and use of diuretics and laxatives are classic for AN.

Loss of appetite and weight are commonly found in a variety of medical illnesses (liver disease, severe infections, and cancer, to name but a few); these must be ruled out by appropriate medical history and tests. Because the symptoms of AN are so distinctive, it is rarely confused with other mental disorders.

Loss of weight and anorexia can be encountered in somatic symptom disorder, but for *that* diagnosis, a patient must show excessive concern about the symptoms—and Marlene's attitude seems the antithesis of concern. Patients with schizophrenia will sometimes have peculiar eating habits, but unless they become dangerously underweight and have the typical distortion of self-image, the diagnoses should not be made together. Hunger strikes are usually brief and occur in the context of trying to influence the behavior of others for personal or political benefit. People with bulimia nervosa usually maintain body weight at an acceptable level. Neither bulimia nervosa nor binge-eating disorder should be diagnosed when bingeing and purging occur only during AN, which is the case with Marlene. However, some patients who initially have AN later become bulimic. Bulimia nervosa may also be diagnosed if there is a history of binge–purge cycles that occur during times the patient does not meet criteria for AN.

Several mental disorders are often associated with AN. Major depressive disorder could be diagnosed if Marlene had symptoms of mood disorder. Panic disorder, agoraphobia, obsessive–compulsive disorder, and substance use may also complicate diagnosis and treatment. Patients with AN may also fear eating in public, though you wouldn't give an additional diagnosis of social anxiety disorder if the anxiety symptoms are strictly limited to eating behaviors. Specific personality disorders have not been related to AN, but some patients may be seen as rigid and perfectionistic. Marlene's history of binge–purge cycles fits the specifier of binge-eating/purging type, which we'll add when coding. Her BMI is under 13, alarming enough to fully deserve the severity specifier of *extreme*. I'd give her GAF score as 45, and her full diagnosis as follows:

F50.02	Anorexia nervosa, binge-eating/purging type, extreme
E44.0	Malnutrition, moderate

F50.2 Bulimia Nervosa

Let's start by sketching an idealized mealtime. Wouldn't it involve the pleasant anticipation of sharing good food with friends, savoring every bite while lingering at the table for fellowship and conversation? That's *so* not the way for people with bulimia nervosa (BN), whose dining experiences tend toward the polar opposite. Typically, in response to feelings of depression or stress, they gobble their food, consuming quantities far greater than for an average meal. Because they're ashamed of their way-out-of-control behavior, they eat alone. And then they head to the bathroom and throw it all up. Their own self-evaluation involves body shape and weight; in that, they resemble patients with anorexia nervosa. What they don't have is the distorted view of being fat when they are not.

Starting in their late teens or early 20s, patients with BN will wolf down prodigious quantities of food once a week or more, often well past the point of uncomfortable satiety. (These binges can be episodic; for example, occasionally one might be interrupted by travel between dining venues.) The fact that patients with BN are generally about average in weight (some are overweight, but not obese) would be surprising, were it not for their compensatory behavior. Besides vomiting, which some do so often that the enamel wears off their lower teeth, they may use laxatives or other drugs; others exercise excessively, just as in anorexia nervosa. Still others fast between binges. But nearly everyone with BN vomits.

BN is slightly more common than anorexia nervosa, affecting (lifetime) about 1.9% of adult women, men much less so; it is more commonly encountered in high-income countries. The crossover rate with anorexia nervosa is in the 10% neighborhood, and it occasionally morphs into binge-eating disorder. People whose professions and activities

TABLE 9.1. Comparison of Three Eating Disorders

	Anorexia nervosa	Bulimia nervosa	Binge-eating disorder
Eats in binges	No	Yes	Yes
Self-perception	Abnormal (perceives self as fat)	Influenced by body weight, shape	Not remarkable
Compensates with exercise, purging	Yes	Yes	No
Body weight is low	Yes	No	No
Feels lack of control	No	Yes	Yes

emphasize slim body lines—gymnasts, figure skaters, dancers, models—are especially likely to have BN. For unknown reasons, the incidence has probably decreased somewhat over the past 20 years. Like patients with other eating disorders, patients with BN often have comorbid conditions—especially mood and anxiety disorders, but also problems with impulse control and substance use.

With time, nearly half of patients with BN recover fully, and another quarter improve. But that final 25% settle into chronic bulimic behavior. Although mortality rates are higher than average for any comparison age group, the condition is less lethal than anorexia nervosa. The suicide rate, however, is also higher than in the general population. Table 9.1 compares features of BN with those of anorexia nervosa and with binge-eating disorder, discussed next.

Note that, as with other eating disorders, DSM-5-TR does not provide a specific duration in judging when a person has improved sufficiently to invoke a specifier of fully or partly recovered from BN. Instead, we are to judge that it has been for "a sustained period of time." In my opinion, that's a tad wishy-washy; just how long is *sustained*, anyway? A sustained downpour could be 3 hours; a sustained siege on a city, 3 months. I prefer the term *substantial*, which puts us on notice to consider not time alone but also the patient's history of starts and stops.

Essential Features of **Bulimia Nervosa**

Patients with BN know that they have lost control of their eating, consuming in binges much more food than would be usual for most people in that time frame. To an extent that is excessive, self-esteem hinges on their weight and body contour. Weight is managed inappropriately by one or more of: fasting, vomiting, excessive physical workouts, and the abuse of laxatives, diuretics, or other medications.

The Fine Print

The D's: • Duration (weekly for 3+ months) • Differential diagnosis (physical disorders, depressive disorders, **anorexia nervosa,** binge-eating disorder, traditional Thanksgiving meal)

Coding Notes

Specify if:

> **In partial remission.** For a substantial period, the patient meets some but not all BN criteria.
> **In full remission.** For a substantial period, no BN criteria have been met.

Specify current severity, based on episodes of inappropriate compensatory behavior per week. Severity level may be increased, depending on functional impairment:

> **Mild.** 1–3 episodes/week.
> **Moderate.** 4–7.
> **Severe.** 8–13.
> **Extreme.** 14+.

Bernadine Hawley

"I eat when I'm depressed, and I'm depressed when I eat. I'm totally out of control." As she tells her story, Bernadine Hawley frequently blots her streaming eyes with a tissue. She is single and 32, and she teaches second grade. She has never before sought mental health care.

Her first 2 years in college, Bernadine had been moderately anorectic. Convinced that she was too fat, she starved and purged herself down to a scant 98 pounds strung out along her 5-foot-5-inch frame. In those years she was always hungry and would often go on food binges, during which she would "clean out the refrigerator—mine or anyone else's." She later admits, "I must have looked pretty sparse." By the time she finished college, her weight had returned to a steady 120 pounds, controlled by self-induced vomiting.

During the intervening 10 years, Bernadine has followed a binge-and-purge pattern. Twice a week on the average, she will come home from work, assemble a meal for three, and consume it. She prefers sweets and starches—at a sitting she might eat two lasagna TV dinners, a quart of frozen yogurt, and a dozen sugar donuts, none of which requires much effort to prepare. Between courses she will vomit up nearly all she takes in. If she doesn't feel like "cooking," she ventures out for fast food, in half an hour wolfing down as many as four Big Macs. What she relishes seems to be not the taste but the act of consumption; one evening she ate a stick of butter she dipped in confectioner's sugar. In a fit of remorse, she once calculated that during a single evening's binge, she consumed and regurgitated over 10,000 calories.

She also frequently purges herself with laxatives. They are effective, but so expensive that Bernadine resorts to theft. To minimize the chances of detection, she carefully shoplifts only one package at a time. Even so, she manages always to keep at least a 3-month supply on the shelf at the back of her closet.

Bernadine is the only child of a Midwestern couple she describes as "solidly dysfunctional." Because her parents never celebrated the anniversary of their marriage, she assumes that it was precipitated by her own conception. Her mother, who then worked in a bank, was cold and controlling; her father, a barber, drank. In the resulting marital strife, Bernadine was alternately censured and ignored.

She's had friends as a child and as an adult, though some of her girlfriends complain that she is overly concerned with her weight and figure. From the few times she tried it in college, she discovered that she has a healthy appetite for sex. But feelings of shame and embarrassment about her bulimia have kept her from forming any long-lasting romantic relationships.

She is often lonely and sad, though these feelings never last longer than a few days. Although Bernadine admits that her weight is currently normal, still, it worries her. She clips low-fat recipes and belongs to a health club. She has often told herself she would give everything she owns to rid herself of the bingeing. Recently she offered a dentist $2,000 to wire her jaws shut. The dentist pointed out the obvious drawback that she might then starve and referred her to the mental health clinic.

Evaluation of Bernadine Hawley

As is true for many patients with BN, Bernadine's disorder began with behavior typical of moderate (can you work out her BMI?) anorexia nervosa. Now, she doesn't qualify for that diagnosis (her weight is within clinical limits for her height, and she doesn't have a distorted self-image—BN criterion E). During her current binge–purge episodes, she loses control and eats far more than usual (criteria A1 and A2). She also maintains her weight by vomiting and using laxatives (B). Friends have pointed out that she focuses excessively on her figure and weight (D). Her episodes occur more often than weekly and have lasted far longer than the 3-month minimum (C).

Shoplifting isn't a criterion for BN, but the two often occur together. Though any history of stealing should raise the possibility of antisocial or borderline personality disorder, Bernadine's history gives no evidence for either. We didn't ask whether she feels a buildup of tension before and relief, or release, after the theft, but we should have. When criteria for kleptomania are met, it should also be diagnosed along with BN.

Rarely, neurological disorders (some epilepsies, Kleine–Levin syndrome) can present with overeating. Excessive appetite can also occur in major depressive disorder with atypical features. Bernadine shows no evidence of any of these conditions. She does not misuse alcohol or drugs, though many patients with BN do.

Bernadine engages in overeating and purging a couple of times per week; this would rate her a severity level of mild. The vignette suggests some interpersonal difficulties as a result of her bulimia; her clinician should dig deeply to learn whether her eating behavior has affected her work and other life experiences. If so, and if markedly so, we'd want to increase the severity level of both her BN (it's permitted under DSM-5-TR guidelines) and her GAF score of 61 (encouraged under my guidelines). Right now, her diagnosis would read:

F50.2   Bulimia nervosa, mild

F50.81 Binge-Eating Disorder

When it comes to food, who among us has never overindulged? (In good conscience, perhaps no one should cast the first scone.) An extra wedge of pie at Thanksgiving, a triple-dip cone after lunch, and we are left, replete and groaning, vowing to sin no more. Heap on extra portions by the plateful, garnish with shame, warm and serve *ad lib*, and you have the recipe for binge-eating disorder (BED).

Overeating behavior usually starts during the teens or early 20s, sometimes on the heels of a diet. The two central features are the rate of consumption (total amounts can be prodigious) and the sense of loss of control of eating behavior. People with BED don't necessarily have specific cravings, and their selections can be both varied and varying with time. Unlike anorexia or bulimia nervosa, BED doesn't usually morph into another eating disorder.

Although BED is a relative newcomer among officially recognized diagnoses, it is the most common of the eating disorders, affecting (lifetime) about 2% of adults and perhaps half that many adolescents. It occurs nearly twice as often in women as in men and is especially prevalent in people with type 2 diabetes. Although it is often associated with obesity, only about one-quarter of overweight patients have BED. However, people who are obese are far more likely than the general population to experience episodes of binge eating; those who do have BED may find it especially hard to lose weight.

This partly heritable condition often begins as a diet winds down. The eating binges typically occur when the person is feeling glum or anxious, and they often involve delicious foods high in fat, sugar, salt, and guilt. Rapid eating forestalls satiety until too much has been consumed, leading to an uncomfortable, overfull feeling. Because of shame and embarrassment, bingeing may occur in secret, which contributes even more than does the fact of obesity to distress and to problems with quality of life.

Essential Features of **Binge-Eating Disorder**

Consuming in binges much more food than is usual for the time frame, patients with BED know they have lost control. During a binge, they will eat too much, too fast until painfully full, yet in the absence of actual hunger. The bingeing causes guilt (sometimes, depression or disgust) and to avoid embarrassment, solitary dining. However, it does not result in behaviors such as vomiting or excessive exercise designed to make up for overeating.

The Fine Print

The D's: • Duration (weekly for 3+ months) • Distress about eating behavior • Differential diagnosis (mood disorders, **anorexia nervosa, bulimia nervosa,** borderline personality disorder, ordinary overweight)

Coding Notes

Specify if:

> **In partial remission.** For a substantial period, the patient eats in binges less often than once a week.
>
> **In full remission.** For a substantial period, the patient has met no criteria for BED.

Specify current severity (level may be increased, depending on functional impairment):

> **Mild.** 1–3 binges/week.
> **Moderate.** 4–7.
> **Severe.** 8–13.
> **Extreme.** 14+.

Monica Hudgens

"I know I'm obese by anyone's standards," Monica Hudgens tells her internist, "and that I'm doing it to myself."

Even as a child, Monica was overweight. Now, at 5 feet 3 inches, she weighs 210 pounds. "I'm 37 now; for years, my BMI has been tracking with my age."

Monica's bingeing started years ago on the heels of a busted relationship. Now, at least twice a week, she will cook supper—she especially loves pasta with roasted hazelnuts. She'll devour one helping, then gobble down another, then another. Even though she is no longer hungry, she'll then have ice cream ("At least two servings—I just scarf it down, no thinking involved") and cookies. Though she feels stuffed ("with nosh and remorse"), she never vomits up what she has just consumed; she's never used laxatives or other drugs to purge. Washing the dishes afterward, she is often surprised to realize that only 30 minutes have elapsed.

"I've always been large. But until the last couple of years, I've dieted pretty hard. Now I just seem to have given up," Monica says as she touches the bran muffin concealed in her purse. She denies any history of substance misuse; other than the obesity, her internist pronounces her healthy.

Born and raised on the West Coast, Monica has been married and divorced. Now she lives with her 15-year-old son, Roland, whose weight is normal. She tends to binge on weekends, when she isn't working. It has worsened since Roland developed his own set of friends and is frequently off doing his own thing.

Monica's self-image is mixed: "I have a terrific sense of humor and a really pretty face, but I know I'm huge. My ex-husband loved hiking in the mountains, but in the end, he decided he didn't want to be married to one."

Monica works as an news reader for the local NPR affiliate. Her "final straw" moment occurred when she was almost offered a better job. "A producer for cable TV heard me on the radio and liked my voice. But when we met for coffee, he lost interest." She looks downcast, but then with just a hint of a smile she adds, "Can't you just see me on TV? It'd have to be widescreen."

Evaluation of Monica Hudgens

In a meal, Monica eats far more than most people do in similar circumstances, and she clearly voices her loss of control ("I've given up . . . no thinking involved" (criteria A1, A2). These binge episodes occur at least once a week and have lasted many months (D). During an episode, she eats rapidly ("gobbles down" her food), feels uncomfortably full, and eats when she isn't physically hungry (B1, B2, B3). She also expresses contempt for her own eating behavior and eats alone (B4, B5); this might be due to embarrassment, though the vignette doesn't make that point explicit. Only three of the B criterion symptoms are required for diagnosis. Her distress (C) is apparent from her first statement to the clinician. Monica doesn't qualify for an alternative eating disorder diagnosis: The absence of purging and other behavior to compensate for her overeating (E) rules out bulimia nervosa, and her weight obviously puts paid to anorexia nervosa. However, she fully matches the essential features of BED.

Some medical illnesses that involve heavy eating have already been mentioned in connection with bulimia nervosa. In addition to those, Monica shows no evidence of Prader–Willi syndrome (caused by deletion of several genes from chromosome 15), in which the patient is often markedly overweight and eats voraciously—a condition usually apparent from childhood and associated with low intelligence. Monica also denies ever using marijuana; cannabis intoxication is sometimes attended by increased appetite.

Patients with BED often have other DSM-5-TR diagnoses, especially mood and anxiety disorders; for many, a substance use disorder is concurrent. Any second diagnosis predicts that the patient will have more severe BED symptoms. Monica should be fully evaluated for major depressive disorder with atypical features, which can involve overeating and weight gain.

Monica binges a couple of times a week, which the severity criteria say should rate her at mild. However, I think I detect a note of desperation in what she tells her clinician. Despite a relatively healthy GAF score of 61, I'm going to assign her a severity level of moderate. Does anyone want to argue?

F50.81   Binge-eating disorder, moderate
E66.9   Obesity

Whereas clearly observable symptoms separate most physical disorders from usual behavior, an astonishing number of mental disorders are basically just everyday behavior writ large. Disordered eating, substance use, depression, anxiety, somatic symptoms, and even personality disorders are made up of bits of behavior that perfectly ordinary people experience at one time or another. DSM-5-TR uses several features to discriminate diagnosable pathology from the everyday.

Number of symptoms. If you occasionally feel a bit anxious, welcome to life in the 21st century! If you have episodes that include marked anxiety, shortness of breath, heart palpitations, sweating, and weakness, you may have panic disorder.

Level of distress. Many DSM-5-TR diagnoses include a statement that the disorder causes the patient (or associates) to feel substantial distress . . .

Impairment . . . and if they're not distressed, the patient is impaired in work, social, or personal contexts.

Time. Other factors being held constant, a minimum *duration* or *frequency* of symptoms may be needed for a diagnosis. For example, consider persistent depressive disorder (duration) and cyclothymic disorder (duration plus frequency).

Severe consequences. These include suicide or suicide attempts, profound loss of weight, and violent acting out.

Exclusions. Most disorders require that we rule out medical illnesses and substance use; for BED, we exclude patients who have anorexia nervosa or bulimia nervosa. Indeed, most diagnoses ask us to consider other mental disorders in the differential.

Some criteria sets get by with one of the above mechanisms; others use a belt and suspenders approach. A few utilize most or all of these categories, in effect adding thumbs through the belt loops for added security.

Additional Eating Disorders

The remaining conditions in this chapter are found primarily in children. Two (pica and rumination disorder) occur during early childhood development. We really don't know how often they occur in adults, but they seem to have relatively little presence in most mental health populations. Ergo, no vignettes.

Pica

Pica, or the consumption of non-nutritional substances, has been commonly reported in young children and pregnant women. The list of consumables is lengthy, and the variety at times astonishing—dirt, chalk, plaster, soap, paper, and even (rarely) feces. One patient from India had consumed quantities of iron nails and glass beads. Pica has been related to iron deficiency, though other minerals (zinc, for one) may be implicated. Of course, various complications can ensue, among them lead toxicity and the ingestion of various parasites that live in soil and other inedible matter. The behavior is sometimes recognized only when the patient comes to surgery for a bowel obstruction.

Patients with autism spectrum disorder and intellectual developmental disorder are especially prone to pica—a risk that increases with the severity of the principal disorder. Affected children may come from a background of low socioeconomic status and neglect. The behavior usually begins by 2 years of age and remits during adolescence, or when the presumed iron (or other mineral) deficiency is corrected. Pica may affect 5% of children who are of school age.

However, the literature is also replete with examples of people whose abnormal dietary intake began when they were already grown. Pica often appears in the family histories of affected adults, whose own history may have begun in childhood. It has traditionally been associated with pregnancy (though a prevalence of only 0.02% was found in a survey of pregnant Danish women) but is also found in patients with schizophrenia.

Medical specialists tend to think of pica as rare, but if you investigate the right populations, you'll find a lot of it. For example, it was diagnosed in most patients who presented with gastrointestinal blood loss that led to iron-deficiency anemia. Pagophagia (ice craving—no, not ice *carving*) is especially common among patients with iron deficiency. In such instances, as well as in cases of schizophrenia, intellectual developmental disorder, and autism spectrum disorder, before you make the diagnosis, you'll have to persuade yourself that the patient's pica needs additional clinical attention.

Borrowed from the magpie, a black-and-white crow whose scientific genus is *Pica,* this term for a type of abnormal eating behavior dates back at least 400 years. Perhaps someone watching actual magpies collect mud for nests assumed that they were eating it.

As long as four millennia ago and across countless cultures, humans have chewed and swallowed clay. Researchers don't know why it happens; hypotheses include a putative detoxifying role of clay and micronutrients absorbed from the clay.

Essential Features of **Pica**

The patient persists in eating dirt or something else that isn't food.

The Fine Print

The D's: • Duration and demographics (1+ months in someone who is at least 2 years old) • Differential diagnosis (**physical disorder, intellectual developmental disorder, autism spectrum disorder, schizophrenia,** nutritional deficits, developmentally typical behavior, anorexia disorder) • Demographic carve-out (not a practice endorsed by the person's culture)

Coding Notes

If pica occurs in the context of another mental or medical disorder or during pregnancy, diagnose it only if sufficiently severe to merit added clinical care.

Specify if: **In remission** (symptoms have been absent for a substantial period).

Code according to patient's age:

> F98.3 Pica in children
> F50.89 Pica in adults

F98.21 Rumination Disorder

During *rumination,* an individual regurgitates a bolus of food from the stomach and chews it again. This occurs by the mechanism of retrograde peristalsis, and it is a normal part of the digestive process for cattle, deer, and giraffes—which are, after all, ruminants. But in humans it is abnormal and potentially problematic, and it is called rumination disorder (RD). It is also uncommon, most often developing in infants after they begin eating solid foods. Boys are more often affected than are girls.

Most people who ruminate will later reswallow the food. Some, however— especially infants and those with intellectual developmental disorder—instead spit it out, risking malnutrition, failure to thrive (in infants), and vulnerability to disease. Mortality rates as high as 25% have been reported. RD can go undiagnosed for years, perhaps because we don't think to ask.

The cause isn't known, though the usual suspects have been suggested. Possible etiologies include the organic (it may be a symptom of gastroesophageal reflux), the psychological (does it reflect a disordered mother–baby relationship?), and the behavioral (perhaps it's reinforced by the attention it attracts).

Of individuals with intellectual developmental disorder who live in institutions, 6–10% are sometimes affected; RD has been reported in an occasional adult without IDD. One study reported it in 1–2% of elementary school children. Ruminating behavior has also been reported in patients with bulimia nervosa, who tend, however, not to reswallow the food. DSM-5-TR criteria explicitly prohibit diagnosis of RD with another eating disorder. In most cases the behavior subsides spontaneously, though it can persist throughout life. Reportedly, one such adult ruminator was Samuel Johnson, the 18th-century lexicographer whose acquaintances commented on his "cudchewing" behavior.

Note that, like pica (and a host of other conditions throughout the chapters of DSM-5-TR), RD that occurs in the context of another mental or medical disorder must be sufficiently severe to warrant additional clinical care.

RD and pica are two of a relative few DSM-5-TR conditions that require no criteria for clinical significance. That is, unless they occur in the context of another mental disorder, there is no requirement for some statement of harm, distress, additional investigation, or impaired functioning to the patient or to other people. Therefore, there isn't any bright line separating the behavior from what's typical.

Pica and RD are now listed with anorexia and bulimia nervosa, which is where they started out in DSM-III. DSM-IV placed them with other disorders that typically begin in childhood. Welcome home, pica and RD!

Essential Features of **Rumination Disorder**

For at least a month, the patient has been regurgitating food; it may be chewed and swallowed again—or not.

The Fine Print

The D's: • Duration (1+ months) • Differential diagnosis (**physical disorders, other eating disorders**)

Coding Notes

If rumination disorder occurs in the context of another medical or mental disorder (such as intellectual developmental disorder), diagnose it only if sufficiently severe to merit added clinical care.

Specify if: **In remission** (symptoms have been absent for a substantial period).

F50.82 Avoidant/Restrictive Food Intake Disorder

Many young children (nearly half) experience some difficulty with feeding, but most outgrow it. Those who don't may have a form of avoidant/restrictive food intake disorder (ARFID), the latest iteration of what used to be called feeding disorder of infancy or early childhood. The current name reflects the fact that we don't really know why some patients eat too little to remain healthy, only that it happens—and not always early in childhood.

The behavior may commence in the context of parent–child conflict centered around eating. Neglect, abuse, and parental psychopathology (depression, anxiety states, or personality disorders, for example) have also been suggested as causes. Physical barriers to the act of chewing and swallowing and hypersensitivity to certain aspects of food such as texture, taste, and appearance have also been suggested. Indeed, DSM-5-TR encourages us to notice that children with ARFID fall into three principal categories: those who just lack interest in eating; those who restrict their diet due to sensory issues (certain foods are unappetizing); and those who don't eat because of an unpleasant experience—perhaps they've choked when trying to swallow. In any case, the consequences of the behavior extend this definition well beyond the everyday picky eater.

Prevalence is probably well under 1%. Most children with ARFID are under the age of 6, but could even an adult ever be so diagnosed? There's nothing in the DSM-5-TR criteria to prevent it, but you won't find examples thick on the ground.

Essential Features of **Avoidant/Restrictive Food Intake Disorder**

With no abnormality of self-image, the patient avoids eating to the point of failing to maintain adequate nutrition or weight (for children, to grow or gain weight normally). Tube feeding or added oral nourishment may be required; social and personal life may be disrupted.

The Fine Print

The D's: • Differential diagnosis (**physical disorders, unavailability of food,** mood or anxiety disorders, autism spectrum disorder, **anorexia nervosa, bulimia nervosa,** psychotic or factitious disorders, obsessive–compulsive disorder, picky eaters) • Demographic carve-out (accepted cultural practices such as religious fasting)

Coding Notes

If ARFID occurs in the context of another mental or medical disorder, diagnose it only if sufficiently severe to merit added clinical care.

Specify if: **In remission** (symptoms have been absent for a substantial period).

F50.89 Other Specified Feeding or Eating Disorder

Numerous people fall outside the definitions of the major feeding and eating disorders; some of them are seriously ill. (It is also critically important to make sure that such a patient doesn't have another definitive condition, such as a mood disorder, schizophrenia, somatic symptom disorder, or any problem caused by another medical condition.) Below are several that can be specified by name, following the "other specified" label and number.

> **Atypical anorexia nervosa.** Some patients lose considerable weight, fear becoming fat, and believe they look fat, even have physiological changes typical of anorexia nervosa, yet their weight remains within normal limits.

> **Binge-eating disorder (of low frequency or limited duration).** The bingeing occurs less than weekly or for under 3 months.

> **Bulimia nervosa (of low frequency or limited duration).** A patient who fulfills most criteria for bulimia nervosa doesn't binge and compensate often or long enough to meet the time criteria.

> **Night eating syndrome.** Episodes of eating occur after the evening meal or upon awakening during the night; the next day, the patient remembers doing so.

> **Purging disorder.** Without binge eating, the patient repeatedly engages in purging behavior (intentionally vomits or uses drugs) to affect weight or appearance.

F50.9 Unspecified Feeding or Eating Disorder

As with unspecified diagnoses in other sections of DSM-5-TR, use unspecified feeding or eating disorder when the patient does not meet full criteria for one of the diagnoses described above, and you do not wish to be more specific.

CHAPTER 10

Elimination Disorders

Quick Guide to the Elimination Disorders

Encopresis. At the age of 4 years or later, the patient repeatedly passes feces into inappropriate places (p. 300).

Enuresis. At the age of 5 years or later, the patient repeatedly voids urine (it can be voluntary or involuntary) into bedding or clothing (p. 298).

Introduction

Encopresis and enuresis usually occur separately, though they can travel together, especially in a child who has been seriously neglected or emotionally deprived. You might encounter either diagnosis as *primary* (symptoms have been present throughout the child's development) or as *secondary* (toilet training was initially successful). Neither of these terms is used in the diagnosis, however. Abnormalities of the genitourinary and/ or gastrointestinal tracts are often suspected but only rarely identified, so that a careful medical history is usually enough to enable the correct diagnosis.

F98.0 Enuresis

By a ratio of 4:1, primary enuresis (the child has never been dry) is more common than secondary enuresis. It is limited to bedwetting; daytime bladder control is unaffected. Parents of children referred to a mental health professional have typically tried the common remedies—fluid restriction before bedtime, midnight toilet use—without success. Because the children typically wet several times a week, they are too embarrassed to sleep over with friends.

In some children, enuresis is associated with non-rapid eye movement sleep, which occurs especially during the first 3 hours of sleep. In others, trauma such as hospitalization or separation from parents may precipitate secondary enuresis, which can occur more than once per night or randomly throughout the period of sleep. Although some enuretic children have urinary tract infections or physical anomalies (then, we *wouldn't* diagnose enuresis), the etiology most often remains unknown. The formal criteria state that the wetting can be done on purpose, but for most children it is accidental and embarrassing.

There is a strong genetic influence: About three-fourths of affected children have a first-degree relative with a history of enuresis. Having two enuretic parents strongly predicts that a child will be affected.

Before age 6, boys and girls are about equally represented (overall, around 5–10% of young children are affected). In older children, enuresis is more frequent in boys. The prevalence falls off with maturation, so that it affects only about 1% of adolescents. An adult who wets the bed will likely continue doing so lifelong.

Shameless advertisement: How do you decide that one event has caused another? Of course, in clinical diagnosis, it's hard ever to be certain, but several features can help you decide with a reasonable degree of confidence that A has caused B. I've discussed these issues (and much more) in my book *Diagnosis Made Easier* (The Guilford Press).

Essential Features of **Enuresis**

Without known cause, a patient recurrently urinates into clothing or bedding—with or without intention. The patient experiences distress or disability, as stated below, or frequency of symptoms, also below.

The Fine Print

The D's: • Duration and demographics (2+ times/week for 3+ months in someone 5 years of age or older) • Distress or disability (work/educational, social, or personal impairment) • Differential diagnosis (**medication side effects** and **physical disorders**)

Coding Notes

Specify the type:

Nocturnal only
Diurnal only
Nocturnal and diurnal

F98.1 Encopresis

Patients with encopresis move their bowels in inappropriate places, such as into their clothing or onto the floor. There are two types. One is associated with chronic constipation, which leads to fissures around the anus. Defecation therefore causes pain, which the child seeks to forestall by delaying the act. Then the stool hardens (which worsens the fissures), and liquid feces leaks from the impacted rectum into clothing and bedclothes.

The less common type, without constipation, is often a matter of secrecy and denial. Children deposit a normal stool in an abnormal location—behind the toilet, in bureau drawers—and then deny knowing how it got there. Encopresis without constipation is often associated with stress and other family psychopathology. Some of these children may have been abused physically or sexually.

Encopresis affects about 1% of elementary school-age children; boys predominate by a 6:1 ratio. When encopresis is voluntary, it may be associated with conduct disorder or oppositional defiant disorder. Note that to receive a diagnosis of encopresis, the person must be at least the developmental equivalent of a 4-year-old.

Essential Features of Encopresis

Whether on purpose or accidental, the patient recurrently defecates in improper locations or into clothes.

The Fine Print

The D's: • Duration and demographics (1+ times/month for 3+ months in someone 4 years or the developmental equivalent) • Differential diagnosis (**laxative use** and **physical disorders**)

Coding Notes

Specify type:

   {With}{Without} constipation and overflow incontinence.

Other Specified Elimination Disorder

Use the other specified elimination disorder category for symptoms of encopresis or enuresis that do not meet the full diagnostic criteria, in cases where you wish to state the reason. Use the following diagnostic codes:

N39.498 With urinary symptoms

R15.9 With fecal symptoms

Unspecified Elimination Disorder

Use the unspecified elimination disorder category for symptoms of encopresis or enuresis that do not meet the full diagnostic criteria, in cases where you do not wish to state the reason. Use the following diagnostic codes:

R32 With urinary symptoms

R15.9 With fecal symptoms

CHAPTER 11

Sleep–Wake Disorders

Quick Guide to the Sleep–Wake Disorders

In this Quick Guide, I have arranged the disorders rather differently from DSM-5-TR's order, to emphasize the most prevalent underlying diagnoses.

Sleeping Too Little (Insomnia)

Insomnia is often a symptom; sometimes it is a presenting complaint. Only occasionally is it a diagnosis independent of another major mental disorder or another medical condition (sidebar, p. 307).

I can't overstate how important it is to evaluate first whether another mental disorder or medical condition could be the cause of insomnia.

Insomnia disorder. It can be comorbid with a medical condition (p. 306), primary (when there's no discernible cause; p. 312), or comorbid with another sleep disorder or mental disorder (p. 309). The last is most often encountered in patients suffering from major depressive episodes (p. 112), manic episodes (p. 123), or even panic attacks (p. 172).

Substance/medication-induced sleep–wake disorder, insomnia type. Most of the commonly misused psychoactive substances, as well as a variety of prescription medicines, can interfere with sleep (p. 351).

Sleep apnea. Although most patients with breathing problems such as sleep apnea complain of hypersomnia, some instead have insomnia. Three principal types are listed: obstructive sleep apnea hypopnea, central sleep apnea, and sleep-related hypoventilation (pp. 323, 327).

Sleeping Too Much (Hypersomnolence)

You might think that the term *hypersomnia* means *only* that a patient sleeps too much. However, it also indicates drowsiness at a time when the patient should be alert. A new word, *hypersomnolence,* has been introduced to keep us alert to both meanings.

Hypersomnolence disorder. Excessive drowsiness or sleepiness can accompany mental or medical disorders, or other sleep disorders; sometimes it's primary (p. 315).

Narcolepsy. These patients experience a crushing need to sleep, regardless of time of day, causing them to fall asleep almost instantly—sometimes, even when standing. They may also have sleep paralysis, sudden loss of strength (cataplexy), and hallucinations as they fall asleep or awaken (p. 319).

Substance/medication-induced sleep–wake disorder, daytime sleepiness type. The use of a substance is less likely to produce hypersomnolence than insomnia, but it can happen (p. 351).

Breathing-related sleep disorders. These disorders commonly result in daytime drowsiness. Three principal types are listed: obstructive sleep apnea (p. 323), central sleep apnea (p. 323), and sleep-related hypoventilation (p. 327).

Circadian Rhythm Sleep–Wake Disorders

There's a mismatch between someone's biological clock and the environment. Five principal types are listed:

Delayed sleep phase type. Falling asleep and waking later than desired (p. 329).

Advanced sleep phase type. Falling asleep and waking earlier than desired (p. 329).

Irregular sleep–wake type. Falling asleep and waking at irregular times (p. 330).

Non-24-hour sleep–wake type. Usually, a progressive drift to sleeping later than desired (p. 330).

Shift work type. Sleepiness associated with changes in work schedule (p. 330).

Jet lag. Feeling sleepy or "hungover" after crossing time zones is no longer considered a sleep disorder; it's a physiological fact of modern life. Nonetheless, I've covered it briefly in a sidebar (p. 330).

Parasomnias and Other Disorders of Sleep

In these disorders, something abnormal happens in association with sleep (or with the stages of sleep), or during the times when the patient is falling asleep or waking up.

Non-rapid eye movement (non-REM) sleep arousal disorder, sleep terror type. These patients cry out in apparent fear during the first part of the night. Often, they don't really wake up at all. This behavior is considered pathological only in adults, not children (p. 339).

Non-REM sleep arousal disorder, sleepwalking type. Persistent sleepwalking usually occurs early in the night (p. 336).

Non-REM sleep arousal disorder, confusional arousals. Patients partially awaken, but they don't walk about and don't appear fearful. This isn't an official DSM-5-TR disorder, but people experience it anyway (p. 341).

Rapid eye movement (REM) sleep behavior disorder. These patients awaken from REM sleep to speak or thrash about, sometimes injuring themselves or bed partners (p. 348).

Nightmare disorder. Bad dreams trouble some people more than others (p. 345).

Restless legs syndrome. The irresistible need to move one's legs during periods of inactivity (especially evenings/nights) leads to fatigue and other behavioral/emotional problems (p. 341).

Substance/medication-induced sleep–wake disorder, parasomnia type. Alcohol and other substances (during intoxication or withdrawal) can cause various problems with sleep (p. 351).

Other specified, or unspecified, sleep disorder. These categories are for problems of insomnia, hypersomnolence, or general sleep issues that aren't covered by any of the preceding groups (p. 354).

Introduction

Sleep is basic behavior for all animals, including humans. Keep in mind these points about the normal sleep of humans:

1. Normality takes in a lot of territory. It includes the amount of sleep, how long it takes to fall asleep and to awaken, and what happens in between.

2. When sleep is abnormal, it can have profound consequences for health.

3. An individual's sleep changes throughout the life cycle. Everyone knows that babies sleep most of the time. As people grow older, they take more time to fall asleep, they require less sleep, and they awaken more often throughout the night. I've heard it said that 9-year-old children sleep the best of anyone. Too bad: Everyone reading this is over the hill, sleepwise.

4. Sleep isn't uniform; it varies in depth and quality throughout the night. The two principal phases of sleep are rapid eye movement (REM) sleep, during which most dreaming takes place, and non-REM sleep. Various disorders can be related to these phases of sleep.

5. Many people who sleep less soundly or more briefly than they think they should do not have an actual disorder of sleep.

6. Even today, sleep disorder criteria are based principally upon clinical find-

ings. EEG and other sleep laboratory studies may be confirmatory, but they are required for diagnosis in just a few of the conditions described here.

Sleep specialists divide sleep disorders into *dyssomnias* and *parasomnias*. A patient with a *dyssomnia* sleeps too little, too much, or at the wrong time, but the sleep itself—what there is of it—is pretty unremarkable. In a *parasomnia,* the quality, quantity, and timing of sleep are essentially normal. But something unusual happens during sleep itself, or during the times when the patient is falling asleep or waking up; motor, cognitive, or autonomic nervous system processes become active during sleep or during the transitions between sleep and wakefulness, and all hell breaks loose.

Consider, for example, sleep apnea (dyssomnia) versus nightmares (parasomnia). Both occur during sleep, but nightmares are usually problematic because they are scary, not because they interfere with sleeping or impair wakefulness the next day—the way sleep apnea does.

Sleeping Too Much or Too Little

F51.01 Insomnia Disorder

What most of us understand by *insomnia* is this: sleep that is too brief or is unrestful. Some people with insomnia may not realize just how tense they are. Some cases may start as insomnia secondary to another medical condition, such as pain from a broken hip. The hip heals, but the patient has become accustomed to the idea of being unable to sleep at night. In other words, insomnia can be learned behavior. Indeed, many medical illnesses can lead to the symptoms of insomnia disorder.

Some people with insomnia may use their beds for activities other than sleeping or having sex—eating and watching TV, for example. These associations condition them to be wakeful when they are in bed; it's part of what sleep clinicians call poor sleep hygiene. These folks may discover the source of the problem when their sleep improves during weekends, during holidays, or on a vacation, when they've escaped their usual habits and habitats. Most patients with insomnia disorder also have some other mental or medical disorder.

Whatever the cause, insomnia can persist forever if it isn't effectively addressed. Insomnia disorder (ID) is found especially in older patients and in women. Many patients complain of unrefreshing (aka nonrestorative) sleep, or of remaining awake when their bed partners swear they have slept all night. For this reason, the statement that insomnia is "sleeping too little" still isn't quite right; rather, insomnia is the *complaint* of sleeping too little. But these patients do have problems that should not be belittled. Giving them time to state what is on their minds is important in seeking the etiology of their difficulties.

Insomnia can be experienced in several different patterns. The most common—especially frequent in older adults—is trouble maintaining sleep (waking during the night, or *interval insomnia*), which accounts for perhaps 60% of insomnia disorders. *Terminal insomnia*—the experience of awakening before it is time to get up and being unable to return to sleep, is less frequently experienced, though it is regarded as classic for severe major depressive disorder. And some people, especially younger adults, complain more of difficulty falling asleep (*initial insomnia*).

Note that the definition of ID requires that the patient experience clinically important distress or disability as a result. Although the distress may be experienced during the nighttime, any resulting disability will most likely be experienced during normal waking hours—reduced effectiveness at work or school, interpersonal conflict at home, daytime fatigue and sleepiness, grumpy demeanor, and the like. Anyone who complains of difficulty sleeping, but who does not experience distress or disability, should not receive the diagnosis of ID. Even with those restrictions, that still leaves up to 10% of the adult population affected by ID (though perhaps a third of all adults complain of trouble sleeping at one time or another). It is a bit more common among women than men.

DSM-5-TR specifies that we should use the diagnosis of ID for any patient who fulfills the diagnostic criteria, whether or not there is a coexisting mental, medical, or other sleep–wake disorder—if the patient's ID is sufficiently serious to require independent clinical attention.

Insomnia Disorder, with Other Medical Comorbidity

Many medical illnesses are associated with sleep problems (mostly insomnia), typically restlessness, increased sleep onset latency, and frequent awakenings during the night. The medical issues cited—which can produce discomfort day or night—include the following:

- Fever resulting from a variety of infections.
- Pain caused by headache (especially some migraines), rheumatoid arthritis, cancer, persistent nocturnal penile erections, or angina.
- Itching caused by a variety of systemic and skin disorders.
- Breathing problems resulting from asthma or chronic obstructive pulmonary disease (COPD), restricted lung capacity (due to obesity, pregnancy, or spinal deformities), or cystic fibrosis.
- Endocrine and metabolic diseases, including hyperthyroidism, liver failure, and kidney disease.
- Sleeping in one position enforced, for example, by wearing a cast.
- Neuromuscular disorders, such as muscular dystrophy and poliomyelitis.
- Movement and other neurological disorders, such as Huntington's disease, torsion dystonia, Parkinson's disease, and some seizure disorders.

Essential Features of **Insomnia Disorder**

Despite having adequate opportunity for sleep, the patient complains of its quality or amount: trouble getting to sleep, staying asleep, or awakening too early in the morning. Occasionally, sleep is just plain unrefreshing.

The Fine Print

The D's: • Duration (3+ nights/week for 3+ months) • Distress or disability (work/educational, social, or personal impairment) • Differential diagnosis (**substance use** and **physical disorders, other mental disorders** such as mood or anxiety disorders, psychotic disorders, posttraumatic stress disorder, sleep apnea and **other sleep–wake disorders,** poor sleep hygiene, too little available sleep time, and just plain normal variation in sleep requirement)

Coding Notes

Specify if:

> **Episodic.** Duration 1–3 months (any shorter-duration insomnia disorder would be coded as other specified insomnia disorder, p. 354).
> **Persistent.** Duration 3+ months.
> **Recurrent.** 2+ episodes in 1 year.

Specify if:

> **With mental disorder.** These include substance use disorders.
> **With medical condition**
> **With another sleep disorder**

In each case, specify the coexisting disorder. You don't need to state which came first; often, you simply don't know.

Nobody knows the frequency of insomnia complaints in a patient who isn't otherwise sick (that is, who has neither another medical nor another mental condition). Such patients are probably a tiny minority of those a mental health professional encounters. Perhaps these people are more likely to seek help from a primary medical care provider. Although texts say that persistent insomnia is fairly common, of over 15,000 mental health patients I have examined, exactly 1 had what I considered primary ID (without another medical or mental disorder).

Hoyle Garner

Hoyle Garner is 58 when he seeks treatment for his insomnia. His wife, Edith, accompanies him to the appointment. Together, they run a mom-and-pop grocery store.

Several years ago, Hoyle learned that he has emphysema. A series of pulmonary function tests had prompted his doctor to ask him to quit smoking. In 3 weeks, he gained 10 pounds and couldn't concentrate well enough to figure how many tins of ham to order at Easter. "I was depressed and uptight, and I couldn't sleep 2 hours without waking up and wanting a cigarette," Hoyle remembers.

"I begged him to start smoking again," says Edith. "When he did, it was a relief for both of us."

Hoyle quit seeing the doctor, and his sleep returned to normal. Within the past few months, however, he's begun awakening several times during the night. Some nights this happens as often as every hour. He feels restless and uncomfortable, with some of the same anxiety he experienced when he'd tried to quit smoking. A few times he has tried sitting on the edge of the bed to have a cigarette, but it doesn't seem to help. And anyway, now Edith complains about the smell of smoke in the night. They still run their grocery, and Hoyle has no trouble at all ordering hams. He never drinks more than a single beer, usually in the afternoon.

"Waking up doesn't bother him much," Edith offers. "He usually goes right back to sleep. He doesn't even feel sleepy the next day. But it leaves me wide awake, wondering how soon he'll wake up again."

Edith's hours awake have given her plenty of opportunity to observe her husband in repose. After he sleeps quietly for half an hour or so, his breathing becomes rapid and shallow. It never stops for longer than a few seconds, and he doesn't snore. They had tried having him sleep with extra pillows (that's what helped her Uncle Will with his heart failure), but it didn't ease Hoyle's sleeping any. Indeed, "it kinda hurt his neck."

"I hope we can get to the bottom of this," Edith concludes. "It doesn't seem to bother him very much, but I've got to get some sleep."

Evaluation of Hoyle Garner

Hoyle's main problem is with sleep, which shows up as frequent awakenings, several times every night, for months (ID criteria A2, C, D) despite sufficient opportunities for sleep (E). Although for him the effects are less than earth-shaking (insomnia due to COPD typically doesn't produce daytime drowsiness), his wife complains quite a lot. And the effect of someone's insomnia on a bed partner or caregiver is one of the symptoms that tells us we have a problem deserving clinical consideration (B).

The features of Hoyle's insomnia would not suggest a severe mood disorder, which could produce early morning awakening. Besides, a mild mood disorder, or adjustment disorder with depressed mood, is typically associated with trouble falling asleep. Based on Edith's observations, Hoyle does not have (F) a variety of narcolepsy or sleep apnea (do check for sleep apnea in any insomnia patient with other medical comorbidity). He was taking no medications at the time, but many patients with medical illnesses will be doing so; then, you'll have to rule out substance-induced insomnia.

Hoyle also has tobacco use disorder, which probably caused the emphysema in the first place; it would be hard to attribute his insomnia to a physiological consequence of nicotine (G). When he was trying to quit smoking, he clearly experienced tobacco withdrawal, and he continued to smoke despite his COPD (p. 470). I'd give him a GAF score of 61. His complete diagnosis would be as follows:

J43.9	Pulmonary emphysema
F17.200	Tobacco use disorder, moderate
F51.01	Insomnia disorder, persistent, with pulmonary emphysema and moderate tobacco use disorder

Note that DSM-5-TR doesn't ask us to specify whether insomnia is "due to" a comorbid physical or mental disorder. It is enough to say that they coexist. That's because it can be extraordinarily difficult to determine whether one has caused the other. We are allowed (indeed, encouraged) to diagnose any disorder with symptoms severe enough to justify independent clinical attention.

Insomnia Disorder, with Non-Sleep Disorder Mental Comorbidity

When it is a symptom of some other mental disorder, insomnia is often directly proportional to the severity of the other diagnosis. And, logically enough, sleep usually improves with resolution of the underlying condition. Meanwhile, patients sometimes abuse hypnotic and other medications. Here's a brief overview:

Major depressive episodes. Insomnia is probably most often a symptom of a mood disorder. In fact, sleep disturbance may be one of the earliest symptoms of depression. Insomnia is especially likely to affect depressed elderly patients. In severe depression, terminal insomnia (awakening early in the morning and being unable to get back to sleep) is characteristic—and a truly miserable experience.

Trauma- and stressor-related disorders. Criteria for acute stress disorder and for posttraumatic stress disorder specifically mention sleep disturbance as a symptom.

Panic disorder. Panic attacks may occur during sleep.

Adjustment disorder. Patients who have developed anxiety or depression in response to a specific stressor may lie awake worrying about it or about events of the day.

Somatic symptom disorder. Many patients with somatic symptom disorder will complain of problems with sleep, especially initial and interval insomnia.

Cognitive disorders. Most patients with neurocognitive disorder have some degree of sleep disturbance. Typically, this involves interval awakening: They will wander at night and suffer from reduced alertness during the day.

Manic and hypomanic episodes. Patients with manic or hypomanic episodes typically sleep less than they do when they are euthymic. However, they don't complain of insomnia. Rather, they feel rested and ready for more activity; it's their families and friends who become concerned (and fatigued). If such patients do complain, it is usually of lengthened sleep onset latency—the time it takes to fall asleep.

Schizophrenia. When they are becoming ill, delusions, hallucinations, or anxiety may keep patients with schizophrenia preoccupied far into the night. Total sleep time may remain constant, but they arise progressively later, until most of their sleeping occurs during the day. DSM-5-TR doesn't provide a way to code a circadian rhythm sleep–wake disorder related to a mental disorder; ID related to schizophrenia (or, perhaps, other specified insomnia disorder) would be about the closest we can come.

Obsessive–compulsive personality disorder. This personality disorder has been cited in association with insomnia.

Anxiety or mania may mask an insomnia that occurs during another mental disorder. Patients may not recognize a sleep deficit until they fall asleep at the wheel or suffer an industrial accident. On the other hand, there's also a risk that clinicians could focus on the problem with sleep and underdiagnose the associated mental problem.

Sal Camozzi

"I'm just not getting enough sleep to play." Sal Camozzi is a third-year student who attends a small college in southern California on an athletic scholarship.

Now it is early November, midway through the football season, and he doesn't think he can maintain the effort. He always keeps regular hours and eats "healthy," but for over a month he has been awakening at 2:30 every morning.

"I might as well be setting an alarm," he says. "My eyes snap open and there I am, worrying about the next game, or passing chemistry, or whatever. I'm only sleeping 5 hours at night, and I've always needed 8. I'm getting desperate."

For a while Sal tried over-the-counter sleeping pills. They helped a little, but mainly they made him feel groggy the next day. He has always avoided alcohol and drugs, and he hates the feeling of chemicals in his body, so he was glad to give them up.

Sal had something of the same problem the previous fall, and the one before that. Then there'd been the same difficulty with sleep; his appetite had fallen off, too. Neither time had things been as severe as now, however. (This year he has already lost 10 pounds; as a linebacker, he needs to keep his weight up.) Sal also complains that he just doesn't seem to enjoy life in general the way he usually does. Even his interest in football and his concentration on the field have diminished.

One summer during high school, Sal had felt listless and slept too much. He'd been tested for infectious mononucleosis and found to be physically well. He was his usual self by the time school started that fall.

Last spring and the one before had been a different matter. When Sal went out for baseball, he seemed to explode with energy, batted .400, and played every game. He didn't sleep much then, either, now that he thinks about it—5 hours a night had seemed plenty. "I had loads of energy and never felt happier in my life. I felt like another Babe Ruth."

The coach notes that Sal was "terrific during baseball season, all hustle, but he talked too much. Why doesn't he put the same effort into football?"

Evaluation of Sal Camozzi

From Sal's history, his sleep disorder isn't related to substance use or to any physical illness. There is similarly no evidence for another sleep disorder.

Sal's sleep difficulty is only the tip of his depressive iceberg. The first thing to look for would be other symptoms of a major depressive episode. Although he doesn't complain of feeling depressed in so many words, he does report a general loss of zest for life. Besides that and the insomnia, Sal also has problems with appetite, interest, and concentration. Together, his symptoms (barely) meet criteria for a major depressive episode. The history doesn't touch on death wishes or suicidal ideas; this needs to be explored.

Besides depression, his diagnosis also needs to account for the obvious episodes of high mood. Sal has had several periods when he feels unusually happy, his energy level increases, he talks a great deal, and his *need* for sleep falls off. Then, and especially in contrast to his present mood, his self-esteem is markedly increased (he notes feeling "like Babe Ruth"). This change in his mood was pronounced enough that others noticed and commented on it. However, it does not appear to compromise his functioning or require hospitalization—if ever it does, we'd need to diagnose manic episode. As matters stand, his symptoms fulfill criteria for a hypomanic episode.

All of this adds up to a diagnosis of bipolar II disorder (p. 135); Sal's current episode is of course depressed. He nearly meets criteria for the specifier *with melancholic features,* but his history of repeated depressions beginning in the same season of the year (fall) and consistently either resolving or switching to hypomania during another season (spring) would be typical for the specifier *with seasonal pattern.* Although in high school Sal may have had an episode of depression that didn't fit this pattern, most of the episodes do, and that meets the requirement. The last 2 years fit the mold exactly.

Sal's sleeplessness would be clinically significant even without the bipolar II diagnosis (ID criteria A, B), since it caused fatigue and occurred several nights a week (C).

But here's the rub: It has persisted for just over a month—perhaps 60 days shy of the 3 months required by DSM-5-TR for ID. Sal does fit the DSM-IV criteria, and Sal hasn't changed; only the criteria have. What to do?

To me, it seems unreasonable that a person who has a disorder that, by definition, is relatively short-lived (patients with seasonal mood disturbance become ill and recover with the seasons) cannot qualify for the additional diagnosis of ID. So, with the understanding that the criteria are only guidelines, not straitjackets, I'm going to stick with my original evaluation. Whether you agree with me or not, his story can still help guide us through the maze of the diagnostic criteria. (If you do disagree, you can code his sleep disorder as G47.09, other specified insomnia disorder, brief insomnia disorder.)

Sal's GAF score would be 55. We are instructed to list the associated mental (or medical) disorder right after the sleep disorder, to make the association clear. I wanted to list first the mood disorder, because it is the more critical to treat, but at least I did put them contiguously. (OK, it's hard to do otherwise when the list includes only two items.)

F31.81	Bipolar II disorder, depressed, with seasonal pattern
F51.01	Insomnia disorder, with bipolar II disorder

To a considerable degree, it's a matter of taste whether to diagnose a sleep disorder that occurs with another mental condition. DSM-5-TR notes that this is appropriate when the problem with sleep is serious enough to justify an evaluation. If the patient's presenting complaint is the sleep problem, I'd consider it evidence of clinical importance. However, these situations are often unclear and usually require judgment. In the example of a mood disorder, any problem with sleep is almost sure to resolve once the depression has been adequately treated. Therefore, no one could be faulted for diagnosing only the mood disorder.

[Primary] Insomnia Disorder

Another type of ID—in which the person has no other apparent condition to which the insomnia can be attributed—is the one least often encountered. Indeed, this type should be one of exclusion, used only after other possibilities mentioned above have been ruled out. In DSM-IV it was called *primary* insomnia disorder.

Of course, the fact that we cannot discern the cause of insomnia doesn't mean there isn't one. Sometimes insomnia may start because a noise or some other stimulus inhibits sleep. (When sleeplessness is due to a noisy surroundings or other conditions not conducive to sleep, it isn't technically insomnia. It's sometimes called, would you believe, environmental sleep disorder? But DSM-5-TR doesn't call it that, leaving that kind of specialization to folks who study sleep.)

Another contributing factor is being active right up until bedtime. Vigorous exercise and arguments are just two of the activities that can promote sleeplessness; people need quiet time to get into the relaxed frame of mind required for efficient sleep onset. Once insomnia is underway, muscle tension from lying awake and thinking negatively ("I'm a terrible sleeper") perpetuates the problem. The result is hours of nighttime frustration, yielding to fatigue and dysphoria the following day.

How often does this type of insomnia occur? No one really knows. Though perhaps a quarter of all adults are unhappy with their sleep, the percentage who would qualify for an ID diagnosis is probably down in single digits. It is especially found in older people and in women. Though over time it may vary, it typically follows a chronic course.

Primary (as in a primary insomnia) is one of those funny words that have taken on meanings different from what most speakers of English understand. In the clinical world, *primary* means an illness or symptom for which no cause can be found. In this context, *primary* doesn't mean that one condition is more important than another, or that one begins earlier than something else. (The World Health Organization also uses *primary* to mean a disorder that attacks the brain directly or preferentially, as opposed to those that attack the brain only as one of several body organs or systems.) DSM-5-TR doesn't use *primary* in any official sense at all, but clinicians do, to differentiate disorders for which we can state a cause from those for which we can't.

Clinicians also use the term *functional* to describe disorders for which there's no obvious basis in brain anatomy, chemistry, or physiology. Most mood disorders and psychoses are called *functional;* that is, we still don't know why or how they have developed. *Functional* has now also officially replaced *conversion symptom.* If you think all this is confusing, consider some of the other words deployed throughout the medical world to mean "I haven't a clue as to the cause": *essential,* as in essential hypertension; *idiopathic,* as in idiopathic thrombocytopenic purpura; *cryptogenic* (literally, "hidden cause") this or that. Sometimes we say *psychogenic,* which gives the illusion that we have found the cause, but then it's often only in our minds—or dreams.

No wonder clinicians in training don't sleep so well.

Curtis Usher

"It's almost spooky. It doesn't seem to make any difference what time I go to bed—9:30, 10:00, 10:30. Whatever, my eyes click open at 2:00 in the morning, and that's it for the rest of the night."

Curtis Usher has had this problem on and off for years. Recently, it's mostly on. "Actually, I guess it's usually at its worst during the week. Whenever I lie there, I'm worrying about work."

Curtis is a project manager at an advertising agency. It's a wonderful job when times are flush, which they haven't been for several years. Curtis's boss is a bit of a tyrant who brags that he doesn't have headaches—he causes them. Curtis doesn't have headaches, but he doesn't get much sleep, either.

At age 53, Curtis is healthy and has regular habits. He has lived alone since his wife divorced him 3 years earlier; she complained that he's dull. Occasionally his current girlfriend stays overnight in his studio apartment, but most evenings he spends lying on his bed watching public television until he drifts off. He never drinks or uses drugs, and his mood is good. Neither he nor anyone else in his family has ever had any mental health problems.

"I don't take naps during the day," Curtis sums up, "but I might as well. I'm sure not getting much done at work."

Evaluation of Curtis Usher

Curtis clearly has trouble sleeping—it would seem to include both initial and terminal components (ID criteria A1, A3)—that has lasted far longer than the required 3 months (D). From what Curtis relates, it occurs several times a week (C) and has reduced his efficiency at work (B). Other than an occasional sleepover with his girlfriend, no other information suggests circumstances that would interfere with his opportunities for sleep (E).

The challenge is to determine whether Curtis's insomnia is stand-alone or whether we need to include in our coding some underlying problem that is destroying his sleep. Although the vignette doesn't cover every possibility, it does touch upon some major points.

Curtis probably does not have another mental disorder (H). His mood has been too good for a major depressive episode. Although he worries about work, we have no information to suggest that he has the wide-ranging anxiety typical of generalized anxiety disorder. He doesn't drink alcohol or use drugs (G); there is no information to exclude a personality disorder, but PDs are probably infrequent as the sole cause of a sleep disorder.

We have only Curtis's own evaluation of his good health to confirm that he does not have another medical condition (also criterion H); his clinician should refer him for a medical evaluation. What about other sleep disorders (F)? Curtis doesn't nap, which would seem to rule out narcolepsy. Sleep apnea also appears unlikely: His former wife complained of dullness, not snoring. Circadian rhythm sleep–wake disorder, delayed sleep phase type would result in awakening late rather than early, and he doesn't get sleepy early, as would be the case with the advanced sleep phase type. The vignette contains no information that would support a parasomnia diagnosis such as nightmare disorder, or a non-REM sleep arousal disorder like sleep terrors or sleepwalking.

Two mechanisms could help account for Curtis's insomnia. His work-related anxiety is one (a demanding boss, tough times in his industry). Alternatively, he often reclines on his bed while watching TV. The association of this waking-related activity with bed (one facet of poor sleep hygiene) could have conditioned him to remain wakeful.

Pending the outcome of a medical evaluation, here's how I'd diagnose Curtis (with a GAF score of 65 and with a Z-code to indicate an area that needs work):

F51.01   Insomnia disorder, persistent

Z72.9   Lifestyle problem (poor sleep hygiene)

Generalized anxiety disorder is important in the differential diagnosis of ID because patients with GAD also sometimes lie awake worrying. The difference is that the anxieties of ID patients are focused on their inability to sleep as well as they think they should. Also watch for "masked depression": Inquire carefully about other vegetative symptoms (diminished appetite, weight loss) of a major depressive episode when you are evaluating patients who present with ID.

F51.11 Hypersomnolence Disorder

Sleep experts have adopted the term *hypersomnolence* in place of the more familiar *hypersomnia*, and here's why: The new term better describes the fact that these conditions can result either in excessive sleep or in a less-than-optimal quality of wakefulness. The latter includes trouble waking up or remaining fully awake, sometimes called *sleep drunkenness* or *sleep inertia*—the sensation of just not being able to fully awaken (or stay that way) when we need to be fully alert. Hypersomnolence disorder (HD) can occur with medical, mental, or other sleep disorders; sometimes it is apparently free-standing.

Patients with HD tend to fall asleep easily and rapidly (often in 5 minutes or less), and they may sleep late the next day. They tend to have trouble awakening in the morning; perhaps 40% feel groggy and report peculiar problems with disorientation, memory, and alertness (sleep inertia). Although total sleep time is likely to be 9 or more hours in 24, they may feel so chronically tired that even after a good night's sleep they take daytime naps. These tend to be long and unrefreshing; they don't improve things much. In their state of reduced alertness, patients with HD may act automatically, performing behaviors they don't recall later.

Although we don't have a lot of information about HD, it probably occurs about equally in males and females and begins when they are relatively young, typically in their teens or 20s. It may affect up to 1% of the general population.

Though the cause of HD isn't always apparent, there are several known associations. Hypocretin (the hormone associated with wakefulness) deficiency occurs less often in cases of HD than in narcolepsy with cataplexy, though on average, its level is less than that for the general population. Also common is a gene allele (HLA DQB1*0602, for anyone who wants *all* the facts), though no one can be sure that HD is strictly a genetic phenomenon. Some patients with HD may be having trouble coping with stress; others may be trying to compensate for a sense of something lacking in their lives. In any event, the outcome is total sleep time that far exceeds the norm, sometimes causing patients with HD to take medications. Central nervous system stimulants can help reduce daytime sleepiness; however, tranquilizers are likely to make matters worse.

HD can occur with or without medical illnesses or other mental disorders, but we should not diagnose it if it occurs *only* with another sleep–wake disorder.

Essential Features of **Hypersomnolence Disorder**

Even after 7+ hours of sleep, the patient complains of severe daytime drowsiness as manifested by one or more of: difficulty remaining fully awake after awakening abruptly, repeated naps or periods of falling asleep that day, or sleeping long (9+ hours at a time) without sleeping well (it isn't refreshing).

The Fine Print

The D's: • Duration (3+ times a week for 3+ months) • Distress or disability (work/ educational, social, or personal impairment) • Differential diagnosis (**substance use disorders, other sleep–wake disorders [e.g., narcolepsy, sleep apnea],** normal sleep variation)

Coding Notes

If the patient has a coexisting disorder, it cannot account for the severity of hypersomnolence symptoms.

Specify if:

> **Acute.** Lasts less than 1 month.
> **Subacute.** Lasts 1–3 months.
> **Persistent.** Lasts 3+ months.

Specify if:

> **With mental disorder**
> **With medical condition**
> **With another sleep disorder.** Don't make the diagnosis at all if hypersomnolence occurs *only* with another sleep disorder.

In each case, code the coexisting disorder.

Specify severity, depending on number of days the patient has trouble maintaining waketime alertness:

> **Mild.** 1–2 days per week.
> **Moderate.** 3–4 days per week.
> **Severe.** 5+ days per week.

Colin Rodebaugh

Ever since he was 15, Colin Rodebaugh dreamed of becoming an architect. He read biographies of Christopher Wren and Frank Lloyd Wright; in the summers, he works around construction projects to learn how materials go together. Now he is 23 and in his second year of architectural school, and he can't stay awake during class.

"I might as well have weights tied to my eyelids," he says. "For the last 6 months, two or three times a day, I just have to take a nap. It could be in class, or anytime. It even happened once when my girlfriend and I were making love. Not after—during!"

Although Colin complains that he is tired all the time, his health appears to be excellent. His father, a family practitioner in Arizona, insisted that he have a complete physical exam. Then, Colin was specifically questioned about any history of sudden weakness, loss of consciousness, or seizure disorder, none of which he has had. His mother practices clinical psychology in Oregon, and she stands ready to vouch for his mental health.

"I get plenty of sleep at night—at least 9 hours. That's not the problem. It's that I hardly ever feel rested, no matter how much sleep I've had. If I do take a nap, I wake up feeling almost as groggy as when I nodded off."

Apart from Colin's sleep problem, school is a frustration. Although he is technically proficient, he's discovered that, unlike some of his classmates, he doesn't have a keen eye for form. Last semester, he realized that what talent he does have lies in drafting, not design. His advisor didn't argue with him when they discussed a possible career change.

Evaluation of Colin Rodebaugh

As with insomnia, the first task in evaluating hypersomnolence is to rule out the many conditions that could be causing it. Although the vignette does not contain all the information Colin's clinician would need, it hits the high points.

Physical illnesses are probably the most important considerations for this differential diagnosis. Based on a recent workup and physical exam, Colin appears to be healthy. Furthermore, he's had no history of sudden weakness or lapses of consciousness that might indicate psychomotor epilepsy. (According to DSM-5-TR criterion F, a patient can have a medical condition and still receive a diagnosis of HD, as long as the medical condition doesn't fully explain the problem with sleep.) We have no information about substance use (E); Colin's clinician would have to evaluate that. At least his mother, who is a mental health professional, feels that there is no indication of another mental disorder (also F). But then, moms are that way.

Narcolepsy is another sleep disorder that causes daytime sleepiness (D). But such individuals are typically refreshed by their brief naps, whereas they leave Colin feeling groggy. His clinician could ask Colin's girlfriend whether he snores or has other symptoms suggestive of sleep apnea. Insufficient nighttime sleep seems so obvious a possibility that it is sometimes overlooked (suspect it in patients who sleep less than

7 hours a night). Colin says he gets plenty of sleep, and at 9 hours a night or more, we wouldn't consider him sleep-deprived (A).

As far as we can tell from the vignette, Colin's sleep disorder has lasted about 6 months, and it occurs nearly every day—certainly every day he has class (B, C). I'd definitely include in his evaluation some mention of the problem he is having with school; it could help point the way to a therapeutic intervention. His GAF score would be about 65.

F51.11	Hypersomnolence disorder, persistent, severe
Z55.9	Inadequate school performance

A teenager who's grumpy and likes to sleep in? Stop the presses!

Well, if the behavior is due to Kleine–Levin syndrome (KLS)—one of myriad disorders subsumed under "HD, with medical condition"—it can be both unusual and distressing. Just how unusual? With a prevalence down around 1 in 1 million, KLS may be the rarest condition mentioned in DSM-5-TR. If ever you encounter such a patient, here's what you should expect to find.

KLS usually begins during the teen years. By 2–3:1, males predominate, though it may be more severe when it occurs in females. All patients experience profound hypersomnolence—sleeping 12–24 hours a day, with a mean and median of 18 hours each. In addition, nearly everyone has altered cognition: derealization, perplexity, perhaps problems with concentration or memory—some patients have complete amnesia for the episodes. These patients become churlish or argumentative and irritable, especially if prevented from sleeping. Four out of five have a change in eating behavior: specifically, voracious overeating (way past the point of feeling full), without, however, the purging behavior that is typical of patients with bulimia nervosa.

In two out of three cases, speech is also abnormal: Patients become mute or lack spontaneous speech; or they speak only in monosyllables; or speech is slow, slurred, or incoherent. Nearly half also experience hypersexuality—some expose themselves or masturbate openly or make inappropriate sexual advances to others. At the same time, nearly half report depressed mood, which usually remits at the end of each episode. Indeed, between episodes, nearly all patients appear completely ordinary.

The cause of KLS is unknown. Sometimes it begins with an infection, perhaps one as mild as a cold; some cases are precipitated by a stroke, a tumor, or another neurological disorder such as multiple sclerosis. Episodes last 1–3 weeks, and typically recur several times a year. This pattern persists for perhaps 8 years, or an average of 12 episodes. Then, for no apparent reason, KLS may simply disappear. Those who continue to have episodes often find them greatly moderated.

If you ever encounter such a patient, write up the case history for publication—and please send me a copy.

Narcolepsy

It's a French word (meaning "to seize with sleep") derived from Greek by a 19th-century French neurologist. Recognized since about 1880, the classic presentation includes four symptoms: sleep attacks, cataplexy, hallucinations, and sleep paralysis. Most people don't have all these symptoms, and patients are sometimes mistakenly diagnosed as having a mental disorder unrelated to sleep.

- REM periods begin within a few minutes of the onset of sleep, instead of the usual hour and a half. (In older patients, sleep latency tends to increase.) Often, they will even intrude upon the normal waking state, resulting in the irresistible urge to sleep. These sleep attacks tend toward brevity, lasting from a few minutes to over an hour. In contrast to the grogginess that patients with hypersomnolence disorder often experience, the sleep of narcolepsy is refreshing—except for children, who may awaken feeling tired. Then there follows a refractory period of an hour or more, during which the patient will remain completely awake. Sleep attacks can be triggered by stress or by emotional experiences (usually "positive" ones, such as jokes and laughter, though intense anger or fear is sometimes the precipitant). The resulting daytime drowsiness is often the earliest complaint of patients with narcolepsy.

- The most dramatic symptom is *cataplexy*—a sudden, brief episode of paralysis that can affect nearly all voluntary muscles, though sometimes just specific muscle groups, such as the jaw or the knees. When all muscles are affected, the patient may collapse completely. If fewer muscle groups are involved or if the attack is brief, cataplexy may go almost unnoticed. Episodes of cataplexy may occur with sleep attacks, but they can be independent, without loss of consciousness. They may be precipitated by intense emotion, such as laughter, weeping, or anger, or even by orgasm. Episodes of cataplexy usually begin within a few months of the onset of hypersomnolence. (Brain lesions such as tumors, infections, or injury can cause some people to experience cataplexy without other symptoms of narcolepsy.)

  Young children, especially those who have been only briefly ill, may not have classical cataplexy; rather, they experience episodes of jaw movement, grimacing, or protrusion of the tongue that can occur even without evidence of emotional triggers. These attacks gradually morph into more classical cataplexy.

- Hallucinations, which are mainly visual, may be the first symptom of narcolepsy. They hint that REM sleep is suddenly intruding upon the waking state, because hallucinations occur when the patient is going to sleep or awakening.

- Sleep paralysis can be frightening: The patient has the sensation of being awake but unable to move, speak, or even breathe adequately. Sleep paralysis is associated with anxiety and fear of dying; it typically lasts less than 10 minutes and may be accompanied by visual or auditory hallucinations.

REM is a relatively shallow stage of sleep. The acronym stands for *rapid eye movement*—behind closed lids, our dreaming eyes track back and forth, as though trying to take in a wide-screen display. This is when most of the dreams that we can recall occur. During REM sleep, our skeletal muscles become paralyzed, which of course we don't notice because we are safely asleep. REM sleep occurs throughout the night, typically beginning about 90 minutes after we first drop off, and it constitutes 20–25% of total sleep time. During REM sleep, heart rate and breathing are irregular; dreams are intense and tend to be remembered; erections of the penis or clitoris occur.

Non-REM sleep is what goes on during the balance of the night. It is of varying depth, defined by EEG patterns, and it is associated with several disorders mentioned elsewhere in this chapter.

A typical history that includes at least three of the four classic symptoms (as described above) is good presumptive evidence for narcolepsy. But because it's a chronic disorder that can be difficult to manage and implies lifelong treatment, the diagnosis should be confirmed by appropriate lab studies. In that regard, the neuropeptide hypocretin (sometimes it's called orexin) has been implicated. Produced in the lateral hypothalamus, it promotes wakefulness. Patients with narcolepsy often have a deficit of hypocretin, probably because some of the neurons that produce it have been destroyed by an autoimmune process. These findings are robust enough that they have crept into the criteria for this disorder.

Strongly hereditary, narcolepsy affects males and females about equally and affects about 1 person in 2,000. It typically starts when the patient is a child or adolescent, but nearly always by the age of 30. Sleepiness is usually the first symptom; cataplexy follows within a year or so. Once begun, it usually develops slowly and steadily. It can lead to depression, impotence, trouble at work, and even accidents in the street or on the job. Complications include weight gain (obesity is frequent) and the misuse of substances to maintain daytime alertness. Mood disorders and generalized anxiety disorder are sometimes comorbid.

The italicized word pairs below are nearly homophones but carefully note the differences in meaning.

Catalepsy (it's from the Greek meaning "to hold down") is the prolonged form of immobility that occurs in catatonia. *Cataplexy* means "to strike down"; it is a brief—typically 2 minutes or less—symptom of narcolepsy precipitated by jokes or laughing and manifested by loss of muscle tone (without loss of consciousness) and leading to brief collapse.

Hypnagogic and *hypnopompic* are two terms widely used to describe events that take place when one is going to sleep or waking up, respectively. They, too, are Greek: *hypn* = "sleep," *agogue* = "leader," *pomp* = "sending away." And note the confusing spellings: hypna and hypno—one more gift from the Greeks.

Essential Features of **Narcolepsy**

The patient cannot resist attacks of waketime sleep, which are associated with cataplexy (defined in the accompanying sidebar), low cerebrospinal fluid hypocretin, or decreased REM sleep latency on nighttime polysomnography.

Cataplexy is often precipitated by strong emotion, such as laughter. Kids may manifest it as episodes of jaw opening and tongue thrusting.

The Fine Print

The D's: • Duration (3+ times/week for 3+ months) • Differential diagnosis (substance use and physical disorders [especially seizures], mood disorders, sleep apnea, too little nighttime sleep)

Coding Notes

Specify:

> **G47.411 Narcolepsy with cataplexy or hypocretin deficiency (type 1).**
>
> **G47.419 Narcolepsy without cataplexy and either without hypocretin deficiency or hypocretin unmeasured (type 2).**
>
> **G47.421 Narcolepsy with cataplexy or hypocretin deficiency due to [a medical condition].**
>
> **G47.429 Narcolepsy without cataplexy and without hypocretin deficiency due to [a medical condition].**

Note: For the last two of the above, first code the underlying medical disorder and then incorporate the name of that disorder into your narcolepsy diagnosis.

Specify current severity:

> **Mild.** Cataplexy under once a week; only 1–2 naps per day; sleep disturbance mild.
>
> **Moderate.** Cataplexy 1–7 times per week; multiple naps per day, moderately troubled nighttime sleep.
>
> **Severe.** Cataplexy that is resistant to medications, with multiple attacks per day and troubled nighttime sleep.

Emma Flowers

"It's been happening like this for several years. Only now it's worse," says Eric Flowers, Emma's husband. He has brought her to the clinic because she no longer feels she can drive safely.

Emma sits slumped in the interview chair next to him. Her chin rests on her chest and her left arm hangs at her side. She has been soundly asleep for several minutes.

"If she hadn't been sitting down, she'd have fallen down," says Eric. "Half a dozen times, I've had to catch her."

As a teenager, Emma had vivid, sometimes frightening dreams that occurred as she was going to sleep, even if it was only a brief afternoon nap. By the time she married Eric, she was having occasional "sleep attacks," when she would experience the irresistible urge to lie down and take a brief nap. Over the next several years, these naps have become more frequent. Now, at age 28, Emma naps for 10 minutes or so every 3–4 hours during the day. Her nighttime sleep seems entirely normal to her, but Eric reflects that she sometimes jerks or restlessly moves around in her sleep.

It was the falling attacks that prompted this evaluation. Initially, Emma noticed only a sort of weakness in her neck muscles when she became sleepy. Over the course of a year the weakness has increased, until now it affects "every voluntary muscle she owns," Eric exclaims. It can happen at any time, but usually it is associated with the sudden onset of sleepiness. At these times, she seems to lose all her strength, sometimes so abruptly that she doesn't even have time to sit down. Then she will collapse, right where she has been standing, though she often retains full consciousness. Today it occurred while she was sitting down. Once it happened while she was trying to park her car. A month ago, she consulted a neurologist, but an EEG revealed no evidence of a seizure disorder and the MRI was normal.

Emma stirs, yawns, and opens her eyes. "I did it again, didn't I?"

"Feeling better?" asks her husband.

"I always do, don't I?"

Evaluation of Emma Flowers

This vignette illustrates most of the typical symptoms of narcolepsy: repeated attacks of irresistible sleep (criterion A) during the day; cataplexy (which does not invariably cause the patient to fall, and during which the patient may remain awake, B1a). Some patients have vivid dreams that occur during the onset of sleep, and sleep paralysis, which also occurs unnoticed during normal REM sleep.

The DSM-5-TR diagnostic criteria don't mention a differential diagnosis; we'll have to help them out. Sleep apnea also causes daytime sleepiness, but it typically occurs in male patients who are middle-aged or older. Differential diagnosis should also include all the other possible causes of excessive somnolence: substance-induced sleep disorders; major depressive episode with atypical features; various cognitive disorders (especially delirium); and a panoply of medical illnesses, such as hypothyroidism, epilepsy, hypoglycemia, myasthenia gravis, multiple sclerosis, and rarer neurological conditions such as Kleine–Levin and Prader–Willi syndromes. Emma's clinician should, of course, consider each of these. Don't disregard plain vanilla insufficient sleep and circadian rhythm sleep–wake disorder, delayed sleep phase type—both staples of adolescence. Although Emma's clinical symptoms fulfill the DSM-5-TR requirements for narcolepsy, for us to determine the coding type, she would have to undergo a lumbar puncture for a measurement of cerebrospinal fluid hypocretin. I'm not sure that she (or many other patients) would willingly submit to the procedure for such limited benefit. Narcolepsy with cataplexy is almost always associated with reduced hypocretin, so, with a GAF score of 60, her diagnosis will almost certainly turn out to be this:

G47.411   Narcolepsy with cataplexy with unknown hypocretin status

---

DSM-5-TR notes that laboratory validators have become increasingly used in evaluating and diagnosing the sleep disorders, to the extent that they are now required for some conditions. One of these, the multiple sleep latency test, is an evaluation done by polysomnography in a sleep laboratory. First described by Dement and Carskadon in 1977, it is the standard by which we now judge hypersomnolence. Here's how it works:

During the patient's usual waking time, in a quiet, darkened room, an EEG is recorded during naps. After 20 minutes, the patient is awakened, then asked to nap again 2 hours later. This is repeated every 2 hours for a total of four or five sessions. To preserve REM pressure for subsequent episodes, each episode of sleep is interrupted as soon as REM is detected. The times until the patient falls asleep (sleep latency) are averaged, yielding the score used for diagnosis. A score of 5 minutes is generally considered significant for the diagnosis of narcolepsy, though average time tends to increase with age.

The multiple sleep latency test is not specific for narcolepsy: Positive scores are found in some people with sleep apnea or sleep deprivation, and even in a few (2–4%) people who have no symptoms at all.

Breathing-Related Sleep Disorders

G47.33 Obstructive Sleep Apnea Hypopnea

Central Sleep Apnea

Apnea is easy: It simply means the absence of breathing. *Hypopnea*—shallow or infrequent breathing—has been variously defined. By convention, it now refers to a period of at least 10 seconds during which airflow is reduced by 30% or more and oxygen saturation of the blood is reduced by at least 4%.

As you have probably guessed, there is also a mixed form. It begins with a central apnea and ends in an obstructive apnea.

Here are two sleep–wake disorders that can kill. For periods lasting 10 seconds to a minute or longer during sleep (never while a patient is awake), airflow through the upper respiratory passages stops completely. Gas exchange falls off, affording a little dose of suffocation every time the patient goes to bed.

In the more common obstructive type, the chest heaves as the sleeper tries to inhale, but tissues in the mouth and pharynx prevent the flow of air. The struggle can rage for up to 2 minutes, culminating in an extraordinarily loud snore. All of this may be inapparent to the patient, but any bed partner is probably well aware. Most patients experience far more than 30 of these episodes per night.

In the less common central type (which comprises a number of possible etiologies), the patient simply stops making any effort to breathe—the diaphragm just takes a rest, so to speak. Snoring can be present, but it is not usually prominent. Affected men may complain especially of hypersomnolence, women of insomnia. Note that patients don't need to have symptoms to qualify for this diagnosis; polysomnographic findings alone will be enough. However, patients typically note that they awaken at night, short of breath, and consequently may feel sleepy the next day. This condition is encountered in chronic use of opioids or with severe neurological or medical illnesses—disorders you are unlikely to find outside a critical care ward. (In Cheyne–Stokes breathing, the person has episodes of taking faster, deeper breaths that gradually tail off into apnea; it occurs in people who have had recent stroke and heart failure.)

Regardless of type, the blood of a person with sleep apnea becomes depleted of oxygen until breathing starts again. Often, they are not aware of these events at all, though some may awaken partly—or even completely. Besides snoring and daytime drowsiness, there are often problems with hypertension and cardiac arrhythmias; patients may also complain of morning headaches and impotence. During the night, some patients become markedly restless, kicking at bedclothes (or bed partners), standing up, or even walking. Other sequelae include irritability and cognitive impairment, as shown by distractibility, problems with perception or memory, or bewilderment. Patients may also experience heavy sweating, hallucinations when going to sleep, sleep talking, or sleep terrors. Nocturia (getting up at night to urinate) is often associated with sleep apnea, though no one knows why.

Although most cases go unevaluated, obstructive sleep apnea hypopnea affects perhaps 5% of the general population, increasing with age to about 20% at 65. Besides old age, risk factors include obesity (shirt collar size over 16½ for adult men), African American ethnicity, male gender, and pregnancy. Enlarged tonsil tissue can put even young children at risk. It is highly familial, with a genetic basis. Central sleep apnea is probably uncommon, more frequent in the elderly and most common in opioid users and people with severe physical illness.

Because sleep apnea is potentially lethal, always consider it in the differential diagnosis of either hypersomnolence or insomnia. Rapid detection and management can save a life. Although an observant bed partner can provide evidence of sleep apnea that is almost definitive, confirmatory polysomnography is now required for diagnosis.

The symptoms are similar for the two types, and discrimination depends on specific polysomnography findings, so I've provided only one vignette.

The criteria make central sleep apnea one of the few DSM diagnoses that you can't substantiate on purely clinical grounds. In fact, no clinical features at all are described. I worry that we may be witnessing the beginnings of change to a world where mental health diagnosis is no longer a clinical discipline, but one that makes its home in the laboratory.

Essential Features of **Obstructive Sleep Apnea Hypopnea**

A patient complains of daytime sleepiness that results from nighttime breathing problems: (often long) pauses in breathing, followed by loud snores or snorts.

Diagnosis requires daytime sleepiness (or fatigue or nonrestorative sleep) and at least 5 apneas or hypopneas per hour as seen by polysomnography. Alternatively, polysomnography reveals 15 apnea/hypopnea episodes per hour, regardless of other symptoms.

The Fine Print

The D's: • Differential diagnosis (physical disorders [asthma], substance use sleep disorders, primary snoring, other sleep disorders).

Coding Notes

Code severity, based on number of apneas/hypopneas per hour:

>**Mild.** Fewer than 15.
>**Moderate.** 15–30.
>**Severe.** 30+.

Essential Features of **Central Sleep Apnea**

For each hour of a patient's sleep, polysomnography shows five or more central sleep apneas.

The Fine Print

The D's: • Differential diagnosis (**other sleep–wake disorders**)

Coding Notes

Specify:

>**G47.31 Idiopathic central sleep apnea.** Because of variability in breathing effort with no evidence of obstructed airway, these patients experience frequent awakenings.

R06.3 Cheyne–Stokes breathing (a pattern of rising and falling depth of breathing, with frequent arousals).
G47.37 Central sleep apnea comorbid with opioid use. First, code the opioid use, unless it is a one-off.

Code severity based on number of apneas/hypopneas per hour and degree of oxygen saturation and sleep fragmentation. DSM-5-TR provides no further guidance.

Roy Dardis

"I guess it's been going on 30 years and more," says Lily Dardis. She means her husband's snoring. "I used to sleep soundly myself, so it didn't bother me. Lately, I've had arthritis that's kept me awake. Roy rattles the windows."

Lying awake nights waiting for the painkiller to take effect, Lily has opportunity for minutely studying her husband's sleeping habits. As someone who sleeps on his back, Roy has always been a noisy breather at night. But every 5 minutes or so, his respirations drop off to nothing. After 20 or 30 seconds, during which his chest will pitch and heave, he'll finally break through with an enormous snort. This is rapidly followed by several additional louder-than-usual snores. "It's a wonder the neighbors don't complain," Lily marvels.

Roy Dardis is a tall man of enormous bulk—a testament to Lily's country cooking. He guesses he's always snored some; his brother, with whom he shared a room as a child, used to tease him about it. Of course, as he jokingly points out, the racket never bothers him because he sleeps right through it. Roy's complaint is that he never feels rested. Whether he's at work or watching TV, he tends to nod off. It leaves him grumpy.

In the mornings, Roy often awakens with a headache that seems localized to the front of his head. Two cups of strong coffee usually fix him up.

Evaluation of Roy Dardis

Lily Dardis presents strong evidence that Roy has sleep apnea: She observes that Roy has many periods when he stops breathing, then resumes with an extra-loud snore. From her description of his struggles to breathe during the apneic periods, this would appear to be an obstructive type of sleep apnea. Roy's bulk, morning headaches, and complaints about dropping off to sleep during the day are also typical of sleep apnea. Clinicians should ask any patient like Roy about hallucinations when going to sleep, changes in personality (irritability, aggression, anxiety, depression), loss of sex interest, impotence, night terrors, and sleepwalking; each of these is encountered with varying frequency in sleep apnea. Patients also often have heart disease, high blood pressure, stroke, and alcohol use, though some of these are undoubtedly complications rather than causes.

Other causes of hypersomnolence should be considered, though they would not seem likely in Roy's case. Daytime sleepiness and hypnagogic hallucinations occur in narcolepsy, but Roy has no episodes of cataplexy, and his daytime naps are not refreshing. Of course, many otherwise healthy people snore, and this should be considered in the differential diagnosis of anyone whose chief complaint is snoring.

Despite Roy's typical history, sleep lab studies must be pursued; in addition to the diagnostic requirement for polysomnography, his blood oxygen saturation during an attack of apnea should be evaluated. Other mental disorders (especially mood and anxiety disorders) and substance-related disorders should be evaluated. Some of these—notably major depressive disorder, panic disorder, and major neurocognitive disorder—may be found as associated diagnoses.

Roy earns a GAF score of 60. We're supposed to use polysomnography results to score severity of sleep apnea. But on clinical grounds I would judge that Roy is at least moderately impaired by his disorder, and that's the level I'll put down—at least until his testing comes back:

G47.33   Obstructive sleep apnea hypopnea, moderate
E66.9   Obesity

Sleep-Related Hypoventilation

Health and comfort demand steady regulation of our blood gases: oxygen (O_2) high, which means 95% or higher; carbon dioxide (CO_2) just right—not too high, not too low—in the range of 23–29 milliequivalents per liter. Our bodies accomplish this balancing act by means of a simple feedback loop: Low O_2 or high CO_2 signals the brain's respiratory center that our lungs need to work harder. In people with sleep-related hypoventilation, however, the chemoreceptors and the medullary (brainstem) neuronal network fail to send the right sort of signal, so breathing remains shallow. When awake, these folks can compensate by intentionally breathing faster or deeper, but during sleep, that strategy fails and breathing becomes shallower still. Symptoms are typically worse during sleep, and periods of apnea—when breathing stops completely—often occur.

This uncommon condition is found especially in people who are severely overweight or who have disorders such as muscular dystrophy, poliomyelitis, amyotrophic lateral sclerosis, and tumors or other lesions of the spinal cord or central nervous system. Most adult patients (typically, men ages 20–50) don't complain of breathing problems, but they do report the insidious development of daytime drowsiness, fatigue, morning headache, frequent nocturnal awakenings, and unrefreshing sleep. They may also show ankle edema and a blue skin tone that indicates oxygen deficiency. Even small doses of sedatives or narcotics can make already inadequate breathing much worse. Tragically, it can affect small children, too (see sidebar).

Despite the many clues, such as daytime sleepiness, fatigue, and morning headache, the DSM-5-TR criteria set rests entirely on results of polysomnography. The syndrome is uncommon, so I've provided no vignette.

Essential Features of **Sleep-Related Hypoventilation**

Polysomnography shows periods of reduced breathing with high CO_2 levels.

The Fine Print

The D's: • Differential diagnosis (other sleep–wake disorders, pulmonary disease)

Coding Notes

Specify:

G47.34 Idiopathic hypoventilation. No identifiable cause.

G47.35 Congenital central alveolar hypoventilation. In newborns, rare.

G47.36 Comorbid sleep-related hypoventilation (due to a medical disorder such as lung disease, obesity, or muscular dystrophy).

Code severity based on CO_2 and O_2 saturation. It's worse if blood gasses are abnormal when the patient is awake.

Even in research reports, sleep-related hypoventilation is sometimes called Ondine's curse. The name refers to the legend of Ondine (sometimes Undine), a European water nymph who falls in love with a knight. Ondine knows that she will lose her immortality should she marry a human and bear him a child. In thrall to love, she takes the plunge anyway; sure enough, she begins to age. Her beauty slips away, taking with it her husband's affection. When she finds him snoring in the arms of another woman, she reminds him that he has sworn "faithfulness with every waking breath." She then utters the curse that he will keep breathing only so long as he remains awake. When he inevitably falls asleep, he dies.

We aren't told how the curse of a now mortal Ondine can have any force, and it remains unexplained why the term is usually attached specifically to the congenital form of hypoventilation. But in roughly 1 of 50,000 live births—traceable to a sporadic mutation of PHOX2B, an autosomal dominant gene on chromosome 4—the child simply doesn't breathe when sleeping. These patients usually die young, though recently, with tracheostomy and nighttime mechanically assisted breathing, some have survived to relatively normal adulthood.

Circadian Rhythm Sleep–Wake Disorders

The word *circadian* comes from the Latin, meaning "about a day." It refers to the body's cycles of sleep, temperature, and hormone production, which are generated in the suprachiasmatic nucleus of the brain's anterior hypothalamus. When there are no external time cues (natural daylight or artificial reminders like clocks), the free-running human cycle is about 24 hours, 9 minutes—a discrepancy too small to cause most of us any serious difficulty. But sometimes a misalignment between our natural body rhythms and the demands of our work or social lives results in unwanted sleeplessness or drowsiness, or both.

The circadian sleep–wake cycle changes throughout life. It lengthens during adolescence, which helps explain a teenager's proclivity for late nights and sleeping in. It shortens again in old age, causing seniors to fall asleep in the evening while reading or watching television, and making both shift work and jet lag a misery.

Circadian Rhythm Sleep–Wake Disorder, Delayed Sleep Phase Type

Because they feel alert and active in the late evening, people with delayed sleep phase—sometimes called "owls" or "night people"—go to sleep late (sometimes progressively later each night) and awaken in late morning or afternoon. Left to their own devices, they feel just fine. But if they must arise early to attend class or get to work (or eat lunch), they feel drowsy and may even appear "sleep-drunk." Irregular sleep habits and the use of caffeine or other stimulants only worsen their plight.

Such patients may account for up to 10% of people who come to the sleep clinic complaining of chronic insomnia. The delayed sleep phase type is by far the most frequent, especially among teens and young adults. A familial component can often be identified.

Note that delayed sleep phase must be distinguished from the lifestyle issues of those who simply prefer going to bed late and sleeping in. Those people may feel quite comfortable with their eccentric schedules, which they don't make much effort to alter. People with the disorder complain of hypersomnolence and would like to change.

Circadian Rhythm Sleep–Wake Disorder, Advanced Sleep Phase Type

Patients with advanced sleep phase are the opposite of those just described; we might call this the "early to bed, early to rise" disorder. Their desired time to sleep is early rather than late, so they feel healthy, wealthy, and wise in the morning but sleepy in the late afternoon or early evening. Sometimes they're referred to as "larks." Advanced sleep phase appears to be much less frequent even than delayed sleep phase, though this could be in part because it causes less discomfort and fewer social problems. It has been reported to increase with advancing age, perhaps affecting 1% of middle-aged adults.

Circadian Rhythm Sleep–Wake Disorder, Non-24-Hour Sleep–Wake Type

The non-24-hour type is also called the free-running type, and it occurs mainly in completely blind people, who of course cannot perceive the light cues that would entrain their biological clocks. About half of blind people may be affected, beginning with the onset of total blindness; most of those with minimal light perception—even the equivalent of a single candle—remain normally entrained. Sighted people who are affected tend to be mainly young (teens and 20s) and male; they often have other mental disorders. The 18-hour schedules that accompany life in a submarine can also lead to a free-running biological rhythm. Most sighted people who undergo a research protocol in which there are no visual time cues will ultimately develop non-24-hour sleep–wake type.

Circadian Rhythm Sleep–Wake Disorder, Irregular Sleep–Wake Type

The pattern here is . . . no pattern. The total sleep duration may be normal, but these patients feel sleepy or wakeful at varying, and unpredictable, times of day. They may take naps, so it's important to rule out poor sleep hygiene. Irregular type may be encountered in various neurological conditions, including neurocognitive disorder, intellectual developmental disorder, and traumatic brain injury. The prevalence is unknown, but it is probably rare. As far as we know, this condition affects the sexes about equally. Age is a risk factor, mainly due to the late-life presence of medical disorders such as Alzheimer's disease.

Circadian Rhythm Sleep–Wake Disorder, Shift Work Type

When workers change from one shift to another, especially when they must be active during their former sleep time, sleepiness sets in and performance declines. Sleep during the new sleep time is often disrupted and too brief. The symptoms, which can affect up to 10% of night shift workers, are worse after a switch to night work, but people vary considerably in the time required for this adjustment. Additional factors include age (older people are more likely to be affected), commuting distance, and whether the individual is naturally a lark or an owl. Symptoms may last 3 weeks or longer, especially if workers try to resume their preferred sleeping schedules on weekends or holidays.

Whatever happened to jet lag? In DSM-IV, it was one of the possible circadian rhythm subtypes, but because it is so common, brief, and (really, when you think about it) pretty darned normal to our jet-setting sensibilities, it has been removed from the pantheon of DSM disorders. Still, it might be useful to mention its symptoms.

You've probably had it yourself. After air travel across several time zones, you experience attacks of intense sleepiness and fatigue. Perhaps, like some people, you feel nauseated or have other flu-like symptoms. But by the second day you begin adjusting to the new time zone, and within a few days you feel just fine.

Most people find that time adjustment is faster and easier after flying westward than the reverse. Perhaps this is because the body's natural cycle is a little longer than 24 hours; perhaps it's because we Americans can keep ourselves awake on the long trip home from Europe, then crash for a truly splendid night's sleep. Studies have shown that adjustment to westward flights occurs at the rate of about 90 minutes per day, whereas adjustment to eastward flights is only about 1 hour per day. This is true regardless of which direction you fly when leaving home. Well, except north or south.

So, if (when) jet lag visits, cope with it as you would with any other normal feature of contemporary life. You are in the remarkable situation of feeling ill without being sick.

Essential Features of Circadian Rhythm Sleep–Wake Disorders

A recurring mismatch between the patient's sleep–wake pattern and environmental demands causes insomnia or hypersomnolence.

The Fine Print

The D's: • Distress or disability (work/educational, social, or personal impairment) • Differential diagnosis (substance use disorders, other sleep disorders, normal sleep variation)

Coding Notes

Specify:

> **G47.21 Delayed sleep phase type.** The patient has trouble falling asleep and awakening on time.
>
> **G47.22 Advanced sleep phase type.** The patient has trouble remaining awake until the desired bedtime and awakens before time to arise.
>
> **G47.23 Irregular sleep–wake type.** The patient's sleep and wake periods vary without pattern throughout the 24-hour period.
>
> **G47.24 Non-24-hour sleep–wake type.** Timing of sleep onset and wakefulness is not entrained to the 24-hour period; each day it gradually drifts (usually later).
>
> **G47.26 Shift work type.** Because of night shift work or frequently changing shifts, patients experience insomnia when they'd like to sleep or hypersomnia during times of preferred wakefulness—or both.
>
> **G47.20 Unspecified type**

Specify if:

Familial. Applies only to delayed and advanced sleep phase types.
Overlapping with non-24-hour sleep–wake type. Applies to delayed type.

Specify if:

Episodic. Symptoms last 1–3 months.
Persistent. Symptoms last 3+ months.
Recurrent. There are two or more episodes within 1 year.

Fenton Schmidt

Remarkably, Fenton Schmidt requested the earliest morning appointment he could get. As he explains to the sleep specialist, "It's partly because I knew I'd be at my worst. I thought you might get a better picture of what I'm up against." He rubs his eyes, which are rimmed with dark circles. "I know, I look like a character in a *Doonesbury* cartoon."

Fenton's trouble began as long ago as high school. "I'd never have made those 8 o'clock classes if my mom hadn't been there for me." He rubs his eyes again and yawns. "Well, *at* me. Couple of times, she dumped a pan of cold water on me. It did get me out of bed."

In college, Fenton tried never to schedule a class before noon. That worked out pretty well because he was living with his father, who had kept the same schedule for 35 years as night shift manager at a convenience store. That was how his dad avoided the hungover feeling of awakening too early. "I saw him once when he got off an early plane. He was asleep on his feet. *His* dad was first-generation American, and the family still speaks a little German. He called it *Schlaftrunkenheit*—sleep drunkenness."

"'Early to bed, early to rise' was written by a sadist," Fenton comments. Several times over the years, he's tried changing his own sleep schedule by going to bed earlier. After a few days, he always gives up. "Lifelong, if I hit the sack before 2 A.M., I just lie there, pissed off."

For a couple of years, Fenton worked the swing shift for an electronics parts fabricator. "That strategy was perfect for me. When I got off at 11:30 at night, I could spend whatever time I needed at home, decompressing. I could go to bed when I wanted, and I only had to get up in time to start my shift at 4. That's P.M."

"So, what is the problem now?" the clinician wants to know.

Now Fenton has begun working at the pancake house managed by the father of his fiancée, Jaylene. "Do you know what time people eat pancakes?" he asks. He and Jaylene both get up early to open the shop. "It works fine for her; she's a lark. But at 5 A.M., this owl doesn't give a hoot."

Evaluation of Fenton Schmidt

Fenton's problem is instantly apparent: His sleeping requirements just don't jibe with those of his job and his social and personal life (criterion A). With no physical illness (such as traumatic brain injury) or substance use problems that would provide an alternative explanation, the resulting hypersomnolence (B) and distress (C) complete the criteria for a circadian rhythm sleep–wake disorder. Of course, his clinician should carefully rule out poor sleep hygiene. The fact that he is genuinely troubled suggests that this is not simply a lifestyle issue.

Fenton's history provides ample evidence that, of the possible subtypes, his would be delayed sleep phase type. There is really no need for further verification by polysomnography. His GAF score would be 62.

G47.21	Circadian rhythm sleep–wake disorder, delayed sleep phase type, familial
Z60.0	Phase of life problem (impending wedding)
Z56.9	Job change

Marcelle Klinger

Marcelle is a 60-year-old registered nurse, one of seven employed by her small community hospital in the northern California hills. The entire facility has only 32 beds, and although there are nursing aides and licensed practical nurses to assist, state law requires that a registered nurse must always be present in the facility. When the nurse who had worked the graveyard shift (11 P.M. to 7:30 A.M.) finally retired, the hospital administrator asked for a volunteer to fill that position.

"Nobody stepped up," Marcelle tells the mental health clinician, "so some genius decided it was only fair that everyone take turns."

This resulted in 4-week shifts. In a year, each nurse would work six of these shifts on days, four on evenings, and two on graveyard. Everyone grumbled, but Marcelle hated it the most. The switch from days to evenings wasn't too bad; she lives close by, so she could be home in bed by midnight. But the graveyard shift was a disaster.

"I'm the only registered nurse there, and I'm supposed to be awake and alert the whole time. Patients depend on me. But my eyes keep squeezing themselves shut, and my brain seems to hum, as if it's going to sleep. Part of the time I feel sick to my stomach. One time I did fall asleep at work, just for 10 minutes or so. When the phone rang, I startled awake, feeling hungover."

Marcelle's physical and mental health are excellent. She's always been a light sleeper, so she finds daytime sleeping nearly impossible. Heavy drapes can keep out most of the light, but traffic noise and the sounds from passersby on the sidewalk outside her bedroom frequently awaken her.

Moreover, the coffee Marcelle drinks to keep awake at work prevents her from going to sleep as soon as she goes to bed. It also gets her up to the bathroom at least once or twice. By late afternoon, when her husband comes home from teaching school, she has seldom slept more than 3 or 4 hours. On weekends, she tries to resume a schedule that allows her to spend time with her family, but this only makes things worse. "I flew to Paris once and felt jet-lagged for a week. Now I'm sick that way for a whole month."

Evaluation of Marcelle Klinger

Several features of Marcelle's condition could contribute to her discomfort:

1. Like many people who must work shifts (criterion A), she tries to *re*-readjust her sleep–wake schedule on the weekends.

2. Cues from outside her window serve to arouse her when she tries to sleep.

3. Because of the physiology of their sleep, older people often have trouble making these adjustments. Marcelle is 60.

4. She drinks coffee to stay awake; the dual effects of the caffeine-induced stimulation and her trips to the loo interfere further with what sleep she does get. Consequently, she suffers from both insomnia *and* hypersomnolence (B), with obvious attendant distress (C).

From her history, we learn that Marcelle has no physical illness, substance use, or other mental disorder. (Although patients with a psychosis such as schizophrenia are sometimes kept up progressively later at night by their hallucinations, mood and anxiety disorders generally produce only insomnia or hypersomnolence.) The vignette provides no evidence for any other sleep–wake disorder: Marcelle's naps are not refreshing, arguing against narcolepsy. She has always been a light sleeper anyway, but light sleep itself is not considered a sleep disorder—except by some light sleepers.

The subtype is obvious; Marcelle's GAF score would be 65.

G47.26	Circadian rhythm sleep–wake disorder, shift work type, recurrent
Z56.9	Varying work schedule

Parasomnias

And here come those disorders where something abnormal happens during sleep. The architecture (as the sleep people say) of sleep itself may be normal, but somehow elements of wakefulness get mixed up with REM sleep or with non-REM sleep.

Non-Rapid Eye Movement Sleep Arousal Disorders

Although awakening to the jangle of a telephone in the dead of night can be a struggle, mostly it's a pretty straight shot from sleeping to fully awake. OK, we don't like it, feel unwell, curse the caller, and turn over to shut out the sound of the ring—but we're awake, all right, and we know it. For reasons largely unclear, however, it doesn't always work that way. For some people, a way station between sleeping and being awake causes reactions that range from bemusement to frank horror.

It all stems from the three possible states of the relationship of body and mind. During wakefulness, they both are working; in non-REM (deep) sleep, both are more or less idling. During REM (dreaming) sleep, though, the mind is at work but the body rests; in fact, our voluntary muscles are paralyzed, so that we cannot move. (The fourth conceivable combination, active body with sleeping mind, is the stuff of zombie films.) During non-REM sleep arousal disorders, people experience simultaneous sleeping and waking EEG patterns; symptoms ensue.

Partial arousals that occur suddenly from non-REM sleep usually occur in the first hour or two of sleep, when slow-wave sleep is most prevalent. Though the behaviors sometimes overlap, there are three main types of abnormal arousal. I've listed them in order of increasing severity:

Confusional arousal < Sleepwalking < Sleep terror

In each of these, events tend to be poorly recalled. Each is more common in children, for whom they are considered generally benign, perhaps caused by a relatively immature nervous system. One of them, confusional arousal, didn't quite make it into the official DSM-5-TR pantheon (sidebar, p. 341).

Some episodes occur spontaneously, but others follow apparent precipitants, which can include stress, irregular sleep, drugs, and sleep deprivation. Although family history is often positive, a genetic causation hasn't been nailed down.

Essential Features of **Non-Rapid Eye Movement Sleep Arousal Disorders**

The person repeatedly awakens incompletely from sleep with sleepwalking or sleep terror events (see Coding Notes). The attempts of others to communicate or console don't help much. The patient has little if any dream imagery at the time and tends not to remember the episode the next morning.

The Fine Print

The D's: • Distress or disability (work/educational, social, or personal impairment) • Differential diagnosis (**substance use** and **physical disorders, other mental disorders** such as anxiety and dissociative disorders, other sleep disorders)

Coding Notes

Specify:

F51.3 Sleepwalking type. Without awakening, the patient rises from bed and walks. The patient stares blankly, can be awakened only with difficulty, and responds poorly to others' attempts at communication.

Specify if:

With sleep-related eating
With sleep-related sexual behavior (sexsomnia)

F51.4 Sleep terror type. Beginning with a terrified scream, the patient abruptly rouses from sleep, showing marked fear and evidence of autonomic arousal, such as dilated pupils, rapid breathing, rapid heartbeat, and sweating.

Sleep paralysis isn't a disorder; it's a normal feature of sleep. But it can be frightening when it occurs right at the start (or conclusion) of sleep, during awareness. Lasting from mere seconds to several minutes, episodes may be accompanied by apparitions of being approached by some sort of "creature" that soon vanishes. Sleep paralysis that's problematic happens in around 8% of young adults. Its frequency is increased by all the usual suspects: sleep deprivation, stress, and keeping irregular hours (such as with shift work). Treatment, other than reassurance, is usually unnecessary.

Non-Rapid Eye Movement Sleep Arousal Disorder, Sleepwalking Type

Sleepwalking behavior tends to follow a fairly set pattern; it usually occurs during the first third of the night, when non-REM sleep is more prevalent. Sleepwalkers first sit up and make some sort of recurring movement (such as plucking at the bedclothes). More purposeful behavior may follow, perhaps dressing, eating, or using the toilet. The person's facial expression is usually blank and staring. If these individuals say anything at all, it is garbled; speaking sentences is rare. Their movements tend to be poorly coordinated, sometimes resulting in considerable danger.

Individual episodes last anywhere from a few seconds to 30 minutes, during which a person will often be hard to awaken, though spontaneous awakening may occur—typically to a brief period of disorientation. Some individuals simply return to bed without awakening. Occasionally a person who goes to sleep in one location will be surprised to awaken elsewhere. Amnesia for the episode is typical, though this varies.

DSM-5-TR lists two subtypes of sleepwalking: with sleep-related eating, and with sleep-related sexual behavior (sexsomnia—yes, even DSM-5-TR calls it that). The former occurs mainly in women, and it's not the same as night eating syndrome, which is a sort of eating disorder wherein the person is awake and remembers it the next day (p. 297). Sexsomnia, which includes masturbation and sometimes sexual behavior with other people, is more common in men. It can have interpersonal and legal repercussions, no surprise.

Sleepwalking may occur nightly, though it's usually less frequent. As with nightmares and sleep terrors, don't diagnose sleepwalking type unless the episodes are recurrent and cause impairment or distress. And, as with so many other sleep disorders, sleepwalking episodes are more likely when a person is tired or has been under stress. In adults, the condition appears to have familial and genetic components.

Perhaps 6% of all children sleepwalk; for them, it isn't considered pathological. It will begin between the ages of 6 and 12 and lasts for several years. Most kids outgrow it by age 15, though perhaps 20% continue to sleepwalk into their adult lives. Sleepwalking affects up to 4% of adult men and women, in whom it tends to be chronic until the fourth decade of life. Although adults who sleepwalk may have a personality disorder, sleepwalking in children has no prognostic significance.

Ross Josephson

"I brought along a video. I thought it might help to explain my problem." Ross Josephson hands a thumb drive to the clinician. Ross lives in a dormitory with two roommates, who provided the video.

Ross walks in his sleep. He supposes it started when he was quite young, though he wasn't fully aware of it until one hot July dawn when he was 12. He awakened in his pajamas, curled up on the porch swing. When he told his mother, she remarked that she and her two brothers had all walked in their sleep when they were young. She guessed that Ross would grow out of it, as they had.

Only he hasn't. In his first year of college now, Ross pursues his nocturnal strolls once or twice a month. At first his roommates were amused; they had lain awake several nights until they caught the complete sequence on their phones. The video was a hit at an impromptu party they had gotten up with some of the girls who live downstairs. Ross took the joke well. In fact, he was fascinated to see how he appears when sleepwalking.

But last week his roommates became alarmed when they caught him stepping through an open window onto the third-floor roof of their building. Other than a low rim around the edge, there was nothing to prevent a nasty 30-foot fall into the grape ivy. They pulled him back inside, but at the cost of a struggle; clearly, the sleeping Ross had resisted guidance. After an interview and physical exam by one of the consultants in the student health service, Ross was pronounced healthy and referred to the campus mental health clinic.

The clinician and Ross watch the video together. The image is grainy and dances around a good deal—perhaps the videographer was trying not to laugh. It shows a pajama-clad Ross sitting up in bed. Although his eyes are open, they don't appear to focus, and his face registers no emotion. At first, he only pulls—aimlessly, it seems—at the sheet and blanket. Suddenly he swings his feet to the floor and stands up. He slips off his pajama top and lets it fall onto the bed. Then he walks through the door into the hallway.

For 2 or 3 minutes, the camera follows Ross. He walks up and down the hall several times and finally disappears into the bathroom, where the camera does not pursue. When he emerges, another young man ("That's Ted, one of my roommates," Ross explains) appears on screen and tries to engage him in conversation. Ross responds with a few syllables, none of which is a recognizable word. Finally, he allows Ted to guide him gently back to his bed. Almost as soon as he lies down, he appears to be asleep. The entire video lasts perhaps 10 minutes.

"When they showed me this the next morning, I was amazed. I hadn't the slightest idea I'd done anything but sleep through the night. I never do."

Evaluation of Ross Josephson

Although sleepwalking is not considered pathological in children, adults with the sleepwalking type of non-REM sleep arousal disorder may have other psychopathology. They should be carefully investigated with a full interview (as should just about everyone who consults a mental health care provider). However, occasional sleepwalking is likely to be more annoying than pathological.

Let's quickly review Ross's relation to the criteria for non-REM sleep arousal disorder. His awakenings are incomplete (almost nonexistent, actually) and recurrent (criterion A1), during which he does sleepwalk, gazing with unseeing eyes. In the video, his roommate doesn't exactly try to comfort him (college roommates tend more toward *Animal House* than *Terms of Endearment*), but he does try to engage Ross in conversation—to no avail. The vignette doesn't specify whether Ross has dream imagery (it should have; criterion B), but it does note that he never has a memory of the episodes the following day (C). Although Ross is not distressed, his roommates are: They wouldn't care to officiate while Ross plunged from a rooftop (D).

The differential diagnosis also includes psychomotor epilepsy, which can begin during sleep and present with sleepwalking. The dissociative condition known as the fugue subtype of dissociative amnesia may sometimes be confused with sleepwalking, but fugues last longer and involve complex behaviors, such as speaking complete sentences. Nighttime wandering can be found in sleep apnea. Ross presents no evidence for substance use (E).

Other nighttime disturbances and sleep disorders can be associated with sleepwalking; these include nocturnal enuresis, nightmare disorder, and the sleep terror type of non-REM sleep arousal disorder. Generalized anxiety disorder, posttraumatic stress disorder, and mood disorders can also occur. However, none of these conditions is suggested by the vignette (F). Ross would have a GAF score of 75; his diagnosis would be as follows:

F51.3   Non-rapid eye movement sleep arousal disorder, sleepwalking type

In the hundreds of years that sleepwalking has been recognized, it has amassed an extensive, if inaccurate, mythology. Also known as *somnambulism* (which means—surprise!—"sleepwalking"), it has been a reliable device for playwrights (paging Mr. Shakespeare) and the authors of innumerable mystery thrillers. One enduring myth is that it is dangerous to awaken a sleepwalker. Perhaps this grew out of the observation that it is *difficult* to do so; in any event, I know of no evidence to support such a belief.

Non-Rapid Eye Movement Sleep Arousal Disorder, Sleep Terror Type

Sleep terror (also known as night terror or *pavor nocturnus*) mostly affects children, with a typical onset during ages 4–12. When it begins in an adult, it is hardly ever after the age of 40. As is true of nightmares versus nightmare disorder (p. 345), only events that are recurrent and produce distress or impairment qualify for a diagnosis of the sleep terror type of non-REM sleep arousal disorder.

A sleep terror attack begins with a loud cry or scream during a period of non-REM sleep, not long after the patient goes to sleep. The patient sits up, appears terrified, and seems to be awake but does not respond to attempts at soothing. There will be signs of sympathetic nervous system arousal, such as rapid heartbeat, sweating, and piloerection (hairs standing up on the skin). With deep breathing and dilated pupils, the person seems ready for fight or flight, aroused but not arousable. An attack usually lasts just a few minutes and terminates spontaneously with return to sleep. Most patients have no memory of the incident the following morning, though some adults may have fragmentary recall.

A single such event in any given night is the rule; there's often a period of days to weeks between sleep terror attacks, though stress and fatigue may increase the frequency. In adults, the disorder is equally common in men and women.

With a peak at age 6, prevalence is around 3% in children; it's less frequent in adults, though hardly rare. In children, sleep terrors are not considered pathological; they almost invariably grow out of them and suffer no medical or psychological consequences later in life. The adult-onset type may be associated with another mental condition such as an anxiety or personality disorder.

Bud Stanhope

Bud Stanhope and his wife, Harriette, have just begun marital counseling. They agree on exactly one thing, which is that many of their problems can be traced to Bud's excessive need for support. They married when each was on the rebound, soon after Bud's first wife divorced him. "I felt so uncomfortable being alone," Bud says.

His chronically low self-esteem means that Bud cannot so much as start a repair project around the house without consulting Harriette. (Once, when she was out of town at a convention, he even phoned his ex-wife for advice.) And because he is afraid to disagree with Harriette, they never resolve anything. "I don't even feel I can tell him how much it bugs me when he wakes me up with those night frights," she says with a sigh.

"Night frights?" says Bud. "I thought those stopped months ago."

As Harriette describes them, Bud's "frights" are always the same. An hour or so after they fall asleep, she'll awaken to his blood-curdling scream. Bud will be sitting bolt upright in bed, a look of stark terror on his face. His eyes wide open, he stares off into a corner. She is never sure if he's seeing something because he never says much that is intelligible—only a babbled random word or two. He seems agitated, plucks at his bedclothes, and sometimes will start to get out of bed.

"The hairs on his arms will be standing straight up. He's breathing fast and perspiring, even if it's cold in the room. Once when I put my hand on his chest, his heart seemed to be beating as fast as a rabbit's."

It takes Harriette 10 or 15 minutes to soothe Bud. He never fully awakens but will eventually lie down. Then he almost instantly falls fast asleep again, while she sometimes lies awake for hours. Bud has one of these attacks every 2 or 3 weeks. Only once has it happened two nights running, and that was during one particularly bad period when he felt sure he was about to lose his job.

Evaluation of Bud Stanhope

Several features of Bud's attacks are distinctive of sleep terrors: the evidence of autonomic arousal (rapid heartbeat, sweating), occurrence soon after falling asleep, Harriette's inability to console him, his lack of full awakening, and his lack of recall the next day. Taken as a whole, this story is virtually diagnostic, but I'll list the important elements anyway. Bud's arousals are both incomplete and recurrent (criterion A). Harriette reports marked difficulty soothing him (A2). If he ever has dream imagery, he does not report it (B), and he has no recall (he was surprised he was still having the terror episodes; C). Without argument (certainly none from Bud or Harriette), the episodes are distressing at the time (D). We'd have to enquire further to make sure that substance misuse plays no role in his history (E). As an exercise, note how each of these features helps to differentiate this disorder from nightmare disorder (p. 345).

Although this did not happen to Bud, sleepwalking (sometimes sleep running) occurs in many patients with sleep terrors. In adults, you may have to distinguish sleep terrors from psychomotor epilepsy, which can also produce sleepwalking. Panic attacks sometimes occur at night, but then the person will awaken completely, without the disorientation and disorganized behavior of typical sleep terrors.

Bud also had significant personality issues. As noted in the vignette, he requires a great deal of consultation and support (he even leaned on his ex-wife for advice during Harriette's absence), and he has trouble disagreeing with others. His low self-confidence, discomfort at being alone, and rush into another marriage when the first one ended provide a strong basis for the diagnosis of dependent personality disorder.

Other patients with different symptoms might qualify for borderline personality disorder. Bud's GAF score of 61 is based more on his ongoing personality traits than on the arousal disorder. Associated conditions in other patients can include posttraumatic stress disorder and generalized anxiety disorder.

F51.4   Non-rapid eye movement sleep arousal disorder, sleep terror type
F60.7   Dependent personality disorder
Z63.0   Partner relationship distress

Confusional arousals occur during the transition from non-REM sleep to wakefulness. The person seems awake but is perplexed and disoriented and may behave inappropriately (hence the term sometimes used, *sleep drunkenness*). It is noteworthy that the person affected by confusional arousal remains in bed.

An episode may be set up by sleep deprivation or by bedtime use of alcohol or hypnotics. Sometimes triggered by a forced awakening, it may begin with physical movements and moaning, then progress to agitation during which the individual (with eyes open or closed) calls out and thrashes about but cannot awaken. There can also occur more complicated behaviors such as sitting up, speaking incoherently, and performing actions that are purposeful though illogical—and, at times, dangerous.

Attempts at comforting the person are met with resistance and may even increase the agitation. The episode typically lasts 5–15 minutes, occasionally longer, before calm is restored and sleep returns. Amnesia for the event is typical; the individual usually doesn't even recall having a dream. If injury occurs, it may be because someone approached or attempted to interfere with a person who was asleep. It is also important—and reassuring—to note that, by a wide margin, most episodes of confusional arousal do *not* involve aggression or violence.

Although this disorder is said to occur mainly in infants and toddlers, it has also been self-reported in 3–4% of people ages 15 and up. Males and females are represented about equally; shift and night workers may be especially vulnerable. The good news: Even though this disorder didn't make the pages of DSM-5-TR, if you encounter it, you can give it an ICD-10 number: G47.51.

G25.81 Restless Legs Syndrome

Restless legs syndrome (RLS) is an evil complaint that clinicians sometimes ignore because it seriously threatens no one; however, it inflicts exquisite torment upon its sufferers. Not usually painful, it's a nearly indescribable discomfort deep within the lower legs that is relieved only by movement, yielding an irresistible urge to shift leg positions every few seconds (trust me on this). Patients will tell you that the sensation feels like itching, tingling, creeping, or crawling, but none of these descriptors quite captures a condition that confers seemingly inconsequential misery unimaginable by someone who's not afflicted.

With a tendency to begin before bedtime, this common disorder can delay onset of sleep; sometimes it awakens the patient during the night. It's associated with disturbed sleep and reduced sleep time. Relief can come in many guises—walking, pacing, stretching, rubbing, even riding a stationary bicycle. The trouble is that each of these stratagems increases wakefulness. Besides causing the person to feel tired the next day, RLS can lead to depression and anxiety. It tends to lessen throughout the night, allowing more refreshing sleep toward morning. Though it may wax and wane over a period of weeks, it overall worsens with time. It's been associated with major depression, generalized anxiety disorder, posttraumatic stress disorder, and panic disorder.

Nobody's sure why RLS occurs, though the neurotransmitter dopamine may play a role. (It's often reported by patients with Parkinson's disease, whose basal ganglia are compromised.) It's also found in neurological conditions such as neuropathy and multiple sclerosis, and in iron deficiency and renal failure. RLS can be exacerbated by medications, including antihistamines, antinausea preparations, mirtazapine (Remeron), and some other antidepressants. The effects of mild obstructive sleep apnea can sometimes look like periodic limb movements, which affect legs (sometimes arms) and occur during sleep and are very frequently encountered in patients with RLS.

If asked, perhaps 2% of people in the general population will complain of RLS serious enough to cause impaired functioning (mostly, disturbed sleep). Women outnumber men about 2:1; a quarter of pregnant women report it, especially in the third trimester. It tends to begin relatively early in life (the teens or 20s); prevalence increases with age. It's more frequent in European Americans, less so in people of Asian descent. Sometimes you'll find a family history positive for RLS; genetic markers have been identified. A simple interview is usually enough to make the diagnosis.

Especially alert (and argumentative) readers may be asking, Why is RLS even a sleep disorder? What does it have to do with sleep? First, RLS has a diurnal component to it, similar to the ebb and flow of other issues regarding sleep. Second, it can delay sleep onset; occasionally, it even awakens patients during the night. Finally, RLS can result in daytime hypersomnolence—often a cause of distress or impaired functioning. If this logic doesn't appeal straight off, I suggest you sleep on it.

Essential Features of **Restless Legs Syndrome**

Unpleasant lower limb sensations cause an impulse to move one's legs, which relieves the symptoms. Legs are more often restless in the evening or later and when the person is resting or inactive.

The Fine Print

The D's: • Duration (3+ times a week for 3+ months) • Distress or disability (work/ educational, social, or personal impairment) • Differential diagnosis (**substance use** and **physical conditions or disorders, other mental disorders**)

Enoch Dimond

Now alone on the set, Enoch Dimond wipes at his makeup as he views for the second time a digital replay of the 10 P.M. news. He cringes at what he sees: a middle-aged anchorman whose Max Factor can barely conceal the deepening worry lines. His wandering gaze seems to resist looking directly at the camera; his hooded eyes betray trouble focusing on the script. He can almost visualize his feet tap-dancing nervously beneath the polished table that serves as his on-camera desk.

In fact, concentration is a big problem: Enoch can so easily drift off into reverie, away from whatever is going on about him. Just last week, the floor director said, "What's the matter, E? Lately you don't seem to be quite with the program—so to speak."

Well, true enough, he supposes. He'd been fine until the last 3 or 4 weeks, but lately he hasn't enough interest to sustain a run on a small bank. (His joke is an outtake from a special they'd recently aired on the financial system.) Always a conscientious performer, now he takes no pleasure in his craft; indeed, he no longer feels good about much of anything. Even sex bores him.

Nothing has seemed to put Enoch off, just the gradual realization that his life isn't moving in a positive direction; he's begun to feel uneasy, a sense that "something terrible is afoot."

Is he depressed? That's what his wife keeps asking, but he doesn't feel depressed. It's not like he goes around crying all the time, for God's sake. He certainly doesn't feel especially good. Food doesn't taste right, so his appetite must seem a bit off. And he's never considered doing himself in. From a network documentary he introduced a couple of months ago, he knows enough to pay attention to thoughts about dying and suicide.

"Well, you sure look depressed to me!" was his wife's latest word on the subject, yesterday. But not, he suspects, her last.

Enoch decides he just needs to be calm. On camera, he is calm. But whenever he starts thinking about himself and his family, his insides roil. He hopes that his public demeanor—artificial smiles and manufactured bonhomie—conceal the misery he feels.

No, what he feels is more like pepless. Fatigued. That's it! So tired he has trouble dragging himself out of bed, even after he's slept his usual 8 hours. Maybe that explains the peculiar sort of tension in his muscles, as if his biceps were coiled springs that never, ever released. Probably because he is just too damned tired and he can't relax, even in his hot tub.

That tension is different from the peculiar sensation he's had in his legs for a couple of years now. He can hardly sit still long enough to get through his half hour on camera. He has worried—could it indicate some weird form of cancer, buried deep within the calf of his leg? Legs, actually, for they both gave him fits. Getting up and walking around, even for a moment, relieves the misery completely, but he can't do that when he's broadcasting. At night in bed, he so often must get up and walk that he feels wiped out the next day. But while working, even the relief of pacing is denied him. "I should have been a weatherman," he's thought more than once. As it is, the only on-air relief from the jittery legs is to try to rub them together under the desk. It's worse when he is lying down, worst of all in the evening. "Or do a morning show."

Strangely (for him, because he isn't really a worrywart), lately he keeps thinking he'll be fired. Not that he has much reason to worry—he lives the risible cliché of being married to the boss's daughter. Of course, that isn't doing him much good, either. They haven't made love for a couple of months; he just doesn't feel interested, in that or much of anything else. He feels ashamed of his physique, though Kristin says she loves the way he looks. Still, he has reflected more than once that someone born Oliver Schmick isn't likely to find jobs in broadcasting thick on the ground.

Evaluation of Enoch Dimond

Enoch has two problems: one with his mood, one with his legs. The former is the more tendentious, so I'll save that discussion for later.

Enoch has all the important symptoms traditionally associated with RLS: The peculiar, uncontrollable sensation in both legs (criterion A), which lead to the irresistible urge to seek relief in movement (A2), is present only when he is inactive or resting (A1) and worsens in the evening (A3). His sleep suffers and he often feels "wiped out" the following day (C). The frequency and duration qualify for the diagnosis (B)—provided that no other diagnosis seems more appropriate (D, E). To that end, we should check his blood chemistries for iron deficiency anemia and renal failure.

And so we come to the matter of Enoch's mood. Here's the problem: He has several depressive symptoms (low interest, lack of pleasure, fatigue), but not enough for a major depressive episode. He also has a feeling of uneasy anticipation combined with tension and worry, though not enough of these to sustain a diagnosis of either panic disorder or generalized anxiety disorder. At one time, the authors of DSM-5 considered a diagnosis of mixed anxiety–depression (which would require a perhaps too-delicate balancing of criteria so as not to meet full criteria for any other mood or anxiety disorder). But that diagnosis was never adopted. Now, if we make any mood diagnosis at all, we'll have to say that Enoch has a form of depression described in DSM-5-TR as other specified depressive disorder. If these symptoms later morph into major depression, we might add the specifier *with anxious distress*.

However, I'd be happy to wait a few days to see whether his depressive and anxiety symptoms will clear up spontaneously. Sometimes we're a tad too ready with a diagnosis when that old, faithful remedy, tincture of time, can sort things out. Being too quick off the mark can lead to diagnosis where none is justified and treatment where none is indicated.

The problem of separating the symptoms of multiple diagnoses occurs pretty often and across every DSM-5-TR chapter. For example, how do we decide whether the peculiar sensation in Enoch's legs is due to an agitated mood disorder or something else entirely? Two principles should guide us away from the former interpretation: (1) Enoch's motor activity is not generalized but limited to his lower extremities; and, (2) more importantly, it preceded the other mood and anxiety symptoms by at least a year. All in all, I'd give Enoch Dimond only the one firm diagnosis, though we should realize that it is not at all a benign one: RLS can lead to insomnia and other complications. I'd also assign a GAF score of 61. If someone demands a coded diagnosis, I'll probably waffle a bit and use other specified depressive disorder, as you can see below. But I'd try to hold out for "wait and see."

| G25.81 | Restless legs syndrome |
| F32.89 | Other specified depressive disorder, depressive episode with insufficient symptoms |

F51.5 Nightmare Disorder

Despite the name, nightmare disorder has nothing to do with lady horses. The mare in question, which dates back at least to the 13th century, was a goblin that sat on your chest and caused awful dreams. (OK, it was a female goblin.) Most contemporary nightmares quickly bring us full awake, so we tend to recall them vividly. They are usually about something that threatens either our safety or our self-esteem. When someone repeatedly has long, terrifying dreams of that sort, a diagnosis of nightmare disorder may be warranted. Daytime sleepiness, irritability, or loss of concentration may be a consequence.

Nightmares develop during episodes of REM sleep, the majority of which occur later in the night. (Onset early during the sleep period is noteworthy enough to earn a specifier.) They can be increased by withdrawal from REM-suppressing substances; these include antidepressants, barbiturates, and alcohol. Although some degree of rapid heartbeat is common, people with nightmares generally have fewer symptoms of sympathetic nervous system arousal (perspiration, rapid heartbeat, increased blood pressure) than do sufferers from the sleep terror type of non-REM sleep arousal disorder.

Childhood nightmares, especially those that occur in young children, have no pathological significance. About half of adults report nightmares at some time or other. The number who have enough nightmares to be considered pathological is unknown, though perhaps 5% of adults claim to have frequent (monthly or more) nightmares. They may be more common in women than in men. To some extent, the tendency to have nightmares may be inherited.

Although many adults with frequent nightmares probably have some psychopathology, there is no consensus among sleep experts as to what it might be. When it is eventually sorted out, the pathology may have more to do with who complains than with the actual nightmare experience. Vivid nightmares sometimes precede the onset of a psychosis. However, most nightmares may be an expected (and hence normal) reaction to stress; perhaps, as some clinicians believe, they help people work through traumatic experiences.

At least half the population has had a nightmare at one time or another. So, do all of these people (that is, do many of *us*) have a sleep–wake disorder? As with so many other conditions, making this decision is a matter of quantity (number of nightmare episodes) and of the reaction patients (and those around them) have to the episodes. These factors must then be filtered through your clinical judgment. Sweet dreams!

Essential Features of **Nightmare Disorder**

Repeatedly, and usually during the second half of the night, the patient instantly and fully awakens from long, terrible dreams concerning danger or survival that are recalled in frightening detail.

The Fine Print

The D's: • Distress or disability (work/educational, social, or personal impairment) • Differential diagnosis (**substance use** and **physical disorders;** non-REM sleep arousal disorder, sleep terror type; REM sleep behavior disorder; PTSD and acute stress disorders, **other mental disorders**)

Coding Notes

Specify if:

> **During sleep onset.** Most nightmares occur more toward morning.

Specify if:

> **With mental disorder.** Includes substance use.
> **With medical condition**
> **With another sleep disorder**

Specify if:

> **Acute.** Has lasted less than 1 month.
> **Subacute.** Has lasted 1–6 months.
> **Persistent.** Has lasted 6+ months.

Specify severity:

Mild. Nightmares occur less than once a week.
Moderate. 1–6 episodes per week.
Severe. Every night.

Keith Redding

"I wouldn't have come at all, but the guys made me." Keith Redding twists his garrison cap in his fingers and looks embarrassed. "Two of them are waiting out in the hallway in case they're needed for information. I think they really stayed to make sure I kept the appointment."

After 6 months in the Army, Keith has just been promoted to private first class. He enlisted right out of high school, thinking he'd become a mechanic and learn a good trade. But his tests showed that he was gifted, so they plunked him into the medics and sent him to school after boot camp. For 2 weeks now, he's been at his new duty station in Texas, living in the comparative luxury of a barracks room with three roommates.

But his sleeping habits make having any roommate a problem. "I have these nightmares," Keith explains. They don't occur every night, but they do occur several nights a week. He typically awakens an hour or two before reveille, whimpering loudly enough to awaken the others. He's had these experiences for several years, so he's more or less used to them. But his roommates, of course, object. The episodes have been worse in the last few months, with the stress of leaving home, moving around, and working at new jobs.

Although Keith's dreams vary, they do have some threads in common. In one, he is lined up for inspection. All the other troops are looking smart in their Class A uniforms, but Keith is buck naked. Though no one has seemed to notice, he keeps trying to cover. In another, he is driving an old cracker-box ambulance. For some reason, he has picked up a wounded gorilla. Maddened with pain, the gorilla is pulling itself forward and stretching a hairy arm out to wrap around him.

"Unfortunately, I have terrific recall. I come instantly awake, and every detail of the nightmare is just as sharp as if I'd seen it on TV. Then I'm awake for an hour or more, and so is everyone else."

The balance of Keith's history is unremarkable. He doesn't use drugs, doesn't drink; his health is excellent, and he hasn't been especially depressed or anxious. He has never had blackouts or seizures, and he doesn't take medications. He loves his job— in the dispensary or on the ambulance—and he believes his commanding officer finds him alert and conscientious. He certainly isn't falling asleep on the job.

"I've met some older guys who've had nightmares after being in combat," Keith says. "I can understand that. But ever since I enlisted, about the worst thing that's happened to me has been a flat tire."

Evaluation of Keith Redding

Keith's nightmares don't bother him much; he has grown used to them. It's his discomfort as regards his roommates that would qualify his nightmares as sufficiently severe to warrant attention (criterion C).

Three aspects of Keith's experience are typical of most nightmares: They occur during the latter part of the night; he awakens instantly and fully (B); and he clearly recalls their content (typically threats to his safety or self-respect—A). Each of these features serves to differentiate nightmare disorder from non-REM sleep arousal disorder, sleep terror type: Sleep terrors occur early during non-REM sleep; they are poorly remembered; and the patient awakens only partially, if at all. Finally, although there may be some vocalization (for Keith, a muffled whine) when the patient is about to awaken, the paralysis of muscles that's a feature of REM sleep prevents the loud scream and physical movements that are typical of sleep terrors.

If the patient complains of daytime sleepiness, other causes should be considered, such as some form of sleep apnea. Keith did not have daytime sleep attacks, though nightmares can be a feature of narcolepsy. Also consider the variety of other disorders in which nightmares can occur: PTSD, mood disorders, schizophrenia, anxiety disorders, somatic symptom disorder, adjustment disorder, and personality disorders (E).

The fact that Keith has been taking no medications is also important to the differential diagnosis because withdrawal from REM-suppressing substances such as tricyclic antidepressants, alcohol, or barbiturates can sometimes increase the tendency to nightmares (D). Seizure disorders (such as partial complex seizures) can occasionally present with bad dreams; abnormal movements noted by a bed partner during the time of the apparent nightmare can be an indication for EEG studies (E). As Keith himself notes, nightmares about a traumatic event are frequently encountered in patients who have PTSD; these may occur in non-REM sleep, which is why patients with PTSD are more likely to scream.

Keith would qualify for a GAF score of 75. His full diagnosis is brief:

F51.5   Nightmare disorder, persistent, moderate

G47.52 Rapid Eye Movement Sleep Behavior Disorder

During REM sleep, our skeletal muscles are paralyzed, which protects us from injury while we're unconscious. But for people with REM sleep behavior disorder (RBD), that mechanism sometimes fails. Then dreams play out as activity; mischief ensues.

Although the motor behaviors in question may consist only of mild twitches, they can escalate to sudden, sometimes violent movements—by punching, kicking, or even biting, people can sometimes seriously harm themselves or a bed partner. Instead of gross motor behavior, or sometimes in addition to it, patients may whisper, talk, shout, swear, laugh, or cry. But the overall prevalence of injury to self or others is over 50%.

Usually, these patients keep their eyes closed—another difference from sleepwalking—and it's rare that they get out of bed. Upon awakening, which they do readily, many patients with RBD report vivid dreams, often of being threatened or attacked by animals or people. Overt behavior may closely reflect their dream content, sometimes called "acting out their dreams." Occasionally, a funny dream can cause smiling or laughter. When severe, these behaviors occur as often as weekly or even greater.

Onset is usually after age 50, so the typical patient is a middle-aged or older man or woman. However, even children can be affected. Up to a third of patients are unaware of their symptoms, and perhaps half don't recall having unpleasant dreams. Overall, the condition affects less than 1% of the general adult population—perhaps greater in those with other mental disorders.

The initial diagnosis can be suspected from the observations of a bed partner; confirmation (with one exception) requires polysomnography. And here's the exception: The patient has symptoms that suggest RBD plus a synucleinopathy condition such as Parkinson's disease and some others (see the accompanying sidebar).

Of patients who present to sleep clinics with RBD, about half will have or will eventually develop one of these illnesses: Lewy body NCD, Parkinson's disease, or multiple-system atrophy. These are collectively referred to as *synucleinopathies,* because their underlying cause is abnormal intracellular masses of the protein α-synuclein. This is the only example I can think of where a mental health disorder is thought to powerfully predict a medical illness whose onset may lie far in the future. We can perhaps feel both encouraged and appalled.

Essential Features of **Rapid Eye Movement Sleep Behavior Disorder**

During periods of arousal from sleep, the patient shouts or speaks or undertakes complex physical actions that can injure self or a bed partner. After such an episode, the patient is completely awake—oriented and alert. Because they occur during REM sleep, these episodes tend to occur after 90+ minutes of sleep, are more frequent later in the night, and don't occur during naps.

The Fine Print

If the person has a typical history as described above, together with a synucleinopathy (such as Parkinson's disease or Lewy body NCD), no polysomnography is necessary. Without this history, there must be polysomnographic evidence of REM sleep with maintenance of muscle tone.

The D's: • Distress or disability (work/educational, social, or personal impairment) • Differential diagnosis (**substance use** and **physical disorders,** other sleep–wake disorders, malingering)

Jackson Rudy

Jackson Rudy attracted considerable clinical attention when he nearly died in the restraint he'd rigged for himself. One November dawn, his wife, Shawna, had to call the paramedics.

For several years, Jackson explains later, he's had really vivid dreams. These are usually benign, but occasionally "I'll dream I'm being chased by big furry animals with slavering jaws. Then they'll turn from biting me to attack Shawna." In his sleep, he will lash out with fists and feet, but of course the only available target is his wife. "I must be thinking I have to keep her safe—but I guess it's from me!"

As a boy, Jackson lived on a ranch where wolves still roamed. Though he'd never seen one attack, more than once he witnessed them prowling around the family's cattle.

Several months ago, when his nocturnal behavior was limited to yelling or some-times jerking his arms and legs around, he consulted his primary care provider. "She suggested I could sleep in the guest room. Shawna and I both thought that was lame." So, Jackson dusted off the leatherworking skills from his ranch days and constructed a tether to restrain his movements. "It was supposed to loop around my arms and chest to keep me from slugging her," he says, "only I sort of got tangled up in it. I nearly hanged myself."

With Jackson's permission, the clinician interviews Shawna. She affirms that his attacks occur mostly in the predawn hours, and that afterward he comes instantly and completely alert. Has he been depressed? Does he drink or use drugs or medication? (Negatives all 'round.) Is his interest good in things generally? In sex?

Shawna smiles. "Even at 60, he's much better at lovemaking than at inventing."

Evaluation of Jackson Rudy

First, let's dispose of the criteria. We know from the history (including Shawna's helpful information) that Jackson's episodes are repeated and physical (criterion A), that they occur while he is dreaming later in the night (not when first falling asleep—criterion B), and that they appear to be a physical enactment of his dreams. He comes fully alert right away (C); and he doesn't use alcohol, drugs, or medications that might cause these behaviors (F). The arrival of the paramedics tells us that the behavior is dangerous and clinically important (E).

Polysomnography can also help with the differential diagnosis of some other dis-orders that entail violence during sleep: both the sleepwalking and sleep terror types of non-REM sleep arousal disorder, nocturnal seizures, and obstructive sleep apnea hypopnea. However, Jackson's history isn't strong for any of these disorders, and I'm comfortable putting them aside. There's no evidence for other medical or mental dis-orders (G).

The remaining criterion (D), verification by polysomnography, isn't quite as vital as DSM-5-TR might lead us to believe. Some experts state that we can omit it in rela-tively mild cases, where there's no significant worry about other disorders. But with the severity of Jackson's lashing out, safety is the better part of evaluation. Jackson probably wouldn't consider himself old yet, but still we need to know that he has none of the degenerative neurological disorders that can be a source of RBD: Lewy body NCD (about 70% of cases are associated with RBD), Parkinson's disease (50%), and multiple-system atrophy (upwards of 90%). RBD is also found in strokes, tumors, and with some medications (beta blockers, certain antidepressants), though it's rare in Alzheimer's disease.

Because of the circumstances in which Jackson nearly died, a few questions about paraphilias would be warranted, and his clinician would want to keep in mind the possibility of a suicide attempt—a red herring here, but something that we must always keep on the diagnostic front burner.

Jackson Rudy's diagnosis is listed below. Although the paramedics were called, I'd say that any danger to himself was a one-off, unlikely to be repeated. I'd put his GAF score at a comfortable 70. As noted, his doctor should observe him carefully for development of an additional disorder.

G47.52   Rapid eye movement sleep behavior disorder

Other Sleep–Wake Disorders

Substance/Medication-Induced Sleep Disorder

As you might expect, substances of abuse can produce a variety of sleep disorders, most of which will be either insomnia or hypersomnolence. The specific problem with sleep can occur during either intoxication or withdrawal.

Alcohol. Heavy alcohol use (intoxication) can produce unrefreshing sleep with strong REM suppression and reduced total sleep time. Patients may experience terminal insomnia and sometimes hypersomnolence, and their sleep problems can persist for years. Alcohol withdrawal markedly increases sleep onset latency and produces restless sleep with frequent awakenings. Patients may experience delirium with tremor and (especially visual) hallucinations; this was formerly known as delirium tremens.

Sedatives, hypnotics, and anxiolytics. These include barbiturates, over-the-counter antihistamines and bromides, short-acting benzodiazepines, and high doses of long-acting benzodiazepines. Any of these substances may be used in the attempt to remedy insomnia of another origin. They can lead to sleep disorder during either intoxication or withdrawal.

Central nervous system stimulants. Amphetamines and other stimulants typically cause increased latency of sleep onset, decreased REM sleep, and more frequent awakenings. Once the drug is discontinued, hypersomnolence with restlessness and REM rebound dreams may ensue.

Caffeine. This popular drug produces insomnia with intoxication and hypersomnolence upon withdrawal (no surprises here).

Other drugs. These include tricyclic antidepressants, antipsychotics, ACTH, anticonvulsants, thyroid medications, marijuana, cocaine, LSD, opioids, PCP, and methyldopa.

Essential Features of Substance/Medication–Induced Sleep Disorder

The use of some substance appears to have caused a patient to have an obvious, serious sleep problem.

For evidence concerning substance-related causation, see sidebar, page 95.

The Fine Print

The D's: • Distress or disability (work/educational, social, or personal impairment) • Differential diagnosis (physical disorders, **delirium, other sleep disorders**)

Use this diagnosis instead of substance intoxication or withdrawal only when sleep symptoms are predominant and require clinical care.

Coding Notes

Coding in ICD-10 depends on the substance used and on whether symptoms are met for a substance use disorder (and, if so, how severe the use disorder is). Refer to Table 15.2 in Chapter 15.

Specify:

> **With onset during {intoxication}{withdrawal}.** This gets tacked on at the end of your string of words.
> **With onset after medication use.** You could alternatively use this if symptoms develop when medication is started, changed, or stopped.

Specify:

> **Insomnia type**
> **Daytime sleepiness type**
> **Parasomnia type** (abnormal behavior when sleeping)
> **Mixed type**

Dave Kincaid

Dave Kincaid is a freelance writer. As Dave explains it to his clinician, "freelance" is the industry's way of calling you unemployed. He's done pretty well for himself, specializing in interviews with people who are unimportant but fascinating. Most of his work is published in small magazines and specialized reviews; he also wrote (and starred in) a couple of podcasts. His novel and a volume of travel essays were remaindered early with good reviews but disappointing sales.

When he has to, Dave supplements his income with temporary jobs. To gather material for his writing, he tries to choose work that's as varied as possible. He has driven a taxi, been a bouncer at a bar, sold real estate, and (in his younger days) served as a guide on the Jungle River Cruise at Disneyland. Now 35, for the last several weeks he has been supporting his third book, a murder mystery, by working in a coffee roastery north of San Francisco. The job doesn't pay much over minimum wage, but neither is it very demanding. Except for the busy 2 or 3 hours around noon, it leaves him plenty of time for blocking out sections of his book to work on at night.

It also leaves Dave time to drink coffee. Besides grinding beans or selling them whole, the roastery serves coffee by the cup. Employees can drink what they want. Dave is a coffee drinker, but he has always limited himself to three or four cups a day. "It sure isn't enough to explain the way I'm feeling now."

How he feels is, in a word, nervous. It's worst at night. "I have this uncomfortable, 'up' sort of feeling, and I want to write. But sometimes I just can't sit still at the word processor. I get that 'live flesh' sensation when your muscles twitch. And my heart beats fast and my gut seems to pour out water, so I spend a lot of time in the bathroom."

Dave seldom gets to sleep before 2 A.M., sometimes after much tossing and turning. On Sundays he sleeps until noon, but on Monday through Saturday he awakens to his alarm, feeling grouchy and in desperate need of a cup of coffee.

Dave's health has been excellent otherwise, which is a good thing because he's seldom had a job with a health plan. Other than early mornings, his mood is good. He has tried marijuana in the past but doesn't like it. He confines his drinking to coffee, but "only three or four cups a day," he says again. He also denies drinking tea, cocoa, or cola beverages. After a moment he adds, "Of course, there are the coffee beans."

When things are slow in the afternoon and Dave is thinking about his novel, he will dip into the supply of candy-coated coffee beans the roastery also sells ($11.95 the half-pound). They come covered in white or dark chocolate; he prefers the dark. They also sell decaffeinated beans, but these are dipped in yogurt, which he doesn't care for at all.

"I don't keep track," Dave says, "but all in all, every afternoon I probably have a few handfuls. Or so."

Evaluation of Dave Kincaid

Although Dave's coffee intake is modest, the coffee itself is strong; it probably contains more than the 250 mg of caffeine usually required for intoxication. He also eats coffee beans; depending on origin, it takes perhaps 70 beans to equal a strong cup of brewed coffee, and he eats chocolate-coated beans by the handful. That way, he may consume the equivalent of one or two additional cups of coffee per day. (In addition, chocolate contains theobromine, a xanthine with effects similar to caffeine.) No wonder he feels nervous! In its proper place (p. 425), we'll discuss Dave's symptoms of caffeinism.

In conjunction with his caffeine use, Dave notes increased latency of sleep onset. He feels tired when it's time to get up, and he requires—coffee!—to get going. Therefore, the basic criteria for substance-induced sleep disorder are all met: Use of a substance causes (criterion B1) a problem with sleep serious enough to require clinical attention (A, E). Of course, caffeine is famously associated with sleeplessness.

Sure, we can think up all manner of other sleep disorders that could cause Dave's symptoms (C, D)—but the rational course would be to eliminate (gradually!) the caffeine use, then reassess the patient's sleep. This is what Dave's clinician sets in motion. In some cases, there can be confusion as to the etiological contributions of physical illness and the medications that are used to treat it. Then, two diagnoses may be warranted.

With the subtype specifiers required in the criteria (and a GAF score of 65), Dave's diagnosis will be as follows:

F15.929   Caffeine intoxication, moderate
F15.982   Caffeine-induced sleep disorder, insomnia type, with onset during intoxication

---

The diagnosis of a substance-induced *anything* rests on deciding that the symptoms are more serious than you'd expect from ordinary substance intoxication or withdrawal. This is a judgment call. In the case of Dave Kincaid, the symptoms are sufficiently prominent to bring him for evaluation.

G47.09 Other Specified Insomnia Disorder

DSM-5-TR gives these examples:

Short-term insomnia disorder. Insomnia lasting less than 3 months.

Restricted to nonrestorative sleep. The patient doesn't feel refreshed by sleep that is otherwise unremarkable.

G47.00 Unspecified Insomnia Disorder

Use unspecified insomnia disorder when a patient's insomnia symptoms do not meet the full criteria for insomnia disorder (or any other sleep disorder) and you decide not to be specific about the reasons.

G47.19 Other Specified Hypersomnolence Disorder

G47.10 Unspecified Hypersomnolence Disorder

Use one of these categories when you've eliminated all other possibilities for a patient's hypersomnolence. The usual guidelines for choosing other specified versus unspecified apply.

G47.8 Other Specified Sleep–Wake Disorder

G47.9 Unspecified Sleep–Wake Disorder

By now, you know the drill.

CHAPTER 12

Sexual Dysfunctions

Quick Guide to the Sexual Dysfunctions

DSM-5-TR addresses three sorts of issues directly tied to sexual functioning. In DSM-IV and before, they were all included in the same chapter; now the sexual dysfunctions, gender dysphoria, and paraphilic disorders are spread out over three different chapters. Except for substance-induced sexual dysfunction, the sexual dysfunctions are gender-specific. DSM-5-TR's organization is alphabetical; I've grouped these disorders by gender and stage in an act of sex at which the dysfunction occurs.

Sexual Dysfunctions

Male hypoactive sexual desire disorder. The patient isn't much interested in sex, though his performance may be adequate once sexual activity has been initiated (p. 358).

Erectile disorder. A man's erection isn't sufficient to begin or complete sexual relations (p. 361).

Premature (early) ejaculation. A man repeatedly experiences climax too soon (p. 364).

Delayed ejaculation. Despite a normal period of sexual excitement, a man's climax is either delayed or does not occur at all (p. 366).

Female sexual interest/arousal disorder. A woman lacks interest in sex or does not become adequately aroused (p. 368).

Genito-pelvic pain/penetration disorder. A woman experiences genital pain during sexual intercourse, often during insertion (p. 371).

Female orgasmic disorder. Despite a normal period of sexual excitement, a woman's climax either is delayed or does not occur at all (p. 374).

Substance/medication-induced sexual dysfunction. Many sexual problems can be caused by intoxication or withdrawal from alcohol or other substances (p. 376).

Other specified, or unspecified, sexual dysfunction. These are catch-all categories for sexual problems that do not meet the criteria for any of the foregoing sexual dysfunctions (p. 377).

Other Causes of Sexual Difficulty

Paraphilic disorders. These include a variety of behaviors that most people regard as distasteful, unusual, or abnormal. Nearly all are practiced almost exclusively by males (p. 580).

Gender dysphoria. Some people have such a strong sense of their gender being different from the sex they were assigned at birth that it causes them discomfort or distress (p. 379).

Nonsexual mental disorders. Many patients develop sexual dysfunctions as a result of other mental disorders. Lack of interest in sex may be encountered especially in somatic symptom disorder (p. 254), major depressive disorder (p. 116), and schizophrenia (p. 63).

Introduction

The sexual dysfunctions usually begin in early adulthood, though some may not appear until later in life—whenever the opportunity for sexual experience arises. Most of them are quite common. Any of them can be caused by psychological or biological factors or by a combination of these. Ordinarily, we wouldn't use one of these diagnoses if the behavior occurs only during another mental disorder.

Also, any of these dysfunctions can be lifelong or acquired. *Lifelong* (also called *primary*) means that this dysfunction has been present since the beginning of active sexual functioning. *Acquired* means that at some time the patient has been able to have sex without experiencing that dysfunction. As you might imagine, lifelong dysfunctions are vastly more resistant to therapy.

Furthermore, most sexual dysfunctions may be either *generalized* or *situational* (that is, limited to specific situations). For example, a man may experience premature ejaculation with his wife but not with another woman. Some dysfunctions may not even require the patient to have a partner; they can occur during masturbation, for example.

DSM-5-TR places tight limits on how much dysfunction is required for diagnosis. The patient must have the symptoms on most occasions (in criteria sets, it is phrased as "almost all or all") of sexual activity over a 6-month period—and those phrases have been explicitly, and confusingly, defined as meaning 75% or more. However, the criteria also specify that they must cause "clinically significant distress," leaving some room for clinician judgment based on how long the problem has existed and the degree to which the problem affects patient and partner. This judgment will be influenced by the circumstances surrounding the particular sex activity—such as degree of sexual stimulation, the amount of that activity, and with whom it occurs. For example, female sexual interest/arousal disorder should not be diagnosed if it occurs only when intercourse is attempted after little or no foreplay.

In addition to these considerations, here are some additional factors to take into account during an evaluation. (Note that in DSM-IV they were subtypes that we added to the official title of each sexual disorder; DSM-5-TR has in effect demoted them to an advisory capacity.)

- Partner factors (such as partner's sexual preferences, problems, or health status)
- Relationship factors (such as poor communication, relationship discord, partners having differing desire for sexual activity)
- Individual vulnerability factors (such as a history of abuse or poor body image)
- Cultural/religious factors (for example, prohibitions against sexual activity)
- Medical factors relevant to prognosis, course, or treatment such as a chronic illness

Although common, the sexual dysfunctions tend to be ignored by clinicians who don't specialize in their evaluation and treatment; too often, we simply fail to ask. An alert clinician may be able to make a diagnosis of one or more of these conditions in a patient who comes for consultation regarding unrelated mental health problems.

F52.0 Male Hypoactive Sexual Desire Disorder

As compared to women, relatively little is known about low sex interest and desire in men. This has partly resulted from the unfounded assumption that it is uncommon. Yet, in a 1994 survey of over 1,400 men, 16% agreed that they had had a period of several months when they were not interested in sex; this is compared with 33% for women. These men tended to be older, never married, not highly educated, Black, and poor. Compared to other men, they were more likely to have been "inappropriately touched" before puberty, to have experienced homosexual activity at some time in their lives, and to use alcohol daily. Even a few percent of younger men (in their 20s) will admit to relative lack of sexual desire, though it seldom rises to the level of male hypoactive sexual desire disorder (MHSDD).

MHSDD can be primary or acquired. The relatively less common primary type has been associated with some sort of sexual secret such as shame about sexual orientation, past sexual trauma, or preference for masturbation over sex with a partner. Such a patient's low sex desire may be masked by the effect of a new romance; this glow typically persists for only a matter of months before frustration and heartache (and more secrecy) set in, for patient and partner alike.

Acquired MHSDD is the more common pattern. It often develops as a consequence of dysfunctions of erection or ejaculation (early or delayed). These in turn can stem from a variety of causes: diabetes, hypertension, substance use, mood or anxiety disorders, sometimes a lack of intimacy with a partner. Whatever the origin, the man's confidence in his ability to achieve or maintain an erection (or to satisfy his partner) yields to a pattern of anticipatory anxiety and failure. He has trouble admitting that his sexual relationship is less than perfect, and so he retires from the fray, so to speak, defeated and uncommunicative.

Such a pattern can begin at almost any stage of life, though about two out of three couples stop having sex by their mid-70s. At any age, when this happens to heterosexual couples, it is overwhelmingly (90%) likely to be at the man's initiative.

And by the way, DSM-5-TR notes that this diagnosis can be applied to a gender-diverse patient.

Essential Features of **Male Hypoactive Sexual Desire Disorder**

A man habitually lacks erotic thoughts and the desire for sexual activity.

The Fine Print

The clinician must judge the deficiency in light of age and other factors that can affect sexual function.

The D's: • Duration (6+ months) • Distress to the patient • Differential diagnosis (substance use or physical disorders, relationship problems or other stressors, other mental disorders)

Coding Notes

Specify:

  {Lifelong}{Acquired}
  {Generalized}{Situational}

Specify severity of distress concerning the symptoms: **{Mild}{Moderate}{Severe}**

Nigel O'Neil

"She's not your typical trophy wife," Nigel O'Neil tells the therapist in confidence. "I love Gemma because she's so competent, so organized—and such a nice person," he adds, almost as an afterthought. "But she just doesn't turn me on the way Bea used to."

At age 53, Nigel is well into his second marriage, solemnized 3 years after his first wife died of malignant melanoma. For several years, Gemma had been his personal assistant in the office where he works for a large publisher of books and periodicals. Around the time Bea died, he turned to Gemma for more than his morning cup of Darjeeling. During his first session, he admits that he still feels guilty about that.

Born in London, Nigel was raised a strict Catholic. "That operationalized to the fact that, before we were married, Bea and I hadn't done much more than a little fooling around," he explains. "We were very young and inexperienced." After the ceremony, he had been able to obtain and maintain an erection satisfactory for intercourse "most of the time, though even then we had our problems, Bea and I." He declines to elaborate, stating only that they seemed minor in comparison.

Gemma is 15 years younger than Nigel. For several months, they pursued an active sex life. "Something else she organized," he remarks. At the office, he appreciates the way she manages his schedule. "At home, not so much." In the last 6 months, when she approaches him for sex, he usually fobs her off with the excuse of being tired or preoccupied. On the few occasions she's persuaded him to try, he couldn't maintain an erection long enough to achieve penetration. The one time they did have intercourse, his attention had "wandered off to the office," and he withdrew before either of them climaxed.

Nigel's internist has checked his testosterone level, which is within the expected range. On his second visit, Gemma tags along. She and Nigel agree that they drink little alcohol and have never used drugs or tobacco. Gemma adds that a few months earlier, in desperation, she subscribed to *Playboy* for him. "He's the only man I know who really does read it for the articles," she comments.

Nigel hadn't seen other women; he doesn't even masturbate. "For months, the magazine's the only thing I've put to bed. I don't even have randy fantasies anymore." The issue doesn't distress Nigel for himself ("It's just not something I ever think about!"), but he becomes almost tearful as he talks about how deeply he cares for Gemma, how he longs for her to be happy—and not abandon him for someone else.

One session when Nigel is in the room, Gemma explains, "Besides books and magazines, our company makes films, mostly about love and lovemaking. Nigel thinks that's a total irony, but I don't think we've finished shooting yet."

Evaluation of Nigel O'Neil

Nigel's history is loaded with indicators of a persistent sexual disorder, including multiple failures of his erection, his interest, his response (to invitations from Gemma), and even his fantasy life (criterion A). His interest in work is good and he denies feeling depressed, so a mood disorder seems unlikely (D), but a thorough review to identify any possible anxiety disorder would seem to be a good idea. The history appears to rule out an etiological role for drugs or alcohol (also D); there isn't any apparent relationship distress—yet, at any rate. The duration meets the 6-month requirement (B), and Nigel's distress is palpable (C).

In addition, Nigel probably will qualify for the diagnosis of erectile disorder. If so, it should also be made (other sexual disorders can coexist with MHSDD). It's just one more issue he and his clinician will need to explore.

Once the principal diagnosis is nailed down, the clinician's real work begins—examining the possible causes of Nigel's lack of sexual interest. Each of these could indicate a therapeutic avenue to explore. As noted in the introduction to sexual dysfunctions, multiple possible contributing factors must be considered. As an exercise (I'm not going to burden you with this list for every patient), let's check out all the possibilities:

Relationship factors—does Nigel resent Gemma's overmanagement of their lives?

Medical factors—does Nigel have, say, diabetes or a cardiovascular condition? (If medical factors were the exclusive cause of his current sexual problems, we wouldn't make this diagnosis at all; see criterion D.)

Cultural/religious scruples—having had sex with Gemma while Nigel was still married to Bea could play a role.

Partner factors—Gemma appears to be healthy, doesn't use substances, and reportedly has a healthy interest in sex.

Individual vulnerability factors—OK, Nigel's clinician needs to dig a little deeper here to determine whether he has had a history of emotional or physical abuse, or any hidden mental disorders.

Clearly in order are further exploratory interviews with both Nigel and Gemma.

Nigel's still unelaborated sexual problems with Bea even make us wonder whether his problem could have been lifelong, rather than acquired. Had his sex interest been on the low side with her, too? Had she complained? Did he fantasize about other women? Men? How affectionate were they as a couple?

In its bare-bones form, Nigel's diagnosis will read as given below, but there's much more work to be done. Despite his difficulties with sex, I'd put his GAF score at a relatively healthy 70.

F52.0   Male hypoactive sexual desire disorder, acquired, generalized, severe

F52.21 Erectile Disorder

Erectile disorder (ED), otherwise known as impotence, can be partial or complete. In either case, the erection is inadequate for satisfactory sex. Impotence can also be situational, in which case the patient can achieve an erection only under certain circumstances (for example, with prostitutes). ED is probably the most prevalent male sexual disorder, occurring at least occasionally in perhaps 2% of *young* men. That number does not improve with age; half or more of men over the age of 70 probably would qualify for this diagnosis. Of the sexual dysfunctions, this is the one most likely to occur for the first time later in life.

A variety of emotions can play a role in the development or maintenance of ED. These include fear, anxiety, anger, guilt, and distrust of the sexual partner. Any of these feelings can so preoccupy a man's attention that he cannot focus adequately on feeling sexual pleasure. Even a single failure may lead to anticipatory anxiety, which then precipitates another round in the circle of failure. The pioneering sex researchers Masters and Johnson also talked about a factor they called *spectatoring,* in which the patient evaluates his performance so constantly that he cannot concentrate on the enjoyment of sex. Such a patient might have an erection with foreplay but lose it upon penetration.

ED should not be diagnosed if biological factors are the principal or only cause. This is unlikely if erections occur spontaneously, with masturbation, or with other partners. Some authorities now estimate that in half or more instances of impotence, there is a biological cause such as prostatectomy for cancer. But when the cause is even partly psychological, the diagnosis can be made.

Note the difference between erectile dysfunction and erectile disorder. In the former, the patient complains that he cannot get and maintain an erection. In the latter, all of the essential features are met.

Like the other sexual dysfunctions, ED can be either lifelong or acquired; the former is rare and hard to treat.

Essential Features of **Erectile Disorder**

The patient almost always has marked trouble achieving or maintaining an erection adequate to consummate sex, or he complains of loss of tumescence.

The Fine Print

The D's: • Duration (6+ months) • Distress to the patient • Differential diagnosis (**substance use** and **physical disorders, relationship problems, other mental disorders**)

Coding Notes

Specify:

   {Lifelong}{Acquired}
   {Generalized}{Situational}

Specify severity of distress concerning the symptoms: **{Mild}{Moderate}{Severe}**

Parker Flynn

"I think I must be over the hill."

If you don't count the three counseling sessions he had while sifting through the wreckage of his first marriage, this is Parker Flynn's first visit ever to a mental health professional. At age 45 he has been a bridegroom for only 7 months, and he's afraid he's losing his sexual potency.

Everything was fine before the wedding, but the first evening of their honeymoon, Parker couldn't get enough of an erection to do either him or his new bride much good. He supposes he'd had too much champagne—usually he doesn't touch alcohol. Pauline had also been married before and knew a thing or two about men. She hadn't criticized; she'd even said it would be all right. But she is attractive and 10 years younger than Parker, and he is worried: Most of the time since, he's been unable to perform.

"Some of the guys warned me, it's what happens when you get older," Parker insists. One friend likes to say, "That which should be easy is hard, and that which should be hard, isn't."

Before he popped the question, he had undergone a complete physical examination. Other than being a few pounds overweight—Parker is devoted to chocolate ice cream—he was given a clean bill of health. The ice cream aside, he denies any other addictions, including alcohol, drugs, and tobacco.

"I get so nervous when it's time to make love," Parker explains. "I can get a pretty good erection when we're fooling around, but when it's time to get serious, I lose it. Pauline's ex was something of a stud, and I keep worrying, how does my performance measure up to his?"

Evaluation of Parker Flynn

Parker's interest in sex seems to be just fine; he gives every indication (vigorous erections) that there is nothing wrong with his excitatory phase. But because he worries about maintaining his erection, he has trouble with just that—maintaining an erection (criterion A2). Stressful enough that he seeks care (C), his problem is exacerbated by the phenomenon of spectatoring, in which his performance is affected by wondering how well he is doing while he's doing it. This situation has been present for 7 months—just meeting the DSM-5-TR time requirement (B, though in obvious cases I wouldn't be too picky: The criterion does say "approximately," after all).

His physical condition is good, pretty much ruling out a causative physical illness (D). Some patients with impotence may suffer from sleep apnea; of course, it is vital to explore this possibility, because of the potentially lethal nature of that disorder. Parker has had no previous mental health problems that would preclude the diagnosis of ED. His difficulty may have begun with an alcohol-related incident, but from his history, substance use plays no role in its maintenance. Also note that, as they age, men may require more stimulation to achieve erection than they once did; such a physiological change does not constitute evidence of ED. Sporadic erectile problems that cause little distress also should not be given this diagnosis.

Parker's problem is not lifelong but acquired; the vignette provides no evidence that it occurs only in specific situations, so neither situational nor generalized type should be specified. With no other obvious specifiers to note (and a GAF score of 70), his diagnosis reads:

F52.21   Erectile disorder, acquired

F52.4 Premature (Early) Ejaculation

As the disorder's name implies, the man climaxes before he wants to—sometimes just as he and his partner reach the point of insertion. However, different studies use widely varying standards for how many minutes constitute early: Is it 7 minutes? Is it 1? Both standards have been proposed, with 2 minutes the current favored standard. Whatever the duration, the climax yields disappointment and a sense of failure for both partners; secondary impotence sometimes follows. Stress in a relationship can exacerbate the condition, which can promote even greater loss of control. However, some women may value premature ejaculation (PE) because it decreases their exposure to unwanted sexual activity or pregnancy.

PE is a commonplace disorder; it affects nearly half the men treated for sexual disorders. It is especially frequent among men with more education—presumably because their social group is sensitive to the issue of partner satisfaction. Whereas anxiety is often a factor, physical illness or abnormalities rarely cause this problem.

Essential Features of **Premature (Early) Ejaculation**

The patient almost always ejaculates before he wants to, generally within a minute of penetration.

The Fine Print a

The D's: • Duration (6+ months) • Distress to the patient • Differential diagnosis (**substance use** and **physical disorders, serious relationship problems** or **other stressors**)

Coding Notes

Specify:

> {Lifelong}{Acquired}
> {Generalized}{Situational}

Specify severity:

> **Mild.** The patient ejaculates 30–60 seconds after penetration.
> **Moderate.** 15–30 seconds after penetration.
> **Severe.** 15 seconds after penetration or less (perhaps even before penetration).

Let's be practical. And honest. The official criteria for premature ejaculation state two standards of time, which boil down to "about a minute" and "too early." DSM-5-TR implies that men can pretty accurately estimate time as long as it's a minute or less, but it seems unlikely in the extreme that, in the heat of the moment, anyone is going to clap a stopwatch on the activity. Therefore, for the vast majority of our patients, we will eschew the clock and accept the statement that "I just flat-out come too soon."

Claude Campbell

Claude Campbell can remember, in embarrassing detail, the first time it ever happened. He was a very young Marine second lieutenant stationed in Vietnam in the last year of the war. Suddenly granted leave to go into town, he had to borrow a pair of Class A uniform trousers from the battalion chaplain.

Claude and two friends were seated at a sidewalk table, drinking a potion that the soldiers called a "Bombs Away," when a prostitute sat down next to him. When she set to work warming her hand between his thighs, it only took a few moments before Claude felt himself lose control. A crimson blush spread across his face as a stain darkened the front of the chaplain's khaki trousers.

"That was one of the worst times, but it sure wasn't the last," says Claude. After leaving the Marines, he finished college, got a job selling computers, and soon married a girl he had dated during high school. Their wedding night, and most of their other nights, were never quite the disaster of the Vietnam bar, but he can never last longer than a minute or so after insertion.

"Not that it bothered her," Claude comments ruefully. "She never enjoyed sex much, anyway. She was always glad to get it over with in a hurry. I know now why she insisted on 'saving it' for after we were married. She never wanted to spend it in the first place."

Claude always hoped that his problems were largely due to his first wife's prudery and disapproval, but several months into his new marriage, things haven't improved much. "She's being very patient," he says, "but we're both beginning to get a little desperate."

Evaluation of Claude Campbell

Claude's difficulty has been with him ever since the dawn of his sex life, and it occurs every time (criterion B). Although a few such incidents might be dismissed in a youngster or in any man with a new partner, in a mature adult (we don't know Claude's age at evaluation) who has been in a lasting relationship with frequent sexual activity, it must be considered pathological (A). Claude's difficulty clearly causes him distress (C); we'd have to enquire further about substance use (D). As noted earlier, physical illness does not play a significant role in the development of PE.

Claude's problem has occurred with two wives and with the sex worker, so it is not situational; as far as we're aware, he's had it forever. I'd place his GAF score at 70.

F52.4   Premature ejaculation, generalized, lifelong, moderate

F52.32 Delayed Ejaculation

Men with delayed ejaculation (DE) achieve erection without difficulty but have problems reaching orgasm. Some only take a long time; others may not be able to ejaculate with a partner at all. Prolonged friction may cause the partners of these patients to complain of soreness. Anxiety about performance may cause secondary impotence in the patients themselves.

Even when it has been present lifelong, the man can usually ejaculate by masturbating (alone or with the help of his sex partner). The personalities of patients with lifelong DE have been described as rigid and puritanical; some patients seem to equate sex with sin. Or the disorder may be acquired from interpersonal difficulties, fear of pregnancy, or a partner's lack of sexual allure. DE is somewhat more common in patients with anxiety disorders.

DE is probably uncommon (under 5%), though it tends to increase with advancing age. Problems with delayed (or absent) climax often have a medical cause; examples include hyperglycemia, prostatectomy, abdominal aortic surgery, Parkinson's disease, and spinal cord tumors. For some, upon orgasm a physical abnormality causes semen to be expelled into the urinary bladder (retrograde ejaculation). Drugs like alphamethyldopa (an antihypertensive) and thioridazine (an antipsychotic), as well as alcohol, have also been implicated. If any of these factors is the sole cause, you wouldn't diagnose DE.

Essential Features of **Delayed Ejaculation**

Almost always, with a partner a man experiences undesired, pronounced delay or infrequency—even absence—of climax.

The Fine Print

The D's: • Duration (6+ months) • Distress to the patient • Differential diagnosis (**substance use** and **physical disorders, relationship problems, another mental disorder**)

Coding Notes

Specify:

   {Lifelong}{Acquired}
   {Generalized}{Situational}

Specify severity, based on amount of distress: **{Mild}{Moderate}{Severe}**

Rodney Stensrud

Rodney Stensrud and his girlfriend, Frannie, come to the clinic seeking relief for Rodney's "performance problem." They have been together for nearly a year, and they disagree as to the extent of the problem.

Rodney is frankly worried. It has always taken him a long time to reach climax, and now, after 40 minutes or so of vigorous intercourse, he sometimes finds himself wilting under pressure. Frannie is more sanguine. Her previous boyfriend had never been able to last longer than 5 minutes, and that often left her feeling frustrated. "Now I almost always come more than once," she says with an air of satisfaction. Recently Rodney has been taking even longer, and she admits that she gets rather sore. "Maybe if we could get it back down to about half an hour," she suggests.

Rodney's parents raised him strictly. Throughout his childhood, he attended a parochial school; as a result, he grew up "pretty clear on the concept of good versus evil." He admits that he feels guilty that he and Frannie are living together without benefit of clergy, but she isn't yet ready to take the next step. She likes to laugh and tell him that she wants to "save something for after the baby comes."

Before meeting Frannie, Rodney's only experience had been with two sex workers he had encountered while he was in the Navy. It had taken him hardly any time at all with either of them. In fact, he felt that the one with the mouth had rather shortchanged him. "There sure wasn't any delay involved," he said. Neither has he experienced any problem masturbating, either as an adolescent or more recently when Frannie was on an extended business trip.

Rodney was referred by a urologist, who found nothing physically wrong. The couple's only drinking is an occasional glass of white wine. At one time, Rodney might have used marijuana at parties, but Frannie is death on drugs, so he's given it up entirely.

Evaluation of Rodney Stensrud

After apparently normal desire and excitation phases, Rodney always takes an inordinately long time to reach climax (criterion A1). From the vignette, this hasn't been a lifelong problem, though now it has lasted for many months (B). The problem causes him enough distress to seek help (C); already he seems headed down the road to secondary impotence.

Rodney's problem is situational; he experienced no ejaculatory delay when with a paid companion or when masturbating. His referring physician notes no physical illnesses that might account for his disorder, and there is no significant substance use. With no evidence of any other mental disorder that might be diagnosed instead, we've exhausted the possibilities of criterion D. His puritanical upbringing reinforces the impression that the basis of his disorder is psychological.

Frannie's reaction to Rodney's disorder is perhaps somewhat atypical. Female partners sometimes complain of discomfort from prolonged intercourse necessary to achieve climax. Would the fact that Frannie found value in Rodney's disorder present a possible issue for therapy? When working with the couple, Rodney's clinician should keep this factor in mind—along with the possibility that he could have an anxiety disorder.

Rodney's GAF score would be about 70. His diagnosis would be as follows:

F52.32   Delayed ejaculation, acquired, situational, moderate

F52.22 Female Sexual Interest/Arousal Disorder

Female sexual interest/arousal disorder (FSIAD) represents the fusion of two older diagnoses: hypoactive sexual desire disorder and female sexual arousal disorder. DSM-5-TR combines them for several reasons. Especially in females, there is a marked overlap between desire and arousal; some authorities think of desire as just the cognitive component of arousal. Moreover, one phase doesn't always precede the other; their relationship really depends on the individual. And treating low desire also improves arousal.

Sexual desire depends upon several factors, including the patient's inherent drive and self-esteem, previous sexual satisfaction, having an available partner, and a good partner relationship in areas other than sex. Sexual desire may be suppressed by long abstinence. It may present as infrequent sexual activity, or as a perception that the partner is unattractive. Some patients become averse to sex, expressing loathing of any genital contact or of aspects of genital sexual contact.

Lack of interest in sex is the most common complaint of women coming to treatment. About 30% of those age 18–59 will admit to experiencing at least several months when they've lacked sexual desire. As a result, perhaps half feel distress, which can affect them and their relationships. Low desire especially affects women who are postmenopausal, either naturally or as a result of surgery. There may be a history of painful intercourse, feelings of guilt, or rape or other sexual trauma occurring in childhood or in a patient's earlier sexual life.

Don't diagnose FSIAD if the problem occurs only in the context of another mental condition, such as major depressive disorder or a substance use disorder. And note that postmenopausal females may need more foreplay to lubricate than they did when they were younger.

FSIAD often coexists with another sexual condition, such as female orgasmic disorder. A woman who doesn't express interest in sex but does respond to sexual activity with excitement would not qualify for a diagnosis of FSIAD. Neither would someone who identifies herself as having been "asexual" her whole life.

In evaluating any patient with a sexual disorder, let's remember to consider the five factors mentioned before (p. 361): partner factors, relationship factors, individual vulnerability factors, cultural/religious factors, and medical factors. And by the way, DSM-5-TR also notes that this diagnosis can be applied to someone who is gender diverse.

Essential Features of **Female Sexual Interest/Arousal Disorder**

A woman's low sexual interest or arousal is indicated by minimal interest in sexual activity or erotic thoughts, response to partner overtures, and enjoyment during sex. She will generally not initiate sexual activity and doesn't "turn on" to erotic literature, movies, and the like.

The Fine Print

The D's: • Duration (6+ months) • Distress to the patient • Differential diagnosis (**substance use** and **physical disorders, relationship problems** or **other stressors, another mental disorder,** insufficient sexual stimulation)

Coding Notes

Specify:

> **{Lifelong}{Acquired}**
> **{Generalized}{Situational}**

Specify severity, based on amount of distress: **{Mild}{Moderate}{Severe}**

Ernestine Paget

"She hardly ever wants to do it," James Paget tells their marriage therapist.

"That's not quite accurate," Ernestine responds. "The truth is, I never want to do it. It's disgusting."

When they got married 3 years earlier, Ernestine had been uninterested in sex, though receptive to its possibilities. "It seemed to mean a lot to him, so I put up with it," she explains. "But he's never satisfied. No matter how often we make love, a few days later there he is, wanting more. It gets old fast."

"It is the usual expectation," her husband remarks dryly, "and it's not my fault how she was brought up."

In Ernestine's family, sex was never discussed, and nudity wasn't allowed. Ernestine could never remember having much curiosity about sex, let alone interest. She was an only child. "I assume her parents only did it once," James offers.

For the first few months, Ernestine would simply lie still and think about other things, enduring what was for her a basically boring activity because it was important to her new husband. Her gynecologist assured her that, as far as her anatomy and hormones were concerned, she was completely normal. Unless she was figuring out whether it was time to start taking her new prescription of birth control pills, she never thought about sex.

"God knows, I never dream about it," Ernestine says. "Maybe if he'd led up to it more, it would have helped. His idea of foreplay is half an hour of *The Late Show* and a slap on the butt." Once, she tried to explain this to James, but he only called her frigid. That was the last word they'd exchanged on the subject.

Now James pretty much ignores Ernestine. She undresses in the closet; they sleep on the extreme edges of their king-sized mattress. She doesn't know where he is getting his sex these days, but it isn't at home and she says she doesn't care.

"At least he doesn't have to worry that I'll try to cut it off, like that Bobbitt woman," Ernestine says. "I don't even like to look at it, let alone touch it with a 10-inch knife."

Evaluation of Ernestine Paget

Ernestine's low sex interest is shown not just by absent interest (criterion A1); she denies even fantasizing (A2) about what is for her a boring activity (A4). This is an important point: Some patients may reject the idea of sex with a partner while still harboring an abstract interest in sex or in sex with some hypothetical person. When Ernestine began her sexual life with her husband 3 years earlier (B), she was merely uninterested. Only with experience did she became intolerant of the very idea of sexual contact, from which we can infer criterion A3. (Three of the six criterion A requirements for FSIAD must be met.) Although she can with equanimity face the prospect of no sex, her husband cannot, and that disparity is causing distress for them both; criterion C is thus satisfied, if by a somewhat circuitous route.

Ernestine's clinician needs to ascertain that she has no other major disorder—such as major depressive disorder, somatic symptom disorder, or obsessive–compulsive disorder—that could explain her antipathy to sex (D). In the presence of any of these, she'd receive the additional diagnosis of FSIAD only if her sexual symptoms persist once the other pathology has been eliminated. Similar arguments would hold for substance use or another medical condition.

The Pagets are also having severe problems with other aspects of their marriage—enough to warrant mention as a spousal relationship Z code. Her abhorrence of sexual contact could also meet the criteria for specific phobia; under the circumstances, however, no such additional diagnosis is necessary.

Ernestine's condition appears to have lasted throughout her sexual life. With our current information, we couldn't determine whether her disorder was generalized or situational. Although we suspect that something in her upbringing may lie at its roots, in DSM-5-TR we have no way to code this putative etiology. With a current GAF score of 61, her diagnosis would be as follows:

F52.22	Female sexual interest/arousal disorder, lifelong, severe
Z63.0	Relationship distress with husband (emotional withdrawal)

Disorders of female sexual arousal and orgasm are often highly correlated. Among health care clinicians, you may encounter less than slavish adherence to the criteria used for these disorders.

F52.6 Genito-Pelvic Pain/Penetration Disorder

Genito-pelvic pain/penetration disorder (GPD), which was new in DSM-5, subsumes the older categories of dyspareunia and vaginismus; these two were combined because they couldn't be reliably differentiated. The old terms will probably retain some currency to describe pelvic pain associated with sex.

Some women experience marked discomfort when attempting to have sexual intercourse. The pain may be experienced as a cramping contraction of the vaginal muscles (vaginismus) that may be described as an ache, a twinge, or a sharp pain. Anxiety can produce tension in the pelvic floor, with resulting pain severe enough to prevent consummation of a relationship—sometimes for years. Soon, anxiety comes to replace sexual enjoyment. Some patients can't even use a tampon; a vaginal exam may require anesthesia.

Up to a quarter of women in the United States will experience recurring pain with intercourse, and at one time or another a robust (though ultimately unknown) percentage of these may fulfill GPD criteria. Infections, scars, and pelvic inflammatory disease have also been reported as causes. Don't diagnose GPD when pain is only a symptom of another medical condition or is due to substance misuse.

Two examples of this somewhat clumsily named condition follow.

Essential Features of **Genito-Pelvic Pain/Penetration Disorder**

A patient has major, repeated pain or other problems with efforts at vaginal intercourse; she may experience anxiety, fear, or pelvic muscle tension.

The Fine Print

The D's: • Duration (6+ months) • Distress to the patient • Differential diagnosis (**substance use** or **physical disorders, relationship problems** or **other stressors,** somatic symptom disorders, inadequate sexual stimulation)

Coding Notes

Note that generalized and specialized specifiers do not apply to patients with GPD.

Specify: **{Lifelong}{Acquired}**

Specify severity, based on amount of distress: **{Mild}{Moderate}{Severe}**

Mildred Frank

Mildred Frank and her twin sister, Maxine Whalen (see next vignette), have been having problems with pain during intercourse. Their symptoms are different and quite personal, but they have always discussed everything with each other. Now they've made the joint decision to seek help. The gynecologist has referred them both to the mental health clinic.

"It's sort of a burning," is how Mildred describes her difficulty. "When it's bad, it feels like your hands do if you're sliding down a rope. It's awful! Even if I use Vaseline, it still bothers me."

The referral letter notes that she's had surgery for a prolapsed uterus but is otherwise healthy. "I could have told you that," she says. "I've hardly ever been to a doctor, except to have my babies."

On close questioning, Mildred admits that the pain doesn't occur often. But during the past year or two she has always been afraid it will hurt, and that invariably makes her tense up when having intercourse with her husband. She's had some vaginal infections, but these have been largely under control during the last few months; the gynecologist doesn't think that they cause the pain she complains of. The letter also notes that her physical exam had been completed easily, with no evidence of vaginal spasm.

"Maybe I do overreact," she says. "At least that's what my husband tells me. He says I'm too excitable, that I should just relax."

Evaluation of Mildred Frank

Many women have sporadic pain with intercourse, in which case the diagnosis of GPD is usually not warranted. But for a couple of years (criterion B) Mildred has experienced pain, tensing, and fear; each is enough to qualify her for the form of GPD once known as dyspareunia (A2, A4, A3). Her distress is manifest (C); as is so often the case, our problem is to rule out other causes.

Mildred describes herself as otherwise healthy, and her gynecologist makes no mention of other medical problems. Although Mildred has had some vaginal infections, the doctor feels that they cannot completely account for her pain. Her clinician would have to determine that there was no substance-induced disorder, though this seems unlikely. Sexual dysfunctions can be expected with a number of mental conditions (anxiety, mood, and psychotic disorders), but her history supports none of these as a possible cause. Painful intercourse famously occurs in patients with somatic symptom disorder, but Mildred claims that she is otherwise healthy, which greatly reduces the likelihood of this diagnosis. All of the foregoing factors should lay to rest our concern about other causes (D).

Although Mildred's pain with intercourse was acquired fairly recently and only occurs occasionally, it did cause her to seek treatment. She has had no partners other than her husband, though nothing in the vignette suggests that she would have fared better with someone else. Although insufficient symptoms were noted to warrant a personality disorder, her clinician should note in the chart any behaviors that seem to justify further investigation. I'd give her GAF score as 71.

F52.6   Genito-pelvic pain/penetration disorder, acquired, mild to moderate

---

In men, the symptom of painful intercourse is rare and almost always associated with physical illness, such as Peyronie's disease (an abnormal bend in an erect penis), prostatitis, or infections such as gonorrhea and herpes. It can cause an inability to complete penetration during sex—or fear that pain will occur. However, at least one study has reported that, contrary to expectation, men with a pelvic pain syndrome experience minimal impact on their interpersonal relationships. Such a situation would obviate a diagnosis of GPD, even were DSM-5-TR disposed to allow it in a man.

Maxine Whalen

Both Maxine Whalen and her twin sister, Mildred Frank, have been having problems with pain during intercourse. As noted above, they made a joint decision to seek help. Finding no anatomical causes for either of them, the gynecologist referred both to the mental health clinic.

Maxine isn't married yet, and she doesn't think she wants to be. "It's not that I don't get horny," she explains. "And I love foreplay. I could do it all night. But every time a man has tried to enter me, something inside clamps down like a trap. I couldn't even get a pencil inside, let alone a penis. I can't even use a tampon."

Maxine relieves her frustration by masturbating, which reliably produces a climax. Oral sex has also worked. "Not many men are likely to be satisfied with that for long," she remarks. "I feel like a freak."

The spasms that contract Maxine's vaginal muscles produce severe, cramping pain. They are so extreme that her gynecologist must use general anesthesia to insert the speculum. The exam reveals no physical abnormalities.

On her second visit, Maxine remembers something that Mildred apparently doesn't know. When the girls were 4, they had been molested in some way. Even Maxine isn't sure exactly what happened. She only knows that some man—she thinks it might be the Uncle Max for whom she is named—had taken the girls to a tavern, stood them on the bar, and encouraged the other patrons to "play" with them.

Evaluation of Maxine Whalen

Maxine's lifelong (criterion B) history of severe pain and obstructed penetration (A1, A2—only one required) suggests the diagnosis. The fact that the spasm is reproduced by the attempted introduction of the gynecologist's speculum is diagnostic. Unless a patient is both unattached and content to refrain from intercourse, it is axiomatic that vaginal spasms will produce distress or interpersonal difficulty (C).

Maxine's history does not indicate that there has ever been a time since she became sexually active when she was free of vaginal spasm (B); therefore, we'll call it lifelong. Her gynecologist found no physical cause (no surprise there because none are usually reported—D). I'd peg her GAF score at about 65.

In DSM-IV, Maxine's diagnosis would have been vaginismus. In DSM-5-TR, it will be:

F52.6   Genito-pelvic pain/penetration disorder, lifelong, generalized, severe

F52.31 Female Orgasmic Disorder

Achieving climax is a problem for a lot of women, though studies have been persistently inconsistent as to just what this means. Perhaps 30% of women report significant difficulties; 10% never learn the trick. A few physical illnesses, including hypothyroidism, diabetes, and structural damage to the vagina, can contribute to the condition; if judged to be exclusively the cause, they foreclose the diagnosis of female orgasmic disorder (FOD). Orgasm can also be inhibited by medications such as antihypertensives, central nervous system stimulants, tricyclic antidepressants, and monoamine oxidase inhibitors. Possible psychological factors include fear of pregnancy, hostility of the patient toward her partner, and general guilt feelings about sex. Age, previous sexual experience, and the adequacy of foreplay must also be considered in diagnosing FOD. A woman who does not achieve orgasm with vaginal intercourse but does with clitoral stimulation would not be given this diagnosis.

Once learned, the ability to achieve orgasm persists, often improving throughout life. But women just don't complain of having premature orgasms the way men do. Although it occurs (shown by surveys), it often doesn't pose a problem. And many women are able to enjoy sex without experiencing climax frequently. FOD is often comorbid with other sexual dysfunctions, especially female sexual interest/arousal disorder.

Essential Features of **Female Orgasmic Disorder**

A woman is troubled by orgasms that are nearly always too slow, too weak, too rare.

The Fine Print

The D's: • Duration (6+ months) • Distress to the patient • Differential diagnosis (**substance use** and **physical disorders, relationship problems, another mental disorder**)

Coding Notes

Specify:

> **{Lifelong}{Acquired}**
> **{Generalized}{Situational}**
>> Or

> **Never experienced an orgasm under any situation**

Specify severity, based on amount of distress: **{Mild}{Moderate}{Severe}**

Rachel Atkins

"I don't think anyone has quite the understanding of frustrating that I do," Rachel Atkins says to her gynecologist.

Her early history was "a sociological nightmare." Her mother was a 16-year-old high school dropout who had gone on to a lifetime of alcoholism and serial marriages. Beginning when Rachel was in middle school, a series of stepfathers had molested her until, when *she* was 16, she'd bolted—into sex work.

"How ironic is that, escaping from abusive sex by going on the game?" she asks. But she was lucky enough to avoid AIDS and, when she was 22, smart enough to jump at a chance at college, financed by a conscience-stricken former client.

As a call girl, Rachel experienced hundreds of men. "It wasn't as bad as you might think," she explains. "I could pick my own johns, and some of them I rather liked—not at all like Mom's assortment of rats." One possible victim of her experiences was her orgasm, which has always been missing in action. "I always figured it'd be there when I really wanted it. Only it never was."

Now a university graduate solidly planted in the academic world (she teaches anthropology at a college in her community), Rachel is nearing 30 and has a boyfriend who wants to marry her. "He knows all about my past, and he's OK with it. But he'd like me to come when we have sex. I think it would reassure him that he's different from all those others. I desperately want to please him, but there's just something missing in me. It's beyond distressing!"

Rachel loves the closeness she feels with Henry, and she lubricates well. "But I can never quite get over the top. It's like when you think you're going to sneeze, you know? And instead, it just dissolves into nothing?" She's tried mood music, alcohol, marijuana, erotic literature, and clitoral stimulation. "But I could be digging pottery shards, for all the good any of it does."

Apart from teenage experimentation and the brief therapeutic flirtation with white wine and marijuana, Rachel has used no drugs. Her general health is excellent, she says.

"I promised Henry I'd always be truthful with him, and I intend to keep that promise. So, I refuse to fake it. I could, though—I've sure had the practice!"

Just why females have orgasms isn't known. Of course, the reason for the male counterpart is obvious: Its absence would leave us bereft of males *and* females. One of the more popular theories is that it developed in parallel with the male orgasm, and there's just been no evolutionary pressure for it to go away. The author of *that* theory must have been a guy.

Discussion of Rachel Atkins

Rachel's problem isn't lack of interest in sex—she looks forward to it with her boyfriend, and she lubricates normally with foreplay. Her difficulty is solely her inability to climax—ever (criterion B). If she had orgasms occasionally, or if she climaxed only with masturbation, she could still receive this diagnosis, according to DSM-5-TR criterion A1; low intensity of orgasm would also qualify (A2). There is no evidence that other medical or mental conditions or substance use contribute in the slightest (D). What she has in abundance is distress (C).

Because she's never experienced a climax, we should add that verbiage to her diagnosis (thereby obviating the other possible specifiers). Because of her overall excellent adjustment, I'd rate her GAF score as very high (95). I would call the severity of her FOD as only moderate, largely because of her composure and well-balanced approach to life. Her FOD troubles her, but it doesn't appear overwhelming.

F52.31   Female orgasmic disorder, never experienced an orgasm under any situation, moderate

Substance/Medication-Induced Sexual Dysfunction

As with physical illness, a variety of psychoactive substances can affect the sexual abilities of men and women. Note that you would substitute the diagnosis of substance/medication-induced sexual dysfunction for a specific substance intoxication diagnosis only when the patient's problems in that area exceed those you would expect in the usual course of substance intoxication.

On average, perhaps half of patients taking antipsychotic and antidepressant drugs will report sexual side effects, though these will not always reach the level of clinical importance. Users of street drugs often have sexual side effects; if they complain less, perhaps they value their drug of choice more highly than sex.

The vast number of possible expressions has persuaded me not to include a vignette for this section.

Essential Features of **Substance/Medication-Induced Sexual Dysfunction**

Substance use appears to have caused clinically important sexual dysfunction.

For evidence concerning substance-related causation, see sidebar (p. 95).

The Fine Print

The D's: • Distress to the patient • Differential diagnosis (physical disorders, **delirium,** other sexual disorders)

Use this diagnosis instead of substance intoxication or withdrawal only when sexual dysfunction symptoms are predominant and require clinical care.

Coding Notes

When writing down the diagnosis, use the exact substance in the title: For example, alcohol-induced sexual dysfunction.

For coding in ICD-10, refer to Table 15.2 (p. 475).

Specify if:

> **With onset during {intoxication}{withdrawal}.** This gets tacked on at the end of your string of words.
> **With onset after medication use.** You could alternatively use this if symptoms develop when medication is started, changed, or stopped.

Specify severity:

> **Mild.** Dysfunction in 25–50% of sexual encounters.
> **Moderate.** 50–75% of encounters.
> **Severe.** 75% or more.

F52.8 Other Specified Sexual Dysfunction

F52.9 Unspecified Sexual Dysfunction

Use one or the other of these categories for patients whose sexual dysfunctions don't qualify for any of the specific sets of criteria spelled out above. Such conditions would include those for whom you conclude that there is a sexual problem, but one of the following obtains:

Atypical symptoms. The symptoms are mixed, atypical, or below threshold for a defined sexual disorder.

Uncertain cause. Insufficient information.

As usual, the *other specified* designation should be used in cases where you choose to state the reasons for not assigning one of the other diagnoses described in this chapter; use *unspecified* when you do not so choose.

CHAPTER 13

Gender Dysphoria

Although this is one of the shortest chapters in the book (containing just a single set of Essential Features), its evolution from one edition to the next demonstrates something important: the change in how we understand this vital aspect of our humanity.

Quick Guide to Gender Dysphoria

Primary Gender Dysphoria

Gender dysphoria in adolescents or adults. Patients have discomfort or distress because their psychological sense of their gender (gender identity) differs from their sex assigned at birth. Some request gender-affirming hormonal or surgical interventions to relieve this discomfort (p. 380).

Gender dysphoria in children. Children as young as 3 or 4 years can feel distress that their own sense of their gender differs from their sex assigned at birth. GD in children is not treated medically before puberty (p. 382).

Other specified, or unspecified, gender dysphoria. Use one of these categories for gender dysphoria symptoms that do not meet full diagnostic criteria (p. 385).

Other Causes of Gender Dissatisfaction or Behavior

Schizophrenia. Some patients with schizophrenia will express the delusion of being another gender (p. 63).

Transvestic disorder. These people have sexual urges related to cross-dressing, but do not experience themselves as the other gender (p. 599).

Introduction

Let's start by defining our terms. As they say on the phone: Our options have changed, so please listen carefully.

Sex, the noun, refers to male and female external genitalia, hormones, chromosomes that contribute to our ability to reproduce—as well as the activities involving sex and associated urges.

Gender is the term used (increasingly over the past 50 years) to indicate the social and cultural roles we inhabit, as distinguished from the biological construct of sex.

Gender dysphoria indicates the negative feelings that occur when a person's assigned gender does not track with the person's experienced gender identity. The language underscores the idea that this is not a disorder; rather, it is the logical outcome of a mismatch of assigned and experienced genders.

Assigned gender is the label, based on appearance of external genitalia, usually given at birth.

Experienced gender replaces "desired gender."

Individual assigned female/male at birth replaces "natal female/male."

Gender-affirming medical procedure is what we now use where we formerly said "cross-sex medical procedure."

F64.0 Gender Dysphoria in Adolescents and Adults

"Push, Mama—one last push!" That command rings out daily across delivery floors and in birthing centers everywhere. Finally, someone exclaims, "Oh! A beautiful baby girl!" Well, of course it's a girl! The joyful parents have known that for months and so has their entire social circle, ever since the gender reveal party.

But not so fast! There could yet be a surprise, perhaps years down the road when the parents discover their "daughter" is actually their son. Gender nonconformity itself is not a mental disorder, but many transgender individuals experience gender dysphoria (GD)—they feel intensely uncomfortable with their assigned gender. They may feel distressed by their primary or secondary sex characteristics. They wish to dress, act, and be treated as members of the other gender (or, for nonbinary people, some combination of both, or something else, including having no gender at all).

Many people don't feel they fit into either gender and may not fulfill the rather demanding criteria for gender dysphoria. These folks are increasingly referred to, and refer to themselves, as nonbinary individuals. You may encounter individuals who refer to themselves as *genderqueer, agender,* or *dual gender. Genderfluid* persons wish to retain a degree of flexibility about their gender identity. I especially like *gender expansive,* which suggests a broad gender spectrum without setting an artificial limit; of course, it isn't my preference that's important. Each term indicates a way of expressing who one is without buying in to the traditional male/female dichotomy. Many but not all nonbinary people also identify as transgender.

The perhaps 1.2 million individuals (in the United States) who identify as nonbinary don't have a set of predictable pronouns they use. Some alternate traditional male/female pronouns; others prefer they/their/them; some use *ze, xe,* or *hir.* The practical approach for the clinician (as for everyone else): Use the pronouns requested by each individual. If unsure, you can ask.

There is no single pathway for gender transition. Social transition may consist of a new name, pronouns, and clothing style. Some transgender individuals undergo hormone therapy to alter secondary sex characteristics, such as voice, breast size, or bodily appearance. Various forms of surgical interventions are also available, but are by no means universal. Most transgender individuals express satisfaction with affirming treatments and live contentedly in their experienced gender.

The outdated term *transsexualism* assumes that all patients with GD desire surgical sex reassignment measures, and is no longer in widespread use. GD is one of the more recently described disorders in DSM-5-TR. Until the 1950s, clinicians did not even recognize the existence of people with GD. It was through the widespread publicity that occurred in 1952, when Christine Jorgensen underwent surgery in Denmark to emerge as a woman, that this condition became generally acknowledged. Even now, GD is pretty infrequent (around 1 in 10,000 for people assigned male and perhaps one-third that for those assigned female). It begins in early childhood (typically, preschool) and appears to be chronic. Causation isn't known for sure. However, there is evidence to support at least a weak genetic component.

Gender identity is not the same thing as sexual orientation. People who are transgender have a variety of sexual orientations, just like people who are cisgender (sex assigned at birth aligns with gender identity).

Posttransition Specifier

The posttransition specifier indicates that the patient now lives exclusively as a person of the experienced gender and has undergone (or is undergoing) one or more gender-affirming medical procedures. These include regimens such as regular cross-sex hormone treatments and reassignment surgery to the experienced gender. Surgery entails orchiectomy, penectomy, and vaginoplasty in a genetic male, mastectomy and phalloplasty in a genetic female.

F64.2 Gender Dysphoria in Children

In the general population, a small percentage of children assigned male at birth (1–2%)—and a smaller still percentage of those assigned female at birth—identify as the other or an alternative gender. It's mainly the former who are ever referred for clinical evaluation, probably because parents worry more about an effeminate son than about a tomboy daughter. Although cross-gender behaviors often begin by age 3, the typical child isn't referred until years later.

Exactly what behaviors are we talking about? From a very young age, these children know they are different. Boys with GD will assume a female role in play and prefer playing with dolls, cross-dressing, and especially associating with a peer group of girls. Girls with GD take the male role in games and strongly reject female activities such as playing with dolls. Of course, all such children, boys especially, risk teasing, bullying, and other forms of peer and family rejection. The 2011 book *Transition*, which describes the childhood struggle with his own gender identity, recounts Chaz Bono's anguish when the development of breasts and onset of menses during puberty caused both physical and emotional torment. The risk of suicide is high in people with GD, especially when they do not have access to gender-affirming treatment.

Of course, GD isn't the only possible explanation for "different" behavior: some boys love beautiful things or just don't like sports or rough games, and some girls, perceiving social advantages in being male, prefer boys' clothing. And, sure enough, follow-up studies of children who have been clinically referred for GD behavior find that, by their late teenage years, most will not qualify for a formal GD diagnosis. On average, those who still are affected (*persisters*, as they are sometimes termed) had as children a greater degree of GD. Girls are somewhat more likely than boys to remain dysphoric.

Prevalence of GD in the general population is probably 1 in 1,000 or less, but ascertainment is often uncertain—the true figure could be higher. It is more common for boys with GD to grow up to become gay men than continue to have GD; a minority become heterosexual as adults; perhaps a few have GD (though the studies vary tremendously as regards percentage). The rate of persisters among girls with GD is higher, but still well under 50%. Ultimate diagnosis in children or adolescents may require prolonged evaluation.

Essential Features of Gender Dysphoria

In Adolescents or Adults

There is a marked disparity between assigned gender and what the patient experiences as a sense of self. This can be expressed as a rejection of one's own sex characteristics or to have those of the other gender. The patient might express the powerful desire to belong to another gender and to be treated as such. Some patients strongly believe that their emotions and responses are typical of another gender.

In Children

There is a marked disparity between assigned gender and what the patient experiences as a sense of self. So, in their powerful longing to be the opposite or an alternative gender, kids may insist that's what they *are*; they prefer clothing, toys, games, playmates, and fantasy roles typical of the other gender while rejecting those typical of their assigned gender. They may hate their own genitalia and powerfully desire the primary and secondary sex features they do not have or will not have without intervention.

Note that in children the number of criteria required (six out of eight) is far greater than for adults (two of six); this is to protect young people who have not yet fully matured.

The Fine Print

The D's: • Duration (6+ months, regardless of age) • Distress or disability (work/educational, social, or personal impairment) • Differential diagnosis (substance use and physical disorders, psychotic disorders, autism spectrum disorder, body dysmorphic disorder, and [in adolescents/adults] transvestic disorder)

Coding Notes

Specify if:

> **With a disorder of sex development** (and code the actual congenital developmental disorder).
>
> **Posttransition** (for adolescents/adults). The patient is living in the experienced gender and has had (or will soon have) at least one gender-affirming surgical procedure or medical treatment (such as a hormone regimen).

The posttransition specifier addresses the fact that patients who have undergone procedures to achieve their experienced gender will no longer meet the criteria for GD; yet they continue to pursue psychotherapy, hormonal treatment, or other remedies for the condition with which they were once diagnosed.

Billie Worth

"I just want to get rid of it. All of it." For the third time in a day, Billie Worth makes explicit this feeling. Neither depressed nor melodramatic, it is a quiet statement of the facts. An early memory is of watching an actress on TV. When she walked, her hand brushed against her skirt, making it appear to dance. Assigned male at birth, toddler

Billie had tried to imitate that walk, to the delight and applause of her mother. For years Billie's father had been imprisoned for forgery.

At age 6, Billie discovered that playing cap pistols and spaceships with boys produced violent headaches. A Barbie doll rescued from a dumpster was a favorite toy, and whenever possible, playmates were chosen from neighborhood girls her age. If they played house, Billie would insist that one of *them* be the dad.

When Billie was a tiny baby, 6-year-old sister Marsha died of meningitis. Afterward, their mother kept Marsha's room just as it had been before she died. Some of Billie's happiest childhood afternoons were spent putting on Marsha's dresses and sitting on Marsha's bed with Barbie. Sometimes, wishing to be a girl, Billie would pretend to be Marsha. Long after her feet had grown too big, she continued to wedge them into Marsha's black patent leather shoes.

As an early teenager, she realized that in fact she *was* a girl. "It suddenly struck me that the only masculine thing about me was these revolting things between my legs," Billie tells one of the clinicians. Claiming to have chronic asthma, she persuaded a physician to excuse her from gym class throughout her 4 years of high school. Although she was a good swimmer, abhorrence of the locker room prevented trying out for the team. Elective courses included shorthand and home economics (four semesters of each). Billie did join the science society, the least gendered club the school sponsored, and one year entered a project in the science fair on using various yeasts to bake bread.

At age 16, Billie bought a bra and panties with money earned babysitting. The first time she put them on, some of the tension that had been present for so long seemed to drain away. Although lingerie was sometimes covertly worn to school, cross-dressing in earnest didn't begin until the start of college. Living off campus, Billie had the privacy in which to experiment with skirts, blouses, and makeup. A sympathetic physician provided estrogens, and as a third-year student, Billie changed the spelling of her name and began to live publicly as a woman.

Two years out of college, Billie requested sex reassignment surgery. By this time, she had had several gay male lovers—unsatisfying experiences, because she did not consider herself to be homosexual. "I'm not a gay man; I feel that I'm a straight woman." By now, thanks to hormones, she had small though well-developed breasts; penis and testicles "just get in the way." To be rid of them, she tells the examining clinician, she would even have the job done in Mexico.

Evaluation of Billie Worth

Billie's early realization of somehow not fitting in with the boys is typical of children with GD. Demonstrating this are several sorts of behaviors, which constitute the principal childhood indicators of this disorder: Pretending to be Marsha, wishing to be a girl (gender dysphoria in children criterion A1); wearing Marsha's dress and shoes (A2). Preferring a cross-gender role, Billie assigned girls to play the dad (A3). Rejection of boys' games (A6), preferring girls' play (A4), and choosing girls to play with (A5) complete the qualifying symptoms.

As an adult, Billie expressed a desire to be a woman (adult criterion A4) and to be rid of male genitalia (A2), a wish to have breasts and a vagina (A3), and the conviction of having the emotions and desires of a straight woman (A6). Only two of these criteria are needed to fulfill the DSM-5-TR definition.

Billie's full realization of being born the wrong sex came in adolescence, ushering in a progression—first dressing as a female, then living as a female and taking hormones—that culminated in the request for sex reassignment surgery. Although the vignette does not expressly state that Billie had no intersex condition, neither does it contain any information suggesting one. (Note that DSM-5-TR will allow patients with a disorder of sex development to be diagnosed with GD. Such a person would receive an additional specifier.) Throughout childhood, adolescence, and into adult life, Billie's distress was way beyond "clinical significance."

The differential diagnosis of GD includes schizophrenia, in which some patients may have delusions of being the opposite gender. Billie shows no evidence of delusions, hallucinations, or any other typical symptoms of a psychotic disorder. The absence of sexual excitement as a reaction to cross-dressing rules out transvestic disorder, though some patients with GD initially have this paraphilia. As you might expect, anxiety and mood disorders are also commonly associated features. Use of substances (alcohol and/or street drugs) may also be a factor, especially in GD patients assigned female.

Billie's diagnosis at the time of evaluation (GAF score of 71) would read as follows:

F64.0   Gender dysphoria in an adult

Interviewed as a child, Billie would have fully met even the rather restrictive DSM-5-TR criteria for children:

F64.2   Gender dysphoria in children

F64.8 Other Specified Gender Dysphoria

Here you could include a patient who has met GD criteria for less than the 6-month minimum.

F64.9 Unspecified Gender Dysphoria

Use unspecified GD for cases of GD symptoms that do not meet full diagnostic criteria and about which you do not wish to be more specific.

CHAPTER 14

Disruptive, Impulse-Control, and Conduct Disorders

The disorders included here comprise emotions and behaviors that cause conflict with other people—often, violating their rights.

Quick Guide to the Disruptive, Impulse-Control, and Conduct Disorders

Primary Disruptive, Impulse-Control, and Conduct Disorders

Conduct disorder. A child patient persistently violates rules or the rights of others (p. 389).

Conduct disorder, with limited prosocial emotions. Use this specifier for child patients whose disordered conduct is callous and disruptive, showing no remorse and no regard for the feelings of others (p. 391).

Oppositional defiant disorder. Multiple examples of negativistic behavior persist for at least 6 months (p. 388).

Intermittent explosive disorder. With no other evident pathology (psychological or general medical), these people have episodes during which they act out aggressively. As a result, they physically harm others or destroy property (p. 392).

Kleptomania. An irresistible urge to steal things they don't need causes these people to do so repeatedly. The phrase "tension and release" characterizes this behavior (p. 398).

Pyromania. People who set fires feel tension and release regarding the behavior of starting fires (p. 395).

Antisocial personality disorder. The irresponsible, often criminal behavior of people with antisocial personality disorder (ASPD) begins in childhood or early adolescence with truancy, running away, cruelty, fighting, destructiveness, lying, and theft. As adults, in addition to criminality they may default on their debts and without remorse engage in irresponsible, reckless, or impulsive behavior. DSM-5-TR lists ASPD in this chapter, though it gives the detailed symptoms with those of the other personality disorders (p. 557).

Other specified, or unspecified, disruptive, impulse-control, and conduct disorder. Use one of these categories for disturbances of conduct or oppositional behaviors that do not meet the criteria for other disorders covered in this group (p. 400).

Other Disorders Associated with Disruptive or Impulsive Behavior

Trichotillomania (hair-pulling disorder). Pulling hair from various parts of the body is often accompanied by feelings of "tension and release" (p. 209).

Paraphilic disorders. Some people (nearly all are males) have recurrent sexual urges involving a variety of behaviors that are objectionable to others. They may act upon these urges to obtain pleasure (p. 580).

Substance-related disorders. There is often an impulsive component to the misuse of various substances (p. 404).

Bipolar I disorder. Patients in an acute manic episode may steal, gamble, act out violently, and engage in other socially undesirable behaviors (p. 126).

Schizophrenia. In response to hallucinations or delusions, these patients may impulsively engage in a variety of illegal or otherwise ill-advised behaviors (p. 63).

Disruptive mood dysregulation disorder. The mood of a child with this disorder is persistently negative between frequent, severe explosions of temper (p. 149).

Child or adolescent antisocial behavior. The code Z72.810 can be useful when antisocial behavior in a young person cannot be ascribed to a mental disorder such as oppositional defiant disorder or conduct disorder (p. 611).

Adult antisocial behavior. Z72.811 is used to describe activities by an adult that are illegal, but do not occur in the context of mental disorder (p. 611).

Introduction

This chapter considers conditions that in other professions might elicit a value judgment of "bad behavior." Fortunately, we do not have to judge them; rather, we can study them to understand why they occur and how we can ameliorate them.

These disorders entail problems with the regulation of behavior and emotions. The behaviors in question may occur on the spur of the moment, or they may be planned; some are accompanied by an effort to resist authority. The acts themselves are often illegal, with consequent injury to the perpetrator or to others.

Each disorder in its own way brings the patient into conflict with social norms. All typically start in childhood or adolescence; in each, males predominate. Some patients may show a progression—for instance, from oppositional defiant disorder (ODD) to conduct disorder (CD) to antisocial personality disorder (ASPD). However, we should not draw the mistaken conclusion that taking one step on the pathway means ultimate arrival at the end of the trail. In fact, most patients with ODD do not go on to develop CD, just as most patients with CD do not progress to ASPD. Still, an important minority of patients do follow that developmental arc.

I usually put child diagnoses toward the end of each chapter. Here I'm going to break my rule, to underscore the (occasional) march from one disorder to the next. Note that it is rare for ODD or CD to manifest for the first time in an adult.

F91.3 Oppositional Defiant Disorder

ODD ushers in a triad of disorders spanning a spectrum of behavior from resistance that is barely outside the norm to acts that are frankly execrable. ODD itself can be relatively mild, with symptoms of negativism and defiance that seem to grow out of any child's normal quest for independence. On the one hand, they are distinguished from ordinary opposition by severity and duration; on the other, they are distinguished from the more problematic CD by the fact that children with ODD don't violate the basic rights of others or age-appropriate societal rules.

The symptoms of ODD first show up around age 3 or 4; diagnosis is typically made within the next few years. Younger children will show oppositional behavior almost every day, whereas for older children, the frequency tends to decline. The effects are worst at home, though relationships with teachers and peers can also be affected. Younger age and more severe symptoms at onset predict a worse outcome. DSM-5-TR does caution us to consider possible modifying factors such as developmental age, culture, and gender; it notes that symptomatic behavior must take place in the context of people other than siblings.

Though ODD runs in families, genetic relationships are not certain. Some authorities attribute ODD to discipline that is harsh or inconsistent, others to imitation of parental behavior. Low socioeconomic status may contribute through the stress of poverty.

Along with CD, ODD is among the most common reasons for referral of a child to mental health professionals. It affects about 3% of all children (boys predominate about 3:2). When it occurs in girls, its expression may be at once more verbal and less obvious; predictions made from its diagnosis may be less robust than for boys.

Over half of those who initially meet ODD criteria will not do so several years later. However, CD will develop later in about a third of patients, especially those whose symptoms begin early and coexist with attention-deficit/hyperactivity disorder; these diagnoses are strongly comorbid. Perhaps 10% will eventually be diagnosed with ASPD. The irritable mood symptoms of ODD predict later anxiety and depression, whereas defiance symptoms point toward CD.

ODD can be diagnosed in an adult, and sometimes it is: It has been reported in 12–50% of adults with ADHD. However, in adults the symptoms of ODD may be obscured by other disorders, or they may appear to constitute a personality disorder.

Essential Features of **Oppositional Defiant Disorder**

Persons with ODD are often angry and irritable, tending toward touchiness and hair-trigger temper. They will disobey authority figures or argue with them, and they may refuse to cooperate or follow rules—if only to annoy. They may accuse others of their own misdeeds; some appear malicious.

If criteria are also met for disruptive mood dysregulation disorder, only diagnose it—not ODD.

The Fine Print

The D's: • Duration and demographics (several symptoms within 6+ months—more or less daily for age 5 and under; at least weekly for older patients) • Distress (patient or others) or disability (educational/work, social, or personal impairment) • Differential diagnosis (**substance use disorders,** ADHD, conduct disorder, **psychotic** or **mood disorders, disruptive mood dysregulation disorder,** intermittent explosive disorder, intellectual developmental disorder, language disorder, adjustment disorder, PTSD, social anxiety disorder, ordinary variability in childhood growth and development)

Coding Notes

Specify severity:

Mild. Symptoms occur in only 1 location (home, school, work, with friends).
Moderate. Some symptoms in 2+ locations.
Severe. Symptoms in 3+ locations.

Conduct Disorder

From as early as 2 years of age, boys usually display more aggressive behavior than do girls. Even beyond this, however, aggressive breaking of rules dominates the behavior of a substantial minority of children. For some, the symptoms of CD may represent only an extreme expression of typical efforts to differentiate themselves from their parents. But note that most CD symptoms, whether they occur in the juvenile years or later, are quite serious and can lead to arrest and other legal consequences. CD is defined in part by the degree to which a child's family, social, or scholastic life becomes affected by such behavior. That can happen as early as age 5 or 6. And, as the child gets older and the disorder progresses, symptoms tend to become more extreme.

DSM-5-TR's 15 listed behaviors constitute four categories: (1) aggression, (2) destruction, (3) lying and theft, and (4) rule violation. Just 3 of the 15 symptoms suffice for diagnosis (they need not be spread across multiple categories). Using these criteria, perhaps 4% of children in the general population will score positive for CD, with rates substantially higher for boys than for girls. Imputed causes include the environment (large families, neglect, abuse) and heredity (substance use, CD, ADHD, psychosis).

About 80% of children diagnosed as having CD have previously had symptoms of ODD. (In fact, some writers question whether ODD and CD are two disorders or one.) But what we really want to know is this: To what degree will such behavior persist into adolescence and beyond?

Children who are highly aggressive by age 7 or 8 are at risk for a serious and constant antisocial/aggressive lifestyle. They are three times as likely as other children to have police records as adults. Indeed, the age of onset—before age 10 years versus at or after—confers enough predictive power that we are encouraged to state it as a specifier. Those with earlier onset (mostly boys) are more likely to be aggressive; half of them will progress to a diagnosis of ASPD. (Later onset predicts an outcome less dire; having especially harmful symptoms foretells a worse outcome.) Girls with early-onset CD are less likely than boys to develop ASPD; rather, they may develop somatic symptom disorder, suicidal behavior, social and occupational problems, or other emotional disorders.

What about CD in adults? As with ODD, the diagnosis is at least theoretically possible, but it is far more likely that an adult will have some other disorder that will obscure the CD symptoms.

The early histories of Milo Tark (p. 559) and Dudley Langenegger (p. 446) illustrate some of the symptoms of CD.

Essential Features of **Conduct Disorder**

In various ways, people with CD chronically disrespect rules and the rights of others. Most egregiously, they use aggression against their peers (and sometimes elders)—bullying, starting fights, using dangerous weapons, showing cruelty to people or animals, even sexual abuse. Also well within their repertoires are intentionally setting fires and otherwise destroying property, breaking and entering, theft with—and without—confrontation, and lying to advance their own goals. Rounding out their list of symptoms may be frequent truancy (beginning at age 12 or younger), repeated runaways, and refusal against a parent's wishes to come home at night.

The Fine Print

The D's: • Duration (symptoms occurring within 1 year, with 1+ symptoms in past 6 months) • Disability (education/work, social, or personal impairment) • Differential diagnosis (ADHD, ODD, depressive and bipolar disorders, intermittent explosive disorder, adjustment disorders) • Demographic carve-out (a person 18 or older must not fulfill criteria for **antisocial personality disorder)**

Coding Notes

Based on age of onset, specify:

> **F91.1 Childhood-onset type.** At least one problem with conduct before age 10.
> **F91.2 Adolescent-onset type.** No problems with conduct before age 10.
> **F91.9 Unspecified onset.** Insufficient information.

Specify severity:

> **Mild.** Has sufficient, but not a lot of symptoms, and harm to others is minimal.
> **Moderate.** Symptoms and harm to others are intermediate.
> **Severe.** Many symptoms, much harm to others.

Specify if:

> **With limited prosocial emotions.** See separate discussion below.

With Limited Prosocial Emotions Specifier for Conduct Disorder

The above-described criteria for CD address the range of behavior of these patients. The specifier *with limited prosocial emotions* asks us to engage with the emotional underpinnings of—or reactions to—that behavior. (The term *prosocial* denotes positive behavior that benefits an individual or society in general.)

CD behavior can take either of two forms. In one, the patient has trouble regulating powerful, angry, hostile emotions. Children with this form of CD tend to come from dysfunctional families that are prone to physical abuse. They are likely to be rejected by their peers, leading to aggression, playing truant, and associating with delinquents.

In the second form, rather than only possessing emotions such as anger and hostility, a minority of patients with CD lack certain qualities such as empathy and guilt. Such persons tend to use others for their own gain. With low anxiety levels and the tendency to become easily bored, they prefer activities that are novel, exciting, even dangerous. As a result, they typically report the four symptoms mentioned in the specifier *with limited prosocial emotions.*

That is, they *might* report the four specifier symptoms. However, candor isn't necessarily the strong suit of these young people, who may be loath to reveal their feelings—and much about their behavior. So it's more important than ever to seek information from collateral resources of long acquaintance with the person.

Reading the Essential Features, you can see why this is sometimes called the *callous unemotional* type of CD. The specifier was renamed because the older label sounded so pejorative. (Use of the CD diagnosis has fallen off in recent years, anyway, partly because it is stigmatizing.) Call it what you will, this subtype of CD, which is more frequent with childhood onset, denotes a patient whose problems of conduct are persistent and severe.

Essential Features of **With Limited Prosocial Emotions Specifier for Conduct Disorder**

Such patients lack important emotional underpinnings. They have a callous absence of empathy (that is, they lack concern for the feelings or suffering of others). They tend to have limited affect and little remorse or guilt, other than regret if caught. They are indifferent to the quality of their own performance.

The Fine Print

To receive the specifier, two or more of these features must be experienced within the past year.

DSM-5-TR doesn't offer you the option of coding a patient who has conduct disorder as *without limited prosocial emotions.* I think this is a mistake—one that clinicians can, and should, correct. After all, no special code number is attached to the *with limited prosocial emotions* designation. It's just verbiage you tack on at the end. So for any patient with CD, you could add instead "without limited prosocial emotions." The double negative conveys valuable information about the patient, whatever the severity status. (Well, I'm assuming that everyone knows what *prosocial* signifies, or even means.)

F60.2 Antisocial Personality Disorder

Last on the path that often connects with ODD and CD comes ASPD, which is the culmination of aggressive, destructive behavior that sets all of society against such patients—whom we soon may be calling *perpetrators.* However, I'll follow DSM-5-TR's lead and defer presentation to its *other* proper place—with the personality disorders in Chapter 17 (p. 557).

F63.81 Intermittent Explosive Disorder

People with IED have periods of aggression that begin suddenly (the classic "hair-trigger temper") on little or no provocation. The stimulus may be quite benign—an offhand comment from a friend, an accidental bump from a passerby on the sidewalk—and all hell breaks loose. The form the particular hell takes may be only verbal, but actual physical violence is a possibility. In either case, the situation may rapidly escalate, sometimes to the point where the individual completely loses control. The whole episode rarely lasts longer than half an hour and may end when the person expresses remorse. Or posts bail.

Patients with IED are mostly young males, and many are relatively undereducated (less than a high school diploma). The condition affects about 4% of Americans lifetime (2% in the previous year); the figures are higher for young people and for those whose education stopped with high school. Reported rates are considerably lower in other countries.

Up to a third of first-degree relatives also have IED; some authorities suggest a strong genetic component. But a history of childhood trauma is also more frequently found in patients with IED than in comparison groups.

IED can be accompanied by other mental conditions, including substance use, mood, and anxiety disorders. The IED usually begins first, by a substantial number of years. (Clinicians note that in the case of patients with bipolar I disorder, it is important to make the IED diagnosis only when the patient is not in an episode of mania.) What's important here is that we should vigorously attempt to rule out all other possible causes of explosive episodes before settling on this disorder.

Whatever you might think of intermittent explosive disorder (IED—yes, the same initials as *improvised explosive device*), it is a condition with a long pedigree. Although it wasn't listed *per se* in the first DSM (published in 1952), the concept was there, hiding in plain sight on page 36. There it masqueraded as *passive–aggressive personality, aggressive type,* whose symptoms were "persistent reaction to frustration with irritability, temper tantrums, and destructive behavior . . ." In DSM-II it was called *explosive personality,* which by DSM-III in 1980 had morphed into the familiar IED. Not the bomb.

Essential Features of **Intermittent Explosive Disorder**

The patient has frequent, repeated, impulsive outbursts of aggression (verbal or physical without damage) *or* less frequent physical eruptions with harm to people, property, or animals. These outbursts are unplanned, have no obvious goal, and are excessive for the provocation.

The Fine Print

The D's: • Duration (aggression without harm 2 times a week for 3 months, *or* aggression with harm at least 3 times in the past year) • Demographics (the patient is 6+ years old, or the developmental equivalent) • Distress or disability (work/educational, social, or personal impairment) • Differential diagnosis (**substance use** and **physical disorders, cognitive disorders, bipolar** or **major depressive disorder, antisocial**

or **borderline personality disorder,** ordinary anger, adjustment disorder for children under age 18, **disruptive mood dysregulation disorder,** conduct disorder, oppositional defiant disorder, autism spectrum disorder, **adjustment disorder** in someone 6–18 years old)

The use of dual tickets of admission for IED (relatively benign aggression twice a week for 3 months versus harmful assault three times in a year) was something new in DSM-5 for this disorder. In fact, it was something new in any DSM for *any* disorder—no other condition features intensity-based versus frequency-based dual qualifiers. Of course, the criteria for nearly every disorder allow for differing degrees of severity, but then they are stated in terms of numbers of criteria met, or the quality or frequency or duration of criteria that are demonstrated.

The justification for this duality is the observation that there are basically two patterns of outburst (high-intensity/low-frequency and the reverse), and that limiting the definition to one group omits from consideration a lot of patients who repeatedly have problems related to their aggressive impulses, but in a different way. In fact, many patients with IED may mix the two patterns of behavior.

DSM-5-TR assures us that, regardless of which pattern a patient shows at intake, outcome and response to treatment will be roughly the same. Isn't it odd, though, that we aren't encouraged to add some sort of specifier that would tell the world just which bar the patient cleared to gain admittance?

Liam O'Brian

Since his teens, Liam O'Brian has had a flash-point temper. He was suspended from 10th grade for using a pair of scissors to assault a classmate who teased him about wearing the wrong colors on Clash Day. The next year, police visited him for breaking a headlamp on the car belonging to the baseball coach—he'd called Liam "out" in a close play at home plate. After he paid for the headlamp, charges were dropped; the coach noted that Liam was "basically a good kid with too much red hair." That year a neurologist reported that his physical exam, EEG, and MRI were all normal.

During his first few years of school, Liam had had difficulty sitting still in class and concentrating on his schoolwork. By the time he entered junior high, these behaviors were no longer a problem. In fact, he earned mostly B's and A's, and in the 2- to 4-month intervals between explosive episodes he was "no more trouble than the average kid."

Since Liam's graduation from high school, his pattern of periodic temper flare-ups has continued pretty much unchanged. After he was fired from two successive jobs for fighting with co-workers, he joined the Army. Within 6 weeks he had received a bad-conduct discharge for assaulting his first sergeant with a bayonet. Each of these incidents was triggered by a trivial disagreement or an exchange of words that could hardly be called provocative. Liam said afterward that he felt bad about his behavior; even the targets of his attacks agree that he "isn't mean, only touchy."

Now 25, his most recent evaluation was ordered by a judge. Liam was arrested in the supermarket by an off-duty policewoman. He had pushed her after she dumped 15 cans of cat food onto the carousel in the express checkout line. The usual examinations, X-rays, and EEG (this time with esophageal leads and sleep recordings) revealed no pathology. He denies ever having delusions or hallucinations. His father, he says, used to rough up his mother when he was drinking, so Liam has always been afraid to try alcohol or drugs.

Liam denies ever having extreme swings of mood, but he does express regret for his unpredictable, explosive behavior. "I just want to get a handle on it," he says. "I'm afraid I just might kill someone, and I'm not mad at anyone."

Evaluation of Liam O'Brian

Liam has a history of many outbursts over a period of at least 10 years (criterion A2). The facts of his behavior are not the issue here; he easily meets the requirements for age (E), frequency, disproportionate rage (B), consequences (marked distress, D) and lack of premeditation (C). Rather, a clinician evaluating Liam should carefully search for evidence of other disorders that might merit precedence for treatment (F).

Liam's mood shows no evidence of either mania or depression, effectively ruling out temper flare-ups of a mood disorder. At wide intervals he has had two neurological evaluations, neither of which revealed evidence for seizures. He never touches drugs or alcohol, and he denies symptoms of psychosis. The presence of any such underlying medical disorder might suggest a personality change due to another medical condition, but there is no evidence for this, either.

Patients with ASPD may act out violently and unpredictably, but unlike Liam, they do not feel remorse afterward. Neither does he show the manipulation, deceit, and callousness that are characteristic of ASPD. Patients with borderline personality disorder will sometimes have temper outbursts and engage in fights, but the generic criteria for personality disorder (p. 546) urge us first to rule out other mental disorders. I'd give Liam a GAF score of 51 along with his diagnosis:

F63.81   Intermittent explosive disorder

F63.1 Pyromania

As with the relationship of kleptomania to shoplifting, pyromania accounts for only a small minority of people who set fires. Only when there is a typical history of yielding with relief to an irresistible buildup of tension can the diagnosis be sustained.

At least 80% of patients are male; often the behavior begins in childhood or adolescence. With their interest in various aspects of fire, they will turn in false alarms, appear as spectators at fires, or collect the apparatus used by firefighters. They may even serve as volunteer firefighters, thereby becoming their own best customers.

Although pyromania is classified as an impulse-control disorder, these patients may make advance preparations, such as searching out a site and collecting combustibles. They may also leave clues, almost as if they want to be identified and apprehended. People who set fires may have low self-esteem and reportedly often have problems getting along with peers. Look for coexisting CD, ASPD, substance misuse, and anxiety disorders in people with pyromania.

As a free-standing diagnosis, pyromania is probably rare, more frequently reported in males.

Essential Features of **Pyromania**

These patients deliberately set multiple fires, but their motivation isn't profit, revenge, terrorism, to cover up a crime, or for any material gain. Rather, theirs is a general interest in fire and its trappings (fire trucks, the exciting aftermath). They feel tense or excited before starting the fire and experience a sense of release or pleasure afterward.

The Fine Print

The D's: • Differential diagnosis (**substance intoxication, mood** and **psychotic disorders, conduct disorder, antisocial personality disorder,** delirium or **neurocognitive disorder, intellectual developmental disorder,** ordinary criminal behavior)

Elwood Telfer

Elwood Telfer's earliest childhood memory is of a candle burning on the kitchen table. He would kneel on a chair as his mother sat in the dark and waited for his father to come home. His father drank, and they often waited a very long time. Periodically, she would put a strand of her own hair into the flame, sending a curl of acrid smoke spiraling toward the ceiling.

"Maybe it's why I've always been fascinated by fire," Elwood tells a forensic examiner when he is 27. "I even have a big collection of firefighting memorabilia—old helmets, a badge from an 1896 fire brigade, and so on. I get them at antique shows."

Elwood set his first fire when he was only 7. He had found an old Zippo lighter that still had some life, and he used it on an oily rag that was lying in a hay field. About a quarter-acre burned in the 20 exhilarating minutes before the fire trucks arrived to put it out. He always remembers the day's excitement as being well worth the beating administered by his father, once he'd sobered up.

Elwood sets most of his fires in fields or vacant lots. Once or twice, he torched an abandoned house, after first making sure that no one, not even a transient, could be inside. "I never wanted to hurt anyone," he tells the examiner. "It's the warmth and the color of the flame and the thrill I like. It never seems to get old."

Elwood has hardly ever had friends. When he entered high school, he was over-joyed to learn that there was a club called the Fire Squad. When he inquired about joining, two upperclassmen laughed and told him that it was an honorary group you could only belong to if you had lettered in football. Elwood felt almost sick with disap-pointment. That evening he started a small brush fire that consumed a neighbor's tool shed. That was the first time he experienced the healing effect of fire.

Months pass when he is inactive and calm. Then he will spot a field or empty build-ing that seems right, and the tension begins to mount. He might deliberately let it build over several days, to enhance the eventual feeling of release that is almost orgasmic. But he indignantly denies that he ever masturbates at a fire scene. "I'm no pervert," he says.

After graduating from high school, Elwood took enough junior college accountancy courses to obtain a job as bookkeeper for a security alarm company. He has worked steadily at that job until the present. He has never married, hasn't even dated, and has no close friends. In fact, he feels uncomfortable around other people. The forensic clini-cian notes no abnormalities of mood, cognition, or content of thought.

Elwood's only arrest ever—the reason for this evaluation—came about because of a change in the weather. It was summertime, and all week the wind had been blowing steadily offshore. Elwood had located a promising field of dry grass and manzanita. On Saturday morning he was off work, and the wind still held. With almost uncontrollable excitement, he used a tin of gasoline to start the fire. But he reacted with horror and panic when the wind suddenly shifted to blow in from the ocean; easily jumping the small service road he had driven in on, the fire gobbled up his car and several coastal dwellings. A firefighter spotted him as he sat on the stony beach, crying quietly.

When the police search Elwood's apartment, they find a huge collection of video newscasts of wildfires.

Evaluation of Elwood Telfer

The phenomenon of "tension and release" required for a diagnosis of pyromania (cri-teria B, D) is well detailed in the vignette. And there's also not much argument that Elwood deliberately sets fires (A) and is fascinated by fire itself and by the trappings of firefighting (C). His clinician's task will be to sort through the differential diagnosis, which is not unlike that for kleptomania.

People with ASPD or other personality disorders will sometimes set fires for profit or revenge. But Elwood has worked at one job for a decade, and his legal difficulties are restricted to fire setting. Through inattention, patients with cognitive disorders will sometimes set their clothing or kitchens ablaze. However, Elwood has symptoms of none of these conditions (F). A person with schizophrenia, manic episode, or other severe mental conditions may sometimes set a fire as a message (for example, to be released from jail, to be returned to a former place of residence). This behavior has been termed *communicative arson*. Another item to consider in the differential diag-nosis is *arson with purpose:* fires set as a matter of political protest or sabotage, or fires set for profit (E). None of these applies to Elwood.

Although Elwood has a great deal of difficulty relating to other people, this vignette includes insufficient evidence to support a diagnosis of avoidant personality disorder. This is not to say that it isn't warranted, only that more information is needed. I'd make a note that he had "avoidant personality features." A very low GAF score (20) reflects Elwood's potential for harming others with his behavior.

F63.1   Pyromania

Among other things, two "manias" are included in this chapter. A third, trichotillomania, can be found at home in the chapter on obsessive–compulsive and related disorders, page 209. In these disorders, the term is not used by itself in the sense of having a manic episode. Rather, appended as a suffix, *-mania* ("madness" in Greek) means having a passion or enthusiasm for something.

F63.2 Kleptomania

In kleptomania, stealing occurs not as the result of need, or even necessarily of desire. When apprehended, people typically have enough money with them to pay for whatever they have taken. Once they have left the scene undetected, they may give away or discard their loot—or even return it to the store. These people recognize that their behavior is illegal and therefore dangerous, but they cannot resist. Fear of apprehension, guilt, and depression are frequent accompaniments.

OK, many otherwise law-abiding people have stolen something—in one study, over a quarter of college students admitted as much. But fewer than 0.5% in the general population meet criteria for kleptomania. (The diagnosis is much more common, up to 8%, in inpatient samples.) It is especially common among younger people; indeed, it typically begins in adolescence. Women outnumber men by perhaps 3:1. Once it begins, often in childhood, it tends to become chronic.

Dating back over 200 years, kleptomania is one of the oldest named disorders in the diagnostic manuals. It is probably also highly overused. Although fewer than 1 in 20 shoplifters can be accurately diagnosed with this disorder, many try to avoid prosecution when they are caught by claiming that they were driven by an irresistible impulse. Look for substance misuse and depression as comorbid diagnoses.

Essential Features of **Kleptomania**

These people repeatedly act on the impulse to steal objects they don't really need. Before the actual theft, they experience mounting tension, which yields to a sense of release when the theft takes place. The behavior is not prompted by anger, revenge, delusions, or hallucinations.

The Fine Print

The D's: • Differential diagnosis (**manic episode** and **psychosis, antisocial personality disorder, conduct disorder,** ordinary criminal activity, major neurocognitive disorder, malingering)

Roseanne Straub

"Fifteen years!" It's how long Roseanne Straub has been shoplifting, but from the expression on her tear-streaked face, you'd think it was the length of her sentence.

Roseanne is 27, and this is her second arrest, if you don't count that time as a juvenile. Three years ago, she was arrested, booked, and released on her own recognizance for walking out of a boutique with a silk blouse worth $150. Fortunately for her, 2 weeks later the shop fell victim to a recession; the owner, otherwise preoccupied, did not follow through with prosecution. Badly frightened, she resisted the temptation to shoplift for several months afterward.

Roseanne is married and has a 4-year-old daughter. She works as a research assistant for a civilian contractor to the military, and a conviction would doom her security clearance and her job. After her previous arrest, her husband, a paralegal, threatened to divorce her and obtain custody of their child if she did it again.

"I don't know why I do it. I've asked myself that question a thousand times." Aside from the stealing, Roseanne considers herself an average person. She has lots of friends and no enemies; most of the time she is quite happy. In every other respect she is honest; she won't even let her husband cheat when he prepares their taxes.

The first time Roseanne ever stole was when she was 6 or 7—on a dare from two school friends. When her mother found the candy she had taken from the convenience store, she had gone with Roseanne and made her return it to the store manager. It was years before she was again tempted to steal anything.

In junior high, she noticed that periodically a certain tension will build up inside her. It feels as though something itches deep within her pelvis where she can't scratch. For several days she will feel increasingly restless, with an excited sense of anticipation. Finally, she will dart into whatever store she happens to be passing, whisk some article under her coat or into her handbag, and walk out, flooded with relief. Years ago, this behavior seemed to be associated with her menstrual periods, but by the time she was 17 her episodes had become completely random events.

"I don't know why I do it," Roseanne says again. "Of course, I don't like being caught. But I deserve to be. I've ruined my life and the lives of my family. It's not as if I need another compact—I must have 15 of them at home."

Evaluation of Roseanne Straub

Whereas Roseanne repeatedly yields to the impulse to take objects she doesn't need (criterion A), ordinary shoplifters plan their thefts and profit from them. And they don't experience the buildup of tension (with subsequent release) that characterize Rose-anne's shoplifting episodes (B, C). People with ASPD or other personality disorders may steal impulsively, but they will also have committed many other antisocial acts; not so with Roseanne (E). When criminals falsely claim to have symptoms of klepto-mania, a diagnosis of malingering may be warranted instead. Patients with schizophre-nia or manic episodes will sometimes experience hallucinations that order them to steal things. Roseanne doesn't hallucinate, and she doesn't seem to be angry or seeking revenge (D).

Anxiety, guilt, and depression are often associated with this disorder. Therefore, watch for diagnoses such as generalized anxiety disorder, persistent depressive disor-der, and major depressive disorder. Kleptomania may also be associated with the eating disorders, especially bulimia nervosa. Patients with substance use disorder may steal to support a drug habit. None of the above, however, applies to Roseanne. With a GAF score of 65, her diagnosis will be:

F63.2   Kleptomania

Tension and release (or *relief*) is a phrase that describes several DSM-5-TR conditions. Among them are pyromania and kleptomania, but it can also be found attached to tricho-tillomania—though it is not a criterion for that disorder. It expresses the typical buildup of anxiety or tension, sometimes for a day or more, until the impulse to act becomes overwhelming. Once the action has been taken, the person experiences a sense of release that may be perceived as relief or pleasure. However, remorse or regret may later come to dominate the emotional landscape.

F91.8 Other Specified Disruptive, Impulse-Control, and Conduct Disorder

F91.9 Unspecified Disruptive, Impulse-Control, and Conduct Disorder

Use one of these two categories to code any problems with the control of impulses or conduct that do not meet the criteria for the disorders described above or elsewhere in DSM-5-TR. As usual, the other specified category should be used when you wish to be specific about a particular presentation; the unspecified category should be used when you do not wish to be specific.

R45.89 Impairing Emotional Outbursts

CHAPTER 15

Substance-Related and Addictive Disorders

Quick Guide to the Substance-Related and Addictive Disorders

Mind-altering substances all yield three basic types of disorder: substance intoxication, substance withdrawal, and what we now call substance use disorder (formerly substance dependence and substance abuse). Most of these DSM-5-TR terms apply to nearly all of the substances discussed; I'll note exceptions as they occur. In addition, because its diagnostic features and some of its physiological features are nearly identical to those of substance use, gambling disorder has been moved into this chapter.

Basic Substance-Related Categories

Substance use disorder. A user has taken a substance frequently enough to produce clinically important distress or impaired functioning, and to result in certain behavioral characteristics. Found in connection with all classes of drugs but caffeine, substance use disorder can even develop accidentally, especially from the use of a medication to treat chronic pain. The discussion, in which alcohol use disorder serves as a model, begins on page 404.

Substance intoxication. This acute clinical condition results from recent overuse of a substance. Anyone can become intoxicated; this is the only substance-related diagnosis likely to apply to a person who uses a substance only once. All drugs but nicotine have a specific syndrome of intoxication, the symptoms of which can be found summarized later in Table 15.1 (p. 412). Using alcohol as the model, a general discussion of substance intoxication begins on page 419.

Substance withdrawal. This collection of symptoms, specific for the class of substance, develops when a person who has frequently used a substance discontinues it or markedly reduces the amount used. All substances except phencyclidine (PCP), the other hallucinogens, and the inhalants have an officially recognized withdrawal syndrome; see Table 15.1

(p. 412). Using alcohol as the model again, a discussion of substance withdrawal begins on page 410.

Specific Classes of Substances

Here are the substances you'll find discussed in the following pages.

Alcohol (p. 406).

Amphetamines and other stimulants (including cocaine) (p. 459).

Caffeine (p. 424).

Cannabis (p. 428).

Hallucinogens (including PCP) (p. 435).

Inhalants (p. 444).

Opioids (p. 448).

Sedative, hypnotic, or anxiolytic drugs (p. 454).

Tobacco (p. 470).

Other or unknown substances (p. 472).

Other Substance-Induced Disorders

Most DSM-5-TR chapters include disorders associated with substance use; every class of substance is represented except nicotine. They can be experienced during intoxication, during withdrawal, or as consequences that endure long after misuse and withdrawal symptoms have ended. They include:

Psychotic disorder (p. 93).

Mood (bipolar or depressive) disorder (p. 151).

Anxiety disorder (p. 192).

Obsessive–compulsive and related disorder (p. 213).

Sleep–wake disorder (p. 351).

Sexual dysfunction (p. 376).

Delirium (p. 493).

Neurocognitive disorder, major or mild (p. 537).

Non-Substance-Related Disorder

Gambling disorder. These patients repeatedly gamble, often until they lose money, jobs, and friends (p. 480).

Introduction

We in the 21st century have access to a growing variety of mind-altering substances, the use of which can lead to serious behavioral, cognitive, and physiological problems. These substances, all of which affect the central nervous system, include medications, toxic chemicals, and illegal drugs. Several substances, however, can be obtained legally without a prescription: alcohol, caffeine, and tobacco, as well as some of the inhalants.

DSM-5-TR lists just over 300 numbered (in ICD-10) substance-related disorders. When all the subcodes and qualifiers are considered, there are hundreds more ways to indicate a patient with a substance-related disorder. For any of these, the clinician must specify the substance responsible, the type of problem, and in some cases the time relationship of substance use to the onset of the problem behavior.

DSM-5-TR uses nine major groupings, plus the catch-all other (or unknown), to categorize substances. These groupings are all artificial, however, and among them we can identify certain similarities:

- Central nervous system depressants (alcohol and the sedatives, hypnotics, and anxiolytics)
- Central nervous system stimulants (cocaine, amphetamines, and caffeine)
- Perception-distorting drugs (inhalants, cannabis, hallucinogens, and phencyclidine [PCP])
- Narcotics (opioids)
- Nicotine
- Other (corticosteroids and other medications)

The terminology keeps changing, but the basic problem remains the same: the fact that people misuse alcohol and drugs. One problem with substance use disorders has been that because they have been so variously defined—by different writers, for different substances, in different eras (and in different DSMs)—there has been substantial disagreement as to exactly what they are and who engages in them.

DSM-5-TR continues the tradition of defining the disorders related to all the substances in terms that are more or less uniform. The trouble is, we keep redesigning the uniform. The definitions now in use replace older words such as *alcoholism, problem drinking, episodic excessive drinking, addiction, habituation, dependence, abuse,* and other (often pejorative) terms applied over the years to people who use mind-altering substances.

Of course, most adults use some substances, but most of us don't use them pathologically. But exactly what is *pathological use?* Let's define it as use beyond the point where negative effects outweigh any positive effects. Often, this point arrives quickly—with first exposure for some users and substances. More typically, pathological use is frequent, heavy, or both, and it always involves physical and emotional symptoms and maladaptive changes in behavior.

Note also that none of the symptoms of substance use explain why users value their chosen substances. In an effort to be objective and consistent, DSM-5-TR criteria ignore many of the nuances of problems with specific substances. Gone, for example, is the descriptive richness of the stages of alcoholism. You can consult mental health textbooks, scientific articles, and even literary works to supplement these criteria.

For a long time now, I've searched for a noun describing substance use disorder that fits comfortably into the current nomenclature. I've finally decided to throw caution to the winds and call it *addiction*. Many substance-use experts bemoan the loss of this term that seems to describe the behavior well and succinctly.

One last note: *Substance-induced* is a DSM-5-TR term used to embrace nearly all drug use disorders—intoxication and withdrawal plus all of the behavioral and mental conditions (such as mood or alcohol disorders) caused by specific chemical agents. *Substance-related* means all of the above plus substance use disorder (what we used to call addiction). This all seems unnecessarily complicated to me, but we're professionals. We can cope.

The Basic Substance-Related Categories, Illustrated by Alcohol-Related Disorders

My approach in this part of the chapter differs somewhat from the DSM-5-TR format. I'll present the Essential Features of substance use disorder, intoxication, and withdrawal, using the example of alcohol for each of these categories. Later, I will discuss whatever intoxication and/or withdrawal syndromes apply to each of the other substance groupings. I'll also briefly mention other disorders related to each substance.

Substance Use Disorder

As noted in the sidebar, clinicians and researchers have argued for years about defining *addiction*. The DSM-5-TR approach is to define *substance use disorder* as the core behavior of those who misuse substances. These criteria specify a type of addiction that includes behavioral, physiological, and cognitive symptoms. As an exercise, let's dissect the language concerning the diagnosis of any substance use disorder:

1. The use is problematic. Though the initial intent may be to cope with other problems, in the end, it only makes things worse for the user—and for the user's relatives and associates.

2. There is a pattern to the use. The use reoccurs in a predictable habit pattern.

3. The effects are clinically important. This usage pattern either has come to the attention of professionals or warrants such attention. (Actually, the official DSM-5-TR language reads "clinically significant." However, the word *significant* has statistical implications that often cannot be sustained in clinical practice. I think *important* works better here. I have sometimes substituted the adjective *material*.)

4. The use causes distress or impairment. This says that the substance use must be serious enough to alter in a negative way the patient's emotions or activities. Substance use disorder is thereby defined in terms similar to those employed for many non-substance-related mental disorders.

5. Interference with the patient's life must be shown by at least 2 symptoms from a list of 11: more use than intended; (mostly futile) attempts to reduce usage; much time spent obtaining or using; craving the substance; shirking of obligations; social problems; reduction in activities important to the user on the job or at play; use despite its physical danger; use despite knowing it has caused physical or psychological health problems; tolerance; and withdrawal symptoms. Severity is judged by counting up the number of these 11 symptoms that are checked off (but see my caveat in a sidebar on p. 410).

Finally, in diagnosing substance use disorder, intoxication, and withdrawal, note that rapidity of onset and of elimination from the body affect the likelihood that a patient will have problems with any given substance. Rapid absorption of a substance (by smoking, snorting, or injection) favors quicker onset of action, shorter duration of action, and greater likelihood of a substance use disorder. A longer half-life (the time it takes the body to eliminate half the substance remaining) reduces the likelihood of withdrawal symptoms but extends the period during which the user could experience them.

Whatever happened to *polysubstance dependence?* DSM-IV used this term to indicate situations in which a patient uses two or more substances but doesn't have enough problems to warrant a diagnosis of addiction to any of them—and yet, in aggregate, does have enough symptoms from substance use to fulfill a "group" diagnosis. That definition was a little complicated and tended to be seldom used. There is also precious little research to indicate that it ever predicted much of anything for anyone.

In DSM-5-TR, any patient who would meet the somewhat Byzantine criteria just mentioned would have to be diagnosed as having an unspecified or other specified substance-related disorder for each substance involved. Perhaps someone can persuade me there's a payoff in *that*.

Alcohol Use Disorder

Although nearly half of all adult Americans at least once in their lives have had some sort of problem with alcohol (driving while intoxicated, missing work due to a hangover), far fewer (about 10%) have had problems sufficient to qualify for a diagnosis of alcohol use disorder. Note that the criteria are the same as for any other substance use disorder, which I've stated below in generic form.

Alcoholism is extremely common: At one time or another, over one in four adult in the United States have had alcohol use disorder, and nearly half of them to a severe degree. The risk for men is greater than for women by a nearly 3:2 ratio. Onset tends to be in the teen years, though older people are not immune. Physiological complications such as withdrawal are likely to appear much later in the disease.

Alcoholism is highly heritable; first-degree relatives have several times the risk of the general population. It has many comorbidities, especially with mood disorders and antisocial personality disorder.

Essential Features of **Substance Use Disorder**

Patients use enough of their chosen substance to cause chronic or repeated problems in different areas of their lives:

- *Personal and interpersonal life.* They neglect family life (duties to spouse/partner, dependents) and even valued leisure activities in favor of using their substance of choice; they may even fight (verbally or physically) with those they care about; and they continue to use despite the realization that it causes interpersonal problems.

- *Employment.* Effort formerly devoted to work or other important activities now goes to obtaining the substance, consuming it, and then recuperating from its use. Result: Patients are repeatedly absent or get fired.

- *Control.* They often use more of the substance or for longer than they intended; they (unsuccessfully) attempt to eliminate or reduce the usage. Through it all, they desperately crave more.

- *Health and safety.* Users engage in behavior that is physically dangerous (most often, operating a motor vehicle); legal issues can ensue. They continue to use despite knowing that it causes ongoing health issues such as cirrhosis or mental problems.

- *Physiological sequels.* Tolerance develops: The substance produces less effect, so patients must use more. And once they stop using, they suffer the withdrawal symptoms characteristic of that substance.

The Fine Print

Tolerance isn't a factor with most hallucinogens, though users may develop tolerance to the stimulant effects of PCP. And there is no category of caffeine use disorder.

Withdrawal isn't a factor with PCP, other hallucinogens, or inhalants.

Don't count tolerance or withdrawal for medications used as prescribed.

The D's: • Duration (the symptoms you count must have occurred within the past 12 months) • Differential diagnosis (physical disorders, primary disorders from nearly every other DSM-5-TR chapter, *truly* recreational use)

Coding Notes

Course modifiers.

In early remission. No criteria (save craving) met for 3–12 months.
In sustained remission. No criteria (save craving) met for 1+ years.
In a controlled environment. The patient's access to the substance is restricted.
On maintenance therapy: Applies only to tobacco.

Severity (modify, with clinical judgment).

Mild. 2–3 symptoms endorsed.
Moderate. 4–5 symptoms.
Severe. 6+ symptoms.

See Table 15.2 (p. 475) for codes.

Quentin McCarthy

"I can get off it, but I can't stay off it." Quentin McCarthy is 43, and he is talking about alcohol. He likes to say that throughout his adult life he has been successful at two things—drinking and selling insurance. Now he's having trouble with both.

Quentin is the second of three sons born to parents who are both attorneys. His brothers were excellent students. Quentin is bright, but he had been hyperactive and the class clown. In school, he had never been able to focus his attention well enough to excel at anything but physical education.

To please his parents, after high school Quentin tried a semester of junior college. It was worse than high school; the only thing that kept him going was guilt. Whereas his older brother was admitted to law school (with honors at entrance), and his younger brother mopped up the prizes at the state science fair, Quentin felt almost joyful when his birthday was that year's fourth pick in the national draft lottery. The following day he enlisted in the Army.

Somewhere in his schooling Quentin had learned to type, so he was assigned to his battalion's administrative section. He likes to say that, throughout 4 years in the military, he never fired his weapon in anger. By comparison with some of the older men's alcohol use, his drinking was moderate. Although he had about the usual number of fights, he managed to avoid serious trouble. When he left the service at age 22, he had held onto his sergeant's stripes through two tours of duty in Vietnam.

After that, life suddenly got serious. Working part time after duty hours in the post exchange, Quentin discovered that he is a natural salesman, so it seemed a logical move to take a job selling life insurance. It also seemed sensible to marry the boss's daughter. When his father-in-law died suddenly 2 years later, Quentin became sole proprietor of the agency.

"The business made me, and it ruined me," he says. "I made a lot of money having lunch with people I could sell large policies to. I told myself that I had to drink with them in order to make a sale, but I suppose that was just rationalization."

As time went on, Quentin's two-martini lunches turned into four-martini lunches. By the time he was 31, he was skipping lunch completely and nipping throughout the afternoon to "keep a glow on." Now, at the end of the day he is sometimes surprised to see how much has disappeared from the bottle of bourbon he keeps in his desk drawer.

The past year brought Quentin two unpleasant surprises. The first came when his doctor informed him that the nagging pain just above his navel was an ulcer; for the sake of his health, he would have to stop drinking. The second, which in a way seemed worse because it injured his pride, occurred one afternoon over lunch. A long-time client of the agency apologetically said that he would be taking his substantial business elsewhere; his wife didn't feel comfortable that he was "doing business with a lush." Thinking back now, Quentin realizes that there have been several other, less blatant instances of customers deserting the fold.

The result has been his resolve to quit, or at least to reduce the amount of his drinking. ("Quitting is easy," he remarks ruefully. "I did it twice in 1 month.") At first, he promised himself he wouldn't drink before 5 P.M.; that proved too restrictive, and he later amended it to "around lunchtime." With the bourbon level in his desk drawer bottle receding as rapidly as ever, Quentin decided he would try Alcoholics Anonymous. "That was worse than useless," he explains. "The stories I've heard from some of those people make me seem like a teetotaler."

A comment made by his wife eventually brought him in for evaluation. "You used to drink to have a good time," she told him. "Now you drink because you need it."

Evaluation of Quentin McCarthy

The Essential Features of substance use disorder (see above) aren't especially complicated, just tedious. Quentin's history of alcohol use illustrates many of them. At least two are needed to qualify for the diagnosis, and they must occur within a 1-year period. This is not to say that they must have begun within the year prior to evaluation, only that the problems must have been present within that time frame. Note that some patients may sporadically present new symptoms and abandon old ones.

- *Using more.* Many people start out consuming relatively small amounts ("just a nip before dinner") but end up skipping dinner and just nipping. As a result, they use more of their substance of choice than they intend. Quentin was sometimes surprised at how much bourbon he had consumed by day's end (criterion A1).

- *Control issues.* When quitting seems too drastic and frightening, people may attempt to reduce their intake by setting rules, as did Quentin (A2). Eventually, realizing he needed help with control, he joined Alcoholics Anonymous—to no avail.

- *Time investment.* This symptom is especially characteristic of those who use substances other than alcohol. Alcohol users often carry on with other activities, sober or not. And like tobacco, alcohol is legal and hence easy to obtain. Quentin spent a good deal of time drinking, which should probably qualify him on this criterion (A3), even though he kept right on working. Other patients, especially those who use drugs other than alcohol, may spend a great deal of time assuring the continuity of their supply. For example, see the story of Kirk Aufderheide (p. 456).

- *Craving* (A4). This criterion, new in DSM-5, is one that many authorities had complained was missing from previous DSMs. It has been linked to dopamine release in substance use and other behaviors such as gambling. We didn't note it in Quentin's vignette, but perhaps the interviewer forgot to ask.

- *Obligations shirked* (A5). Many patients with alcohol use disorder abandon their responsibilities at home, in the community, or at work in favor of drinking. Quentin gets a pass on this one.

- *Worsening interpersonal/social relations.* The patient continues to use, though it causes fights or arguments with close associates. You could argue (I would) that Quentin's customers' taking their business elsewhere presents such an example (A6).

- *Reduction of other activities* (A7). Patients with substance use disorders commonly ignore work and social activities. This was not the case with Quentin, who devoted the necessary time to work (though some clients objected to his drinking).

- *Physical dangers ignored* (A8). Driving while under the influence is by far the most common, but many others, such as operating heavy industrial machinery, can also occur. The vignette doesn't indict Quentin on physical danger.

- *Psychological/medical warnings ignored.* Quentin drank despite the danger from ulcers (A9). Other patients may ignore physician warnings about liver disease (cirrhosis or hepatitis) or esophageal varicose veins, which can rupture after prolonged retching. Those who use drugs intravenously often continue to share needles, despite the well-known risks of HIV and hepatitis. Most substances can also exacerbate suicidal ideas, mood disorders, and psychoses—which are likewise ignored.

- *Tolerance.* When a substance has been used so extensively that the user's body has grown accustomed to the chemical effects, we say that tolerance has developed. This is especially apparent as regards alcohol, opioids, and sedatives, but it can be found in all substance groups apart from hallucinogens. With tolerance, the patient either requires more of the substance to obtain the same effect or feels less effect from the same dose. Or both. Quentin was experiencing some of this when he discovered to his surprise how rapidly the level in his bottle had declined (A10).

• *Withdrawal* (A11). This criterion can show up either as a symptom picture that is characteristic for the class of substance, or as use of the substance to avert or treat these symptoms. Quentin drank through the afternoon to keep his glow on, so we can't give him this one—yet. We'll discuss substance withdrawal next.

To sum up, Quentin qualifies for at least 5, possibly 6, of the 11 criteria for alcohol use disorder. The next vignette will reveal whether he also meets the criteria for alcohol withdrawal.

DSM-5 was the first manual to include severity criteria specific for substance use disorders. In part, that was necessitated by the deletion of the substance abuse category—a staple of previous DSMs since 1980 and misunderstood by many clinicians as a sort of "substance use lite." Numerous studies determined over the years that the substance abuse criteria failed as regards both validity and reliability. The diagnosis of alcohol abuse, when made at all, was typically based on one criterion, driving while intoxicated—a behavior that, while dangerous, is a weak reed on which to prop a diagnosis. But most of all, the abuse diagnosis simply didn't predict enough to make it worthwhile.

The idea of severity criteria is a good one, but its implementation does sow the seed of discontent, partly because we determine severity simply by totaling the number of criteria met. The seed is, not all criteria are created equal: Some imply far more disability and distress than others. For example, either tolerance or withdrawal suggests that the individual has been using heavily and for an extended period (in most cases, many months, and probably for years).

Other criteria may have far less serious import. Arguments with a spouse or partner, while not trivial (as most of us can testify), depend not only on the person's actual use, but on the other person's perception of use and, yes, tolerance for the behavior. Craving may be found even in individuals who don't meet other criteria for a substance use disorder. Fortunately, these are issues that are solvable with more research and experience. Maybe in DSM-6.

Substance Withdrawal

Withdrawal symptoms develop as the concentration of a substance decreases in the brain of a frequent user. The generic criteria for substance withdrawal are simple: They require only that the patient experience specific symptoms after quitting a substance that has been used heavily for a specified time. Stress or impairment must result, and no physical illness or other mental disorder must better explain the symptoms.

The symptoms that develop during substance withdrawal are specific to the substance used and are described in the relevant sections of this chapter. However, certain symptoms are found in withdrawal from many substances:

- Alteration in mood (anxiety, irritability, depression)
- Abnormal motor activity (restlessness, immobility)
- Sleep disturbance (insomnia or hypersomnia)
- Other physical problems (fatigue, changes in appetite)

Check out Table 15.1 for a more complete listing.

For a substance to cause withdrawal symptoms, a patient must first become tolerant to it. This requires frequent use for a period of time that depends on the specific substance. Heroin may require only a few injections, whereas for alcohol, weeks of heavy drinking are usually needed to produce clinically important tolerance. Most patients who are dependent on a substance that is suddenly denied them will experience withdrawal.

Some substances don't produce withdrawal. Hallucinogens, for example, can induce an addiction, yet no withdrawal syndrome has been reported. On the other hand, DSM-IV listed no caffeine withdrawal syndrome—a serious gaffe, as any coffee drinker who switches suddenly to decaf will testify. Fortunately, DSM-5 put that one right.

The time course of withdrawal depends on the drug's half-life—the time it takes for the body to eliminate 50% of the substance. Withdrawal symptoms typically begin within 12–24 hours after the last dose is consumed and persist no longer than a few days. A powerful urge to resume use of the substance often accompanies the withdrawal symptoms.

Analysis of blood, breath, or urine can attest to the patient's substance use, but more often evidence is obtained from history. Denial may color self-report, so histories are often more reliable if a relative or friend—anyone but the patient—augments the information. As a rule of thumb, many clinicians mentally double the amount of a substance a patient claims to have used.

Essential Features of **Substance Withdrawal**

After using a substance heavily and at length, the patient suddenly stops or markedly reduces intake. This yields a substance-specific syndrome that causes problems.

The Fine Print

The D's: • Duration to symptom onset (generally hours to days) • Differential diagnosis (physical disorders, primary mental disorders)

You can find the specifics of each substance withdrawal syndrome in Table 15.1 (p. 412).

TABLE 15.1. Symptoms of Substance Intoxication and Withdrawal

		Substance intoxication								Substance withdrawal					
		Alcohol/sedatives[a]	Cannabis	Stimulants[b]	Caffeine	Hallucinogens	Inhalants	Opioids	PCP	Alcohol/sedatives[a]	Cannabis	Stimulants[b]	Caffeine	Tobacco	Opioids
Social	Impaired social functioning			×											
	Inappropriate sexuality	×													
	Social withdrawal		×												
	Interpersonal sensitivity			×											
Mood	Labile mood	×													
	Anxiety		×	×		×				×	×			×	
	Euphoria		×	×			×	×							
	Blunted affect, apathy			×			×	×							
	Anger			×							×			×	
	Dysphoria, depression					×		×		×	×	×	×	×	×
	Irritability										×		×	×	
Judgment	Impaired judgment	×	×	×		×	×	×	×						
	Assaultiveness, belligerence					×			×						
	Impulsivity								×						
Sleep	Insomnia, sleeplessness			×						×	×	×		×	×
	Bad dreams									×	×				
	Hypersomnia											×			
Activity level	Aggression	×									×				
	Agitation, increased activity		×	×			×	×		×		×			
	Tirelessness			×											
	Restlessness			×							×				×
	Decreased activity, retardation			×		×	×					×			
Alertness	Reduced attention	×						×							
	Hypervigilance			×											
	Stupor or coma	×		×			×	×	×						
	Time seems slowed		×												
	Poor concentration												×	×	

[a] This grouping also includes hypnotics and anxiolytics.
[b] Cocaine and amphetamines

		Substance intoxication								Substance withdrawal					
		Alcohol/sedatives[a]	Cannabis	Stimulants[b]	Caffeine	Hallucinogens	Inhalants	Opioids	PCP	Alcohol/sedatives[a]	Cannabis	Stimulants[b]	Caffeine	Tobacco	Opioids
	Confusion			×											
	Drowsiness							×					×		
Perception	Ideas of reference					×									
	Fears of insanity					×									
	Persecutory ideas					×									
	Perceptual changes					×									
	Brief hallucinations/illusions					×				×					
	Depersonalization/derealization					×									
Autonomic	Dry mouth		×												
	Constricted pupils							×							
	Dilated pupils			×		×									×
	Sweating			×		×				×	×				×
	Piloerection														×
Muscle	Muscle weakness			×			×								
	Muscle twitching				×										
	Muscle aches												×		×
	Muscle rigidity								×						
Neurological	Dystonia, dyskinesia			×											
	Nystagmus	×					×		×						
	Tremors					×	×			×	×				
	Blurred vision					×	×								
	Double vision						×								
	Impaired reflexes						×								
	Seizures			×					×	×					
	Numbness								×						
	Headache										×		×		
Gastrointestinal	GI upset, diarrhea				×										×
	Nausea, vomiting			×						×			×		×

(cont.)

TABLE 15.1 (cont.)

		Substance intoxication								Substance withdrawal					
		Alcohol/sedatives[a]	Cannabis	Stimulants[b]	Caffeine	Hallucinogens	Inhalants	Opioids	PCP	Alcohol/sedatives[a]	Cannabis	Stimulants[b]	Caffeine	Tobacco	Opioids
	Abdominal pain										×				
	Increased appetite/weight gain		×									×		×	
	Decreased appetite/weight loss			×							×				
Motor	Incoordination	×	×			×	×								
	Unsteady gait	×					×								
	Stereotypies			×											
	Trouble walking								×						
	Lethargy						×								
	Trouble speaking								×						
	Slurred speech	×					×	×							
Cardiovascular	Chest pain			×											
	Irregular heartbeat			×	×	×									
	Slow heart rate			×											
	Rapid heart rate		×	×	×	×			×	×					
	Blood pressure up or down			×					×						
General	Depressed breathing			×											
	Dizziness					×									
	Red eyes		×												
	Chills			×							×				
	Fever										×				×
	Reduced memory	×					×								
	Nervous, excited				×						×				
	Rambling speech				×										
	Hyperacute hearing								×						
	Red face				×										
	Increased urination				×										
	Fatigue											×	×		
	Tearing, runny nose														×
	Yawning														×

414

Alcohol Withdrawal

Heavy drinking for days or longer is required to produce alcohol withdrawal. (Drinkers can tolerate greatly varying amounts of alcohol, so it's hard to be precise.) Symptoms begin a few hours after drinking stops and coincide with a rapidly declining blood alcohol level. Nearly all patients will show evidence of central nervous system overactivity, such as sweating, racing pulse, or heightened reflexes (see sidebar). The most common symptom is tremor; nausea and vomiting may also occur. Some patients may have brief hallucinations that last 12–24 hours. After 2 or 3 days, a few may even have seizures.

Perhaps half of alcohol use disorder patients will ever experience withdrawal. Often relatively mild (sometimes it is called *uncomplicated withdrawal*), it is usually brief, lasting but a few days and peaking on the second. However, the accompanying anxiety, irritability, and sleeplessness may persist a good deal longer.

The heavier the drinking has been, the more likely symptoms will be severe; "uncomplicated" withdrawal then shades into other, more serious syndromes. The best known of these is delirium, which affects only about 5% of those hospitalized for withdrawal. When delirium occurs during severe alcohol withdrawal, it is commonly called *delirium tremens* (DTs). When a patient has both seizures and delirium, the seizures almost invariably come first. Rodney Partridge, a patient with alcohol withdrawal delirium, is described later (p. 494).

Another alcohol withdrawal syndrome is alcohol-induced psychotic disorder with hallucinations. Formerly known as *alcoholic auditory hallucinosis,* it is an uncommon (though not rare) disorder whose symptoms can almost exactly mimic schizophrenia. Danny Finch, a patient with this disorder, is described in Chapter 2 (p. 95).

The number 100 can serve as a useful reminder when looking for physiological signs of alcohol withdrawal: pulse over 100 beats per minute; temperature over 100°F; diastolic blood pressure approaching 100 mmHg. Rapid respirations may serve as another sign—though I hope they're nowhere near 100 per minute.

Essential Features of **Alcohol Withdrawal**

After heavy, lengthy use of alcohol, the person suddenly stops or markedly reduces intake. Within hours to days, this yields symptoms of increased nervous system and motor activity such as trembling, sweating, or rapid heartbeat; anxiety; agitation; sleeplessness; nausea or vomiting; short-lived illusions or hallucinations; or grand mal convulsions.

The Fine Print

The D's: • Duration to onset (a few hours to a day or more) • Distress or disability (work/educational, social, or personal impairment) • Differential diagnosis (**physical illness;** psychotic, mood, and anxiety disorders; **other substance withdrawal**)

　　The specifics for alcohol withdrawal are listed in Table 15.1 (p. 412).

Coding Notes

Specify if: **With perceptual disturbances.** The patient has auditory, tactile, or visual illusions without delirium or hallucinations, and with intact insight (that is, realization that the perceptual symptoms are unreal and caused by the substance use).

　　Coding in ICD-10 depends on the presence of perceptual disturbances; see Table 15.2 (p. 475).

Quentin McCarthy Again

By the time Quentin seeks help, he is drinking the equivalent of nearly a pint of hard liquor per day. He declines the offer of a brief hospitalization to detoxify, and instead begins an outpatient withdrawal regimen of decreasing doses of a benzodiazepine. He is asked to return in 3 days.

On Quentin's next visit, he looks gray and unhappy. He signs in at the registration desk with a wobbly scrawl, and his hand trembles as he reaches out an arm to have his blood pressure and pulse evaluated. Both vital signs are elevated.

For 3 days Quentin has consumed no alcohol at all. Beginning the second morning, he has felt increasingly anxious—a sensation reminding him of his first night in Vietnam, when he awakened to the booming of howitzers. His anxiety grows throughout that day. By bedtime he is exhausted, but he hardly sleeps at all. When he arrives 4 hours early for this next clinic appointment, he admits that he has taken none of the medicine he was given. "I wanted to do it myself," he explains.

Now Quentin adheres faithfully to his medication plan. Over the next several days, his withdrawal symptoms abate. Within 2 weeks, he no longer needs the pills. ("For real, this time," he offers with a touch of chagrin.) However, because he feels strongly tempted to drink when having lunch with clients, he requests disulfiram (Antabuse) therapy.

Three months later, Quentin is still taking disulfiram and hasn't touched alcohol. He attends at least one Alcoholics Anonymous meeting every day. He has rescued his insurance agency from the doldrums and has even persuaded two of his former clients to return with their business. However, he admits that he occasionally feels angry when he wants a drink.

Further Evaluation of Quentin McCarthy

When he stops using alcohol (alcohol withdrawal criterion A), Quentin develops typical alcohol withdrawal symptoms (see Table 15.1, p. 412). They include rapid pulse, insomnia, anxiety, and tremor (criteria B1, B3, B7, and B2—though only two are required for diagnosis). They combine to make him so uncomfortable that he hurries back to the mental health clinic (C). Going longer without medication might have put him at serious risk for withdrawal seizures or perceptual disturbances such as auditory or visual hallucinations. Then he might have qualified for other diagnoses—for example, alcohol-induced delirium or alcohol-induced psychotic disorder with hallucinations. Of course, Quentin's withdrawal symptoms further substantiate his primary diagnosis of alcohol use disorder.

Could any physical or other mental disorder have caused these symptoms (D)? The differential diagnosis for withdrawal symptoms is long and substance-specific. For opioid withdrawal, it includes flu-like syndromes. Patients withdrawing from cocaine and amphetamines typically have symptoms of depression. But both Quentin's history and symptoms are so typical for alcohol withdrawal that other diagnoses would seem highly unlikely.

At this point his diagnosis would read:

F10.230   Severe alcohol use disorder, in withdrawal, without perceptual disturbances

But now, we must consider the matter of course modifiers for substance use disorder.

Can someone go into substance withdrawal without having substance use disorder? If you scrutinize the criteria and do the math, it's theoretically possible. The criteria don't say it cannot happen, but aside from patients who are medically habituated (not to alcohol, we'll stipulate), it must be a rare event.

Course Modifiers for Substance Use Disorder

After at least 3 months with no substance-related symptoms other than craving, the patient can be considered for a course modifier. The choices are *early remission* and *sustained remission*. The standard for early remission is 3 months to 1 year; for sustained remission, it is 1 year or longer. To either period can be added a further specifier: *in a controlled environment*, if the patient is living in a facility that prevents access to substances. Such an environment would include jails and prisons (well, in theory), locked hospital wards, and therapeutic communities.

Essential Features of **Substance Use Disorder Course Modifiers**

These designations are straightforward and self-explanatory. Remission and controlled environment specifiers apply to use disorder for each category of substance.

Remission

Remissions are divided into early versus sustained. Until a patient has been clean (or sober) for 90 days, no designation of remission is possible.

> **In early remission.** *Early remission* begins after 3 months clean and sober for that substance (and without any of the substance use disorder symptoms—with one allowed exception: craving). It can last until the person has been sober for 1 year.
>
> Patients are especially vulnerable to relapse during the first year of sobriety. So, after a full year has elapsed, they may qualify for . . .
>
> **In sustained remission.**

In a Controlled Environment

Someone who is in early or sustained remission and lives in an environment that restricts access to the substance may be given this modifier. Good control of contraband would characterize such an environment—a well-run jail, therapeutic community, or locked hospital ward.

In a controlled environment can apply to these classes of substance use: alcohol; cannabis; hallucinogens; inhalants; opioids; sedatives, hypnotics, or anxiolytics; stimulants; other (or unknown); tobacco.

On Maintenance Therapy

A patient who takes a medication designed to reduce the effects of a substance may be described as *on maintenance therapy*. It is listed as a specifier for both opioids and tobacco, when the patient currently has no symptoms of the substance use disorder.

Severity

> **Mild.** Presence of 2–3 criteria substance use disorder criteria.
> **Moderate.** Presence of 4–5 criteria.
> **Severe.** Presence of 6+ criteria.

There's an interesting question implied in the statement concerning the specifier *on maintenance therapy:* Why does it apply *only* to tobacco and opioids? Why not to alcohol (Antabuse)? Or anything else for which an effective maintenance treatment is devised? Of course, the specifier is only a set of words, so you can apply it wherever you like. If your patient is doing well on Antabuse, say so.

Evaluation of Course Modifiers for Quentin McCarthy

When he first came to the clinic, Quentin had been alcohol-free for only a few hours; at that point, his diagnosis of alcohol use disorder would not qualify for a course modifier other than severity (which was indeed severe—we've counted 5 or 6 criteria). On his return to the clinic after 3 days, moreover, he would also have qualified for a diagnosis of alcohol withdrawal. But at his reevaluation, 3 months into recovery, he has no symptoms of alcohol use disorder (other than perhaps craving); his withdrawal symptoms have abated; and he is still taking disulfiram.

The occasional episodes of anger, when a patient would like a drink, are typical for alcoholism recovery; patients themselves sometimes refer to them as "dry drunk" experiences. That's what is happening with Quentin, and I would simply note it in the diagnostic summary.

According to Table 15.2 (p. 475), Quentin's diagnosis (finally!) at 3 months would read as given below. His GAF score on admission would be 40; at 3-months, GAF would be 70. Although the official manual doesn't say I can do so, I tacked on the "on disulfiram" to impart additional information. So far, no one's complained.

F10.20   Severe alcohol use disorder, early remission, on disulfiram

Substance Intoxication

Anyone can get drunk. Anyone can inhale toxic fumes. Although most people who become intoxicated do so voluntarily, people can also be affected accidentally (for example, through exposure to industrial chemicals or drinking a spiked punch). Regardless of intent, for a diagnosis of substance intoxication to be appropriate, the central nervous system effects of the substance must cause psychological changes or behaviors that don't work well for the individual. Note that substance intoxication is almost always reversible. When there are permanent effects of substance use, look instead to another diagnosis (for example, substance-induced cognitive disorder).

The behavior of an intoxicated person changes in disadvantageous ways; that is, the changes cause problems. (DSM-IV called them *maladaptive*, which I think is a useful term we should keep.) These include work/educational or social problems, abnormally labile (unstable) mood, impaired thinking, defective judgment, and belligerence. This criterion is important because it helps to discriminate patients who are only intoxicated in the physiological sense (excessive digitalis, for example) from those whose behavior impairs functioning. A person who drinks a 6-pack of beer and then goes quietly to bed without disturbing anyone may well be intoxicated in the physiological sense but has not earned the mental health diagnosis of alcohol intoxication. (Going to bed is a behavioral change, but not usually maladaptive. Quite the opposite, actually.) So, to diagnose someone as having substance intoxication requires both hurtful behavioral changes *and* physiological symptoms and signs.

As for the signs of physiological impairment that will be noted, these tend to be substance-specific, though there are certain common themes:

- Agitation or loss of motor coordination
- Loss of ability to sustain attention
- Impaired memory
- Reduced alertness (drowsiness, stupor)
- Effects on the autonomic nervous system (dry mouth, heart palpitations, gastrointestinal symptoms, changes in blood pressure)
- Mood changes (depression, euphoria, anxiety, and others)

You'll find more in Table 15.1 (p. 412).

Then there remains the ubiquitous requirement that all physical illnesses and other mental disorders must be ruled out. As a rule, symptoms of intoxication (or withdrawal) that last longer than about 4 weeks may point to another mental or physical disorder. For example, a drinker who still has depressive symptoms a month after drying out should be evaluated for major depressive episode.

Essential Features of **Substance Intoxication**

Shortly after using a substance that can affect the central nervous system, the patient develops characteristic physical symptoms and clinically important behavioral or psychological changes that are maladaptive.

The Fine Print

The D's: • Duration to symptom onset (shortly after) • Differential diagnosis (physical disorders, intoxication from other substances, other mental disorders)

You can find the specifics of each substance intoxication syndrome in Table 15.1 (p. 412).

Alcohol Intoxication

The picture of acute alcohol intoxication is so familiar that it seems almost unnecessary to describe it here. However, we should make several observations.

There is a great deal of variability in the blood levels of alcohol different people can tolerate without appearing drunk. The range may be as great as fivefold (from 0.3 to 1.5 mg/mL), even though many jurisdictions now set the sobriety level for driving at 0.8 mg/mL and will probably be setting it even lower in the future. Furthermore, the symptoms of alcohol intoxication are usually more prominent when the blood level is rising (during the early part of the drinking period) than when it is falling and the person is sobering up. Levels of alcohol in the body can be measured in urine, blood, breath, or even saliva.

Alcohol intoxication should only be diagnosed when there is evidence (typically historical) that the patient has drunk enough, rapidly enough, that most people would be having the effects—and that these behaviors pose a real problem for the drinker. It is such a rite of passage for youth that much of the general population would probably qualify—if they ever came to the attention of medical personnel or legal authorities. In borderline cases, the diagnosis may mean factoring in the drinker's weight, age, and general state of health.

Essential Features of **Alcohol Intoxication**

Shortly after drinking alcohol, the patient becomes disinhibited psychologically or behaviorally (such as rapid mood shifts, sexual or physical aggression, impaired judgment). There is also evidence of neurological impairment (imbalance or wobbly gait, unclear speech, poor coordination, jerking eye movements called nystagmus, reduced level of consciousness or diminished memory or attention span).

The Fine Print

The D's: • Differential diagnosis (**physical disorders, intoxication from medications** or **other substances, other mental disorders**)
You can find the specifics of alcohol intoxication in Table 15.1 (p. 412).

Coding Notes

See Table 15.2 (p. 475) for codes.

Dolores McCarthy

In one of Dolores McCarthy's earliest memories, she is 4 years old and sitting on her grandfather's lap. She rests her head against his soft old cotton sweater. He wraps his arms securely around her as she clings to his neck. Also clinging to him is a particular smell that she has always associated with her grandfather. Not until she was a teenager does she realize what the smell is: beer.

By the time Dolores turned 10, she had watched in horror as, by degrees, the old man died of cirrhosis. Then, in her teens, she saw how her father's drinking wrecked her parents' marriage. In college, when she discovered that two glasses of wine would ease her chronic sense of tension, she promised herself that she would use alcohol and never let it use her.

Accordingly, she evolved a set of rules to control her consumption. She allowed herself only one drink before dinner, and never more than three in a day (except on weekends and vacations, when she could have four). From her father's unfortunate example, she had learned: Regardless of the occasion, never drink during work and never allow "extras." Even on her 22nd birthday—which was also the day she married Quentin, the young salesman in her father's office—she had only four glasses of champagne (just enough to cast a comfortable glow over the occasion).

Despite her control, Dolores has had two lapses. The first occurred 12 months ago, when she became pregnant for the first and only time. Although she wanted a child, she took the precaution of having an amniocentesis. When it revealed that she was carrying a baby with Down syndrome, she gulped several extra drinks and drove around while deciding what to do. A Breathalyzer-measured blood alcohol level of 1.2—courtesy of the police officer who watched her run a stop sign—landed her in traffic court just 1 week after the abortion.

Her second arrest for driving while intoxicated occurred 6 months later, when she lost her self-control once again after her mother died of Alzheimer's disease. The day Quentin entered treatment was therefore only the third time he had ever known his wife to be drunk.

Now Dolores accompanies her husband to his second clinic appointment. She has been worried about Quentin for several months, and when his agitation kept them both awake most of that night, she went down to the kitchen and poured them each a drink. When he refused his, she drank it for him. Then she lost count and had a couple more.

"Anything was besher—was better than what he was going through," Dolores tells the clinician that morning. After correcting herself, she speaks slowly and deliberately.

On the spur of the moment, Dolores decides that she should accompany Quentin to his appointment, to be sure he doesn't get into trouble. They take her car; she insists on driving. (Quentin was never a fighter, so he doesn't dare remind her of what happened on the other occasions she drove after drinking.) Fortunately, traffic is light and she only needs two extra tries when parking in an unusually generous space at the curb.

As Dolores enters the clinic building, however, she stumbles and might have fallen, but someone grabs her elbow and steadies her as she wobbles into the waiting room. She fumbles with the large buttons of her coat until her husband undoes them for her. She then slumps into a chair where, with her coat thrown over her, she dozes until they are called into the clinician's office.

Evaluation of Dolores McCarthy

We'll first address the question of alcohol use disorder. Although Dolores drinks more than the average adult, she has had few problems from her alcohol use—saved by her vigilance and the unfortunate examples of the men in her family. She has never drunk enough to develop tolerance or withdrawal symptoms, and her control has been almost unwaveringly iron-fisted. When it slipped, she's tumbled into legal problems: two arrests for driving under the influence of alcohol within a 12-month period. Drunk driving qualifies as using alcohol when it's dangerous to do so (criterion A8 for alcohol use disorder). In other patients, such evidence might include fights or arguments with family or friends, lapses in business judgment, or embarrassing behavior such as making sexually inappropriate remarks.

That's one criterion met for alcohol use disorder, but Dolores needs two to qualify, even minimally. As we scan the list, we see that her qualifications are not extensive. She has certainly never experienced tolerance or withdrawal, and there is no evidence of interference with her work or personal life. You might think that all her efforts at control would qualify her, but they were almost completely *successful*. OK, persistent desire to control alcohol use works (A2); so does a persistent strong desire to use (A4), which barely gain her admittance to the alcohol use disorder ballpark. Still, she will earn a severity rating of only *mild*.

However, Dolores can claim several criterion C symptoms of alcohol intoxication, any one of which will qualify her for that diagnosis. Shortly after drinking (A), her judgment is impaired (she drove the car—B). She slurs her words, walks unsteadily, and has difficulty even *un*buttoning her coat (C1, C3, C2). When she finally enters the office, she lapses into a doze, but that's hardly a (C6) coma, is it?

A clinician attending Dolores will have to consider whether a history, physical exam, or laboratory data are needed to be sure her symptoms are not due to another medical condition (D). However, her typical symptoms and history of recent alcohol use make that seem unnecessary. A diagnosis of alcohol-induced delirium would not be warranted in Dolores's case: Although her reduced attention span and lowered state of consciousness came on quickly, the vignette contains no evidence of cognitive changes such as disorientation, memory loss, perceptual disturbance, or language problems (though she slurs her words, her thought processes seem intact).

Although Dolores had an abortion and experienced the death of her mother, neither of these events occurred recently, and so seem unlikely to affect the course of her treatment; we don't need to give them a Z-code. With a GAF score of 75, Dolores' diagnosis would be as below. To get the code, we can use Table 15.2 (p. 475) to pinpoint intoxication with mild use disorder.

F10.120   Mild alcohol use disorder, with alcohol intoxication

Other Alcohol-Induced Disorders

Table 15.2 (p. 475) lists other alcohol-induced disorders with their codes. I've provided other additional alcohol-related vignettes elsewhere: Danny Finch (p. 95), Barney

Gorse (p. 220), Rodney Partridge (p. 494), Mark Culpepper (p. 537), Charles Jackson (p. 539), Jack Weiblich (p. 570), and at least one patient in Chapter 20.

F10.99 Unspecified Alcohol-Related Disorder

Use unspecified alcohol-related disorder to categorize alcohol-related symptoms that cause clinically important impairment or distress but do not meet full criteria for any of the disorders described above. One example would be *alcohol idiosyncratic intoxication*. Some people react strongly to a very small amount of alcohol (too little for most people to appear intoxicated). For instance, a person who is ordinarily withdrawn and unassuming may become hostile and belligerent after a single glass of wine. This condition occurs within minutes of the drinking and lasts a few hours at most. Predisposing factors may be advancing age, fatigue, and brain injury, such as that which might result from trauma or infection. This phenomenon has also been called *pathological intoxication;* in DSM-III-R, it had a code number of its own. In DSM-5-TR, assuming it is serious enough to cause problems, code it here.

Caffeine-Related Disorders

Caffeine, the most widely used psychoactive substance in the world, is present in coffee, cola beverages, tea, chocolate, and a variety of prescription and over-the-counter drugs. Perhaps two-thirds to three-quarters of all adults frequently consume at least one of these. Although tolerance and some degree of withdrawal are undeniably associated with caffeine, few people would ever experience enough social problems to qualify for caffeine use disorder; in any case, DSM-5-TR provides no such criteria set.

Black coffee has long been used as a folk remedy to sober up people who have consumed too much alcohol. However, caffeine does nothing to relieve their symptoms. Rather, it only adds agitation to the mix for someone who was formerly "only" inebriated.

I had planned to point out that caffeine is the only substance in this chapter that carries no legal restrictions anywhere. But that would be wrong.

Australia is probably the strictest country of all: The limit is up to 32 mg per 100 mL of liquid, which means that a standard can of energy drink can contain no more than the equivalent of cup of instant. In the United States there is a legal limit on carbonated beverages—you can have up to 71 mg in a 12-ounce drink. But there is no limit on the caffeine content of other foods. Red Bull gives you 80 mg in 8 ounces.

Although there are no age limits on the consumption of caffeine-containing drinks, as with so many things we love, just because it's legal doesn't mean it's a good idea.

F15.920 Caffeine Intoxication

Symptoms of the sort caused by "Mr. Coffee Nerves"—the now-retired antihero of newspaper comic-page advertisements for Postum, which was once sold as a hot drink alternative to coffee—may seem too familiar to rate much space. However, it has been estimated that about 7% of adults may at some time have symptoms of caffeine intoxication, also known as caffeinism. The symptoms are much like those of generalized anxiety disorder (p. 190). The person feels "wired," excessively energetic, excitable, and driven. Loud speech, irritability, and jitteriness are also commonly associated with caffeine intoxication.

The effects are determined by several factors. Of course, individual tolerance is important, but so is the amount ingested. A new user might experience symptoms from as little as 250 mg of caffeine—just a couple of cups of strong brew. However, even an experienced coffee drinker who takes in more than 500 mg per day risks intoxication. Other individual characteristics, such as age, fatigue, physical condition, and expectations, can also play a role. A diagnosis of caffeine intoxication is not usually made in people who are younger than 35; perhaps it takes years even to develop awareness that there is a problem.

I have not included a separate vignette in this section, but Dave Kincaid, whose substance-induced sleep disorder was described in Chapter 11, illustrates caffeine intoxication as well. For Dave's full story, see page 352. We'll evaluate Dave's caffeinism below.

Essential Features of Caffeine Intoxication

Shortly after consuming caffeine, the person develops symptoms of increased nervous system and motor activity, such as feeling jittery or excited, restless, trouble sleeping, rapid or irregular heartbeat, twitching muscles, intestinal upset, excess urination, agitation, red face, rambling speech, periods of not getting tired.

The Fine Print

The D's: • Duration to symptom onset (recent) • Distress or disability (work/educational, social, or personal impairment) • Differential diagnosis (**physical disorders, intoxication from other substances, other mental disorders** [such as caffeine-induced anxiety and sleep disorders])

You can find the specifics of caffeine intoxication in Table 15.1 (p. 412).

Evaluation of Dave Kincaid's Caffeinism

Dave Kincaid works at a coffee-roasting store while he is writing his novel. He has free access to the rich, thick coffee they serve there. He also snacks on quite a few chocolate-covered coffee beans. In all, he probably consumes over 1,000 mg of caffeine per day (criterion A for caffeine intoxication), so he has reason to feel "up" (B3). He can't sit still when he is trying to type (B1), and at night he lies awake with insomnia (B4). Rapid heartbeat, abdominal upset, and nervousness (B10, B7, B2) are also typical symptoms that can be encountered even with relatively mild caffeinism—which Dave's was not.

Most of the DSM-5-TR symptoms can be found after as few as two cups of coffee, though perhaps not in full concert, as with Dave. Muscle twitching ("live flesh," as Dave calls it—B8), agitation, and periods of tirelessness require substantially greater caffeine intake (1 gram of caffeine or more per day). In all, he has at least six symptoms; DSM-5-TR criteria requires only five. No wonder he's distressed (C)!

Because its symptoms are sometimes confused with other mental disorders, it is important to keep caffeine intoxication in mind. If we assume that Dave includes his mental health when he says that he has been well, he probably won't have a previous history of disorders such as anxiety disorders (especially generalized anxiety disorder and panic disorder), mood disorders (especially with manic or hypomanic episodes), and various sleep disorders. At one period in his life, he smoked a little marijuana, but he has never used other substances whose effects might be confused with caffeinism. These would especially include the central nervous system stimulants: cocaine, amphetamines, and related substances.

Ruling in or out caffeine-induced anxiety disorder and caffeine-induced sleep disorder requires some clinical judgment. For these disorders, the symptoms must be more severe than are typically found in plain caffeine intoxication, and they must be serious enough to need independent clinical attention.

F15.93 Caffeine Withdrawal

Way back in *DSM-IV Made Easy*, I noted that caffeine withdrawal wasn't an official DSM diagnosis, but that it should be. A lot of other clinicians apparently had the same idea, for the clamor to move it into The Good Book began years ago.

Caffeine withdrawal may be especially likely during changes in a person's social schedule, as during vacations, over weekends, and the like. Then that person is likely to encounter fatigue, headache, and sleepiness. Somewhat less frequent symptoms include impairment of concentration and motor performance. DSM-5-TR notes that migraine and viral illness are examples of possible physical disorders to rule out.

Essential Features of **Caffeine Withdrawal**

Someone suddenly stops or markedly reduces the extended, daily intake of caffeine, yielding headache, symptoms suggesting flu (nausea or vomiting, muscle pain), and central nervous system depression (fatigue, dysphoria, poor concentration).

The Fine Print

The D's: • Duration to symptom onset (3+ symptoms within 1 day) • Distress or disability (work, social, or personal impairment) • Differential diagnosis (**physical disorders, other substance intoxication** or **withdrawal, other mental disorders**)
   You can find the specifics of caffeine withdrawal in Table 15.1 (p. 412).

You

How many coffee drinkers have had an experience like this one? You have come to stay with friends who, you realize upon awakening the first morning, eschew coffee—there isn't a bean in the house. After frantic, futile foraging for even a jar of instant, you decide, "This isn't worth the effort. I'll get along without it for a change."

And for the first few hours, you get along just fine. But as lunchtime inches around, you find you aren't feeling quite so well. Last night you were eager to see old friends and new places; now you've only the strength to crawl back into the old sack. Because your stomach is fomenting revolution, you wonder, "What intestinal horror could I have been exposed to on the plane?" As your headache, which for a couple of hours has been hanging back at the edge of your skull, now asserts itself, you can only growl when your hosts suggest it's a lovely day.

Finally, in desperation, you make your painful way to the Starbuck's down the street. An espresso and a double latte later, your headache scurries for the exit, the day brightens, and you depart renewed, leaving the astonished barista a truly world-class tip.

Evaluation of You

Look, this isn't astrophysics. You've suddenly been cut off from your quotidian coffee fix (criterion A), whereupon you develop classic symptoms of caffeine withdrawal: headache, fatigue, irritability, and physical complaints that resemble the flu (B1, B2, B3, B5; only three criterion B symptoms are required). You feel so lousy you'd risk the distress and social embarrassment of alienating good friends you rarely see (certainly not recently enough to remember that they don't stock your beverage of choice—C).

Of course, you might have the flu or another medical condition, or maybe it's jet lag. Yes, you'd need to rule out other, competing causes for your symptoms (D), but this shouldn't prove too onerous: With your GAF score of 85, you hardly need a physical exam. Rapid improvement with a shot of the Elixir of Life confirms that the diagnosis for You is:

   F15.93   Caffeine withdrawal

I have an ulterior motive for choosing *You* as the example of caffeine withdrawal: It demonstrates how easily just about anyone can sneak into the DSM.

Many books and articles comment on the countless Americans (and, by extension, perhaps billions of ordinary people the world over) who could eventually be diagnosed with a mental or behavioral disorder. Even a decade ago, 46% of Americans were diagnosable by DSM-IV criteria.

If I sound preachy here, I apologize—without feeling especially sorry—but I do want to underscore the extent to which we've pathologized some of our most cherished behaviors. For if even *You* can inhabit the pages of DSM-5-TR, who couldn't?

Other Caffeine-Induced Disorders

Caffeine use disorder has been included in Section III of DSM-5-TR as a subject for further study. That's partly because quite a few long-time caffeine users develop symptoms of a substance use disorder. These especially include making multiple attempts to stop using and continuing to use despite knowing that it is creating medical problems for them—and withdrawal symptoms. You will find a complete listing of caffeine-induced disorders in Table 15.2 (p. 475).

F15.99 Unspecified Caffeine-Related Disorder

Cannabis-Related Disorders

Cannabis is the generic name of the hemp plant, *Cannabis sativa,* whose active ingredient is tetrahydrocannabinol (THC). Depending on the variety of hemp and where it is grown, the leaves and tops may contain anywhere from 1% to about 10% THC; the potency has been rising for several decades. (In some California locales, careful nurturing of selected cultivars has produced the latter figure and higher—a dubious triumph of U.S. agriculture.) Hashish, which is a resin produced from the leaves of the hemp plant, contains about 10% THC.

Cannabis is the most widely used illicit substance (OK, in some jurisdictions it is now somewhat licit) in the United States, and indeed in the world. Perhaps 25% of all Americans who use cannabis will at some time experience use disorder. Since 2007, its popularity is once again on the rise, and it has been legalized or decriminalized in over half the United States. Unsurprisingly, it is more popular among younger people, especially males.

Use of cannabis more often than weekly increases the likelihood of addiction. People who suddenly quit after heavy use may experience mild physiological symptoms that can last several weeks; these include anxiety, sleeplessness, and other symptoms similar to those of sedative withdrawal. The serious behavioral and psychological consequences seen in those withdrawing from other substances (cocaine, opioids, alcohol, and the like) are less problematic with cannabis. Therefore, for the first time, DSM-5 included criteria for cannabis withdrawal. Heavy users may learn with surprise that they have developed tolerance. Relative to other substance use disorders, the development of cannabis use disorder can take a long time. It tends to occur in the context of social use, which may be more common than with other drugs of abuse. Eventually, the familiar symptoms of substance use disorder emerge.

Flashbacks are rare. So is depression, which, when present, is usually temporary and mild. Some patients experience paranoia that can last up to several days. Using cannabis may worsen the psychosis of someone who already has a psychotic disorder.

Cannabis may be one of the most difficult substances for some patients to stop using, simply because it causes relatively few of the medical complications that help motivate the cessation of other, more dangerous substances. Although cannabis is usually smoked, THC can be absorbed from the gastrointestinal tract—hence the (often true) stories you hear about marijuana brownies. Because absorption can be erratic, THC that has been swallowed is especially dangerous.

Some clinicians believe that there is also a syndrome of chronic cannabis use. Though variable, the symptoms are said to include mild depression, reduced drive, and decreased interest in ordinary activities—the so-called *amotivational syndrome*. Adolescents are especially likely to experience cognitive effects from heavy use. These include decreased memory, attention, and thinking, which can persist beyond the period of acute intoxication and worsen with long years of habitual use.

Cannabis Use Disorder

The characteristics of cannabis use disorder are like those of nearly every other specific substance use disorder. The criteria are identical to those for a generic substance use disorder (p. 404). DSM-5-TR also mentions *cannabinoid hyperemesis syndrome*, wherein people complain of nausea and vomiting that appear related to frequent cannabis use. For coding, see Table 15.2 (p. 475).

Cannabis Intoxication

Devotees of cannabis value it for the relaxation and elevation of mood it confers. It causes their perceptions to seem more acute; colors may appear brighter. Adults can fancy they see the world afresh, much the way a child does. Their appreciation for music and art is enhanced. Their ideas flow rapidly; they may find their own conversation especially witty.

The effects of cannabis are many and varied, with both negative and positive reactions strongly influenced by setting and frame of mind. Time sense often changes—a few minutes may seem like an hour. Users may become passive and drowsy; mood drifts into apathy. Motor performance suffers (cannabis notoriously impairs driving performance). Cannabis also produces red eyes and a rapid heartbeat. Indeed, most users have probably experienced intoxication at one time or another.

Often a user will appear unaffected, even when highly intoxicated. Illusions may occur, but hallucinations are rare. Users generally retain insight; they remain unconvinced by their own misperceptions and may even laugh about them.

Especially in first-time users, intoxication can begin with anxiety, which may progress to panic. In fact, the most common untoward reaction to cannabis is an anxiety disorder. Some people fear that the body distortions they perceive mean impending death.

Essential Features of **Cannabis Intoxication**

Shortly after using cannabis, the patient develops symptoms of motor incoordination or altered cognition (anxiety or euphoria, poor judgment, isolation from friends, a sense of slowed time) plus 2+ of telltale red eyes, dry mouth, rapid heart rate, and hunger.

The Fine Print

The D's: • Duration to symptom onset (minutes to hours, depending on route of administration) • Differential diagnosis (**intoxication from other substances, other medical** or **mental conditions**)

You can find the specifics of cannabis intoxication in Table 15.1 (p. 412).

Coding Notes

Specify if: **With perceptual disturbances.** The patient has auditory, tactile, or visual illusions without delirium or has hallucinations with intact insight. (Intact insight means the realization that the perceptual symptoms are unreal and caused by the substance use. Hallucinations without insight would suggest a diagnosis of cannabis-induced psychotic disorder.) Coding in ICD-10 depends on the presence of perceptual disturbances; see Table 15.2 (p. 475).

The criteria for cannabis intoxication do not require that recent use produce distress or disability, but do require clinically important, troublesome psychological or behavioral changes. It would be hard to argue that social withdrawal and defective judgment are anything but clinically significant, but euphoria? Suppose a person reports feeling really, really happy and nothing comes of it? Then is that person not intoxicated? Some diagnostic criteria work better than others. Some still leave much to the interpretation of the individual clinician.

Russell Zahn

"You got a candy bar on you?" Russell Zahn shambles into the interviewer's office and slumps onto the sofa. He flicks a lock of hair back across one shoulder of his torn denim jacket. "I know it's only an hour since breakfast, but I'm really hungry."

At age 27, Russell lives on general relief and is often homeless. In the hills of northern California where he grew up, the principal cash crop is marijuana. For the first several years since leaving high school, he worked at its cultivation and marketing; more recently, he has been just a consumer. Now he has been referred to the mental health clinic by a judge grown weary of his repeated courtroom appearances for possession of small amounts of marijuana. Russell volunteers that he has enjoyed a joint in the alley outside, just before coming in for his appointment.

Russell isn't especially unhappy about being evaluated; he just doesn't see much need for it. He requires very little to live on. Whatever his relief check doesn't cover, he earns by begging. He has his own corner in the business section of town, where for 6 hours a day he lounges behind a cardboard sign requesting contributions. Every couple of hours he will walk back to the alley and sneak a toke. "I don't smoke on duty," he says. "It's bad for business."

All in all, life seems a lot better now than when he was a kid. When he was 6, both of Russell's parents died in an automobile accident. For the next 2 years, he was passed around among grandparents, aunts and uncles, and a cousin; no one really wanted him. Ultimately, he terminated a 6-year tour of various foster homes by running away when he was 14.

The alternative lifestyle of the northern California marijuana industry suited Russell just fine—until he discovered that no industry at all suits him even better. It has been years since he's worked at anything, and he supposes he never will again. His mood is always good. He has no health care needs. He's tried all the other drugs ("Except smack; that's death!"), but he doesn't really care for any of them.

Russell stands and stretches. He rubs his already brick-red eyes. "Well, thanks for listening."

The interviewer asks where he is going and points out that his appointment isn't over. "You've only been here about 20 minutes."

"Really?" Russell slouches back into his chair. "It seems more like an hour. I've always had a lousy sense of time."

Evaluation of Russell Zahn

Russell's time distortion (typically, time seems to crawl) fulfills the DSM-5-TR requirement for maladaptive behavior or psychological changes (criterion B for cannabis intoxication) due to recent cannabis use (A). It is not clear how clinically important this is for Russell, but the interviewer certainly notices. Red eyes (C1) and heightened appetite (suggested by his desire for a midmorning candy bar—C2) provide the two physical indicators necessary to make the diagnosis. For coding purposes, note that he has no evidence of disturbed perception (such as illusions or hallucinations).

Of course, possible use of other substances (notably alcohol and hallucinogens, if perceptual problems are noted) should be considered in the differential diagnosis of cannabis intoxication. History and the odor of alcohol can be important to this differentiation and to ruling out mental disorders such as anxiety and mood disorders (D).

Does Russell have a cannabis use disorder? He has smoked it for years, but even coupled with long duration, frequency doesn't force an automatic yes. Although he might have greater tolerance for the drug than the average user (substance use disorder criterion A10), there is no evidence that he uses more than he intends or that he has ever tried to exercise control. (DSM-5-TR lists a withdrawal syndrome for cannabis; stay tuned for more of Russell's history.)

Russell does spend considerable time procuring and using marijuana (A3), and his homeless, aimless life may be partly due to the use of the drug (A7). (Alternatively, you could argue that a personality disorder has caused these problems and the cannabis use, but that seems to me a bit speculative.) The vignette does not suggest any physical or psychological problem caused by cannabis. Still, considering Russell's relaxed work ethic, the time he spends using, and his probable tolerance to the drug, a diagnosis of cannabis use disorder (moderate, regardless of symptom number: I'm claiming clinician's privilege on this one) seems warranted. However, I'm also willing to entertain arguments.

In any event, with no evidence of perceptual changes such as hallucinations or illusions, we can use Table 15.2 (p. 475) to arrive at a preliminary diagnosis. (ICD-10 gives us different numbers to use, depending on the presence of perceptual disturbances.)

F12.220   Moderate cannabis use disorder, with intoxication, without perceptual disturbances

Cannabis Withdrawal

As recently as the debut of DSM-IV, some researchers still wondered whether cannabis withdrawal even existed. Now it is known that a huge percentage (a third to nearly all) frequent users will experience withdrawal at some time. Perhaps the diagnosis simply took time to emerge from the haze created by a relatively weak available drug combined with relatively few truly heavy users. In the past several decades, however, much evidence has accumulated that cannabis withdrawal is real—that at one time or another, perhaps a third of users experience this uncomfortable state. I need to repeat that, as for certain other drug classes, withdrawal that stems from medical use should not be counted as a criterion for cannabis use disorder. This is becoming ever more relevant in our era of medical availability of marijuana in so many jurisdictions, and legal recreational pot in some.

Half or more of those who experience withdrawal mention craving the drug, with dysphoria and restlessness. Some report vivid, often unpleasant dreams or nightmares. Symptoms can be about as severe as for nicotine withdrawal; in fact, some users substitute tobacco (or alcohol) to combat their withdrawal symptoms. The whole experience lasts for a few days to a couple of weeks, with the physical symptoms decreasing sooner than psychological symptoms do. In several studies, withdrawal symptoms were a strong predictor of relapsing use.

Essential Features of **Cannabis Withdrawal**

After stopping heavy, long-lasting cannabis use (several months or longer), the patient experiences symptoms such as troubled sleep, poor appetite or weight loss, depressed mood, anxiety or a feeling of nervousness, restlessness, and physical discomfort from shakiness, sweating, chills/fever, headache, or abdominal pain. Increased irritability may appear as anger or aggressive behavior.

The Fine Print

The D's: • Duration (heavy, daily use for months; onset within a day or two of stopping use) • Distress or disability (work/educational, social, or personal impairment) • Differential diagnosis (**physical disorders, other substance-use intoxication** or **withdrawal, other mental disorders**)

You can find the specifics of cannabis withdrawal in Table 15.1 (p. 412).

Coding Note

Note that ICD-10 (Table 15.2, p. 475) allows only one code for withdrawal (there must be a use disorder, which can only be moderate or severe).

Russell Zahn Again

Russell is taken into custody a couple of days after his evaluation. A bored judge quickly agrees that he should remain incarcerated, then departs for the long Labor Day weekend.

Russell's first few hours in jail aren't too bad. That day and the next, he talks to a friendly guard and plays cribbage with his cellmate. But he sleeps fitfully, and by Sunday he is boisterous and agitated, hitting the bars of his cell with a spoon—which is about the only good he gets from his dinner tray. "I'm just not hungry, OK?" he snaps, as the guard removes the untouched meatloaf.

Russell lies awake nearly the entire night. He feels sweaty and has chills, headache, and a cramping abdominal pain that doubles him over on his bunk. "It's like the worst flu you ever imagined," he whines to the nurse practitioner making rounds even though it's a weekend. In response to his agitated complaint, he's checked with a touchless thermometer: no fever. Finding nothing physically wrong, the nurse practitioner tells the guard, "Just a pothead coming unglued. A couple of weeks will put him right."

Further Evaluation of Russell Zahn

Can we stipulate that Russell's experience with cannabis has been both long-lasting and heavy (criterion A for cannabis withdrawal)? Abruptly deprived of weed, Russell experiences nearly every criterion in the cannabis withdrawal list, including anger (B1), anxiety (B2), insomnia (B3), anorexia (B4), agitation (B5), and abdominal pain (B7)—certainly enough to provoke the distress required for diagnosis (C). We'll take the nurse practitioner's word that these aren't due to the flu or some other physical ailment (D).

The symptoms for cannabis withdrawal are a lot like those of withdrawal from other substances (alcohol, sedatives, stimulants, and tobacco), each of which we'll have to include on our list of differential diagnoses. But the history makes Russell's diagnosis crystal clear; to his previous use disorder symptoms, we will append withdrawal. With all that we've now learned, I'd upgrade his cannabis use disorder to a level of severe, regardless of how many symptoms we can count.

Russell's GAF score would be 50 (about his highest level in the past year). Using Table 15.2 (p. 475), we'd give Russell (no longer intoxicated) a diagnosis reflecting withdrawal and his use disorder. And somewhere in the summary I wrote up, I'd want to stress the importance of further investigating the possibility of a personality disorder. Right now, there's too little information and too much pot to allow any sort of reliable personality assessment.

F12.23	Severe cannabis use disorder, with withdrawal
Z59.01	Homeless, currently in jail
Z56.9	Unemployed
Z65.3	Repeated arrests

Other Cannabis-Induced Disorders

You will find a complete listing of cannabis-induced disorders in Table 15.2 (p. 475). Two possibilities deserve special mention:

Cannabis-induced psychotic disorder, with delusions. This disorder involves delusions that are often persecutory. It lasts only a day, several days at the most. In the United States, it is rare and most often encountered in juveniles. But in other countries and cultures (for example, some in West Africa), it may be more common. Most U.S. patients who have delusions associated with cannabis probably have other diagnoses as well, such as schizophrenia and drug–drug interactions.

Cannabis-induced anxiety disorder. See the case history of college student Bonita Ramirez in Chapter 4 (p. 193).

F12.99 Unspecified Cannabis-Related Disorder

Hallucinogen-Related Disorders

Also called *psychedelic* or *psychotomimetic* drugs, hallucinogens as a rule produce illusions, not hallucinations. From long usage, however, the misnomer has stuck. Two such drugs that occur naturally are psilocybin (obtained from certain mushrooms) and peyote (cactus, though probably not the one growing in a flower pot near your kitchen sink). On the other hand, phencyclidine (PCP) is a manufactured hallucinogen that has toxic effects similar to those that occur in cacti and 'shrooms. I also discuss lysergic acid diethylamide (LSD) and some others. (A withdrawal syndrome hasn't been established for this drug class, so the substance use criteria include only 10 criteria, not the customary 11.)

Phencyclidine

PCP used to be listed in its own separate section; since DSM-5, reason has prevailed, and it is now bundled in with the other hallucinogens—though the respective criteria for use disorder and intoxication remain distinct. Called *angel dust* on the street, PCP is a hallucinogen with both stimulant and depressant qualities. In its typical street dose of 5 mg, this highly potent substance produces psychotic symptoms so convincing that they are hard to distinguish from schizophrenia. A person with a genetic predisposition to schizophrenia who takes it risks activating serious pathology.

PCP was originally developed as an anesthetic agent; harmful side effects caused it to be scrapped for human use in the mid-20th century, and even its use in veterinary medicine has been halted. Its less potent analogue, ketamine, is used as an anesthetic agent and to treat severe depressive disorders. However, because PCP is cheap and easy to produce (it can be mixed up almost literally in a bathtub), it is still sometimes used by young people who value it for the euphoria it produces.

Despite lack of a withdrawal syndrome in humans, PCP's addictive potential is pronounced—as dangerous as that of cocaine and heroin, some say. When it is swallowed, symptoms begin within an hour; smoking reduces that to a few minutes. A high lasts from 4 to 6 hours and may be repeated in runs lasting several days.

The use of PCP is seemingly limited only by the user's resourcefulness—by snorting, by swallowing, or by injection. It can even be absorbed vaginally. However, it is typically smoked in cigarettes, which are preferred because the effects occur so quickly that the user can titrate them with some precision, perhaps averting emergency room visits for overdose.

PCP and ketamine are both used by relatively small numbers of individuals—especially by males in their teens and 20s.

LSD and Other Hallucinogens

The classic example of a manufactured hallucinogen is LSD, which in the 1960s was embraced as the first new mind-altering substance to be developed in generations. In the United States, legal manufacture of LSD has long since vanished; all supplies currently come from illicit labs, largely in northern California. Newer synthetics—MDA, MDMA (3,4-methylenedioxymethamphetamine, aka ecstasy), and others—continue to turn up. These are sometimes called "designer drugs" because they are created by tweaking their chemical structure. They thereby resemble the pharmacological properties of known hallucinogens but can, for a time, evade illegal status. Then, there are the venerable natural substances—mescaline, psilocybin, and lysergic acid amide (similar to LSD and found in morning glory seeds and elsewhere in nature)—each of which is generally a less potent hallucinogen than LSD or PCP.

During the past 20 years or more, LSD appears to have fallen out of fashion; it is now used by under 1% of college students. However, designer drugs (especially MDMA, which combines hallucinogenic and stimulant qualities; see sidebar, p. 461) may have increased in popularity. Most users consume other substances, as well. In many cases, drugs sold on the street are quite different from what is promised. Lacking a quality control ethic, vendors freely substitute cheap for dear, available for rare. Thus, for example, so-called psilocybin may in fact be ordinary mushrooms onto which some entrepreneur has sprayed LSD or PCP.

Tolerance to LSD occurs so rapidly that an individual will rarely use it more than once a week. More frequent use simply doesn't produce an effect worth the trouble. No withdrawal syndrome from LSD or other hallucinogens is defined, though some people reportedly crave them after stopping. MDMA is especially likely to produce a use disorder.

Because one hallmark of successive DSMs has been renaming disorders in the interests of greater descriptive accuracy, it is astonishing that the hallucinogens *still* retain their mendacious label. (I emphasize *still* because, 2 decades ago with DSM-IV, I was similarly appalled.) Typically, they do not produce hallucinations at all, but illusions; some writers have referred to them as illusionogens. There's been a movement afoot to replace the term *psychedelic* ("mind-manifesting") with *entheogen*, used to denote a substance that evokes a religious or spiritual effect. I don't think it has a prayer.

Phencyclidine Use Disorder and Other Hallucinogen Use Disorder

The characteristics of the use disorder for both PCP and other hallucinogens are nearly identical to those of every other substance use disorder in the manual. Except for the symptom of withdrawal, which doesn't appear to occur with most hallucinogens, the criteria are a straightforward adaptation of those for a generic substance use disorder (p. 404). I discuss them as they apply to the two vignettes that follow. Code numbers are given in Table 15.2 (p. 475).

Phencyclidine Intoxication

With much variability, the effects of PCP are related to dose. Besides euphoria, PCP can produce lethargy, anxiety, depression, delirium, and behavioral problems that include agitation, impulsivity, and assault. Even catatonic symptoms and suicide have been reported. Some users experience violent, exaggerated, unpredictable responses to light or sound; as a result, clinicians may recommend sensory restriction for intoxicated patients. Physical symptoms include high fever, muscle rigidity, muteness, and hypertension. Heavy doses can result in coma, convulsions, and death from respiratory arrest.

Essential Features of **Phencyclidine Intoxication**

Shortly after using PCP or something similar, the patient develops serious symptoms of behavioral disinhibition—impulsivity, hostility, agitation, aggression, poor judgment. With it, there are signs of neurological impairment and muscle dyscontrol: jerking eye movements called nystagmus, trouble walking or speaking, rigidity of muscles, numbness, coma, or seizures. Pulse rate and blood pressure can be high; some people become abnormally sensitive to loud noises.

The Fine Print

The D's: • Duration to onset of symptoms (within 1–2 hours) • Differential diagnosis **(physical disorders; intoxication from other substances; other mental disorders)** You can find the specifics of phencyclidine intoxication in Table 15.1 (p. 412).

Coding Notes

See Table 15.2 (p. 475) for codes.

Jennie Meyerson

At age 24, Jennie Meyerson has been troubled half her life. When she was 12, her father walked out on the family in the midst of the worst argument she can ever remember between her warring parents. The divorce preoccupied her mother and the aftermath drove Jennie's older sister from home, leaving Jennie pretty much on her own.

By the time she was 14, she had begun smoking marijuana after school—and sometimes between classes. Within a year, smoking had replaced classes. The morning she turned 18, her mother kicked her out of the house. Then she lived with a succession of boyfriends, each of whom introduced her to a new recreational drug. She has been in and out of mental hospitals and is a double alumna of the local Betty Ford clinic.

Jennie's latest interviewer is Reggie Polansky, a young police officer. One Saturday afternoon, he is called to the sixth floor of a run-down apartment building where a young woman is sitting on a ledge high above the street. The sweetish smell of marijuana smoke assails Polansky as he walks through the room to the window.

The ledge just outside the window is perhaps 10 inches wide. About a yard to his left sits Jennie, barefoot and bare-legged, wearing a cotton blouse and a thin skirt that flutters in the breeze. She sits quietly, her face tilted up to the late summer sunshine. On the pavement 80 feet below, a crowd has gathered.

Gripping the windowsill, Patrolman Polansky pokes his head out. "What are you doing out there?"

"Jes' ress—just res-ting." With effort, she finally pronounces the words. She doesn't open her eyes or turn her head. "I'm gonna fly."

"You don't want to do that. Come on back in here!"

"You c'mon out . . . here! I'm Amelia Earhart. We can both fly." Jennie giggles, and they converse for several minutes. OK, she's joking about being Amelia Earhart, but she does think she can learn to fly. It came to her in a flash this morning, after she "got dusted." She's been using angel dust off and on for the past several months, she tells him.

Patrolman Polansky points to her hand. The webbing of skin between her thumb and forefinger is bleeding. "You've cut yourself."

Jennie says she must have done it on the jagged window cornice as she was climbing out. Perhaps it's a message from God. That must be it, she says, because she hasn't felt it at all. It's like God's wounds. Instead of pain, she feels happy, strong, and light. She feels like practicing for the Labor Day air show on Monday.

"Look how close the ground is," she says. "It seems like I can just step down there." She stands, raises both arms, and steps lightly onto the wind.

Evaluation of Jennie Meyerson

Jennie's recent use of angel dust and badly affected judgment amply meet criteria A and B for phencyclidine intoxication. Of the physical symptoms required, two are documented in the vignette: trouble speaking (slurred speech—C5) and reduced pain perception (she hasn't noticed the torn skin of her hand—C3). Two are what's required.

Jennie also had an illusion (the ground looked close to her, rather than six stories down). Such perceptual distortions can also be the work of intoxication with other drugs, including stimulants, opioids, and cannabis. The odor in the room suggests marijuana to Patrolman Polansky; PCP users often spray their drug onto something they can smoke (marijuana or tobacco, sometimes parsley). When reliable information is lacking, a definitive diagnosis often depends on a toxicology report.

The vignette gives no information as to the extent of Jennie's problem with PCP, so we can't confirm a diagnosis of phencyclidine use disorder. The vignette clearly indicates that Jennie had, at a minimum, previous occupational (school) problems resulting from her use of a variety of substances. Further diagnosis would depend on additional information about her usage patterns within a 12-month period. All things considered, a *provisional* diagnosis of moderate to severe phencyclidine use disorder seems justified. Considering the outcome, I think that the severity code I've given is correct, regardless of how many symptoms we can conjure.

Jennie's statements that she can fly and that she has stigmata ("God's wounds") don't seem firmly held; I wouldn't consider them delusional. This would discount schizophrenia and any other psychosis. There is no evidence that her disorder is due to a physical illness (D). In other patients, rapid resolution (often without treatment) may help differentiate intoxication due to hallucinogens from other conditions such as mood and anxiety disorders. Hallucinogen users should also be evaluated for personality disorders and the use of other mind-altering substances.

Jennie's postmortem diagnosis would be as below. Of course, her GAF is nil, and we'll never have the chance to explore the possibility of a personality disorder.

F16.220   Severe phencyclidine use disorder (provisional), with
             phencyclidine intoxication

Other Hallucinogen Intoxication

The first symptoms of other hallucinogen intoxication are typically somatic. Patients may mention dizziness, tremor, weakness, or numbness and tingling of extremities. Perceptual changes (usually illusions) include the apparent amplification of sounds and visual distortions (such as of body image), as well as *synesthesias* (in which one type of sensory experience produces the sensation of another—for example, a professor I know of saw red, white, and blue upon hearing a C-E-G chord played on the piano).

Hallucinations, if they occur at all, may be of vivid geometric forms or colors. Auditory hallucinations can also occur. Many people experience intense euphoria, depersonalization (that is, a sense of detachment from oneself), derealization (a sense of unreality in one's perceptions), dreamlike states, or the impression that time speeds up or slows down. Attention may be impaired, though most users retain insight.

The specific features are greatly influenced by setting and by a person's expectations. Some users find the experience pleasant; others become extraordinarily anxious. A "bad trip" usually includes feelings of anxiety and depression; panic attacks may occur. These reactions will occasionally be prolonged, characterized by fears of becoming psychotic. Typically, acutely negative reactions subside within 24 hours—the time it takes to excrete all the drug.

LSD is an extremely potent agent; just a few micrograms (an amount that can be soaked onto a postage stamp) can produce significant symptoms. It is absorbed from the gut, and action begins within an hour. The effects tend to peak at 2–4 hours and may last half a day. Like PCP, LSD and other hallucinogens can be lethal.

Essential Features of **Other Hallucinogen Intoxication**

Shortly after using a non-PCP hallucinogen, the patient develops behavioral or psychological symptoms such as intense depression or anxiety, paranoid ideas, poor judgment, fears of insanity, and ideas of reference. Although fully awake and alert, there will be sensory changes such as colors appearing more intense, illusions, depersonalization/derealization, or hallucinations. There may even be synesthesias, in which a sensory stimulation produces an effect of a different sensory output—such as, ringing a bell causes the person to see colors. Finally, there will be physiological symptoms such as dilated pupils and blurred vision, sweating, rapid or irregular heartbeat, trembling, or poor coordination.

The Fine Print

The D's: • Duration until onset of symptoms (usually 1 hour or less) • Differential diagnosis (**other substance intoxication, other mental disorders, other medical conditions,** hallucinogen persisting perception disorder)
    You can find the specifics of other hallucinogen intoxication in Table 15.1 (p. 412).

Coding Notes

In recording your diagnosis, use the specific name, rather than *other hallucinogen*.
    See Table 15.2 (p. 475) for codes.

Wanda Pittsinger

She's 26, but Wanda Pittsinger still works at the cinema. She started there on a part-time basis in her last year of high school; after graduation, she moved to full time and stayed on. The pay is minimum wage, but making change and popcorn isn't demanding, and she gets to see a lot of first-run movies—though maybe not in start-to-finish order.

Wanda's job has lasted longer than her marriage. The year she was 22, she was married to Randy for almost 10 months. Other than a pregnancy, which she also terminated, the main thing she got from the relationship was an introduction to LSD. She still sees Randy occasionally, but by now they are not much more than friends; about the only activity they pursue together is tripping, which almost invariably wipes out their sex drive.

Wanda has tried other drugs. Marijuana gives her headaches; cocaine makes her nervous. The one time she snorted heroin, she threw up. But acid seems just about right. It always raises her spirits and makes her feel giddy. Apart from the colored shapes and change in the size of things, sometimes when she looks into a mirror, she seems to see herself melting. This doesn't bother her; you expect weird things to happen when you drop acid. She thinks that LSD can reveal new meanings or insights, and values that sensation of thinking deeply. The experience is almost always worth the palpitations and blurred vision that constitute her only side effects.

Acid even gives Wanda a better feeling about Randy. Occasionally she'll still trip with him on a day off, and he continues to supply her with the little squares of blotting paper impregnated with LSD. As a present, he once gave her two movie tickets that had been soaked in the stuff. She keeps them tucked into the corner of her dresser mirror.

Evaluation of Wanda Pittsinger

While using LSD, Wanda's psychological and behavioral changes are minor, with the pluses and minuses pretty much a wash. They help her tolerate Randy, but she loses interest in sex. One can argue whether these are clinically important—they aren't enough to get her into treatment, as a "bad trip" might (criterion B). But she has additional symptoms of other hallucinogen intoxication: She notes the usual side effects of blurred vision and palpitations of her heart (D5, D4). She also has some typical perceptual changes: illusions of lights, patterns, and shapes (C), and the sensation of possessing special insight. Moreover, she feels euphoric—another common experience with this drug.

The differential diagnosis of other hallucinogen intoxication includes delirium, neurocognitive disorder, epilepsy, and schizophrenia. Beyond her illusions, none of Wanda's symptoms suggest these disorders. However, her clinician would need a complete workup, including a mental status evaluation, to rule out other disorders. Hypnopompic imagery (visual imagery experienced when awakening) can take on the aspect of a flashback, but Wanda's illusory experiences occur at times when she is fully awake.

DSM-5-TR allows a diagnosis of other hallucinogen use disorder, but it is pretty rare. Like Wanda, most users take LSD infrequently; rapid tolerance (loss of effect) results from use more often than once or twice a week. There is no evidence that she has lost control over the use of this substance or that its use alters the way she approaches her job or social life.

OK, it's problematic whether Wanda qualifies for a diagnosis of other hallucinogen intoxication (F16.920). I'll give a fuller diagnosis a bit later.

F16.983 Hallucinogen Persisting Perception Disorder

We call it a *flashback* when a patient reexperiences some of the same symptoms as during intoxication—and the hallucinogen isn't currently present to provide a stimulus. Symptoms of flashback can include seeing faces, geometric forms, bursts of color, trails, afterimages, and halos; micropsia (in which things look small) and macropsia (they look huge) also occur. Was Alice having a flashback when she fell down the rabbit hole? Diminished interest in sex may be a feature. The patient usually retains insight into what is happening.

Flashbacks can be triggered by stress, by entering a dark room, or by using marijuana or phenothiazines. Although flashbacks that last but a few seconds are common—over half of hallucinogen users have them—only a small percentage report that they have enough of these symptoms to be distressing or to interfere with their activities. These experiences tend to decrease with time; however, they can occur weeks or months after use and persist for years.

Essential Features of **Hallucinogen Persisting Perception Disorder**

After stopping the use of a hallucinogen, the patient again experiences at least one of the misperceptions that occurred during intoxication.

The Fine Print

The D's: • Duration to symptom onset (variable) • Distress or disability (work/educational, social, or personal impairment) • Differential diagnosis (**physical disorders, delirium, other mental disorders, hypnopompic imagery**)
   You can find the specifics of hallucinogen intoxication in Table 15.1 (p. 412).

Coding Notes

See Table 15.2 (p. 475) for codes.

Wanda Pittsinger Again

Wanda comes for help because she sometimes finds herself tripping when she hasn't dropped acid for several days.

"I noticed it one night at work when I walked into the auditorium just before the main feature. I saw my own face on the screen, first all in green, and then rather sparkly. Then my image seemed to sort of dissolve, and I saw that it was only a trailer for a Woody Allen film that was scheduled in 2 weeks."

When Wanda told Randy about this the next day, he called it a flashback and said that it was "cool." Despite Randy's reassurance, these experiences worry her. She has stayed home from work for a day or two, because she feels she can't cope with the flashbacks *and* with her job. She hasn't used drugs of any sort since.

In the nearly 2 months since she last used LSD, Wanda has experienced several flashbacks. Mostly she sees "trails"—spooky afterimages of people or objects that ghost across her field of vision. A couple of times she has seen Randy's face on the ceiling of her bedroom. Once the kitchen table seemed to grow so high that she thought she'd never be able to reach it to eat her breakfast. But never again has she viewed her own image on the silver screen.

Further Evaluation of Wanda Pittsinger

Though the details had changed, when Wanda walked into the darkened theater on the occasion that eventually triggered her clinic visit, she experienced a recurrence of the illusions she had had during LSD intoxication (criterion A). Flashbacks of some degree or other are common; perhaps one-quarter of LSD users have them. Wanda's wouldn't qualify for a diagnosis at all if they hadn't upset her so (B).

As in hallucinogen intoxication, Wanda's clinician must rule out delirium, neurocognitive disorder, schizophrenia, epilepsy, and space-occupying lesions in the brain (C). She won't qualify for a diagnosis of hallucinogen-induced psychotic disorder because she has insight that her misperceptions are caused by substance use. The previous history of LSD use and the typical presentation make secure her current diagnosis. Her GAF score would be 70.

F16.983   Hallucinogen persisting perception disorder

Note that the description of hallucinogen persisting perception disorder doesn't distinguish it all that sharply from substance-induced psychotic disorder. Indeed, the principal bulwark separating the two is the verbiage asserting that flashbacks must be neither due to another medical condition nor better explained by another mental disorder. The requirement, like so many others, invokes your judgment as the clinician; your decision must rest on the patient's degree of insight and the history of substance use. The criteria won't help you a lot here; you'll need to depend on your diligent evaluation.

Other Phencyclidine-Induced or Hallucinogen-Induced Disorders

You will find a listing of PCP-induced and other hallucinogen-induced disorders in Table 15.2 (p. 475). Here are several that merit special mention:

Hallucinogen-induced mood disorder. Depression or anxiety is relatively common; euphoria is rare. Sleep is often decreased. Patients may be restless and experience feelings of guilt. They may express fear that they have destroyed their brains or gone crazy. Hallucinogen-induced mood disorder may last relatively briefly, or it may endure for months.

Hallucinogen-induced personality change. Chronic or one-time use may lead to character change, such as the development of magical thinking or a basic change in attitude.

Hallucinogen-induced persisting psychosis. Occasionally a hallucinogen seems to trigger a psychosis that may last a long time, perhaps forever. There has been a good deal of controversy over whether this is "only" an underlying psychosis that might eventually have developed, even if the patient had never used drugs.

F16.99 Unspecified Phencyclidine-Related or Hallucinogen-Related Disorder

Inhalant-Related Disorders

Accidentally inhaled, a volatile hydrocarbon-based substance is called a toxin; used on purpose to produce intoxication, it's an *inhalant*. Intentional users will breathe almost anything that evaporates or can be sprayed from a container. Inhalants include glue and gasoline (which are perhaps the most popular), solvents, thinners, various aerosols, typewriter correction fluid, and refrigerants. Preference may be guided more by availability than by effect.

Users value inhalants for several reasons. They relieve boredom and concern. They alter ideas, moods, the sense of time, and perceptions (producing changes in color, size, or shape of objects, and sometimes frank hallucinations). Inhalants are also cheap and, like everything else that is absorbed through the lungs, quick to take effect.

Neurological damage from prolonged use of inhalants is quite variable. Encephalopathy and peripheral neuropathy are widely experienced. Also, there can be ataxia, symptoms of parkinsonism, loss of vision, and involvement of the fifth and seventh cranial nerves, producing numbness and paralysis of the face. Chronic users may experience weight loss, weakness, disorientation, inattentiveness, and loss of coordination. Death, while rare, can result when a patient uses a bag or mask that excludes oxygen from the mixture being breathed. Fetal malformations are another potential complication of use.

Three groups of patients use inhalants. Boys and girls experiment with them, often as a group activity; the incidence peaks at around age 14, though popularity has been declining through the first years of the 21st century. Adults (mostly men) can become dependent on them. Finally, they are used by individuals who are also chronic users of other drugs. Many inhalant users come from underprivileged social groups. Personality disorders, especially antisocial personality disorder, are common among inhalant users.

Let's see, nitrous oxide aka laughing gas. That term was coined by Sir Humphry Davy, a British chemist who in 1800 noted that it promotes anesthesia and the giggles. Curiously, although nitrous oxide can produce intoxication and is inhaled, it isn't classified as an inhalant. That's apparently because someone decided an inhalant must be carbon-based, which kicks nitrous off the bus. (ICD-11, which looms in the near future, does include nitrous oxide among the inhalants.) But to classify a patient who has problem with nitrous oxide in DSM-5-TR, you must use the "other (or unknown) substances" categories. Me?—I'd've just tweaked the definition of inhalant and called it a day.

Inhalant Use Disorder

The characteristics of inhalant use disorder are like those of nearly every other substance use disorder. They are identical to the generic criteria (p. 404), except that, as with the hallucinogens, you won't find withdrawal among the symptoms of inhalant use disorder. (OK, there may be some mild withdrawal symptoms, but DSM-5-TR doesn't consider them serious enough to list withdrawal as a criterion.) Score according to the usual rules (see Table 15.2, p. 475).

DSM-5-TR notes that it's sometimes not possible to determine exactly which volatile hydrocarbon is responsible for inhalant use disorder; then you can use the general term *inhalant use disorder*. Of course, if the principal volatile component of, say, glue is toluene, you'd go with *toluene use disorder*. Nitrous oxide and any of the nitrites (amyl, butyl, isobutyl) are considered other (or unknown) substances, and a use disorder involving any of these is coded accordingly.

Inhalant use disorder is uncommon, even among the primary user group: teenage boys. It tends to remit spontaneously, giving way to other substances and various other mental disorders. And of course, for some the end stage is death from a breathing-related calamity.

Inhalant Intoxication

People with inhalant intoxication are rarely found in emergency rooms or medical offices (though they're occasionally encountered in morgues). Many of their symptoms are similar to those experienced by people with alcohol intoxication. Early symptoms include drowsiness, agitation, lightheadedness, and disinhibition. Later on, ataxia, disorientation, and dizziness may develop. More severe intoxication produces insomnia, weakness, trouble speaking, disruptive behavior and, occasionally, hallucinations. After a period of sleep, a user will often feel lethargic and hungover. Probably, just about anyone who's used inhalants very much has at some time experienced intoxication.

Toluene, a widely used solvent, is a principal component of many of the substances abused. It is associated with headache, high mood, giddiness, and cerebellar ataxia (irregular, uncoordinated movements often accompanied by poor balance, walking with feet wide apart, and staggering). Small doses may yield fatigue, headache, inhibited reflexes, and tingling sensations.

Inhalants are usually absorbed by *bagging* or by *huffing*. When bagging, people spray, squeeze, or pour the contents into a bag from which they can inhale the vapors. They huff by breathing through substance-soaked rags placed into their mouths. Either method can evoke a high that lasts for hours.

When you evaluate someone you suspect of using inhalants, be sure to ask carefully about all other substance classes. The use of multiple substances is common in these patients, whose symptoms may be due in part to the use of alcohol, cannabis, hallucinogens, or tobacco. The only sure way to determine what a patient has been using is chemical analysis for substances in the patient's blood or urine.

Essential Features of **Inhalant Intoxication**

Upon inhaling a chemical substance, the person experiences such emotional or behavioral symptoms as poor judgment, hostility, aggression, apathy, or other behavior changes. In addition, to a clinically important degree there will be various other symptoms, such as unsteady walking, euphoria, dizziness, slow or weak reflexes, trembling, weakness, blurred or double vision, drowsiness, poor motor coordination, stupor or coma, jerking eye movements called nystagmus, unclear speech, psychomotor retardation.

The Fine Print

The D's: • Duration to onset (within moments) • Differential diagnosis (**physical disorders, other mental disorders, intoxication with other substances**)

You can find the specifics of inhalant intoxication in Table 15.1 (p. 412).

Coding Notes

See Table 15.2 (p. 475) for codes.

Dudley Langenegger

From the age of 12, Dudley Langenegger had been in trouble for running away, for breaking and entering, and for something he didn't understand called "incorrigibility." Days before his 18th birthday, the judge gave him a choice: "Jail or the military." Now he's been in the Army for 6 months, long enough to finish basic training.

Even when he is clean and sober, which is far from the rule, Dudley is never a model soldier. Often insolent, he only complies enough to spend most of his weekends confined to base rather than the stockade. When his unit boards a ship for its joint operation with the Navy, Dudley goes along.

So, apparently, do several tubes of model airplane cement. At least, that's what Dudley says he was huffing in the galley at midnight. As he tells his story, he requires several sharp commands and at least one good shaking from the first sergeant to keep him from wandering off the subject or falling asleep. His breath smells like a paint shop.

For about 3 years, Dudley has been inhaling various vapors, mainly organic solvents. Where he grew up, a lot of the guys do this; the stuff is easy to get, cheap, even legal. He admits that the issue of legality doesn't weigh heavily, but cost and ease of acquisition are key.

Airplane glue produces a quick, reliable high; Dudley likes it because it raises his mood and makes long hours seem to flash by. Tonight, he's having his own private party. Everyone else has gone to bed, and he wants to boost himself out of the low mood he's been in. It works so well that he thinks it might be a good idea to throw pots and pans around in the galley, which is how the military police find him.

The sea is calm as they escort Dudley to the brig, but he stumbles, sways, and almost falls onto the bunk. He rubs his eyes, which are already brick red. He seems to be trying to determine where he is. "It can't be the barracks," he says with a giggle, "there's no Playmate posters on the wall."

"I never use it more than once or twice a week," he explains with another giggle. "Too musha stays vits s'posed, uh, bad for your brain."

Evaluation of Dudley Langenegger

As a result of sniffing glue, Dudley has the bad judgment (criterion B) to cause a commotion in the galley; the inopportune giggling suggests maladaptive emotional changes. In addition to the obvious ill timing of his drug use, he has several physical symptoms of inhalant intoxication. These include slurred speech (C4), lethargy (his first sergeant had to keep him awake during the interview—C6), and poor coordination (C3). The giggling would suggest euphoria (C13), but we'd want a direct question about his mood to be sure. His eyes are irritated, and he smells of solvents. (A physical examination might well reveal nystagmus and depressed reflexes as well; however, only two of these numerous symptoms are required for a diagnosis.)

The differential diagnosis includes use of other drugs such as alcohol; the history is usually sufficient to discriminate these causes, and the odor of glue on Dudley's breath is a dead giveaway. Various neurological conditions (such as multiple sclerosis) also require ruling out (D).

Dudley comes close to fulfilling criteria for inhalant intoxication delirium. When apprehended and interviewed, he is obviously less than fully alert and cannot sustain attention without a lot of direction. He is also disoriented (he doesn't know where he is), and he can't speak clearly. However, we'll only diagnose delirium if his impairment lasts longer than expected for an intoxication and if it requires independent clinical attention.

Does Dudley qualify for a diagnosis of inhalant use disorder? That judgment requires some extrapolation. Huffing has certainly interfered with Dudley's work (substance use disorder criterion A4), but there is little direct evidence for other criteria. His problems with fights, poor work performance, and the legal system might be related to his use of inhalants, but they could also be attributed to a personality disorder. (There isn't enough information for any of those diagnoses, either. The possibility should be explored later.) No one seems to have thought to ask him whether he craves inhalants. Although we might infer a strong desire to use them from his behavior, it remains just that: an inference, not evidence. He has continued to use these drugs despite evidence of psychological or physical problems, but does he know this? Again, we can only infer, as we would with the question of how much time he spends obtaining and using inhalants.

All in all, the farthest I'd go is to call Dudley's a provisional case of inhalant use disorder. After all, the criteria are meant to guide, not impede us as we navigate the diagnostic shoals. Dudley's 3-year history, with attendant difficulties, would seem enough to sustain the diagnosis. With too few definite criteria nailed down, however, I'd call it of moderate intensity—and interview him hard, once he's improved, for more information. I'd note in the case summary that I could make no diagnosis of a personality disorder, but that he had antisocial personality traits. He's also had some symptoms suggestive of conduct disorder, but they'll require further exploration, too.

If we knew that toluene, for example, is the solvent used in the airplane glue, we'd use that word in the diagnosis (toluene intoxication). We don't, so Dudley's full diagnosis (with a GAF score of 40) is as follows:

F18.220   Moderate inhalant use disorder (provisional), with inhalant intoxication
Z65.3   Arrested by MPs

Other Inhalant-Induced Disorders

You will find a complete listing of inhalant-induced disorders in Table 15.2 (p. 475).

F18.99 Unspecified Inhalant-Related Disorder

Opioid-Related Disorders

Years ago, opioids were the most feared of the mind-altering substances. For a time, cocaine assumed that distinction, but now the scourge of oxycodone (notoriously, Oxycontin) and other synthetic opioids are back in the lead. And in terms of human wastage and criminal activity, opioids remain among the costliest of illegal drugs. Users can spend several hundred dollars a day on their habits, mostly obtained through criminal activity. Of the opioid drugs, heroin, once the worst of a bad lot, has often taken second place to oxycodone in terms of usage and consequent physical harm.

Heroin has several times the power of morphine to produce euphoria and to blunt the perception of pain, to the point that users become indifferent to pain. And fentanyl has about 50 times the power of heroin. Carfentanyl, legally sold to tranquilize elephants and other huge animals, is more powerful still.

Some users, especially those who are middle-class and middle-aged, may start to abuse opioids during medical treatment. Ready access to drugs places health care professionals at special risk for opioid use. However, most problematic users begin in their teens or 20s because of peer pressure. Opioid use is generally preceded by the use of other drugs, such as alcohol or marijuana. In this group, risk factors for opioid use include low socioeconomic status, residence in an urban area, divorced parents, and relatives who abuse alcohol.

Opioid users value their drugs because of the high, which they experience as euphoria and diminished concern for the present. First-time opioid users, on the other hand, often experience vomiting and dysphoria. But some degree of tolerance to any opioid drug develops within the first few doses; then the lives of users quickly become dominated by the pursuit and consumption of the drug. It remains unclear why some people exposed to narcotics become addicted and others do not. Once hooked, however, users may go to nearly any length to obtain drugs. They will steal, lie, plead, and promise you just about anything in the world.

Overall, there is about a 4% lifetime prevalence of opioid use (mostly prescription opioids) in the adult population, with rates falling off in older age groups. Actual use disorder is nearly an order of magnitude less. Males outnumber females by about 3:2. Even after detoxification, once opioid users return to familiar environments, many begin to use again—typically within 3 months. The risk of death (especially from overdose) runs 6–20 times that of the general population. Of those who live long enough, a substantial number eventually shake off their addiction.

Most users of heroin inject the drug intravenously, and half or more of these users test positive for HIV or hepatitis C. These are important considerations for clinicians who work with this population. Needle marks indicate the injection of heroin or "speedballs" (mixed heroin and cocaine). From all sources (overdose, violence, and associated illness), the overall mortality among active heroin users approaches 2% per year. And synthetics such as fentanyl now account for nearly three-quarters of all opioid deaths.

Some writers interpret the fact that users of hard drugs often begin with alcohol and marijuana as denoting what they call a "gateway effect," meaning that the latter drugs lead to opioid addiction. That conclusion might be correct, but after years of research, no one yet is sure whether it is. It is still entirely possible that some hereditary or environmental precursor leads to a variety of behaviors, including the use of alcohol, marijuana, and opioids.

Opioid Use Disorder

The characteristics of this disorder are similar to those of all other specific substance use disorders. For its features, see those for a generic substance use disorder (p. 404); I've provided details of coding in Table 15.2 (p. 475).

Opioid Intoxication

When an opioid drug is injected, its effects are felt almost immediately. This "rush," which has been compared to an orgasm, is rapidly followed by euphoria, drowsiness, the perception of warmth, dry mouth, and heaviness in the extremities. Some users experience a flushed face and itching nose. In contrast to cocaine intoxication, violence is rare during opioid intoxication.

Opioid intoxication can sometimes be confused with sedative or alcohol intoxication. The typical presence of extremely constricted (pinpoint) pupils can help make the distinction; however, in severe (perhaps lethal) overdose, pupils can dilate. Once again, a urine or blood test may be necessary to differentiate among the various possible causes of an individual's symptoms.

Although opioid users often become tolerant to enormous quantities, overdose with opioids is always a medical emergency. It can produce clouding of consciousness (including coma), severe respiratory depression, shock, and ultimately death from anoxia. Opioid overdose can be treated effectively with intravenous naloxone, a potent opioid antagonist.

People who use opioid drugs often wear dark glasses. Sometimes this is a cultural fashion statement; some do it to hide their constricted pupils. When you interview opioid users, ask them to remove dark glasses. Other physical stigmata of opioid use include scarring of the arms and of just about any other location where a vein is prominent enough to inject drugs. The subcutaneous route of administration, called "skin popping," is a last resort for those who have already destroyed their accessible veins thorough years of needle use.

Essential Features of Opioid Intoxication

Shortly after using an opioid, the patient experiences mood changes such as dysphoria or elation followed by apathy, increased or reduced psychomotor activity, or poor judgment. Then come constricted "pinpoint" pupils (or dilated pupils, if in severe overdose) plus evidence of impaired functioning: lethargy (or even coma), unclear speech, wandering attention, or poor memory.

The Fine Print

The D's: • Differential diagnosis (**physical illness, other mental disorders,** including **another substance intoxication**)

You can find the specifics of opioid intoxication in Table 15.1 (p. 412).

Coding Notes

Specify if: **With perceptual disturbances.** The patient experiences hallucinations, during which insight is retained, or illusions. This unusual state must be discriminated from delirium. Coding in ICD-10 depends on the presence of perceptual disturbances; see Table 15.2 (p. 475).

Herm Cry

Herm Cry is admitted to the detox unit 24 hours after he last shot up. The junk was good-quality—he knows, because afterward he slept nearly 8 hours. But then he awakens to the all-too-familiar aching muscles and runny nose that tell him it is time to go out and earn his next fix. He's had no regular job for at least a year, but he knows some ways of getting money that don't involve the inconvenience of a paycheck.

At a young age, Herm became familiar with the symptoms of withdrawal. His father's drinking was well known in their working-class St. Louis neighborhood. By the time he was 10, Herm had watched his father suffer through at least two episodes of DTs. Alcohol never did much for Herm. He doesn't care for the taste, and he certainly doesn't need the hangover. His mother, a public health nurse, has had her own problems with Demerol.

Off and on since he was 12, Herm has smoked marijuana. But it wasn't until a neighborhood block party the night he turned 16 that he first snorted heroin. "All of a sudden," he tells his most recent clinician, "I knew I'd found the way."

Within a few minutes, Herm felt happier than ever before in his life. It was as if a warm bath had drained away all the anger, depression, and anxiety he had ever contained. For a few hours, he even forgot how much he hated his old man. All he had left was an overwhelming sense of tranquility that gradually gave way to drowsy apathy. The following day, using a sterile syringe he stole from his mother, Herm injected heroin for the first time. Almost immediately, he vomited; this was followed at once by a sense of pleasure that seemed to race through his limbs to the tips of his fingers and toes. Rubbing his itching nose, he fell asleep. When he aroused himself, several hours had passed. He injected again, using a smaller quantity of the drug (all he had left). When he awakened this time, he briefly considered stopping. His next thought was the realization that, more than anything else he could remember, he wanted to use heroin again.

Evaluation of Herm Cry

The sense of tranquility and peace that Herm experienced (opioid intoxication criterion B) after injecting heroin (A) is what causes people to return to the drug after the first time, even if it has made them sick. Of course, after they have used it for a few days, they no longer need a positive reason; simply avoiding the curse of withdrawal is motivation enough to continue. That's what makes even euphoria "clinically problematic," as noted in the criteria.

Herm also has at least one typical neurological aftereffect of opioid intoxication: profound drowsiness that lasts for several hours after injecting (intoxication—C1). (The runny nose and aching muscles are symptoms of the impending withdrawal. See the next vignette, which continues Herm's story.)

Criterion C also requires pinpoint pupils, which are sometimes so pronounced that the person cannot see clearly. Patients are unlikely to complain about this feature, so the diagnosis of opioid intoxication requires us to observe it. Assuming that Herm had constricted pupils and that no other mental disorder or physical illness better explained his symptoms (D), criteria for opioid intoxication would be fulfilled.

Most opioid users meet criteria for a comorbid mental disorder. These include mood disorders (up to 75%), alcohol-related disorders (about 30%), antisocial personality disorder (25%), and the anxiety disorders (12%). Up to 13% of opioid users attempt suicide—small wonder, considering their predicament.

Because there is very little material in this first vignette pertaining to the issue of personality disorder, we'd have to defer that diagnosis for Herm. I'd phrase my note in the summary to alert future clinicians to the possibility, while trying not to prejudice them as to its nature. He would also seem a likely candidate for problems with the legal system, but the first vignette includes no such evidence.

Although we already have evidence of craving, much of the material that would qualify Herm for a diagnosis of opioid use disorder is contained in the next vignette. So at this point, for coding purposes, we'll pretend he has no use disorder. With no perceptual disturbances (see Table 15.2, p. 475), his diagnosis would be simply this:

F11.920   Opioid intoxication

Opioid Withdrawal

Although some symptoms of opioid withdrawal may appear after a very few doses, it takes a week or two of continuous use to produce the typical withdrawal syndrome. Opioid withdrawal strongly resembles a flu-like viral illness: nausea and vomiting, dysphoria, muscle aches and pains, watery eyes and runny nose, fever, and diarrhea. Another symptom of autonomic nervous system activation that occurs during withdrawal is *piloerection:* small hairs stand up, producing "goose flesh." This is the origin of the phrase "going cold turkey."

How rapidly symptoms of withdrawal appear depends principally on which drug is used; consult a reference on opioids or search the Internet for information about the half-lives of specific drugs. Even after most of the symptoms have abated, some patients may suffer a protracted abstinence syndrome, characterized by anxiety and low self-esteem, that can last as long as 5 or 6 months. Perhaps 60% of heroin users will at some time experience withdrawal.

Essential Features of **Opioid Withdrawal**

After cutting back from several weeks of heavy opioid use, the patient develops characteristic symptoms of rebound excitation—they include dysphoria, nausea/vomiting, diarrhea, aching muscles, tearing (runny nose), yawning, fever, sleeplessness, and autonomic symptoms such as dilated pupils, and (less frequent) sweating and piloerection.

The Fine Print

If withdrawal is induced by administering an opioid antagonist such as naloxone, signs and symptoms will begin within minutes.

The D's: • Duration to symptom onset (within several days) • Distress or disability (work, social, or personal impairment) • Differential diagnosis (**physical illness, other mental disorders, withdrawal from other substances**)

You can find the specifics of opioid withdrawal in Table 15.1 (p. 412).

Coding Notes

See Table 15.2 (p. 475) for codes.

Herm Cry Again

Sixteen hours after his last fix, Herm still hasn't scored. His usual suppliers have refused to extend credit. He tries to borrow money from his mother, but she refuses, and the earrings he liberated from her dresser have proven worthless. Although the abdominal cramps are worsening and he feels nauseated, he manages to make it to the apartment of a former girlfriend for whom he had briefly pimped. But she has just shot up the last of her own stash and is asleep. He appropriates her used syringe for his own use later, in case he scores.

Ducking into a restroom in the bus station, Herm narrowly avoids the disastrous consequences of explosive diarrhea. As he is about to emerge from the stall, he suddenly retches into the grimy toilet bowl. He sits down on the cool tile floor and tries to rub away the goose flesh on his arm, then dabs at his runny nose with a bit of toilet paper. He is too weak, he realizes, to hustle. He will have to enter detox for a few days, until he feels stronger.

Then he can go out and acquire what he really needs to get well.

Further Evaluation of Herm Cry

Herm awakened to muscle cramps and a runny nose—typical early symptoms (criteria B3, B4) of opioid withdrawal. As the day progresses and he cannot obtain more heroin (A1), he develops gastrointestinal symptoms of vomiting and diarrhea (B2, B6). He has goose flesh (B5), and by the time he's admitted, a clinician could probably find dilated pupils (B6). (Just three symptoms from criterion B are needed for a diagnosis of withdrawal.)

Based on Herm's symptoms related in the two vignettes, now we can talk about opioid use disorder. Of course, he suffers from withdrawal (substance use disorder criterion A11). Herm's most notable behavioral symptom is the impairment in his functioning (for a year or more, he has forsaken work for criminal activities—A7). He spends a great deal of time trying to obtain heroin (A3), and he has had no job for a year or more (A6), in part because his drug habit fully occupies his time. Craving for the drug is almost universal in addicted individuals who have, like Herm, suddenly stopped using (A4); we've noted it in the first vignette. He may meet other criteria for opioid use disorder as well, such as tolerance and attempts to quit, but these are not addressed in the vignette. Even so, I think we can agree that, in all probability, Herm is severely dependent. Table 15.2 (p. 475) spells out the coding for ICD-10. Because it is the main reason for Herm's entering treatment, opioid withdrawal is listed first in his diagnostic summary.

Herm's personality diagnosis would not change. He has several characteristics (thievery and pimping) of antisocial personality disorder, but we don't know that these ever occur outside the context of his substance use. However, ASPD is well represented among other users of opioids. I'd give him a GAF score of 55.

F11.23   Severe opioid use disorder, with withdrawal

Other Opioid-Induced Disorders

You will find a complete listing of opioid-related disorders in Table 15.2 (p. 475).

Sedative-, Hypnotic-, or Anxiolytic-Related Disorders

Sedatives, hypnotics, and anxiolytics are prescribed for different purposes but share many features. Those most relevant to mental health are the symptoms of intoxication and withdrawal they have in common. The terms applied to these substances are somewhat confusing, and not always precisely used. A *sedative* is anything that reduces excitement and induces quiet without producing drowsiness. A *hypnotic* helps the patient get to sleep and stay there. And an *anxiolytic* is one that, well, reduces anxiety. Depending on dose, however, most of the drugs discussed in this section can have any of these actions.

The major drug classes covered in this section are the benzodiazepines, such as diazepam (Valium) and alprazolam (Xanax), and the barbiturates, such as pentobarbital (Nembutal); other classes include the carbamates (such as meprobamate, once notorious as Miltown) and some other barbiturate-like hypnotics. Users value the barbiturates and benzodiazepines for the disinhibition they produce, which means that they induce euphoria, reduce anxiety and guilt, and boost self-confidence and energy. There are two main patterns of abuse, which can be summarized roughly as follows.

Some people get started with a prescription obtained to combat the effects of insomnia or anxiety. Then, to varying degrees, they increase the dose. Although they would probably have withdrawal symptoms if they abruptly stopped using the drug, many of these people would never meet the behavioral criteria for a generic substance use disorder (p. 404). They may not even recognize, or admit to, cravings.

A more frequent route to misuse occurs when (mainly young) people employ these drugs to produce euphoria. This is the history we classically associate with the misuse of most of these substances. In the past, this has been especially true of the use of barbiturates and specialty drugs such as methaqualone and glutethimide. In recent years, however, the legitimate manufacture of these drugs has been either greatly curtailed (barbiturates) or banned altogether (methaqualone). Physicians' prescribing practices have also changed. Government regulation has been an important catalyst for these changes.

Only infrequently are benzodiazepines the primary substances misused, but they are often employed to mitigate the undesired effects of other drugs—for example, to calm the jitters induced by central nervous system stimulants. Benzodiazepines are also sometimes employed to boost the high of methadone or to ease the symptoms of opioid withdrawal. In the early 2000s, use during the previous year of sedatives and tranquilizers was about 3 out of 1,000 persons in the general population. The benzodiazepines preferred by users are diazepam, alprazolam, and lorazepam; users will pay premium prices to be sure they are getting the real thing. Other than those with substance use disorder, mental health patients have a very low rate of abusing, say, benzodiazepines.

Sedative, Hypnotic, or Anxiolytic Use Disorder

The characteristics of this disorder are similar to those of other specific substance use disorders. The criteria are those for a generic substance use disorder (p. 404). Note, however, that when a drug is prescribed for medical purposes, tolerance and withdrawal are not to be used as symptoms of a use disorder. See Table 15.2 (p. 475) for coding.

Sedative, Hypnotic, or Anxiolytic Intoxication

As with most drugs, the effects achieved using sedatives, hypnotics, or anxiolytics depend strongly on the setting where they are consumed and the expectations of those who use them. Mood is often labile, with case reports ranging from euphoria to hostility and depression. Loss of memory like that occurring in heavy alcohol consumption has also been reported with flunitrazepam (Rohypnol), notorious as the "date rape" drug. Other common effects include unsteady gait, slurred speech, nystagmus, poor judgment, and drowsiness. In very high doses, these drugs produce respiratory depression, coma, and death, though these outcomes are far more likely with barbiturates than with the benzodiazepines. DSM-5-TR criteria are nearly identical to those for alcohol intoxication.

Essential Features of **Sedative, Hypnotic, or Anxiolytic Intoxication**

Shortly after using a sedative, hypnotic, or anxiolytic drug, the patient becomes disinhibited psychologically or behaviorally (such as rapid mood shifts, sexual or physical aggression, impaired judgment). There is also evidence of neurological impairment (imbalance or wobbly gait, unclear speech, poor coordination, jerking eye movements called nystagmus, stupor or coma, or diminished memory or attention span).

The Fine Print

The D's: • Differential diagnosis (**physical illness, intoxication with a different substance** (alcohol), **other mental disorders,** cognitive disorders)

You can find the specifics of sedative, hypnotic, or anxiolytic intoxication in Table 15.1 (p. 412).

Coding Notes

See Table 15.2 (p. 475) for codes.

Kirk Aufderheide

When the forklift load of galvanized iron pipe crushed his pelvis, Kirk Aufderheide promised himself that he would never complain about anything else again, if only he could regain the use of his legs. Four months later, on the day he hobbles out of the hospital using an aluminum walker, he begins trying to fulfill that promise. But he hasn't reckoned on the muscle spasms.

Despite the insulin-dependent diabetes he's lived with for 15 years, Kirk considers himself a healthy 35-year-old. His only previous hospitalization was for febrile convulsions as a child. The combination of his diabetes and a strict religious upbringing have helped him avoid street drugs, alcohol, and tobacco. Until his accident, he prided himself on never taking so much as an aspirin.

But the muscle spasms change all that. They've probably been there ever since the accident, but Kirk didn't notice them until the first day he was allowed out of bed. Thereafter, any time he is up and about, he is likely to be seized with excruciating cramps in his lower back. Reluctantly, he accepts a prescription for diazepam. A 5-mg tablet four times a day, his doctor assures him, will help relax the spasms.

Miraculously, it works. For nearly 2 weeks Kirk can move around in relative comfort, if not pain-free. When the spasms return and his doctor tells him that 20 mg a day is the maximum he should take, he seeks out another doctor. Within months, Kirk is seeing four physicians and taking between 60 and 80 mg of diazepam every day. He visits one doctor under an assumed name (where Kirk lives, the prescription of benzodiazepines is tightly controlled). Physicians three and four work across the state line, just a few miles from his house. A fifth doctor notices his low mood and warns him not to take too much of the drug; it's the last time Kirk sees that physician.

What with waiting for his appointments and driving to distant pharmacies, Kirk occupies hours each week just obtaining his supply. Much of the balance of his time— he hasn't yet returned to work, so he stays home and keeps house for his wife and two daughters—he spends in front of the television set; he recalls little of what he watches. His wife complains that he has changed: He's moody, and he seems unable to follow the thread of a conversation.

Evaluation of Kirk Aufderheide

Kirk's wife describes him as moody, which is the sort of psychological change you'd expect from diazepam intoxication (criterion B). He has an unsteady gait and poor memory (for the television he watches), two of the symptoms specific for intoxication (C3, C5); the diagnosis requires only one.

Although the present criteria are almost exactly those for alcohol intoxication, historical information and the absence of alcohol smell on the breath can help discriminate (D). Kirk has no history to implicate alcohol. However, a different patient might need a blood test to identify which was being used.

Does Kirk qualify for a diagnosis of diazepam use disorder? His degree of tolerance (substance use disorder criterion B9) causes him to take four times the maximum dose recommended—far more than any one of his physicians would prescribe. He spends considerable time traveling to four different doctors and pharmacies to obtain his supply (B3). He also continues to use diazepam, even though one physician says that high doses could harm him (B8).

With a GAF score of 25, Kirk's diagnosis at this point would be as follows:

F13.220	Moderate diazepam use disorder, with intoxication
Z87.828	Fracture (crush) of pelvis, healed
E10.9	Type 1 diabetes without complications
Z56.9	Unemployed

Sedative, Hypnotic, or Anxiolytic Withdrawal

When a patient stops using or markedly reduces the high dose of a sedative/hypnotic drug, the result is much like the abrupt cessation of alcohol use; indeed, the criteria for withdrawal are nearly identical for the two classes of substance. (In this context, a high dose means several times the therapeutic dose—for example, 60 mg or more of diazepam.) However, the time course will vary with the half-life of the drug. You can read a pharmacology text or Google the specific drug for information about its half-life.

One diagnostic challenge is to distinguish withdrawal symptoms from the reemergence of those symptoms that led to treatment in the first place (anxiety, agitation, and insomnia play a prominent role in each). The time course can help: Any symptoms that remain (or appear) 2–3 weeks after the drug has been discontinued are probably old symptoms reemerging.

Essential Features of **Sedative, Hypnotic, or Anxiolytic Withdrawal**

After lengthy use of a sedative, hypnotic, or anxiolytic drug, the patient suddenly stops using or markedly reduces intake. Within hours to days, this yields symptoms of increased nervous system and motor activity such as trembling, sweating, nausea/

vomiting, rapid heartbeat, agitation, sleeplessness, anxiety, short-lived hallucinations or illusions, convulsions.

The Fine Print

The D's: • Duration to onset (a few hours to several days) • Distress or disability (work/ educational, social, or personal impairment) • Differential diagnosis (**physical illness, other mental disorders, intoxication** or **withdrawal from alcohol,** essential tremor, delirium)

Specify if: **With perceptual disturbances.** The patient has auditory, tactile, or visual illusions without delirium or hallucinations with intact insight (that is, realization that the perceptual symptoms are unreal and caused by the substance use).

You can find the specifics of sedative, hypnotic, or anxiolytic withdrawal in Table 15.1 (p. 412).

Kirk Aufderheide Again

Four days short of the first anniversary of his accident, Kirk's wife receives notice that she is being transferred to a branch office in the interior of the state. The family has to move. At their new location, Kirk encounters tighter controls on the prescription of benzodiazepines, coupled with far fewer compliant physicians and pharmacies. Once they settle into their new home, he realizes that he has no choice but to reduce his intake of diazepam.

Although Kirk intends to taper his usage, he puts it off until he has nearly run out. So, on a warm summer morning he finds himself suddenly facing the prospect of taking only 4 tablets; the day before, he downed 16. At first, he is surprised at how little it bothers him. For several days he experiences insomnia, but he expected that. (With no job to go to, he's had time to read some magazine articles about the effects of substance use.)

But at 4 A.M. on the third day, Kirk awakens to a sense of anxiety that borders on panic. He feels nauseated and his pulse is racing. For 2 days his agitation mounts, to the point that he cannot even sit still long enough to eat the meal he has prepared. On the fifth day, his wife arrives home to find him having a grand mal seizure.

Further Evaluation of Kirk Aufderheide

With a marked decrease in intake of diazepam (criterion A), Kirk notes some of the classic withdrawal symptoms (two are required): racing pulse, insomnia, and nausea (B1, B3, B4). (Diazepam's relatively long half-life means that it can take quite some time—up to a week—for withdrawal symptoms to develop.) Childhood febrile seizures might have made him more susceptible to withdrawal seizures. Kirk's occur within a few days (B8)—the fate of perhaps a quarter of people who abruptly withdraw from these substances. The fact of his impairment goes almost without saying (C).

Anxiety and panic attacks commonly occur as rebound phenomena; therefore, anxiety disorders form an important part of the differential diagnosis (D). When hallucinations occur during withdrawal, they can be mistaken for a manic episode or various psychotic disorders. Delirium is also a relatively common complication. Antisocial personality disorder is often encountered among patients who obtain these medications illegally.

Kirk has no illusions or hallucinations that would qualify for the specifier of *with perceptual disturbances*. Because the seizure was the focus of treatment on admission, I've listed it first. The rest of his diagnosis remains as it was before.

R56.9	Withdrawal seizure
F13.230	Moderate diazepam use disorder, with withdrawal, without perceptual disturbances

Other Sedative-, Hypnotic-, or Anxiolytic-Induced Disorders

You will find a complete listing of these disorders in Table 15.2 (p. 475). I'll briefly mention one of these:

Sedative, hypnotic, or anxiolytic withdrawal delirium. Any delirium will usually occur within a week of the patient's discontinuing a drug. Like delirium due to other causes, it features reduced attention span and problems with orientation, memory, perception (visual, auditory, or tactile hallucinations or illusions), or language disturbance. It is typically preceded by insomnia.

F13.99 Unspecified Sedative-, Hypnotic-, or Anxiolytic-Related Disorder

Stimulant-Related Disorders

Stimulants (sometimes called psychostimulants) affect mental or physical functioning, or both. For example, these drugs typically enhance—at least for a time—alertness, mood, and activity levels. Worldwide, some stimulants are used by prescription to ameliorate the effects of both mental and physical disorders. In addition, many are used, and misused, recreationally. Although caffeine is also a stimulant, it occupies its own niche among psychoactive drugs and is considered elsewhere.

DSM-5-TR mentions two main types of stimulants: amphetamines and cocaine. These two drug classes occupied separate sections in editions prior to DSM-5, though their symptoms for intoxication and withdrawal are identical. Now, with commendable logic, they have been combined. Still, their patterns of use are different enough that

I've continued to provide two sets of vignettes as illustrations. Oh, yeah, and they retain their separate numbers—for all substance-related health problems.

Amphetamines and Related Compounds

Abusers value amphetamines (the international spelling is amfetamines) for the euphoria, appetite suppression, and increase in energy they provide. Although many people begin amphetamine use by snorting, blood vessel constriction in the nose makes absorption unpredictable, so other routes are sought. Smoking or injection produces a rapid effect, such that binge users take the drug repeatedly for half a day to 2–3 days. Effects of the drug fall off rapidly as tolerance develops. It is almost inevitable that a period of nonuse will occur, during which users remember how "wonderful" the drug is (that's the euphoria talking) and want more. This institutes a cycle of use and withdrawal that will last about 10 days.

Amphetamine users tend to look sleep-deprived and anorectic. Physical signs include circles under the eyes, poor hygiene, and dry, itchy skin that is prone to acnelike lesions. Users who inject can get vasoconstriction at the site, with dead patches of skin. Those who inhale may develop nosebleeds, even a perforated nasal septum. Toxic symptoms include chest pain, palpitations, and shortness of breath.

For decades after they were first synthesized in 1887, no regulations limited amphetamine use. Through the middle years of the 20th century, it was commonplace to see them recommended for weight control, depression, and nasal stuffiness; they were widely abused in the 1960s and into the 1970s. More recently, tight controls and changing prescription practices have greatly reduced their availability. Virtually their only legitimate uses now are to treat obesity, narcolepsy, some depressive disorders, and attention-deficit/hyperactivity disorder.

Amphetamines are sometimes used intermittently at relatively modest doses by truckers, students, and others (mostly young men) who want something beyond caffeine to keep them awake. Some use these drugs to produce euphoria, often leading to "speed runs" that can last for weeks. These runs may produce episodes of delirium and, when the supply runs out, "crashes." Some people use stimulants to counterbalance the effects of sedatives and other drugs of abuse.

Only about 2% of emergency room drug-related visits are due to amphetamines and their ilk. The prevalence of use among high-school-age youngsters is around 2 per 1,000—close to that for cocaine. Some data suggest that those dependent on amphetamines may stop using them after a decade or so. The substances related to amphetamine that are available by prescription include methamphetamine (Desoxyn), dextroamphetamine (Dexedrine), amphetamine combinations (Adderall), diethylopropion (Tenuate), and methylphenidate (Ritalin). Illicit methamphetamine can be synthesized in small batches, but much of the product available in the United States is made in laboratories, either domestic or Mexican.

Ecstasy (MDMA) has structural similarities to both amphetamines and mescaline, one of the hallucinogens, and its effects are both stimulant and mildly psychedelic. It's been around for over a hundred years; nearly 4% of Americans have tried it. Rarely used every day, its typical use occurs at "raves" and in other social situations. Although it has a terrible reputation for causing physical harm and addiction, it rates somewhere near the lower end of the scale, according to a study published in *The Lancet* in 2007.

Cocaine

Cocaine now fills a good part of the niche once occupied by amphetamines. The effects of cocaine are nearly identical to those of amphetamines, but its half-life in the body is much briefer. Toxic symptoms therefore are of briefer duration than for amphetamines. All of this may explain cocaine's greater appeal and addicting power. With a short half-life, cocaine creates powerful craving; use occurs more frequently than with amphetamines. The symptoms of severe intoxication include convulsions, heartbeat irregularities, high fever, and death. Paranoid thinking can increase as the binge goes on. Delusions (often of plots against or attack upon the user) are usually self-limited and brief—a matter of hours. Perceptual distortions occur, but actual hallucinations are rare.

Cocaine that has been heated with bicarbonate yields a white lump that is not destroyed by heating. It produces a popping sound when smoked, hence the name crack. The availability of crack accounted for much of the rise in cocaine use during the latter part of the 20th century; however, the number of users may have declined somewhat early in the 21st century.

Most users of cocaine begin by taking it intermittently but will rapidly progress to runs similar to those of amphetamines. Because almost no tolerance to cocaine develops, runs can continue for several days, though a day or less is more usual. Addiction to crack cocaine occurs after just a few weeks.

Note that the cross-sectional evaluation may not adequately discriminate patients who use cocaine from those who use amphetamines or related drugs. Even history can be unreliable: What is sold on the streets often doesn't match what's advertised. Even the more reliable suppliers have little control over impurities or contaminants. The only sure way to determine what substance a patient is using is to obtain a urine or blood specimen for toxicology.

Long out of fashion after a brief spurt of popularity in the early 1900s, cocaine enjoyed a resurgence during the 1970s when the U.S. government clamped down on the manufacture and distribution of amphetamines. Since then, plummeting cost and rising availability have made it, behind marijuana, the second most frequently used illicit drug in the United States and worldwide. In recent years, about a quarter of drug-related visits to emergency rooms have been due to cocaine. Men more than women tend to be afflicted by this scourge, which is concentrated among younger people (age 15–34). Users have four to eight times the expected mortality of their nonusing peers.

Khât

An African plant called khât contains an alkaloid, cathinone, which breaks down into ephedrine, a central nervous system stimulant with a variety of medical uses. Indigenous people (in Yemen, for example) chew the leaves for the effect of euphoria and excitement, similar to a strong brew of coffee. A mild withdrawal syndrome can occur. Khât ranks near the bottom of the stimulants for physical harm and addiction potential, though mild psychoses and hypomanic states have been reported. DSM-5-TR includes this in the other and unknown section of the manual; I think it belongs with the stimulants. In the end, perhaps it doesn't matter that much—it's only a number. Just describe the patient well.

"Bath Salts"

Relatively new are so-called "bath salts," often marketed "not for human consumption" to evade state and federal drug laws. These compounds, variously named and sold online or in head shops as an alternative to cocaine, often contain a version of cathinone that's been chemically fiddled with. The powerful inhibition of monoamine reuptake leads to a variety of physical and mental symptoms—delirium, hallucinations, paranoid delusions, agitation, rapid heartbeat, blood pressure elevation, fever, and seizures. Withdrawal may produce profound craving; overdose can mean death. Users tend to be male and relatively young (20s). Since 2012, bath salts have been illegal in the United States.

Stimulant Use Disorder

The characteristics of stimulant use disorder are like those of nearly every other specific substance use disorder. The criteria are those for a generic substance use disorder (p. 404). I've listed the coding in Table 15.2 (p. 475). But you probably know that by now.

Stimulant Intoxication

DSM-5-TR has mashed together amphetamine and cocaine use syndromes, but there are enough differences that they deserve to be discussed separately. The Essential Features of intoxication and withdrawal are the same for both, however.

Essential Features of **Stimulant Intoxication**

Shortly after using a stimulant drug, the patient exhibits altered behavior (stereotypies, hypervigilance) and symptoms of mood/affect (anger, anxiety, euphoria or depression, blunted affect) as well as impairment in judgment or psychosocial functioning (increased or decreased sociability). There will also be physical and neurological changes: lowered or raised blood pressure, heart rate, and motor activity; dilated pupils; chills or sweating; nausea/vomiting; evident weight loss; and muscle weakness, chest pain, respiratory depression, or irregular heartbeat. And finally, there can be confusion, convulsions, coma, dyskinesia (lost control of voluntary muscles), or dystonia (muscle cramping or spasms).

The Fine Print

The D's: • Duration to onset of symptoms (within minutes) • Differential diagnosis (**physical illness, other mental disorders** including other causes of intoxication)
    You can find the specifics of stimulant intoxication in Table 15.1 (p. 412).

Coding Notes

Specify if: **With perceptual disturbances.** Auditory, tactile, or visual illusions or hallucinations with intact insight (the patient recognizes that the symptoms are unreal, caused by the substance use). Hallucinations without insight suggest a diagnosis of stimulant-induced psychotic disorder.
    When recording, specify the stimulant by name.
    Coding depends on the presence of perceptual disturbances; see Table 15.2 (p. 475).

Amphetamine Intoxication

Amphetamine injection leads rapidly to feelings of euphoria, confidence, and well-being. Users experience a "rush" of energy and euphoria; they find their own thoughts profound, and their sexual interest picks up. However, they pay the price of anorexia and agitation. When the intoxication is severe, they become confused and their speech rambles.

    With extended use, the person may begin to withdraw from other people and focus on obtaining and using drugs. Hallucinations (auditory, or perhaps haptic—bugs crawling on the skin—or paranoid ideas) can develop; violence can ensue. Some people adopt stereotyped behaviors: ritualistic reenactments of things they ordinarily enjoy, such as assembling and dismantling electronic equipment. Any of these syndromes can resemble schizophrenia, but the alert clinician will focus on the longitudinal history as obtained from informants. Laboratory studies help confirm the toxic origins of the behavior.

Freeman Cooke

"I was hyperactive when I was a child," says Freeman Cooke to the interviewer. "My mother used to give me coffee to slow me down."

Moving restlessly around the office, Freeman looks as if he's just had several cups too many. He has already twice excused himself to the bathroom, where he nearly vomits. The nurse who checks him notes that his blood pressure is high, and that his pulse is racing along at 132 beats per minute. He admits that he snorted a half gram of "crystal meth" not long before coming to the clinic.

Freeman is the oldest of four children. His mother was an unhappy, nervous woman who always seemed unwell. His father made good money as a finish carpenter, but his appetite for vodka grew as his family expanded. When still a child, Freeman promised himself that he would avoid alcohol and treat his wife, if he ever had one, with more respect than his father had done. He managed to keep half his promise. After completing high school, Freeman got married and obtained a job as a helper with a long-distance moving company. The pay is good, but the hours are awful.

When he and his boss are on the road, they sometimes work 18 hours straight. Like many truckers, he uses dextroamphetamine to pep him up and keep him awake. At first, he took them only when he was working. When he came home from a 10-day trip, he would "crash and burn," sometimes sleeping for 20 hours at a stretch. But by the time he had enough seniority and experience to buy his own rig, he was using amphetamines recreationally, too.

Freeman started snorting powdered methamphetamine ("meth"), but he soon switched to smoking because it gave him a better "flash." When high, he feels insanely happy, tireless, and powerful. "Like I could lift a grand piano, all by myself," he explains. Then, he also likes to indulge his talent for argument; he will sometimes keep his wife up late at night with a tirade about matters that the next day even he finds trivial. After a few hours, as the effect of the high begins to wear off and only the memory remains, he feels driven to smoke meth again and again. But with each use during a run, it takes more of the drug to produce the flash. Eventually, either his supply or his constitution gives out, and he will once again crash. When he struggles back to consciousness, he is often astonished at how much of the stuff he has consumed.

When Freeman awakens after an unusually memorable 2-day run, he finds a note from his wife: She is leaving him. For the first time, he realizes how exactly like his father he has become.

Evaluation of Freeman Cooke

Like all other types of substance intoxication, stimulant intoxication must be documented with marked, detrimental behavioral or psychological changes (criterion B). For Freeman, that will be easy: His recent use (A) has led to arguments with his wife, culminating in her departure. Of the physical signs and symptoms (two required), he has elevated pulse and blood pressure (C1, C3) as well as agitation and nausea (C7, C5). At evaluation, he had no hallucinations or illusions that would qualify for the perceptual disturbances specifier.

Freeman also qualifies for a diagnosis of amphetamine use disorder. Requiring more of the drug to achieve a high on successive occasions of use, he clearly experiences tolerance (stimulant use disorder criterion A10). He sometimes uses more methamphetamine than he intends (A1), and he spends lots of time and energy using and recovering from the effects (A3). I base my judgment that his use pattern is severe partly on evidence of amphetamine withdrawal (A11), discussed below, though I would also claim clinician's privilege in asserting that he is seriously dependent. I'd give him a GAF score of 55.

F15.220	Severe methamphetamine use disorder, with intoxication
Z63.0	Separated from wife

Cocaine Intoxication

Cocaine is probably the strongest pharmacological reinforcer yet devised. Laboratory animals will choose it in preference to food, water, and sex; given free access, they will use it again and again until they die.

Humans ingest it by snorting, injecting, or smoking. Smoking crack can produce a rush of euphoria and a feeling of well-being that begins within seconds. The user feels alert and self-confident and has increased sexual desire. These positive feelings last for a few minutes, then give way to dysphoria (anxiety, depression, fatigue) and an intense craving for more of the drug. With continuing use, the euphoric effects lessen, and the dysphoria takes over. Motivation bends to a single goal: obtaining more cocaine.

Behavioral changes associated with cocaine intoxication include aggression and agitation, often leading to fighting and hypervigilance. Cocaine postpones fatigue, and the resulting increase in energy breeds impaired judgment and an increased willingness to take risks. Violence and crime are frequent products of the cocaine-intoxicated state.

Mental symptoms include delusions, feelings of omnipotence, ideas of reference (beliefs that external events have a special meaning unique to oneself), and tactile hallucinations. Other symptoms include irritability, increased sensory awareness, anorexia, insomnia, and spontaneous ejaculation. If the intoxication is severe, there may be rambling speech, perplexity, anxiety, headache, and palpitations of the heart.

Amanda Brandt

Since her graduation from college at age 22, Amanda Brandt has worked as a futures trader on the Chicago Stock Exchange. It is a fast-paced, high-pressure life, and she loves it. "I was an economics major in college," she explains, "and what can you do with that? Teach?"

Futures trading exactly suits Amanda's temperament. Since early high school she has been energetic and outgoing. Her job introduces her to a lot of young people who are as bright and well paid as she.

Amanda's father is a Baptist minister; he and her mother are both teetotalers. Though both of her grandfathers are long dead, Amanda thinks they suffered from alcoholism, which she supposes might have something to do with her parents' attitude toward alcohol. "I'm sure they didn't dream I smoked pot in college," she says. "But it never seemed to bother me, and it was the social thing to do."

What's social in her corner of the Exchange, she soon discovers, is cocaine. She and her fellow traders earn more than enough money to afford quantities of the powdery stuff, though perhaps not as much as they use. The advent of crack brought a price decrease, and Amanda's use has soared. She's always hated the pain of needles; snorting seems gross, so she's learned to smoke it.

"Within a few seconds of lighting up, you feel—what's better than wonderful? It's like a total body climax," she says. "I feel like even my lungs are coming."

The rush of the intense high blasts her with a pleasure that obliterates any concern she might have about the agitation and pounding heartbeat. For 15 minutes or so, she knows she's incalculably witty; she loves and controls the world. While she orbits, she doesn't need people, sex, food, water—not even air. For that quarter of an hour, she feels she could live forever.

Evaluation of Amanda Brandt

Amanda's use of cocaine produces profound behavioral and psychological changes, including alterations in her judgment and social life (criterion B). She thinks that the pleasure produced by the drug is worth its side effects—in her case, rapid heartbeat and a sense of agitation (C1, C7). An outside observer would probably notice other symptoms of acute intoxication mentioned in the criteria, but two suffice for diagnosis. Her subjective sensations give some inkling of why people become addicted to cocaine.

Besides amphetamine intoxication (the symptoms are of course the same as for cocaine), some of the other mental disorders that feature hyperactivity or mood instability should be considered, such as bipolar I disorder. Physical illnesses such as hyperthyroidism are of course a priority in the differential diagnosis. Phencyclidine intoxication can involve perceptual distortions similar to cocaine intoxication. Patients who become psychotic or delirious when intoxicated must be discriminated from those with schizophrenia and other psychotic disorders, and from delirium due to various medical conditions (D).

We'll have a fuller diagnosis later, but from the information given in this vignette, Amanda's principal diagnosis now is:

F14.920   Cocaine intoxication

Stimulant Withdrawal

As with intoxication, the Essential Features of amphetamine and cocaine withdrawal are identical, so I've given them only once.

Essential Features of **Stimulant Withdrawal**

After lengthy use of a stimulant, the patient suddenly stops or markedly reduces the intake. This yields symptoms of dysphoria plus evidence of physiological changes: intense dreams, sleep and motor activity that can be either increased or decreased; feeling hungry, feeling tired.

The Fine Print

The D's: • Duration to onset of symptoms (hours to a few days) • Distress or disability (work/educational, social, or personal impairment) • Differential diagnosis (**physical illness, other mental disorders,** including **intoxication** or **withdrawal from other substances**)

You can find the specifics of stimulant withdrawal in Table 15.1 (p. 412).

Coding Notes

Name the specific stimulant responsible for the withdrawal with the code.

See Table 15.2 (p. 475) for codes.

Amphetamine Withdrawal

A few hours after the last use of amphetamines, there comes the crash: agitation, anxiety, depression, and exhaustion. The user experiences an intense craving that may later wane in the face of oncoming depression, fatigue, and insomnia (which is accompanied by the ironic craving for sleep). Still later, voracious appetite may develop. The fatigue and apathy worsen in the 12 hours to 4 days following the crash; some symptoms can last 7–10 days or even longer. Suicide attempts may result. In short, the user becomes a patient.

Freeman Cooke Again

When he checks into detox, Freeman is still wired from the last half gram of meth he smoked this morning. Coming off a 2-day binge, he knows from experience that if he is going to do something about his habit, he must take the plunge when he's still intoxicated. If he waits until he crashes, he won't do anything but sleep. Then he'll start looking for drugs again.

Freeman declines lunch and is playing cards with three other patients at a table in the corner of the day room when he feels himself beginning to slip. He notes, almost with amusement, that he's like an old, wind-up turntable, running slower every moment. With each hand, it's harder to play the cards; they might have been made of lead. Suddenly, he is overwhelmed with depression so profound that, tired as he is, he has to try to escape. His body aches for some speed.

Back in his room, he starts to pack his few possessions. When the gym bag is half full, he puts it aside and collapses onto the bed. He realizes that he utterly lacks the energy to go out and hustle. The drug craving gradually gives way to the need for sleep, but his eyes remain resolutely open. He is doomed to lie there for hours, paralyzed by fatigue but locked in wakefulness. It's going to be a long night.

Further Evaluation of Freeman Cooke

After he stops ingesting amphetamines (stimulant withdrawal criterion A), Freeman rapidly becomes depressed (B). He also suffers from fatigue (B1), psychomotor slowing (B5), and insomnia (B3), even though he badly wants to sleep. This more than fulfills the two symptoms required. His typical, profound craving for speed is not a criterion for stimulant withdrawal, though it is for stimulant use disorder.

The differential diagnosis of Freeman's condition includes bipolar I disorder (because of his fluctuating moods) and other substance-induced disorders, such as cocaine withdrawal and phencyclidine intoxication. Patients who develop psychosis during intoxication may be mistakenly diagnosed as having a schizophreniform disorder or some other psychotic disorder. None of these must better explain his symptoms (D). That, together with the misery his symptoms cause him (C), fully qualify Freeman for the diagnosis of stimulant withdrawal.

Even after most of the acute effects of withdrawal have dissipated, mood symptoms can last for weeks or months. If that happens to Freeman, I'd consider a diagnosis of methamphetamine-induced mood disorder.

Now we can exchange Freeman's previous diagnosis for the following:

F15.23   Severe methamphetamine use disorder, with methamphetamine withdrawal

Cocaine Withdrawal

After the acute intoxication phase, blood cocaine levels drop rapidly. Unless more drug is immediately consumed, a rapid crash into depression occurs. The patient may also experience irritability, suicidal ideas, fatigue, loss of interest, and a decreased ability to experience pleasure. Panic attacks are common; the need for cocaine is intense. Most of these symptoms will tend to increase for 2–4 days, then abate, but the depression can linger for months. Suicide attempts are fairly common; some of them succeed.

About half of those who have problems with cocaine use also have mood disorders, often bipolar or cyclothymic. This sets them quite apart from individuals with opioid-related disorders.

Amanda Brandt Again

In the aftermath of her intoxication, Amanda dies—or so it seems, as she feels suddenly, incurably depressed. The supreme self-confidence she enjoyed moments ago is shoved aside by an anxious uncertainty that over the next day or two will gradually overwhelm her. The only remedy is to smoke another lump of crack, then another, and another, until her supply runs out. Then she will be left sleepless and exhausted, while every cell in her body remembers exactly how exhilarating it feels to be high—and craves to experience it again.

By her fourth year on the Exchange, Amanda's life is unraveling. Compared to the importance of using cocaine, work now seems irrelevant. She calls in sick for several days in a row; when she does go in, her mind is focused on when and how she can score her next vial of crack. When she is finally fired, she moves to a smaller apartment and sells her BMW. Now that she can devote all of her time to obtaining and using crack, it requires just 2 months to smoke her life savings and the proceeds from selling what she owns.

It is her final binge that brings Amanda to treatment. After smoking her last pipeful, she roams the hallway in her apartment building, weeping and knocking on doors. When anyone answers, she tries to push her way in. Someone calls the police, who take her to the emergency room. There she becomes enraged and strikes out with her fists. Ultimately, she is restrained and admitted to a mental health inpatient unit.

Further Evaluation of Amanda Brandt

Amanda's history makes it painfully clear that cocaine is the source of her disorder. When she runs out of it (criterion A), she shows (by weeping and anxiety) the requisite dysphoria and several of the physical symptoms listed in the criteria: insomnia, fatigue, and speeded-up psychomotor activity (B3, B1, B5). For any withdrawal syndrome to be diagnosed by DSM-5-TR criteria, it must produce marked distress or greatly affect the patient's life (C); no one conforms to this more closely than Amanda. Not included in the criteria, but typical nonetheless, are her eidetic memory for the crack experience and her crushing desire for more.

At this point, we have enough information to give Amanda another substance-related diagnosis: cocaine use disorder. She spends nearly all of her time (substance use disorder criterion A3) satisfying her craving (A4) for crack cocaine, which has consumed her car and her job (A7). Already tolerant to the drug (A10), she finally develops withdrawal symptoms (A11).

Several other cocaine-related disorders are listed in DSM-5-TR. Some of these occur frequently; others, not so much. If Amanda's depression persists substantially longer than the period of withdrawal, cocaine-induced mood disorder might be added to her list.

Other patients may have associated mental conditions, such as gambling disorder, antisocial personality disorder, and posttraumatic stress disorder. With a GAF score of 35 and her extensive history, I'm going to rate Amanda as severely ill; you can count up symptoms—if you wish.

F14.23	Severe cocaine use disorder, with withdrawal
Z56.9	Unemployed

Other Stimulant-Induced Disorders

You will find a complete listing of amphetamine-related disorders in Table 15.2 (p. 475); some are described more fully at other points in this book. I'll briefly mention three here:

Stimulant-induced psychotic disorder, with delusions. These patients often, though not always, develop paranoia with ideas of reference and well-formed delusions. Their awareness of the environment is accentuated. They may watch other people closely and later "notice" that others are watching them. They may also overreact to any perception of movement; some hallucinate. The delusions can last a week or longer. When well developed, this disorder may resemble schizophrenia in all but the time course.

Stimulant-induced psychotic disorder, with hallucinations. Patients with this type of psychotic disorder may scratch excessively if they think they see bugs crawling on their skin.

Stimulant intoxication delirium. Some users experience an agitated delirium associated with intoxication. They may perform remarkable feats of strength; their wild, irrational behavior occasionally results in someone's severe injury or death.

F15.99 or F14.99 Unspecified Stimulant-Related Disorder

The coding depends on whether the substance is related to amphetamines (or similar drugs, F15) or to cocaine (F14).

Tobacco-Related Disorders

Because tens of millions of Americans are dependent on tobacco, the potential for withdrawal problems is enormous. Owing in part to the intense craving tobacco induces, it has been called the most widely used addictive drug in the United States. (And percentagewise, fewer Americans—about 20% of adults—smoke than is the case for citizens of most other countries.) Men outnumber women perhaps 3:2. Each year, tobacco is responsible for 5 million deaths worldwide; that's at least 60 times greater than for heroin.

It is hard to find clear evidence of primary reinforcers for tobacco. That is, its chemical effects do not include the direct production of euphoria, elevated self-esteem, or the enhancement of energy—the effects so valued by those who use, say, cocaine or opioids. Rather, tobacco produces nausea, vomiting, and anxiety, especially in the novice smoker. (Although it has been reported to reduce anxiety, this is probably the effect of "curing" the user's tobacco withdrawal.) So why do people smoke? In a nutshell, social factors get them started, and then they are hooked.

In 2013 it was reported that people with mental illness are 70% more likely to smoke than are those without. There is a strong positive correlation between addiction to tobacco and alcoholism, schizophrenia, and other mental disorders. When you interview mental health patients, always ask about tobacco use.

Like caffeine, tobacco is legal, easy to obtain, and cheap (well, relative to heroin). Most people can use it without interfering in any material way with their other, non-substance-related pursuits. But in a single year, they may repeatedly try to stop, suffer from withdrawal symptoms, and eventually return to smoking despite the knowledge that they are courting a cardiovascular catastrophe.

Look, I *know* it's actually nicotine that people are hooked on. And that's what the DSMs called it—nicotine-related disorders—up to 2013. The change was made because it's tobacco, with its tars and nitrosamines, that are actually causing the physical harm. With the advent of vaping, people can easily develop a nicotine habit without touching a cigarette or can of chewing tobacco or snuff. However, though *we* know the name of the responsible substance, this time we'll just go with the flow.

Tobacco Use Disorder

The characteristics of tobacco use disorder are similar to those of other specific substance use disorders. The criteria are those for a generic substance use disorder (p. 404), and coding is given in Table 15.2 (p. 475).

F17.203 Tobacco Withdrawal

Someone who is withdrawing from tobacco often complains most bitterly not of the specific symptoms listed in these criteria, but of yearning for a cigarette. This persistent craving can overwhelm the ability to focus on other, more substantive (but less pressing) issues. The result is a moody, anxious person who sleeps poorly and eats too much, knowing that everything could be fixed by one dose of a perfectly legal substance that is being used every day by over a billion people worldwide. No wonder these folks are irritable! Onset of withdrawal symptoms occurs within a day of last use and is often detectable within a few hours. Withdrawal will occur in about half those who stop using.

I've provided no separate case vignette for tobacco withdrawal. However, Hoyle Garner (Chapter 11) had a sleep disorder due to chronic obstructive pulmonary disease that was caused by smoking. He was also diagnosed as having tobacco use disorder and had at one time experienced tobacco withdrawal. His story begins on page 308.

Essential Features of **Tobacco Withdrawal**

After daily use for several weeks or more, the person suddenly stops or markedly reduces regular tobacco use. This yields multiple symptoms of crankiness (irritability, anger, easy frustration), anxiety, depression, restlessness, trouble concentrating, problems with sleep, and hunger.

The Fine Print

The D's: • Duration to onset of symptoms (within 24 hours) • Distress or disability (work/educational, social, or personal impairment) • Differential diagnosis (**physical illness, other mental disorders** that include **other substance intoxication** and **withdrawal**)

You can find the specifics of tobacco withdrawal in Table 15.1 (p. 412).

Other Tobacco-Induced Disorders

The other tobacco-induced disorders are listed in Table 15.2 (p. 475).

F17.209 Unspecified Tobacco-Related Disorder

Other (or Unknown) Substance-Related Disorders

The category of other (or unknown) substance-related disorders covers disorders linked to substances not included in the groups already described in this chapter. The generic criteria for substance use disorder (p. 404), substance intoxication (p. 419), and substance withdrawal (p. 410) given earlier, and the criteria for substance-induced disorders described in other chapters (example: substance-induced bipolar disorder) are applied here when appropriate.

Here are some examples of the substances that could be included in this category:

Anabolic steroids. The value to users of the anabolic steroids derives from athletic ability and perceived enhanced physical attractiveness. For body builders and other athletes, this desire can be a powerful motivator to use these drugs. Besides the obvious effects on the physique, users report euphoria, increased libido, and at times aggression (so-called 'roid rage). Steroid use has been implicated in the killing of 16 civilian Afghanis by U.S. Army Sergeant Robert Bales in 2012—but then, so has the antimalaria drug mefloquine. Anabolic steroids are often used in a social context, and this use may continue unabated for months or years. Like other substances of misuse, people take them longer than initially desired, cannot stop, spend excessive time using or trying to get them, and use them even though they know they cause harm—factors that will be familiar to anyone who has read the generic criteria for a substance use disorder. Cessation can also cause withdrawal symptoms, such as depression, fatigue, restlessness, insomnia, loss of appetite, and reduced interest in sex. Some users develop an intense drug craving.

Nitrous oxide. Nitrous oxide is an anesthetic inhalant that produces lightheadedness and mild euphoria; hence its ancient nickname, "laughing gas." It is used as a propellant in cans of whipped cream and cooking sprays—except when it is employed to produce a high. Then it can result in a degree of depersonalization/derealization and dizziness, with some distortion of sound. First used recreationally late in the 18th century, it may be the world's oldest artificially produced substance of abuse. I've already ranted about its exclusion from the inhalant drugs (p. 444).

Over-the-counter/prescription drugs. Over-the-counter and prescription drugs that can result in addiction include antiparkinsonian drugs, cortisone and its derivatives, antihistamines, and others.

Betel nut. People in many cultures (Bloody Mary in *South Pacific*) chew betel nut to achieve a mild high or sensation of floating.

Kava. Made from a pepper plant that grows in the South Pacific, kava causes sedation and loss of coordination and weight.

Other (or Unknown) Substance Use Disorder or Intoxication or Withdrawal

Symptoms of other (or unknown) substance use disorder, intoxication, and withdrawal are identical to those described for generic substances. Coding is given in Table 15.2 (p. 475).

F19.99 Unspecified Other (or Unknown) Substance-Related Disorder

Recording and Coding Substance-Related Disorders

OK, Table 15.2 is *really* fussy. You can just accept the fuss, or you could instead try to understand this stuff as it's printed in DSM-5-TR. But that way lies madness. The table encompasses most of what occupies 42 pages in DSM-5-TR. It can help you a lot, but you'll have to devote some time to it.

Follow through some of the examples given. Read over the footnotes so you understand that the numbers in parentheses have different meanings, depending on which column they are in. It may also help to remember that in these directions and in this table, "use" is a noun, not a verb.

We can utilize Table 15.2 to code three sorts of problems:

A. Substance use disorder

B. Substance intoxication or withdrawal

C. Substance-induced mental disorder

Note that "B" and "C" depend on first knowing whether there is a use disorder, and what its severity is; that makes determining the presence or absence of "use disorder" the first order of business. (The criteria are listed on p. 404.)

If your patient has substance use disorder, intoxication, or withdrawal, but no additional substance-induced mental disorder, code from one of the first three columns ("Just use; no I or W," "Intoxication," and "Withdrawal") as follows:

A. For substance use disorder (with no intoxication or withdrawal and no associated mental disorder)

   1. Determine the substance and write down the F number. For alcohol (as an example), that would be F10.

   2. For *current* substance use that is either mild or moderate/severe, select the appropriate row just under the F number. Now read across one column to the "Just use; no I or W" column. Write down the first decimal you encounter, the one with no parentheses—and you are done. Well, except that you would append some words, such as:

   F10.20   Moderate alcohol use disorder

   3. If the use isn't current—that is, this patient is in remission (either early or sustained), use the number in parentheses. A person with mild alcohol use disorder, who hasn't had a drink in a year or more, you'd write down:

   F10.11   Mild alcohol use disorder, in sustained remission

TABLE 15.2. ICD-10-CM Code Numbers for Substance Use Disorder, Substance Intoxication, Substance Withdrawal, and Substance-Induced Mental Disorders

Substance name and use disorder (or no use disorder)	Substance use/intoxication/withdrawal			Substance-induced disorders									
	Just use; no I or W	Intoxication	Withdrawal	Psychotic I/W	Mood[a] I/W	Anxiety I/W	OCD	Sleep I/W	Sex. I/W	Delirium I/W	NCD major	NCD mild	Unspecified
Alcohol F10													.99
mild use dis.	.10 (11)[b]	.120	.130 (132)[c]	.159	.14	.180		.182	.181	.121 (131)[d]		.188	
mod./severe use dis.	.20 (21)[b]	.220	.230 (232)[c]	.259	.24	.280		.282	.281	.221 (231)[d]	.27 (.26)[e]	.288	
no use dis.		.920	.930 (.932)[c]	.959	.94	.980		.982	.981	.921 (.931)[d]	.97 (.96)[e]	.988	
Caffeine F15						I		I/W					.99
mild use dis.													
mod./severe use dis.													
no use dis.		.920	.93			.980		.982					
Cannabis F12				I		I		I/W		I			.99
mild use dis.	.10 (11)[b]	.120 (122)[c]	.13	.159		.180		.188		.121			
mod./severe use dis.	.20 (21)[b]	.220 (222)[c]	.23	.259		.280		.288		.221			
no use dis.		.920 (.922)[c]	.93[g]	.959[g]		.980[g]		.988[g]		.92[g]			

(cont.)

Note. dis. = disorder; I = intoxication; mod. = moderate; NCD = neurocognitive disorder; OCD = obsessive–compulsive and related disorder; Sex. = sexual dysfunction; Sleep = sleep–wake disorder; W = withdrawal.

[a]Same numbers are used for substance-induced bipolar and depressive disorders. But you can use words to specify.

[b]Second numbers (.11) and (.21) indicate a use disorder in early or sustained remission [same number for both early & sustained].

[c]Two numbers in a cell indicate separate codes for either intoxication or withdrawal without (or with) perceptual disturbances.

[d]For delirium, first number = intoxication; (second number) = withdrawal.

[e]Alcohol-induced major NCD can occur without or with confabulation and amnestic syndrome. The number in parentheses denotes the latter.

TABLE 15.2 (cont.)

Substance name and use disorder (or no use disorder)	Substance use/intoxication/withdrawal			Substance-induced disorders									
	Just use; no I or W	Intoxication	Withdrawal	Psychotic	Mood[a]	Anxiety	OCD	Sleep	Sex.	Delirium	NCD major	NCD mild	Unspecified
Phencyclidine F16				I	I	I				I			.99
mild use dis.	.10 (.11)[b]	.120		.159	.14	.180				.121			
mod./severe use dis.	.20 (.21)[b]	.220		.259	.24	.280				.221			
no use dis.		.920		.959	.94	.980				.921			
Other hallucinogen F16			.983[h]	I	I	I				I			.99
mild use dis.	.10 (.11)[b]	.120		.159	.14	.180				.121			
mod./severe use dis.	.20 (.21)[b]	.220		.259	.24	.280				.221			
no use dis.		.920		.95 [g]	.94[g]	.980[g]				.921[g]	0		
Inhalant F18				I	I	I				I			.99
mild use dis.	.10 (.11)[b]	.120		.159	.14[f]	.180				.121	.17	.188	
mod./severe use dis.	.20 (.21)[b]	.220		.259	.24[f]	.280				.221	.27	.288	
no use dis.		.920		.959	.94[f]	.980				.921	.97	.988	
Opioid F11					I/W	W		I/W	I/W	I/W			.99
mild use dis.	.10 (.11)[b]	.120 (.122)[c]	.13		.14[f]	.188		.182	.181	.121 (.188)[d]			
mod./severe use dis.	.20 (.21)[b]	.220 (.222)[c]	.23		.24[f]	.288		.282	.281	.221 (.288)[d]			
no use dis.		.920 (.922)[c]	.93[g]		.94[f,g]	.988[g]		.982[g]	.981	.921[g] (.988)[d,g]			

476

				I/W	I/W	W		I/W	I/W	I/W		I/W	
Sed./hyp./anx. F13													.99
mild use dis.	.10 (.11)[b]	.120	.130 (.132)[c]	.159	.14	.180		.182	.181	.121 (.131)[d]		.188	
mod./severe use dis.	.20 (.21)[b]	.220	.230 (.232)[c]	.259	.24	.280		.282	.281	.221 (.231)[d]	.27	.288	
no use dis.		.920 (.922)[c,g]	.930 (.932)[c,g]	.959[g]	.94[g]	.980[g]		.982[g]	.981[g]	.921[g] (.931)[d,g]	.97	.988	
Amphet/ stimulant F15							I			I			.99
mild use dis.	.10 (.11)[b]	.120 (.122)[c]	.13	.159	.14	.180		.182	.181	.121		.188	
mod./severe use dis.	.20 (.21)[b]	.220 (.222)[c]	.23	.259	.24	.280		.282	.281	.221		.288	
no use dis.		.920 (.922)[c,g]	.93	.959[g]	.94	.980[g]		.982[g]	.981[g]	.921[g]		.988	
Cocaine F14							I			I			.99
mild use dis.	.10 (.11)[b]	.120 (.122)[c]	.13	.159	.14	.180		.182	.181	.121		.188	
mod./severe use dis.	.20 (.21)[b]	.220 (.222)[c]	.23	.259	.24	.280		.282	.281	.221		.288	
no use dis.		.920 (.922)[c]	.93	.959	.94	.980		.982	.981	.921		.988	
Tobacco F17						W							.209
mild use dis.	Z72.0		—										
mod./severe use dis.	.200 (.201)[b]		.203			.208							
no use dis.													
Other (unknown) F19													.99
mild use dis.	.10 (.11)[b]	.120 (.122)[c]	.130 (.132)[c]	.159	.14	.180		.182	.181	.121 (.131)[d]	.17	.188	
mod./severe use dis.	.20 (.21)[b]	.220 (.222)[c]	.230 (.232)[c]	.259	.24	.280		.282	.281	.221 (.231)[d]	.27	.288	
no use dis.		.920 (.922)[c,g]	.930 (.932)[c]	.959[g]	.94[g]	.980[g]		.982[g]	.981[g]	.921[g] (.931)[d,g]	.97	.988	

[f] Inhalants and opioids can have only depressive mood disorders, not bipolar ones.

[g] For intoxication or withdrawal or a disorder induced by medication, use this number and append the words, "prescribed medication taken as directed."

[h] This code is for hallucinogen persistent perception disorder (p. 441). I couldn't find a better place to put it. Tables have their limits.

4. If the patient doesn't qualify for a use disorder, you'd of course select the "no use disorder" row:

> F10.920   Alcohol intoxication

B. For a patient who is currently intoxicated or experiencing withdrawal

1. Select the substance and its F number.

2. Use the appropriate row: mild use disorder, moderate/severe use disorder, or no use disorder, and read across to the I or W column. Write down the decimal you find there:

> F10.920   Alcohol intoxication
> F10.120   Mild alcohol use disorder, with intoxication

3. If you find two numbers in the cell: The first indicates a patient *without* a perceptual disturbance; the second (in parentheses) is for one *with* a perceptual disturbance. And here are the words you would use:

> F10.232   Severe alcohol use disorder, with withdrawal, with
> perceptual disturbances

4. For someone who is intoxicated on or withdrawing from a medication taken as prescribed, you would select the "no use disorder" row and append the words "with prescribed medication taken as directed."

> F15.93   Amphetamine withdrawal, with prescribed medication
> taken as directed
> F15.922   Amphetamine intoxication, with perceptual
> disturbances, with prescribed medication taken as
> directed

5. And a patient who has a delirium gets yet more specific numbers for intoxication and withdrawal.

> F10.121   Mild alcohol use disorder, with intoxication delirium
> F10.131   Mild alcohol use disorder, with withdrawal delirium

C. If your patient has a substance-induced mental disorder (such as one of mood, anxiety, or sleep).

1. Select the substance and its F number.

2. Choose the appropriate column of the 10 listed under the "Substance-induced disorders" heading.

3. Determine whether there is a use disorder for that substance. If so, is it mild or moderate/severe?

4. If there's no use disorder, read across the row "No use disorder" for that sub-stance. Record decimal and number from the column under the substance-induced mental disorder in question. Combine the F number with the decimal to create the whole code. If the patient has been intoxicated or withdrawing, then add the appropriate words "with onset during intoxica-tion" or "with onset during withdrawal."

F10.980   Alcohol-induced anxiety disorder, with onset during intoxication

5. If there is a use disorder, select the line for either mild or moderate/severe use disorder, and read across to the appropriate substance-induced disor-der column. Add the appropriate intoxication or withdrawal verbiage, as in step 8.

F10.281   Severe alcohol use disorder, with alcohol-induced sexual disorder, with onset during intoxication

6. Finally (!), for a mental disorder caused by a medication taken as prescribed, code according to the row labeled "No use disorder." So, an opioid-induced mood disorder would be F11.94; one for sedative/hypnotic/anxiolytic would be F13.94, and so forth. And add the verbiage.

F11.94   Opioid-induced depressive disorder, with prescribed medication taken as directed

You may have noticed that we sometimes lose data in coding (for example, F12.21 codes either moderate or severe use disorder in either early or sustained remission). But we can gain it back again with the words we attach to the numbers; for example:

F21.21   Severe cannabis use disorder, in early remission.

Beyond the numbering, there's a prescribed order for laying down the words involved in a substance-related diagnosis. Rather than a template, I've provided some examples.

F10.920   Alcohol intoxication
F10.232   Severe alcohol use disorder with alcohol withdrawal, with perceptual disturbance
F10.14   Mild alcohol use disorder with alcohol-induced bipolar disorder, with onset during intoxication
F10.24   Moderate alcohol use disorder with alcohol-induced depressive disorder, with onset during withdrawal
F10.121   Mild alcohol use disorder with alcohol-induced intoxication delirium, acute, with mixed level of activity

F10.26   Severe alcohol use disorder with alcohol-induced major
              neurocognitive disorder, persistent, amnestic–confabulatory type,
              with behavioral disturbance

If two or more substances have caused a disorder, you'll need to create a string of descriptors (as above) for each substance. And it's conceivable that a patient could have both intoxication (or withdrawal) *and* a substance-induced mental disorder. Then you'd end up with two sets of codes, each of which indicates the substance use disorder status.

Finally, I *know* some of these number are inconsistent. Don't blame me. Don't even blame DSM-5-TR; the process is controlled by the good people of ICD-10-CM.

Non-Substance-Related Disorder

F63.0 Gambling Disorder

Gambling is an extremely common behavior that, like so much else in life, becomes a disorder only when pursued to excess. There are striking similarities between pathological gambling and the use of substances, not least of which is that they both activate reward centers (ventral striatum) of the brain; dopamine is implicated. This helps explain why DSM-5-TR includes gambling with substance use disorders.

During an episode, most gamblers report feeling high or aroused—behavior that usually takes several years to become pathological. Initial success leads to increased gambling; at some point, "the big win" of an amount that may exceed the gambler's yearly earnings produces overconfidence. And that encourages more risk. From here on, because all games of chance are weighted toward the house, it is an easy (if painful) spiral into crushing loss, desperate attempts to get even, broken ties of family and friendship, and eventual ruin. Attempts at suicide are a frequent complication, sometimes an endpoint.

In the United States, gambling disorder affects about 6 adults in 1,000 (lifetime). Males outnumber females by about 3:1; women develop gambling problems later than men and seek treatment earlier. Some people only become symptomatic at certain times, such as when their sport of choice is in season. So, a person who quite literally bets the farm on college football during the fall of each year may have minimal problems with gambling at other times of the year. Some use gambling to combat feelings of depression, anxiety, or isolation; others may be affected chronically. Some gamblers will eventually cast off their addiction and enter remission.

Clinicians need to be sensitive to the broad range of gambling activities, from convenience store scratch tickets to bingo to casual sports, slot machines, poker, dice, dogs, and the ponies. Gamblers are unlikely to seek treatment voluntarily, so listen to the reports of friends and families.

Essential Features of **Gambling Disorder**

Gambling so takes over the lives of people with this disorder that they will borrow, lie, and otherwise jeopardize important relationships or opportunities. Indeed, plans for gambling—and memories of past experiences—consume their thoughts. As they try to maintain the excitement or recoup their losses, they may risk more money; repeated (and futile) efforts at control yield irritability and restlessness. Some gamble as a way of coping with stress. Some borrow or steal from others to relieve their increasingly desperate financial straits.

The Fine Print

The D's: • Duration (a year or more; qualifying criteria must all be present within a 12-month time span) • Distress or disability ("clinically significant") • Differential diagnosis (substance use disorders, **manic episode,** professional gambling, social betting, use of dopaminergic medication [such as for parkinsonism])

Coding Notes

Specify if course is:

> **Episodic.** Symptoms subside for months at a time.
> **Persistent.** Symptoms are continuous for years.

Specify if: **In {early}{sustained} remission.** No criteria for gambling disorder are met for {3–12 months}{over 1 year}.

Specify severity:

> **Mild.** Meets 4–5 criteria
> **Moderate.** Meets 6–7 criteria.
> **Severe.** Meets 8–9.

Randy Porter

The Christmas he was 12, Randy Porter's parents gave him a roulette wheel. It was handmade from shiny ebony, and it had mother-of-pearl inlaid numbers. The layout was printed on green felt; the ball was ivory. "Best quality you'll find outside of Monte Carlo," his father bragged when Randy opened the box. Throughout high school, Randy loved operating a casino for his friends. Once or twice some adults drifted in from his parents' bingo night; then they played for real money.

Now Randy is 25, divorced, and broke. He had a good job managing a restaurant near the Las Vegas strip. He can't honestly say he took it to be near the action, but it had seemed a godsend after he'd flunked out of college in the wake of too many all-night bridge sessions (penny a point). It was an easy 5-minute walk to two of the most glittering casinos in town—a walk that Randy used to take frequently on his lunch hour. "I know everybody there," he reports. "I used to have accounts all over town. But nobody's let me run a tab for years."

Randy's early encounters with a real roulette table seemed harmless enough. At noon, he would stroll over to watch the action and place the odd bet. He won a few dollars and lost a few more. All in all, he found that he could take it or leave it, mostly take it—he relished the adrenaline surge when he had money in play. He could afford modest losses; by then, he was married, and his wife was making good money dealing blackjack at a different casino. Then one Saturday afternoon when his wife had to work, black came up seven times in a row, and he walked away from the table with over $55,000 in his pocket. Later he said, "It was maybe the unluckiest day of my entire life."

In subsequent weeks, Randy lost himself (not to mention the 55 grand) in gambling fever. His lunch hour soon stretched to two as he returned to the table again and again to recoup his losses. After he was caught "borrowing" from his employer, he tried Gamblers Anonymous; he quit because "I don't believe in a higher power." Over the next 2 years he became "totally obsessed," as his wife put it on more than one occasion, with the idea of scoring another big win so that he could quit when he was ahead. Tired of being ignored and lied to about their finances, she finally left him.

"She said she might as well be married to a one-armed bandit," Randy remarks sadly.

Attentive and pleasant, Randy sits quietly throughout his interview. Though he expresses remorse for the difficulties he has caused himself and others, he describes his mood as neither depressed nor ecstatic, but "in the middle." His speech is clear and goal directed. His cognition and reasoning are excellent.

As his wife was departing, Randy had begged her to stay, promising to reform. "I wouldn't bet on it," she'd said as she turned the doorknob.

Evaluation of Randy Porter

Like many other nascent gamblers, Randy got his start as an adolescent through gambling activities in his home. In a few years, he became thoroughly preoccupied with gambling (criterion A4); unsuccessfully tried to control it (A3); lied, stole, and eventually lost his wife and his job (A7, A9, A8). In an effort to recover, he chased his losses (A6) with more betting—the long-term symptom that so powerfully defines gambling disorder. He therefore amply meets the symptomatic criteria (only four are required) for gambling disorder, provided that his behavior was not better accounted for by a manic episode (B). However, Randy shows no symptoms of mania, no depression, and no evidence of periodicity in his gambling behavior—so we can safely rule out mood disorder. Social gamblers set limits on their losses and gamble in the company of friends; professional gamblers respect the odds and maintain strict self-discipline. Randy's behavior fits neither pattern.

The real challenge in evaluating any patient who gambles excessively is to determine whether there is an associated mental disorder. Commonly associated conditions include mood disorders, panic disorder, obsessive–compulsive disorder, and agoraphobia. Also look for problems with substance use (which can either precede or accompany gambling behavior) and suicide attempts (which may result from it). When present, any comorbid mental disorder is likely to have begun first.

Of course, people with antisocial personality disorder can become heavily involved in gambling, and research has also identified borderline personality disorder in people with gambling disorder. Randy, however, shows none of the behaviors that would be diagnostic of those personality disorders. Neither has he demonstrated evidence that his behavior is episodic, and he certainly isn't in remission (the other possible specifier, besides severity), so his full diagnosis would be—uh, wait a minute. Let's talk about severity. According to DSM-5-TR criteria (which require counting symptoms), Randy barely qualifies for a severity level of moderate. But here's a fellow whose addiction (let's not be afraid to call it that) has essentially ruined his life. I don't know where he's working now, but I doubt that it's for his original employer, and he's probably sleeping in his car. I'd give him a relatively low GAF score of 55, and I don't call this a moderate anything. Once again, I'm going to assert clinician's prerogative and say that his level of severity should be—severe.

F63.0	Gambling disorder, severe, persistent
Z63.5	Divorced

CHAPTER 16

Cognitive Disorders

Here's why I'm departing from the DSM-5-TR name for this group of disorders: When I was rereading this chapter prior to publication, I noticed that *I* was growing confused. The current accepted name for what we used to term dementia is *neurocognitive disorder*, whereas the name for the collected cognitive disorders is *neurocognitive disorders*. In some passages, I had trouble deciding exactly what I had meant—one disorder or the whole collection. If it gave me trouble, surely it would puzzle others, too. So, after much thought and consultation, I decided to stick with the DSM-IV title for the chapter, and reserve *neurocognitive disorder (NCD)* for the conditions we used to call dementia.

Quick Guide to the Cognitive Disorders

With a structure simplified since DSM-5, classification of the cognitive disorders is logical, though the details can be pretty darned complicated.

Delirium

A *delirium* is a rapidly developing, fluctuating state of reduced awareness in which all of the following are true:

- The patient has trouble with awareness (operationally defined as orientation) and shifting or focusing of attention, *and*
- There is at least one deficit of memory, orientation, perception, visuospatial skills, or language, *and*
- The symptoms are not better explained by coma or another cognitive disorder.

One of the following causes can be identified:

Delirium due to another medical condition. Delirium can be caused by trauma to the brain, infections, epilepsy, endocrine disorders, toxicity from medications, poisons, and various other diseases affecting almost any part of the body. I have listed many of these conditions in the "Physical Disorders That Affect Mental Diagnosis" table in the Appendix (p. 661). Occasionally more than one cause for delirium will be identified in the same patient.

Substance intoxication delirium, substance withdrawal delirium, and medication-induced delirium. Alcohol and other sedative drugs of abuse, as well as nearly every class of street drug, can cause delirium in both intoxication and withdrawal. Medications can also be implicated (p. 493).

Delirium due to multiple etiologies. Delirium can have multiple causes in the same patient (p. 496).

Other specified, and unspecified, delirium. Use one of these categories when you don't know the cause of a patient's delirium or when it doesn't fully meet diagnostic criteria (p. 498).

Major and Mild Neurocognitive Disorders

A major or mild neurocognitive disorder (NCD) differs from delirium in several ways:

- The time course is relatively slow. Delirium develops across hours or days, an NCD across weeks and months.
- Although patients with NCDs can have impaired ability to focus or shift attention, it isn't prominent.
- The cause of an NCD can usually be found within the central nervous system; the cause of delirium is often elsewhere in the body.
- Some patients recover from an NCD, but this isn't the usual course.

DSM-5-TR distinguishes between major NCD (which was called dementia in DSM-IV and earlier) and mild NCD. In mild NCD, any of the etiologies listed below can be implicated in relatively mild effects on patient's ability to function independently. Discerning the boundaries between major and mild NCD can be problematic, however.

One of the following types of NCD will be identified:

Major or mild NCD due to Alzheimer's disease. This is the most common cause of NCD. It begins gradually and progresses inexorably. A bit more than half of all major NCDs are of the Alzheimer's type (p. 512).

Major or mild vascular NCD. Due to vascular brain disease, these patients experience loss of memory and other cognitive abilities. Often this is a stepwise process, with relatively sudden onset and a fluctuating course. Some 10–20% of major NCDs are vascular (p. 530).

Major or mild NCD due to other medical conditions. A large number of illnesses can cause NCDs (again, see "Physical Disorders . . ." in the Appendix, p. 661). Some of the most noteworthy include brain tumor, Creutzfeldt–Jakob disease (infection by a slow virus, or prion disease), traumatic brain injury, HIV, Huntington's disease, Parkinson's disease, and frontotemporal NCD (formerly Pick's disease). The most common toxins causing NCDs are those resulting from kidney and liver failure.

Substance/medication-induced major or mild NCD. Some 5–10% of NCDs are related to prolonged use of alcohol, inhalants, or sedatives (p. 537).

Major or mild NCD due to multiple etiologies. Like a delirium, an NCD can have multiple causes in the same patient (p. 541).

Unspecified NCD. This category is useful when you know the patient's cognitive status is impaired, but you don't know why (p. 543).

Other Causes of Cognitive Symptoms

Dissociative disorders. Profound, temporary loss of memory may occur in patients who suffer from dissociative amnesia (p. 243) or dissociative identity disorder (p. 240).

Pseudodementia. With their apathy and slowed responses, some patients often look as if they have the severe memory loss and other symptoms of neurocognitive disorder. But careful clinical evaluation and psychological testing reveal severe major depressive disorder (p. 116) and cognitive functioning that is relatively intact, though they may have problems with attention and concentration. Pseudodementia accounts for about 5% of older patients referred for a dementia workup. Pseudodementia is a useful term DSM-5-TR uses only once, in quotes, in reference to major depressive disorder.

Malingering. Some patients will intentionally exaggerate or falsify cognitive symptoms to obtain funds (insurance, workers' compensation) or to avoid punishment or military service (p. 616).

Factitious disorder imposed on self. Some patients may feign cognitive symptoms, but not for direct gain (such as gaining money or avoiding punishment). Their motive often appears to be a desire to be hospitalized or otherwise cared for (p. 272).

Whatever happened to age-related cognitive decline? This DSM-IV diagnosis referred to the fact that older patients often report trouble remembering names, telephone numbers, or places where they put things. On testing, they tend to appear ordinary, and DSM-5-TR just considers it a part of what's normal, deserving of no special coding. It takes objective evidence of impairment in at least one cognitive domain to cause DSM-5-TR to sit up and take notice.

Introduction

Cognition refers to the mental processing of information—more specifically, memory and thinking in the storage, retrieval, and manipulation of information to achieve knowledge. A clinician obtains information about these processes by observation during an interview and by asking the patient to perform certain tasks during the mental status evaluation.

The cognitive disorders (major, mild, and delirium) are abnormalities of these mental processes that are associated with temporary or permanent brain dysfunction. Their main symptoms include problems with memory, orientation, language, information processing, and the ability to focus and sustain attention on a task. A cognitive disorder is caused by substance use or other medical condition that leads to defects of brain structure, chemistry, or physiology. However, the underlying cause cannot always be defined.

With early recognition and adequate treatment, many cognitive disorders (especially deliriums) are reversible. Ignored, some may spontaneously improve, but often they cause permanent disability. Moreover, though the criteria are relatively simple, their associated symptoms can cause cognitive disorders to mimic virtually any other mental condition. For example, delirium can present with symptoms of depression and anxiety; major neurocognitive disorder can show up as psychosis. Whatever your patient's history or symptoms, it is therefore vital to consider neurocognitive etiologies near the top of your differential diagnosis. If you forget about cognitive disorders, emotional symptoms can all too easily obscure an underlying delirium, or you might diagnose a primary psychotic disorder when the patient's problem is actually neurocognitive.

Depending on the underlying cause, cognitive disorders can begin at any age. They are extremely common, especially in a hospital setting. They may constitute up to one in five of all mental health admissions.

Delirium

Although the brain itself can be involved directly (as with a brain tumor or seizure disorder), most deliriums are caused by disease processes that begin outside the central nervous system. These include endocrine disorders, infections, drug toxicity or withdrawal, vitamin deficiency, fever, liver and kidney disease, poisons, and the effects of surgical operations. (A more complete listing is given in the "Physical Disorders . . ." table, p. 661.)

We can easily state the basic features of delirium:

- In just hours to several days, the patient develops . . .
- Reduction in awareness and attention, accompanied by . . .

- Some sort of additional *cognitive deficit,* such as problems with orientation, memory, language, perception, or visuospatial capability.

- The intensity of these symptoms tends to fluctuate throughout the course of a day.

Inattention is often the first symptom you might notice. During an interview, you identify difficulty focusing on the topic at hand; the patient's experience may be of drowsiness or somnolence. Thought processes slow down and appear vague; there may be trouble with reasoning and solving problems. You may have to ask questions several times before the patient responds. On the other hand, inattention may instead appear as a hyperalert distractibility, with rapid shifting from one focus to another.

Any of several areas can constitute the additional cognitive deficit; two or more may occur at the same time.

Language. You will recognize problems with language in speech that is rambling, disjointed, pressured, or incoherent, or speech that leaps from one topic to another. Some patients will have trouble writing or naming things. Speech that is merely slurred, without demonstrating incoherent thoughts, suggests intoxication, not delirium.

Memory. Delirious patients nearly always have trouble remembering things. Recent events are always affected first; older memories (especially those from childhood) are usually the last to go.

Executive functioning. The patient has difficulty in planning, organizing, sequencing, or abstracting information. In practice, the patient has trouble making decisions, taking steps that break a habit pattern, correcting errors, or searching for the source of a problem (troubleshooting). Obviously, novel or complicated situations will be fraught for these patients.

Orientation. Many patients will be disoriented, sometimes so severely that you cannot examine them adequately. Disorientation is most likely to be for time (date, day, month, year); next comes disorientation for place; lastly, patients fail to recognize relatives and friends (disorientation for person). Only the most severely ill patients become unsure of their own identities.

Perception. Patients with even mild or early delirium don't perceive their surroundings as clearly as usual: Boundaries are fuzzy, colors are abnormally bright, images distorted. Some patients misidentify what they see (illusions), whereas others experience false perceptions (hallucinations are especially likely to be visual). If they later experience false beliefs or ideas (delusions) grafted onto their hallucinations, these delusions are typically incomplete, changing, or poorly organized. Confronted by visual misperceptions, patients may not be able to tell whether they are dreaming or awake. Those who accept their hallucinations as reality may feel quite anxious or fearful.

Other areas often revealing disturbance in delirium include the following:

Sleep–wake cycle. A change in a patient's sleep cycle (insomnia, day–night reversal, vivid dreams, nightmares) almost invariably occurs.

Psychomotor activity and behavior. Sometimes physical movements may be slowed, especially if the delirium is due to metabolic problems; these patients can appear sluggish. Others may experience increased motor activity (agitated behavior, picking at bedclothes). A flapping tremor of the hands is common. So are vocalizations, which are sometimes no more than muttering or moans, though some patients may weep or call out. Those who feel threatened may strike out with fists or attempt to escape.

Mood. Depression and fear are common emotional reactions to the experiences mentioned above; mood often becomes unstable, perceived by others as lability of affect. (Dysphoria can sometimes be the presenting symptom in delirium; then there is a danger of misdiagnosing the patient as having a major depressive disorder.) Some patients will only react with perplexity; still others will exhibit bland, calm acceptance, or perhaps even intense anger or euphoria.

Delirium usually begins suddenly, and its intensity often fluctuates. Most patients will be more lucid in the morning and worse at night—a transient phenomenon called *sundowning*. When you suspect delirium, try to interview the patient in sessions several hours apart. Because the symptoms of delirium so often fluctuate with time of day, unremarkable or marginal findings at noon may give way to clear evidence of illness in the evening. If multiple visits are not practical, nursing staff (or chart notes) may provide the needed information.

Though symptoms can persist for days to weeks, most deliriums last a week or less and then resolve, once the underlying condition has been relieved. Some, however, will evolve into neurocognitive disorder. After delirium resolves, most patients recall the experiences incompletely; they may have amnesia for certain (or all) aspects, and that which is recalled may seem dreamlike. Delirium is common on medical wards, where it may be mistaken for other mental disorders, including psychosis, depression, mania, "hysteria," or personality disorder.

Delirium has the overall highest incidence of all mental disorders. By some estimates, up to half of hospitalized elderly patients become delirious. It is more common in children and elderly people than in young and middle-aged adults.

Delirium has many aliases. Neurologists and internists call it *acute confusional state*. Other terms sometimes used for delirium include *toxic psychosis, acute brain syndrome,* and *metabolic encephalopathy.* These terms are useful to know when you are discussing a delirious patient with clinicians who do not specialize in mental health.

Some clinicians regard delirium as a state of agitated mental confusion during which the patient experiences visual hallucinations that are unusually vivid. This would be the case for delirium tremens. However, DSM-5-TR uses the term *delirium* in a much broader sense, to encompass conditions with the more varied symptoms mentioned in the Essential Features.

Essential Features of **Delirium**

Over a short time, the patient develops problems with attention that wanders and with reduced environmental awareness. Additional cognitive changes (memory, use of language, disorientation, perception, visuomotor capability) set in. Severity often fluctuates during the day. History, physical examination, or laboratory findings directly implicate a physical condition, substance use, toxicity, or some combination as the physiological cause.

The Fine Print

For tips on identifying substance-related causation, see sidebar, page 95.

The D's: • Duration (onset is hours to days; once established, it is typically brief, though it can endure) • Differential diagnosis (**another neurocognitive disorder,** psychotic disorders, factitious disorder, malingering)

Coding Notes

Specify if:

Hyperactive. Agitation or otherwise increased level of activity.
Hypoactive. Reduced level of activity.
Mixed level of activity. Normal or fluctuating activity levels.

Specify duration:

Acute. Lasts hours to a few days.
Persistent. Lasts weeks or longer.

Specify whether delirium is:

Substance intoxication delirium (diagnose rather than substance intoxication

> if delirium symptoms are predominant and severe enough to need clinical attention).
>
> **Substance withdrawal delirium** (diagnose rather than substance withdrawal if delirium symptoms are predominant and severe enough to need clinical attention).
>
> **Medication-induced delirium** (diagnose when delirium symptoms are side effects of medications that have been taken as prescribed).
>
> Code numbers for substance- (and medication-) caused delirium are given in Table 15.2 (p. 475). Footnotes there indicate the order to use in coding.

F05 Delirium Due to Another Medical Condition

Delirium can have many causes, related in part to the patient's age group. In children, fever and infection are the most common causes; in young adults, drugs; in middle-aged adults, withdrawal from alcohol and head injury; in older patients, metabolic issues, cardiovascular failure, and excessive medications. Delirium in an older patient will often have multiple causes (p. 496).

Because it may be caused by a disease that can lead to neurocognitive disorder or even kill outright, any delirium is a true emergency. When you suspect one, immediately obtain appropriate medical consultation or testing; often evaluation by a neurologist will be required. However, formal (neuropsychological) testing can be difficult in patients who cannot adequately sustain attention on a task. Therefore, the diagnosis of delirium may sometimes depend on a bedside evaluation.

Again, the "Physical Disorders . . ." table in the Appendix (p. 661) lists some of the more frequently encountered medical causes of delirium.

Harold Hoyt

After rheumatic heart disease had led to years of gradually worsening fatigue and shortness of breath, Harold Hoyt, a 48-year-old bricklayer, finally consents to a mitral valve replacement. Warning him that open heart surgery can cause delirium, his surgeon recommends a mental health consultation as a preventive measure.

"I ain't crazy," Harold replies by way of refusal.

The procedure goes well, but right away the recovery room staff notices that Harold seems withdrawn and uncommunicative. He ignores his wife and daughter during their brief bedside visits. When he speaks or writes notes, it is to complain about the tube in his nose or the impossibility of sleep in the brightly lighted ward.

On the third postoperative day, Harold becomes increasingly restless. After he pulls out his nasogastric tube, he is quieter for a time, but in the evening, they find him crying and trying to get out of bed. He asks a nurse why he is there; he's incredulous when told that he's had heart surgery. As they speak, his voice trails off and he seems to forget that anyone else is present. When he speaks again, he asks about the outcome of a football game he had watched the week before.

The following morning Harold carries on a routine, though brief, conversation with the dietary aide who brings breakfast. But by nightfall he is again talking to himself and must be restrained from pulling out his IV. However, he can give the date accurately.

A mental health consultant diagnoses a "classic postcardiotomy delirium" and recommends that family members sit with Harold to provide stimulation and reality checks. Within 36 hours he is fully oriented and conversing with his family, and his improved physical condition allows a move out of the recovery unit. He remembers nothing of his behavior of the previous 2 days and expresses surprise that he ever needed restraints.

Evaluation of Harold Hoyt

In the hours after surgery, Harold's problem with attention causes him to have difficulty even expressing a thought (his voice trails off in midsentence, and he veers into a discussion of football); the fact that he is also unaware of his surroundings (he forgets others are present, doesn't know why he is in the hospital) completes the requirement for delirium criterion A. His cognitive problems develop rapidly and fluctuate with time of day, increasing in the evening and at night (sundowning—criterion B). He has further problems with short-term memory (among other things, he even forgets that he's had surgery), and on at least one occasion he is disoriented to time; either of these issues passes muster for criterion C. He isn't comatose, and he has no preexisting neurocognitive disorder that would better explain his symptoms (D). His recent history of heart surgery provides evidence of a direct link to his delirium; indeed, his surgeon warned him it might happen (E).

We need to consider a differential diagnosis, even though the criteria do not describe one beyond a different cognitive disorder. When his delirium was first developing, Harold was withdrawn and seemed irritable. These features suggest a depressive disorder, which is only one of many mental disorders sometimes confused with the cognitive disorders. Because hallucinations are so common, schizophrenia and other psychotic disorders also appear in the differential diagnosis, though the history of an operation and rapid fluctuations in cognition are pretty reliable (but hardly infallible) giveaways. Occasionally a patient (especially one who has previous experience with health care) will feign the symptoms of delirium to obtain money or some other material benefit. This sort of deception can be difficult to detect; when it is found, malingering is the typical designation (though I tend to be *really* parsimonious with this Z-code). When you cannot identify any practical motive for deception, consider factitious disorder imposed on self. Harold becomes somewhat agitated and tries to get out of bed; perhaps this was due to anxiety at finding himself in a strange place without knowing why. But there are plenty of people who have anxiety symptoms without having an anxiety disorder.

The variety of potential causes of delirium is vast; although many of them are included in the "Physical Disorders . . ." table in the Appendix (p. 661), the list there is by no means comprehensive. As Harold's consultant noted, cardiotomy is a classic precipitant of delirium (experienced by about 25% of patients after open heart surgery). Somewhat ironically for Harold, the strongest preventative measure against postcardiotomy delirium is a mental health consultation before surgery.

When coding a delirium, be sure to include the medical condition(s) responsible. Harold's GAF score at consultation is a low 40; by discharge, it has improved to a relatively robust 71.

Z95.4   Presence of prosthetic heart-valve replacement
F05   Delirium due to prosthetic heart-valve replacement surgery, acute, hyperactive

"Delirium Due to Medical Cause Often Misdiagnosed." That headline in an online report described a paper presented some years back at a geriatric psychiatry meeting. Of 112 consecutive patients admitted with the diagnosis of a mental health disorder, 27—nearly one-quarter—were ultimately found to be suffering from a delirium due to some underlying physical disorder. The most frequent diagnosis was a urinary tract infection. Other conditions affecting more than one patient included drug usage and poor control of blood sugar. Mostly, the patients were at first diagnosed as having a different cognitive disorder, but psychoses and mood disorder diagnoses were also prevalent.

Substance Intoxication Delirium, Substance Withdrawal Delirium, and Medication-Induced Delirium

People who abuse street drugs or alcohol are at serious risk for developing delirium. Many drugs can produce intoxication delirium, but heavy use of sedatives such as alcohol and barbiturates, when suddenly discontinued, is notorious for causing withdrawal delirium. The most notorious is alcohol withdrawal delirium, popularly called delirium tremens, or DTs. Its hallmarks are agitation, tremor, disorientation, and vivid hallucinations. In someone who has suddenly stopped after many weeks of heavy drinking, DTs can occur within a few days. DTs can also appear when a substance-misusing patient develops a medical illness (such as liver failure, head trauma, pneumonia, or pancreatitis); alcohol users are at special risk for each of these conditions. Alcohol withdrawal delirium isn't especially common, even among the heaviest users of alcohol, but it is severe; if it goes untreated, up to 15% of patients will die. This makes it an extremely important mental health event.

Delirium—especially intoxication delirium, but also the withdrawal type—can also be caused by prescribed medications. High doses aren't necessary; in combination with other drugs or illnesses, low doses can cause delirium, especially in older people.

Drugs with anticholinergic effects (such as antiparkinsonian agents and antidepressants) are probably the most likely offenders. Although intoxication delirium can occur within minutes of taking cocaine or hallucinogens, for many other substances it will occur only after drug levels have built up over several days or longer.

Rodney Partridge

A barroom knife fight leaves Rodney Partridge with a severed artery in his arm that requires several units of whole blood and a 2-hour surgical repair. But apart from a slight tremor, when Rodney awakens from the anesthesia late Sunday morning, he feels almost as good as new. By evening he is eating voraciously and enjoying the attentions of the nursing staff. On Monday, however, when his surgeon comes around to make sure the dressing is still dry, the head nurse confides in a worried whisper: "He's been awake most of the night, demanding to be released. The last hour or two, he's been trying to pick things off his sheets."

When the mental health consultant appears in his doorway, Rodney is propped up in bed; he is restrained by a canvas halter around his chest and by leather cuffs on his ankles and left wrist. His free hand tremulously roams the bedclothes, pausing occasionally to pinch up a bit of air and fling it to the floor. Suddenly, Rodney throws a triangle of dry toast at the curtain rod over his window.

"Got him! Cheeky bugger."

"Got who?" the consultant wants to know.

"Oh, my God!" Startled, Rodney lurches against his chest restraints and drops a second piece of toast. Leaving it on the sheet, he plucks some more at his bedclothes.

"Got who?" repeats the consultant.

Rodney's gaze returns to the curtain rod. "It's those guys up there. One of them mooned me."

The guys are about 4 inches tall and wear short pants, green jackets, and pointed caps. For half an hour they have been parading around on the curtain rod, making obscene gestures and throwing multicolored caterpillars onto Rodney's bed. Whenever a caterpillar lands, it begins crawling toward him, munching a swath across the sheet as it advances.

Although he isn't exactly frightened, Rodney is far from placid. With his gaze constantly darting around the room, he seems to be watching for other predators. He insists that the guys (and caterpillars) are real, but he has no idea why they are there. He is also vague about his orientation. He knows he's in a hospital—"never been told the name"—thinks he was admitted a week ago, and misses the date by nearly 5 months. When asked to subtract sevens from 100, he responds: "Ah, 93 . . . 80 . . . um . . . there's a purple one."

With a little urging and a lot of Librium for sedation, Rodney admits that he has been a heavy drinker most of his adult life. Too many vodka sours have landed him currently between jobs (and wives), and for the last 3 months he has spent most of his waking hours consuming a quart or more of hard liquor per day. Although his morning shakes often require "a hair of the dog," he has never before had hallucinations. He agrees that he is "probably an alcoholic"—in fact, several times he's started with Alcoholics Anonymous, but could never stay the course.

Evaluation of Rodney Partridge

Several points in Rodney's history suggest some sort of cognitive disorder. First, his orientation is poor (he's unclear about the date and has no idea what hospital he is in—reduced awareness of the environment). The second tip-off to delirium is his reduced attention span (he has difficulty focusing on his conversation with the mental health consultant). Together, these two features constitute criterion A for a delirium. The symptoms began rapidly and appear to be a change for Rodney (B); time would tell the extent to which they might have fluctuated had Rodney's consultant not intervened with treatment.

Criterion C requires at least one of these cognitive disturbances—perceptual changes, problems with memory, language, visuospatial capability, or other orientation problems; Rodney has rather dramatic hallucinations (perceptual changes, C). The hallucinations of alcohol and other withdrawal deliriums are classically visual, but auditory or tactile hallucinations can also occur. The content of delusions, if any occur, is often related to hallucinations.

Rodney has several other symptoms typically associated with delirium. He has become so hyperactive (increased startle response) and agitated (trying to get out of bed) that he must be restrained. His tremor is evident. Although Rodney seems only bemused, many patients are badly frightened by hallucinations, which can be grotesque beyond belief. His symptoms are clearly more severe than you'd encounter in simple alcohol withdrawal; by themselves they would warrant clinical attention.

Hallucinations could suggest schizophrenia, a mistake careful clinicians avoid by asking informants how long the patient has had psychotic symptoms. (See the sidebar on p. 496 for some points that discriminate causes of psychosis.) As with any delirium, other conditions to rule out include other psychotic disorders, malingering, and factitious disorder. Rodney's history provides ample evidence for a causal relationship between his drinking and his symptoms (E).

Although Rodney Partridge meets the criteria for alcohol withdrawal, alcohol withdrawal delirium better explains his symptoms, which are serious enough to require care. We need to choose among the specifiers for acuteness and activity level. And here's another issue: Because they occur only during a delirium, we don't need a separate diagnosis for his psychosis—a principle that applies to disorders of mood, anxiety, sleep, and sex, any of which can become problematic during a delirium.

Of course, Rodney also qualifies for a diagnosis of alcohol use disorder: In addition to withdrawal (A11), he has tried Alcoholics Anonymous without success (A2), and he prefers drinking to working (A5). Although the number of substance use symptoms we've identified isn't high by actual count, I'd still code as severe just about any patient who's had DTs. In any event, the presence of alcohol use disorder helps determine his two mental health diagnoses, which I've looked up in Table 15.2 (p. 475). His GAF score on admission would be a strikingly low 30.

F10.231	Severe alcohol use disorder, with acute alcohol withdrawal delirium, hyperactive
S45.119A	Laceration of brachial artery
Z56.9	Unemployed
Z63.5	Divorced

When psychotic symptoms turn up in patients with NCD, delirium may be the cause. Of course, that's important to know, because treatment of the delirium can greatly ameliorate the discomfort (to all) of the hallucinations and, sometimes, delusions. But studies show that delirium is often underdiagnosed in patients with NCD, and that the two disorders often occur together. Here are a few points that help discriminate delirium from NCD:

Delusions. In delirium, they are more likely to concern dangers in the immediate environment. In NCD, they are typically of being robbed or abandoned.

Hallucinations. In delirium, visual hallucinations and illusions are common. In Alzheimer's disease, they are not so common (though they are somewhat more frequent in NCD with Lewy bodies).

Flow of thought. Delirious people are likely to have thought processes that are illogical, perhaps with derailment. A patient with NCD is more likely to have poverty of thought.

Attention. It's affected in delirium, though relatively spared in Alzheimer's disease. However, attention is deeply affected in Lewy body NCD.

F05 Delirium Due to Multiple Etiologies

Probably more patients than we recognize have multiple causes for their delirium. Many such diagnoses are undoubtedly missed because one cause is predominant and obscures the others. The signs and symptoms do not differ from those in the foregoing examples, but of course, successful treatment can hinge heavily upon accurate identification of all contributing factors.

Delirium due to multiple etiologies is not really a disorder—it is a collection of two or more diagnoses occurring in a single patient. I include it here as a reminder of its importance to adequate treatment. It is especially common among older people, who are likely to have numerous medical problems.

Emil Brion

At age 72, Emil Brion already has such severe emphysema that he requires oxygen day and night. "I always warned him about smoking, but he was actually proud of being a three-pack-a-day man," says his wife. "Now, if he takes the oxygen off to smoke, he gets goofy and scared."

She means that Emil will see things: A light cord resembles a snake; a pile of clothes on the chair becomes a lion ready to spring. He might wake up whimpering from a nightmare. Sometimes he seems so distracted that she can hardly persuade him to put the oxygen back on. But all things considered, he is doing pretty well. He can even drive a little, as long as he uses his oxygen.

Then, on the Fourth of July, Emil strolls barefoot through the back yard and slices the outer sole of his heel on a broken piece of glass. The cut doesn't hurt much, so he forgets to clean it up, several days go by before either he or his wife notices how red and swollen the injured area has become. By that time, according to the specialist in infectious diseases who admits him to the hospital, he has developed a severe septicemia.

Despite continuous IV antibiotics, for 3 days Emil's temperature hovers above 102 degrees. Even with nasal oxygen running, his arterial oxygen saturation is low. During much of the day he sleeps; at night he lies awake, mumbling to himself and groaning. When he speaks clearly enough to be understood, he complains that he is a miserable old man who wishes he were dead.

On Emil's seventh hospital day, his fever finally breaks. He removes the oxygen tube and whispers to the nurse, "Wheel me outside so I can have a smoke."

Evaluation of Emil Brion

Emil's wife notes that when he goes without his oxygen, he is sometimes so distracted that he can't even focus on restarting it. With a second disorder (systemic infection) added to the anoxia, he rapidly (delirium criterion B) becomes somnolent (A). His other cognitive difficulties (C) include illusions (the light-cord snake) and nightmares, and he begins to mumble (language difficulties).

Several other symptoms typically associated with delirium are also apparent. There is a change in his sleep pattern (drowsy during the day, awake at night). He becomes depressed and even wishes himself dead; perhaps at times he recognizes how desperately ill he is. As to preexisting cognitive conditions (D), the only one would be the possibility of another delirium.

Even before the infection sets in, Emil has fluctuating states of consciousness and attention with occasional hallucinations, suggesting a persistent delirium caused by anoxia. But his mental condition has more than one cause, as shown by the fact that the infection makes him even sicker, despite the oxygen. That either of these could cause delirium, and that both precede it, satisfies criterion E.

Once the infection in his bloodstream resolves and his fever breaks, his cognition suddenly improves. However, a complete evaluation of his mental status would be needed to be sure that no residual symptoms suggested NCD or a depressive disorder. We wouldn't confuse his perceptual problems with schizophrenia because they developed so rapidly—and at an advanced age.

Note that in the coding of Emil's delirium, a separate code for each specific cause is entered on a separate line, though in his case the numbers remain the same. His GAF score on admission was only 25; it is 80 at discharge.

J43.9	Emphysema
A41.9	Septicemia
F05	Delirium due to anoxia, persistent, hypoactive
F05	Delirium due to septicemia, acute, hypoactive

F05 Other Specified Delirium

F05 Unspecified Delirium

Use other specified or unspecified delirium as a catch-all category for any delirium that does not meet the criteria for one of the previously described types. For other specified delirium, DSM-5-TR specifically mentions:

Subsyndromal delirium. Called attenuated delirium syndrome in DSM-5, the cognitive symptoms are not sufficient for a more specific diagnosis.

Symptom Domains

Although we can organize our thinking about them in different ways, over the years some consensus has developed of what constitutes the domains important to what DSM-5-TR calls major and mild neurocognitive disorders (NCDs). Here are descriptions of those considered central to the understanding of all cognitive disorders, but especially to major NCD.

The folks who write (and do research) about cognitive matters often refer to neurocognitive domains. However, they never quite define just what they mean by *domain*. DSM-5-TR has carried that tradition forward, even to the extent of ignoring it; furthermore, it has done away with the glossary—Oh, right, the glossary in DSM-5 ignored it, too. Anyway, lets us have a go at a definition.

The *Oxford English Dictionary* says that a *domain* is "a sphere of thought or action," a dimension of thought or a field of knowledge. Therefore, we can regard a neurocognitive domain as a group of functions that pertains to one aspect of thinking, perception, or memory.

And, wouldn't you know, even domains can have domains (well, sometimes they are called facets). For example, the domain of language includes naming, grammar, receptive language, fluency, and word finding. And just where DSM-5-TR's facets belong is also a bit fraught. Depending on the expert you consult, you can find working memory located as an aspect of memory and learning, a component of complex attention, or a subdivision of executive functioning. Good luck.

Complex Attention

Complex attention means the ability to focus on tasks in such a way that their completion isn't derailed by distractions. It is more than the simple attention span you evaluate when you ask a patient to repeat a string of digits or spell *world* backward. It also involves processing speed, holding information in mind, and being able to attend (more or less) to multiple tasks at once, like writing a grocery list while listening to the radio. In mild NCD, a patient may be able to perform tasks when a lot is going on, but it will take extra effort.

> Pauline has begun to have trouble using her computer. If a phone call interrupts her, she may spend minutes trying to determine where she left off. She used to read the newspaper and write email online, with an open window for each; now she must limit herself to one task at a time, so as not to become confused.

> Jason's daughter-in-law complains (for him) that in the past several months, he's had increasing difficulty dressing himself. "If I'm talking to him, he gets distracted and is likely to leave a shoe untied. A year ago, he could listen and talk and dress, but there might be some hesitation. It was as though he needed to restart himself between tasks. Now, I have to restart him."

> Jason's attention span and processing capability were no longer up to the task of coping with the need for divided attention. A year ago, Jason could complete his task by putting forth some extra effort, compatible with a diagnosis (then) of mild NCD. Now, of course, his cognition has fallen further behind, and he is operating at the level of an actual—and *major*—NCD. Pauline is now, of course, where Jason was last year.

Learning and Memory

Memory exists in many variations. Just a few years ago (it seems), we spoke mainly of long- and short-term memory. Now there's a congeries of terms that we must, um, remember. A good, simple categorization is summed up by the mnemonic PEWS:

- *Procedural memory.* That's the sort of memory we need for skills such as typing and playing the flute (ahem!) and riding a bicycle. It allows us to learn a sequence of behaviors and repeat them, without having to expend conscious effort.
- *Episodic memory.* This is the memory for events the individual has experienced

as personal history—the night Mom died, where you went on your last vacation, your dessert choice when you went out to eat yesterday. Episodic memory always takes our personal point of view; it is often visual.

- *Working memory.* By this we mean the very short-term storing of data that we are actively processing. We test it by asking the patient to do mental arithmetic or spell words backward. It is often regarded as synonymous with immediate memory and regarded as an executive function.

- *Semantic memory.* This is the type of memory we mean when we speak of general knowledge—in short, facts and figures. This is where most of what we learn ends up, because we no longer associate it with anything concrete in our lives, such as where we were when the learning took place.

In each division except working memory, memories tend to endure for up to many years—though episodic tends to be shorter than semantic. Working memory, however, is brief (spanning but a few minutes, if even that).

As memory deteriorates, the time it takes to process information increases. So, a person might have trouble performing mental arithmetic or repeating back a story that was just related or holding in mind a telephone number long enough to dial it. With declining cognitive ability, the little assists that once helped lose their punch.

Just before Christmas, 74-year-old Sarah spends 2 days searching the house for the presents she has hidden. She and her son, Jon, finally find them in the storage shed. But her problems are only beginning. She has always prided herself on her ability to remember telephone numbers, but since February, when Jon was assigned a new extension number at work, she can never seem to recall what it is or where she has written it down. After several days of frustration, Jon finally pastes the new number onto the base of her landline phone. However, it's the two fires she starts while cooking that lead to this evaluation. When asked to name the president of the United States, she says, "That's what you should know for yourself. I don't feel like helping you anymore."

By the time Audrey turns 80, she may sit idle in the senior care day room until someone reminds her to put some more stitches into the sampler she is making. Some days, she doesn't even recognize her daughter when she comes to call. But she can still play her favorite songs on the piano.

Perceptual–Motor Ability

Perceptual–motor ability is our capacity to assimilate visual and other sensory information—and use it. That use is usually motor, though also included would be facial recognition, which lacks a motor component. Note that, in a perceptual–motor deficit, the sensory abilities themselves are just fine: The person can see about as well as ever, but has difficulty navigating the immediate environment, especially when perceptual cues are reduced (as at twilight or nighttime). Handwork and crafts take extra effort; copying a design onto a sheet of paper can pose a real problem. As with other attributes of cognitive functioning, problems in this domain exist on a continuum from nil to mild to major.

> When Jeanne moved into her senior living apartment 3 years ago, she relied on the sign on her door—"Jeanne's Room"—to tell her where to point her walker. Now, however, she shuffles right on past the sign, unless someone is there to direct her.

> Agnes has an *agnosia:* She cannot recognize or identify familiar objects (such as the parts of a ballpoint pen), even though her sensory functioning is intact.

Perceptual–motor ability requires contributions from other domains—executive functioning, for example—so that there is a great deal of confusion, even among researchers who study the subject, as to exactly what domain is meant. Overlearned motor behaviors such as the use of a fork and knife are typically preserved until late in the course of a neurocognitive disorder. Many different tests have been recommended, each of which is subject to various interpretations, depending on the expert you consult. Copying a simple design is one just about everyone accepts.

Executive Functioning

Executive functioning is the set of mechanisms people use to organize simple ideas and bits of behavior into more complex ones on the way to a goal, such as dressing or finding their way around town. When executive functioning is affected, patients have trouble interpreting new information and adapting to new situations. Planning and making decisions become difficult. As mental flexibility is lost, behavior becomes driven by habit rather than by reason and feedback error correction.

> Sarah looks a good 10 years younger than her stated age of 75, but again today she got a phone call while dressing and forgot to finish buttoning her silk blouse. Now she's trying to sort the laundry, but several times she just picks up an item and moves it to a different countertop.

> Marcus has always done the cooking in his household. (His wife is an attorney who still earns most of their money.) At age 67, he is having more and more trouble in the kitchen. He used to plan a different menu for each day of the week, but now he sticks pretty much to mac and cheese. Even so, he sometimes leaves out the salt. Twice last month he forgot the pan on the cooktop, and a small fire started.

Language

The *language* domain includes both receptive language (understanding) and expressive language. The latter includes naming (the ability to state the name of an object such as a fountain pen), fluency, grammar, and syntax (structure) of language. Some patients may use circumlocutions to get around words they can't remember. Increasingly, they may come to depend on clichés; they may become vague, circumstantial, or in the end, completely mute.

> Several years into his dementia, Jerome now mixes up words such as *table* and *chair*.

> Marcelle has developed a naming *aphasia:* She says the word "thingy" for an increasing variety of objects she encounters.

Social Cognition

Social cognition refers to the processes that help us recognize the emotions of other people and respond to them appropriately. It includes decision making, empathy, moral judgment, knowledge of social norms, emotional processing, and *theory of mind*—the ability to imagine that other people have beliefs and desires, and to recognize that others may have ideas different from our own. A person with social cognition deficits may have difficulty recognizing the emotion portrayed in a scowling (or smiling) face. These patients, who have damage to the amygdala, may be overly friendly toward others. Some, however, don't adhere to accepted standards of propriety or conventional social interaction.

> Eileen has begun to criticize the morals of her two grandkids—to their faces; they just roll their eyes and ignore her. She has distanced herself from others in her large extended family and eats many of her meals alone in her bedroom. The others laugh and say she's had a "personality transplant."

> A lifelong atheist, lately Harold utters loud blasphemies even when passing a church on Sunday. He may greet parishioners with an open fly because he often neglects to zip up.

Confusion is a term often used to describe slowed thinking, loss of memory, perplexity, or disorientation in people with NCDs. Of course, you're familiar with it, because other health care providers (neurologists and internists), as well as patients and the general public, use it. DSM-5-TR even sneaks it in occasionally. However, the term is inexact and, well, confusing; in all my writing, I've avoided it whenever possible. Except if I get confused.

Major and Mild Neurocognitive Disorders

Whatever the underlying etiology, patients with NCD share a number of features that serve as criteria for diagnosis. Then the difference between the major and mild forms of NCD boils down to severity of the symptoms. Before getting into specific requirements, let us review these several important points.

Decline

NCD implies loss; there is always a decline from a previous level in one or more areas of functioning. People who have always functioned at a low level (intellectual developmental disorder) do not necessarily have an NCD. However, like anyone else, such a person can develop an NCD. In fact, many people with Down syndrome develop an Alzheimer's type of NCD when they are middle-aged. Even a child who suffers a decline, perhaps due the lasting effects of a traumatic brain injury, may be said to have suffered NCD.

Every patient with NCD will have a deficit in at least one of the cognitive domains discussed just above. Most patients, however, especially early in the course of a disease, won't have them all. Whereas loss of memory is paramount in Alzheimer's and some of the other degenerative disorders, it may be less prominent in patients whose underlying condition is vascular disease. Other patients may first develop problems with language, executive functioning, perceptual–motor functions, or social cognition. But there's always decline.

Overall prevalence for NCD depends on exact definition and the study quoted. As of 2013, they ranged from about 2% at age 65 to the neighborhood of 5–10% at age 75 to 15–30% at age 80 and above. (Actually, a Rand study in 2013 reported 15% at age 71.) Recent research suggests, however, that lifestyle changes (increased exercise, decreased smoking, improved diet) may be helping to reduce the prevalence of NCDs in older people.

Not Exclusively a Delirium

NCD cannot be diagnosed if the symptoms occur only when the patient is in the throes of a delirium. However, these two conditions can (and often do) coexist, as when a patient with NCD due to Alzheimer's is given medication that produces a substance intoxication delirium.

Not Accounted for by Another Mental Disorder

Decline of cognitive ability is sometimes associated with, for example, schizophrenia (which was once called *dementia praecox*—early dementia). The NCD criteria state that such causes of cognitive decline must be ruled out before an NCD can be diagnosed.

Confirmed by Testing

NCD criteria require that testing confirm the patient's decline. Of course, formal tests of the appropriate cognitive domain(s) are preferred, but for many patients that's simply not going to happen. Then, bedside estimates of ability will have to suffice. Formal testing may be especially important for patients who present as "the worried well." As people age, they notice little lapses of memory or quirks of behavior that make them wonder, "Am I losing it?" (Trust me on this.) Then the results of objective testing can provide the reassurance they, their relatives, and their health care providers all need to enable them to get on with their lives.

There is at least one instance in which testing alone can lead us astray. That is the case of a high-functioning person whose formal testing reveals functioning at an average level, or even better. But for this person, who would formerly have tested off the charts, functioning at a normal level represents a substantial decline. That's partly why DSM-5-TR now emphasizes a combination of two requirements—testing plus concern on the part of those who know the patient.

Impairment

And here's the big difference between a mild NCD and a major one: In the case of a major NCD, the loss of cognitive ability must be severe enough to have a definite impact on the patient's work or social life. This impact doesn't have to be severe; some patients will be able to function satisfactorily with some help—paying bills or shopping, for example. People with mild NCD, on the other hand, can continue to function *independently* if they put forth more effort. The difference between major and mild NCD, then, is one of degree. Take special note of this: Many patients with mild NCD will *not* progress to major NCD. The trouble is, we might not be able in advance to tell one group from the other.

The onset of NCD is often gradual though, of course, this depends a lot on the cause. The first indication may be loss of interest in work or leisure activities. Or family and friends may note a change in long-standing personality traits. When executive functioning is affected, judgment and impulse control suffer. Loss of the social graces ensues, as shown when a previously refined person starts making crude jokes or neglects personal appearance and hygiene. Stripped of the ability to analyze, to understand, to remember, and to apply old knowledge to new situations, the patient may have only a skeleton of habit to rely on.

Patients with NCDs become increasingly vulnerable to psychosocial stresses: What might have been a minor problem a few years earlier now grows to monumental proportions. Some become apathetic, some irritable; others may ignore the interests or desires of their group. Another might try to compensate for a failing memory by compulsively making lists. The misperceptions (hallucinations or illusions) so common in delirium are often absent, especially early in the process. As major NCD worsens, paranoid ideas and delusions of infidelity may lead to abusive, even assaultive behavior.

On the other hand, some patients are placid, especially early in the illness as apathy ushers in a gradual reduction in activity. Those who retain some insight may become depressed or anxious. Later, a person who becomes frustrated or frightened may experience outbursts of anger. Restlessness and pacing can lead to wandering from home; patients with NCD sometimes remain lost for hours or days. A person in the final stage of major NCD may lose all useful speech and self-care, and end up confined to bed, unaware of attendants or family.

Although most cases of NCD are found in older patients, it can be diagnosed any time after the age of 3 or 4, which is when a person's cognitive functioning becomes reliably measurable. The course depends on the underlying cause. Most often it is one of chronic deterioration; however, some NCDs can become static, or even remit. Remission is especially likely in NCD due to hypothyroidism, subdural hematoma, or normal pressure hydrocephalus. When one of these causes is diagnosed early and successfully treated, full recovery can occur.

The suspicion of NCD demands medical and neurological evaluation to confirm its source and, whenever possible, to intervene with treatment. In many cases, a biological cause can be identified. These include primary diseases of the central nervous system, such as Huntington's disease, multiple sclerosis, and Parkinson's disease; infectious diseases, such as neurosyphilis and acquired immune deficiency syndrome (AIDS); vitamin deficiencies; tumors; trauma; various diseases of the liver, lungs, and cardiovascular system; and endocrine disorders. (A fuller listing is given in the "Physical Disorders . . ." table in the Appendix, p. 661.) However, some NCDs must be diagnosed not on the basis of demonstrated pathology, but by inference from clinical features and by ruling out other nonorganic causes. This is often the case with NCD due to Alzheimer's disease or frontotemporal degeneration.

Dementia is the term formerly applied to patients with major NCD, which in some situations is preferable to the older term. A good example is a young person whose cognitive problems stem from traumatic brain injury—you want to call attention to a significant problem without using the pejorative term *dementia*. Another might be the patients we once diagnosed as having amnestic disorder, whose problems with thinking are generally focused on a single cognitive area. However, the terms *dementia* and *demented* are still understood—and used—by most of the world. For convenience, not to mention my own sanity, I'll continue to use them occasionally in the rest of this chapter, but only when referring to *major* NCD.

Essential Features of {Major}{Mild} Neurocognitive Disorder

Someone (the patient, a relative, the clinician) suspects that there has been a {marked} {modest} decline in cognitive functioning. On formal testing, the patient scores below accepted norms by {2+}{1–2} standard deviations. Alternatively, a clinical evaluation reaches the same conclusion. The symptoms {materially}{do not materially} impair the patient's ability to function independently. That is, the patient {cannot}{can} negotiate activities of daily life (paying bills, managing medications) by putting forth increased effort or using compensatory strategies such as keeping lists.

The Fine Print

One standard deviation below norms would be at the 16th percentile; two would be at the 3rd percentile.

The D's: • Duration (symptoms tend to chronicity) • Differential diagnosis (delirium, normal aging, **another mental disorder** (especially **major depressive disorder** [pseudodementia], **schizophrenia**)

Coding Notes

Specify if:

With behavioral disturbance [specify type]. The patient has clinically important behaviors such as apathy, agitation, or responding to hallucinations or mood problems.

Without behavioral disturbance. The patient has no such difficulties. The wording and actual codes are given in Tables 16.1 and 16.2.

For major NCD only, specify current level of severity:

Mild. The patient requires help with activities of daily living, such as doing housework or managing money.

Moderate. The patient needs help even with such basics as dressing and eating.

Severe. The patient is fully dependent on others.

Recording Major Neurocognitive Disorders

For most of the etiologies in Tables 16.1 and 16.2, list first (with code number) the etiological agent. The exceptions: Unknown etiology (rather obviously) and vascular disease—which is just an arbitrary rule. *Don't worry; this will become clear soon.*

Any of the five etiologies in Table 16.1 can be due to either *probable* or *possible* disease, depending on the criteria that are met. In all other etiologies (Table 16.2), there should be sufficient certainty about the cause (lab testing, imaging) that a *possible* diagnosis isn't necessary. Select the "F0" number appropriate for your diagnosis. For major probable, these will be F02; for major possible, F03. Vascular major is F01. *Remember, keep calm.*

Now the fun part. Note that most of the Major NCD diagnoses have *.xy* appended.

TABLE 16.1. Probable and Possible Etiologies for Major/Mild NCDs

Presumed etiology	Major NCD due to probable	Major NCD due to possible	Mild NCD due to probable	Mild NCD due to possible
Alzheimer's disease	G30.9 Alzheimer's disease F02.*xy*	[no etiology code] F03.*xy*	G30.9 Alzheimer's disease F06.70 w/o behavioral symptoms or F06.71 w/ behavioral symptoms Add codes for specific symptoms[a]	[no etiology code] G31.84 (and state w/ or w/o behavioral disturbance— words only)
Frontotemporal degeneration	G31.09 Frontotemporal degeneration F02.*xy*	[no etiology code] F03.*xy*	G31.09 Frontotemporal degeneration F06.70 w/o behavioral symptoms or F06.71 w/ behavioral symptoms Add codes for specific symptoms[a]	[no etiology code] G31.84 (and state w/ or w/o behavioral disturbance— words only)
Lewy body disease	G31.83 Lewy body disease F02.*xy*	[no etiology code] F03.*xy*	G31.83 Lewy body disease F06.70 w/o behavioral symptoms or F06.71 w/ behavioral symptoms Add codes for specific symptoms[a]	[no etiology code] G31.84 (and state w/ or w/o behavioral disturbance— words only)
Parkinson's disease	G20 Parkinson's disease F02.*xy*	[no etiology code] F03.*xy*	G20 Parkinson's disease F06.70 w/o behavioral symptoms or F06.71 w/ behavioral symptoms Add codes for specific symptoms[a]	[no etiology code] G31.84 (and state w/ or w/o behavioral disturbance— words only)
Vascular disease	[no etiology code] F01.*xy*	[no etiology code] F03.*xy*	I67.9 cerebrovascular disease F06.70 w/o behavioral symptoms or F06.71 w/ behavioral symptoms Add codes for specific symptoms[a]	[no etiology code] G31.84 (and state w/ or w/o behavioral disturbance— words only)

Note: Major NCD coding for x and y decimal places:

x (first digit after decimal point): A = mild; B = moderate; C = severe.

y (second/third digits after decimal point): .x2 = with psychotic disturbance; .x3 = with mood symptoms; .x4 = with anxiety; .x11 = with agitation; .x18 = with other behavioral or psychological disturbance; .x0 = without accompanying behavioral or psychological disturbance. If multiple symptoms, two or more of these codes may be needed.

[a]Specific clinically important mental/behavioral symptoms attached to the disorder for mild NCD. See Table 16.3.

TABLE 16.2. Additional Major and Mild NCD Etiologies

Presumed etiology	Major NCD	Mild NCD
Traumatic brain injury	S06.2XAS diffuse traumatic brain injury with loss of consciousness or unspecified duration, sequela F02.*xy*	S06.2XAS diffuse traumatic brain injury with loss of consciousness or unspecified duration, sequela F06.70 w/o behavioral symptoms or F06.71 w/ behavioral symptoms Add codes for specific symptoms[a]
HIV infection	B20 HIV infection F02.*xy*	B20 HIV infection F06.70 w/o behavioral symptoms or F06.71 w/ behavioral symptoms Add codes for specific symptoms[a]
Prion disease	A81.9 Prion disease F02.*xy*	A81.9 Prion disease F06.70 w/o behavioral symptoms or F06.71 w/ behavioral symptoms Add codes for specific symptoms[a]
Huntington's disease	G10 Huntington's disease F02.*xy*	G10 Huntington's disease F06.70 w/o behavioral symptoms or F06.71 w/ behavioral symptoms Add codes for specific symptoms[a]
Another medical condition; multiple etiologies (including probable causes)	[Code #s] Medical conditions [but no code # for cerebrovascular disease] F02.*xy* [If vascular, F01.*xy*]	[Code #s] Medical conditions (include I67.9 for cerebrovascular disease) F06.70 w/o behavioral symptoms or F06.71 w/ behavioral symptoms Add codes for specific symptoms[a]
Unknown etiology	[no etiology code] F03.*xy*	G31.84 (and state w/ or w/o behavioral symptoms—words only)
Substance/ medication induced	See Table 15.2 (p. 475) for code numbers State in words only: severity of NCD (mild, moderate, severe); with psychotic disturbance, with mood symptoms, with anxiety, with agitation, with other behavioral or psychological disturbance, without other behavioral or psychological disturbance	

Note: Major NCD coding for *x* and *y* decimal places:
x (first digit after decimal point): A = mild; B = moderate; C = severe.
y (second/third digits after decimal point): *.x2* = with psychotic disturbance; *.x3* = with mood symptoms; *.x4* = with anxiety; *.x11* = with agitation; *.x18* = with other behavioral or psychological disturbance; *.x0* = without accompanying behavioral or psychological disturbance. If multiple symptoms, two or more of these codes may be needed.
[a]Specific clinically important mental/behavioral symptoms attached to the disorder for mild NCD. See Table 16.3.

The table footnotes tell us that the *x* after the decimal point is for the NCD severity code, with A = mild, B = moderate, and C = severe. *Easy does it.*

You will then use the *y* part after the decimal to signify whatever behavioral or psychological symptoms accompany the NCD. There are potentially six of these, and they are listed in the footnotes. You might have to list more than one of these. *Don't despair; Read the examples.*

If the cause is use of a substance, you must consult Table 15.1 (p. 412) for coding. You won't use the ABC's to indicate severity, and you will state the behavioral/psychological symptom in words only—no code is attached.

Wherever applicable, the *possible* and the *probable* labels should come just before the name of the etiological disorder, not before the NCD. After all, the reasoning goes, the fact of the NCD isn't at question—it's the cause that's a bit uncertain. *Breathe slowly.*

OK, here are some examples.

A patient whose probable Alzheimer's disease has moderate major NCD with symptoms of depression:

G30.9	Alzheimer's disease
F02.B3	Major NCD due to probable Alzheimer's disease, moderate, with depressive symptoms

A patient whose possible Alzheimer's disease has led to a severe major NCD with anxiety and depression:

[note that no etiology is stated]

F03.C4	Major NCD due to possible Alzheimer's disease, severe, with anxiety
F03.C3	Major NCD due to possible Alzheimer's disease, severe, with depression

A patient's severe barbiturate use disorder has led to a severe NCD with anxiety. Table 15.2 has codes for neither NCD severity nor for the behavioral symptoms, so we'll just state them in words:

F13.27	Severe barbiturate use disorder with barbiturate-induced NCD, severe, with anxiety

And, this patient has had well-documented strokes leading to a severe major NCD with psychosis:

[note that no etiology is stated]

F01.C2	Severe major NCD probably due to vascular disease, with psychosis

And, suppose you don't know the cause, but your patient has severe anxiety symptoms along with major NCD. You would record:

F03.C4   Severe major NCD due to unknown etiology, with anxiety symptoms

For examples of NCD due to multiple etiologies, see page 541.

Recording Mild Neurocognitive Disorders

For the *probable* causes listed in Table 16.1 and for most of those in Table 16.2, first write down the causative agent with its unique code number. These are mild NCDs, so no further severity codes are needed.

Next, write down

F06.71   Mild NCD with behavioral symptoms, *or*
F06.70   Mild NCD without behavioral symptoms

If it is the former, you can describe accompanying behavioral/psychological symptoms with codes and words. I've listed them in Table 16.3; you may need to use more than one code.

For mild NCDs due to *possible* causes (and unknown etiologies), you won't code the causative agent (because, the cause being only possible, you aren't all that certain).

TABLE 16.3. Clinical Problems That Can Accompany NCD

F06.0	Psychotic disorder [due to X medical condition] with hallucinations
F06.1	Catatonic disorder [due to X medical condition]
F06.2	Psychotic disorder [due to X medical condition] with delusions
F06.3	Mood disorder [due to X medical condition]
F06.31	Mood disorder [due to X medical condition] with depressive features
F06.32	Mood disorder [due to X medical condition] with major depressive episode
F06.33	Mood disorder [due to X medical condition] with manic features
F06.34	Mood disorder [due to X medical condition] with mixed features (or with hypomanic-like features)
F06.4	Anxiety disorder [due to X medical condition]
F06.8	Other specified disorder [due to X medical condition]
F07.0	Personality change [due to X medical condition], labile, disinhibited, aggressive, apathetic, paranoid, other, combined or unspecified type

Rather, just write down G31.84 and state, in words only, whether or not there are any behavioral or psychological symptoms.

And here are the examples:

A patient with gradually failing memory and issues with attention span who can still manage activities of daily living and personal care with the help of reminders and a really up-to-date calendar has no accompanying behavioral or psychological symptoms. Both parents were diagnosed with Alzheimer's. Here is how you would describe this patient:

G30.9   Alzheimer's disease
F06.70   Mild NCD due to probable Alzheimer's disease, without behavioral symptoms

Now we've discovered that this patient has been having both anxiety and manic-like symptoms associated with the Alzheimer's NCD.

G30.9   Alzheimer's disease
F06.71   Mild NCD due to probable Alzheimer's disease, with behavioral disturbance
F06.4   Anxiety disorder due to mild NCD
F06.33   Bipolar and related disorder due to mild NCD, with manic features

Suppose instead, this patient had no family history and no genetic evidence for Alzheimer's, but you judge there to be steady, progressive decline in memory and learning with no evidence of mixed etiology. In short, you diagnose possible Alzheimer's. Then you would record:

[note the absence of etiology code]
G31.84   Mild NCD due to possible Alzheimer's disease, without behavioral symptoms

Now, suppose a different patient's years-long, heavy inhalant use appears the cause of a severe NCD that includes depression and anxiety. Then you would write down:

F18.27   Heavy inhalant use disorder with inhalant-induced severe major NCD, with anxiety and depression

Finally, what about a patient who has some cognitive symptoms but not enough to make a diagnosis of NCD or delirium?

R41.9   Unspecified neurocognitive disorder

Mild NCD is a newish name (DSM-5) that comes with a lot of built-in synonyms. They include *mild cognitive impairment, age-associated memory impairment,* and *nondementia cognitive impairment.* These patients do not have full-fledged NCD, but they aren't exactly well, either. Although they have symptoms, their functional abilities are largely intact, but follow-through requires extra effort. Don't confuse mild NCD with *age-related cognitive decline,* which is normal (where did I put my keys?) for the person's age—and which in ICD-10 no longer has diagnostic status. And don't, please, overinterpret it—although some patients who can be diagnosed with mild NCD will later develop the major form of the disorder, by no means will all do so.

Here's an additional quibbling note about mild NCD. The Good Book tells us that if we use this term, we are not to write down a code for the presumed causative agent. I find myself pushing back against this stricture. Surely, if we know that a person has had, for example, a traumatic brain injury, and that the result is a mild NCD, then we are allowed (heck, I'll say *obligated*) to indicate as much. It is information that could be valuable to the next clinician who sees the patient, and hence it may be of considerable value to the patient. As I understand it, the authors of DSM-5-TR wanted to be consistent in not writing down causes when the clinician may be uncertain about etiology, which with mild NCD is often the case. But when we have pretty darned strong evidence, our duty is to the patient, not to a book.

Neurocognitive Disorder Due to Alzheimer's Disease

The most common cause of what was once called senility, NCD due to Alzheimer's disease, has been recognized since the early 1900s. Alzheimer's accounts for well over half of all patients with neurocognitive disorder; the majority of elderly patients in nursing homes have this degenerative disorder. Patients with Down syndrome who are over 40 are also at high risk. Indeed, any clinician who treats older patients is bound to encounter it frequently. Patients with early-onset Alzheimer's disease are especially likely to have relatives with the same disorder.

NCD due to Alzheimer's disease is also important because so many other disorders, both cognitive and otherwise, can be mistaken for it. Despite our diagnostic advances, it is *still* a diagnosis of exclusion that should only be made once all other causes (especially those that can be treated) have been ruled out.

Patients with Alzheimer's disease often, perhaps usually, first experience the behavioral and psychological symptoms that will eventually be described as "behavioral disturbance." Existing personality traits may be accentuated: The person may become more obsessional, secretive, or sexually active. Other early indicators of dementia can include apathy, emotional lability (sudden weeping or temper outbursts), or the loss of a previously acute sense of humor. Eventually, nearly all patients with Alzheimer's will have some of these symptoms, which exacerbate disability and may herald rapid decline and early death.

Eventually, however, as in other dementias, memory loss will come to the fore. Recent memory (the ability to recall information that was learned within the previous few minutes) is usually the first aspect to be involved; remote memory is affected later on, as patients forget familiar names or repeatedly ask questions that have just been answered. To compensate, some write themselves notes or compile lists. Although a sense of self is generally preserved until late in the disease, severely demented patients may fail to recognize their relatives or long-time friends, and ultimately may even fail to answer to their own name.

Loss of executive functioning (usually attributed to frontal lobe damage) can be tested directly by asking the patient to identify similarities and differences or to carry out a sequence of steps, as on the MMSE. But executive functioning is often best evaluated from the history or from observation of some of these behaviors: closely trailing the clinician or a companion (imitation behavior); frozen expression until prompted (lack of spontaneity); putting on more than one pair of trousers (perseveration); or repeatedly getting lost on the ward, though oriented at home (environmental dependency). The emerging picture may be that of a person who can navigate and function reasonably well in a fixed, familiar environment, but who has difficulty adapting to changing circumstances. Some patients are referred for evaluation only when they cannot cope with the unfamiliar surroundings of a new residence. As is true of most of us, patients with Alzheimer's may do better when they are rested.

Language functions may be manifested at first by trouble finding words (aphasia). The vocabulary contracts as clichés and stereotyped phrases are substituted for real communication, and the patient stops using complex sentences. Reading and writing may deteriorate; conversation rambles.

Many patients with Alzheimer's disease will also have perceptual issues such as illusions or hallucinations. Some may become inordinately suspicious and develop paranoia. About 20% become depressed; even those who are not depressed often experience insomnia or anorexia. Therefore, it is important to consider Alzheimer's (or other causes of NCD) in the differential diagnosis of any older patient who presents with symptoms that suggest a depressive disorder.

The typical patient lives 8 or 10 years after the onset of Alzheimer's disease. The clinical course, though variable, is typically a steady decline through three stages:

1. From 1 to 3 years of growing forgetfulness.

2. Then, 2 or 3 years of increasing disorientation, loss of language skills, and inappropriate behavior. Until they reach advanced stages, most patients appear grossly normal, though physical exam may reveal typical "frontal release signs" such as the palmomental reflex—pursing of lips when the palm is stroked. (However, some elderly people develop frontal release signs without having

evidence of dementia.) Hallucinations and delusions may appear during this stage.

3. A final period of severe dementia, during which there is disorientation for person and complete loss of self-care.

Insight is almost always absent, and sooner or later judgment becomes impaired. At the end may come complete muteness and lack of response. Patients with Alzheimer's tolerate physical illness poorly; infection or reduced nutrition that a person without the disease would shrug off may trigger a superimposed delirium.

Alzheimer's disease is found in 11% of people 65 and over and in a third of those over 85. It accounts for well over half of all dementia cases. Although Alzheimer's disease is all too common, the etiological relationship must usually be inferred from the absence of other possible causes. Because some of these are treatable, and because Alzheimer's disease has such a dismal prognosis, it is vitally important to rule out all other possible alternatives. (DSM-5-TR lists NCD due to Alzheimer's first, as do I; don't let this lead you astray.)

Nearly every patient with neurocognitive disorder will have problems with memory and learning, but it is only one of the six cognitive domains that can be affected. In DSM-5-TR, however, a defect of memory is a requirement for the diagnosis of NCD due to Alzheimer's.

Essential Features of **Neurocognitive Disorder Due to Alzheimer's Disease**

The patient has a {major}{mild} neurocognitive disorder (p. 503) that begins slowly and progresses gradually. Two or more of these symptom domains must be involved: complex attention, learning and memory, perceptual–motor ability, executive functioning, language, social cognition (p. 498).

The Fine Print

The D's: • Duration (chronic) • Differential diagnosis (delirium; age-related cognitive decline; intellectual developmental disorder; **other physical, mental, neurological disorders; substance use; other causes of NCD,** especially **cerebrovascular** and Lewy body diseases and frontotemporal degeneration

There are two ways to arrive at a diagnosis of probable major NCD due to Alzheimer's disease, and one way each to a diagnosis of possible major, probable mild, or possible mild NCD due to Alzheimer's. See the chart below.

	Major NCD due to Alzheimer's		Mild NCD due to Alzheimer's	
	Probable	**Possible**	**Probable**	**Possible**
	Meets criteria for {major}{mild} NCD			
	Insidious onset, gradual progression of disability			
# domains affected	Two or more		One or more	
Positive genetic evidence (testing or family history) for Alzheimer's disease	Major NCD due to probable Alzheimer's disease	—	Mild NCD due to probable Alzheimer's disease	No evidence
Steady, gradual decline; no extended plateaus No evidence of mixed causes[a] Decline in memory and learning + 1 more domain	All 3 factors present: Major NCD due to probable Alzheimer's disease	If any of these 3 factors is missing: Major NCD due to possible Alzheimer's disease	—	Steady, gradual decline with no extended plateaus; no evidence of mixed causes;[a] decline in memory and learning: Mild NCD due to possible Alzheimer's disease

[a]Any evidence for mixed causes forces a diagnosis of NCD due to multiple etiologies.

Coding Notes

Record the diagnoses and code numbers from Table 16.1 (p. 507).

Hank Altig

Two years before he moves to Sunny Acres, Hank Altig takes a job as greeter with a big box store. He has been retired for several years, and at the age of 66, he wants more activity. "I just don't feel like sitting around idle any longer," he tells the screener at his preemployment physical exam. "I've still got some good years in me." Though he gives his address, Social Security number, and new cell phone number from memory, still he wonders aloud why he occasionally walks into a room and then can't remember why he is there. "Don't we all?" comes the response.

Hank worked nearly 40 years as an accountant, a profession that requires concentration and a high tolerance for boredom; being a greeter requires only his presence and a willingness to smile. These he gives in good measure. "Eighty percent of success is just showing up," he quotes.

For months, every time Hank shows up, he has shaved carefully and paid meticulous attention to his clothes, his shoes—even his hair and nails. "I want to be the greeter's greeter," he tells his daughter. Sandy lives just down the street and is the principal informant at his clinical assessments.

Nearly a year into the job, Hank begins to have problems. When first he'd hired on, he memorized the location of half the items in the store. But every few days, something gets moved to a different shelf, and now he can't seem to keep the changes in his head. Sandy buys him a tiny Moleskine notebook in which he can keep track of the items people ask about most. He also uses it for his appointments—mostly these are dinner dates with Sandy—and other important information. Whenever Hank has trouble remembering something, Sandy will smile and say, "Where's Moley?" Often Hank can look up what he wants to know.

Now 18 months have passed, and Sandy has begun to worry. "There's been no dramatic change," she says, "just a steady slide." Once or twice when waiting for Hank to get off work, she notices that he seems at first unaware when someone asks for assistance. She knows that several times he's been late going in; sometimes he arrives without bothering to shave. If she points it out, he just shrugs and turns away.

Now they are back at the clinician's office. Sandy reports that Hank has stopped cooking. Mostly he eats cold cereal unless she fixes something for him and brings it over. "I'm so worried," Sandy says. "No one in the family has had anything like this."

"Where do you like to shop for groceries?" asks the interviewer. With no response forthcoming, Sandy prompts, "Where's Moley?" But Hank just looks blank, and the little notebook never leaves the pocket of his cardigan.

Evaluation of Hank Altig

Even when Hank first sought employment as a greeter, he was concerned about his memory. Concern (on the part of the patient or someone else) is necessary but not sufficient for a diagnosis of any NCD. Hank's early concern was based on a common occurrence that had no clinical significance, as his clinician noted at the time. The requirement for a diagnosis is that there be concern about a decline plus *objective evidence*—the kind that can only be obtained by actual neuropsychological testing or by a bedside evaluation such as the MMSE. (We're at something of a disadvantage in this discussion because we don't have the results of testing; we'll have to interpolate a bit.)

In any event, we can be reasonably confident that Hank didn't have any important cognitive deficit at the time he started his job. He not only quoted Woody Allen accurately, but his executive abilities were intact: He got himself to work on time and nicely groomed, and he committed to memory the locations of numerous items in the store. However, after several months, he began to falter.

First evaluation. Hank is at this point concerned, as is Sandy (NCD criterion A1), that he has difficulty learning new material. His memory isn't quite what it once was: He appears to have lost some of his former ability to memorize and recall the new locations of products in his store. However, he can compensate with the little notebook that Sandy gave him (B), setting us up for a diagnosis of mild NCD. To complete the evaluation, we'd need objective evidence of cognitive decline—formal testing of some sort, whether a cognitive evaluation or just the MMSE completed in the office (A2). The remaining criteria, that neither a delirium (C) nor some other mental disorder such as depression or schizophrenia (D) is present, are fulfilled in the vignette.

Now his clinician should complete the evaluation with a formal mental status evaluation, or at least a bedside evaluation of cognitive ability such as the MMSE. That, plus a neurological exam and enough laboratory (especially radiological) testing to pinpoint the cause of his decline. In an elderly person, you'd want to rule out a traumatic brain injury by the absence of history of blows to the head; a substance-induced NCD would (of course) feature a prominent history of substance or medication use. Physical exam would reveal no evidence of Parkinson's disease, and history and preserved affect would eliminate pseudodementia due to a depressive disorder. Skull X-rays and MRI could rule out brain tumors and normal pressure hydrocephalus; blood tests could exclude hypothyroidism and vitamin B_{12} deficiency as possible causes. The steady rather than stepwise decline renders unlikely a vascular disease etiology, which is a common cause of neurocognitive disorder in older patients. As far as we can tell from the vignette, Hank has none of the core or suggestive features that would suggest NCD with Lewy bodies or frontotemporal degeneration.

All this seems to leave NCD due to Alzheimer's disease as the disorder of exclusion—but would it be "probable" or "possible"? DSM-5-TR criteria are a little finicky about this discrimination, but we can puzzle our way through them. Let's start with the time that Hank first begins to have problems.

The criteria for mild NCD due to Alzheimer's disease would allow a probable (the stronger) diagnosis reserved for patients who have positive evidence from genetic testing or family history; neither of these applies to Hank. So let's examine the other evidence summarized in that fussy table in the Essential Features. His decline appears to be steady; at least we have no evidence of a stepwise decline or that he has ever reached some sort of plateau. Next, we should look for evidence of other possible etiologies for his symptoms. Lo and behold, we discarded them all just a couple of paragraphs ago. Finally, his principal symptoms are decline in his memory and in his ability to learn. Therefore, at that time he fulfills the criterion (C) for mild NCD due to possible Alzheimer's disease. Whew!

The second evaluation. Now let's move on to his subsequent history. By the time more months have passed, Sandy notices that Hank's attention wanders while he is on the job and that he has begun showing up for work less well-groomed than before—presumptive evidence for markedly reduced executive functioning. And even with reminders, he is no longer able to compensate for his memory problems by using his pocket notebook. The result, as we infer from the fact that he subsequently moves to Sunny Acres, is a decline that is gradual (his entire story spans nearly 2 years) and in important ways interferes with Hank's capacity to pursue independently the activities of everyday life (B). We need formal testing to confirm our impression; I'm going to declare that this was done and that it did demonstrate a significant decline in Hank's cognitive performance.

There's *still* no genetic or family history to help us out. But as noted just above, Hank does have a gradually progressive course of declining memory and learning, with no evidence for mixed causes. And this time, we can find evidence of impairment in other cognitive domains—executive functioning and attention. We have now collected the evidence to support a diagnosis of major NCD due to probable Alzheimer's disease (also criterion C).

But before we wrap up, what about behavioral disturbance? Hank doesn't really respond to Sandy's last question, and he has lost interest in cooking and shaving. I'd interpret this as apathy, which by the liberal DSM-5-TR definition (which also allows depression, psychosis, and agitation) constitutes behavioral disturbance. Other than giving Hank's GAF score (twice), this is where we'll stop.

First evaluation (GAF = 65):

G31.84   Mild neurocognitive disorder due to possible Alzheimer's disease, without behavioral disturbance

Second evaluation (GAF = 40):

G30.9   Alzheimer's disease
F02.B18   Major neurocognitive disorder due to probable Alzheimer's disease, moderate, with apathy

Neurocognitive Disorder with Lewy Bodies

One of the newer NCD diagnoses in the book, NCD with Lewy bodies (I'll refer to the major form as dementia with Lewy bodies, or DLB) was until the mid-1990s only a gleam in the eyes of a few researchers and clinicians. Now DLB is recognized as the second largest cause of neurocognitive disorder—it accounts for up to 10% of patients with NCD, as against 60–75% for Alzheimer's. There are currently well over a million such patients in the United States alone.

Discovered a full century ago, Lewy bodies are spherical bits of protein (α-synuclein) found in the cytoplasm of brain cells located especially in the brainstem nuclei, substantia nigra, and locus ceruleus. Patients with DLB also frequently have amyloid plaques that are typical of Alzheimer's disease; these people have clinical features of both Parkinson's and Alzheimer's diseases as well. Those similarities probably explain why DLB remained obscure for so long.

- *Fluctuating attention.* Early on, patients with DLB tend to experience less of the early memory loss that is typical for patients with Alzheimer's. Most affected are attention span and alertness, which in fact tend to wax and wane over minutes, hours, or even days in over half of patients with DLB. This fluctuation of symptoms constitutes the first of the principal ("core") features.

- *Hallucinations.* The second core feature is well-formed visual hallucinations, which occur early and tend to persist. Typically, they are of animals or intruders. They can occur with or without insight and may be accompanied by delusions that are sometimes systematized.

- *Later onset of Parkinson's-type symptoms.* Typical motor symptoms of Parkinson's disease—immobile face, hand tremor, shuffling gait—constitute the third core feature, but they must not predate the cognitive decline. If they do, the diagnosis is not DLB at all, but rather Parkinson's disease with NCD. The rule of thumb: DLB symptoms must begin at least a year before motor symptoms appear.

Patients with DLB are also prone to dizziness, falls, and unexplained fainting spells. Depression is common, as is autonomic dysfunction (orthostatic hypotension, incontinence of urine). REM sleep behavior disorder (p. 348) is sometimes noted and may be an early symptom. Early diagnosis is especially important in DLB, because these patients can be exquisitely sensitive to antipsychotics, relatively low doses of which cause muscle rigidity, fever, and other symptoms of neuroleptic malignant syndrome (p. 614).

DLB typically begins around age 75; men are affected somewhat more often than are women. After diagnosis, the typical patient lives about 10 years.

It isn't at all clear that Parkinson's NCD and DLB are different entities; some authorities believe that they exist on a continuum. They both involve α-synuclein protein and degeneration of the substantia nigra of the brain. Both feature Parkinson's motor symptoms, though with different timing: For a diagnosis of DLB, the movement disorder must show up only after cognitive symptoms have been present for a year or more. Preexisting movement disorder shifts the diagnosis to Parkinson's NCD.

Of course, this creates something of a dilemma for the clinician who needs to make a diagnosis *now,* using as a criterion something that hasn't occurred yet. Not all of these patients do develop the motor symptoms of parkinsonism, and you only need two of the core features to diagnose the probable form of the disease. Finally, there can be no definitive diagnosis without pathological verification.

Essential Features of **Neurocognitive Disorder with Lewy Bodies**

The patient has a {major}{mild} neurocognitive disorder (p. 503).

Beginning slowly and progressing gradually, the disease has these core features: wide fluctuation in attentiveness; elaborate, clear hallucinations; and symptoms of parkinsonism that begin a year or more after the cognitive symptoms.

Some patients have features that *suggest* DLB: REM sleep behavior disorder, marked sensitivity to antipsychotic drugs.

The Fine Print

The D's: • Duration (tends to chronicity) • Differential diagnosis (delirium; **substance-related disorders; other mental disorders** (especially depressive or psychotic disorders); **physical disorders,** other causes of NCD—especially Alzheimer's and **vascular** diseases and frontotemporal degeneration)

See the accompanying chart for guidance in arriving at a diagnosis.

		Probable NCD with Lewy bodies	Possible NCD with Lewy bodies
Core features	Fluctuating alertness and attention	One core feature plus one or more additional core or suggestive features	One core or suggestive feature
	Repeated, vivid, detailed hallucinations		
	Parkinsonism that begins only *after* the cognitive decline		
Suggestive features	REM sleep behavior disorder (p. 348)		
	Exquisite sensitivity to antipsychotics		

Coding Notes

Record the diagnoses and code numbers from Table 16.1 (p. 507).

You can't code **with behavioral disturbance,** but if you note it's there, you should mention it in writing anyway.

Sheila Wilton

"Dr. Brantleigh said she has schizophrenia," Sophia reports. Sophia is Sheila Wilton's grown stepdaughter, and she provides most of the historical information. The shape of her lips says she doesn't for 1 minute believe Dr. Brantleigh.

The problems began about 3 months earlier, when Sheila had trouble finding her way back from the store. She's shopped at Safeway on the corner for many years, but twice now she's apparently turned left instead of right and wandered many blocks astray. The first time, a policeman brought her home. The second, a neighbor recognized her and called Sophia, who came to collect her. "At first, she seemed fuzzy, confused," Sophia laments, "but when I asked her later to tell me our address and such, she responded with all the facts."

A few days later, Sophia found Sheila sitting on the edge of her bed, talking to a vivid hallucination of her husband standing beside her. "He was motioning to me to get up and fix breakfast," Sheila could finally relate. "Dad's been dead for 7 years," Sophia finishes up.

They consulted their local medical provider, who, finding nothing wrong, referred Sheila for psychological evaluation. A tentative diagnosis of schizophrenia and another trip to the doctor netted a prescription for haloperidol, "and then all hell broke loose." Sheila's quiet little hallucination turned hostile. Still using mime, her phantom husband now threatened her, sometimes with a closed fist, sometimes with his heavy walking stick. She responded at first with agitation, then with fury that ultimately dwindled into a perplexity that would wax and wane. Within a day or two, she became overly sedated, then rigid—so stiff she could hardly walk. "Now they're saying she's catatonic and needs shock treatments," Sophia says. "I don't understand it. No one in her family has ever had any sort of mental illness."

Off and on during the day, Sheila will be confused, at times not even knowing where she is. But in the doctor's office she is fully oriented, missing the correct date by only 2 days. "That's about as well as I can do," remarks Sophia. "But it's so typical of the way she's been—first she's out of it, then she's back in it. Brantleigh implied that she was doing it for the attention I was giving her. He used the word *malingering*."

Evaluation of Sheila Wilton

Let's for a moment put aside the hallucinations and focus instead on the domains of Sheila's other cognitive symptoms. These are perceptual–motor (aside from the hallucinations, she couldn't find her way home) and complex attention (she has fluctuating awareness). We'd need formal testing to put a number to the extent of her decline, but from this and the other information in the vignette, I'd judge her clinically as being moderately impaired, thereby earning a diagnosis of major NCD. Her symptoms interfere with her independence—at least for such important activities of daily living as working around the house and managing money. It appears that she can still feed and dress herself, so her current level of severity would be mild. (Note the distinction: She would have mild *major* NCD, not *mild* NCD. The semantic nightmare is bound to cause some clinicians heartburn.)

And while we're talking about the basic NCD diagnosis, let's consider the specifiers. Sheila does have rather pronounced hallucinations, which earns her the qualifier *with behavioral disturbance*.

Though we could mount a cogent argument for a neurological consultation, there wouldn't appear to be other medical disorders, and certainly not other mental disorders (the diagnosis of schizophrenia is obviously bogus) that could better explain her symptoms. In short, she appears to have some sort of a major neurocognitive disorder. But which one? First, a couple of facts—sobering for those who like to achieve certainty while life endures. For many patients, only the fullness of time (read: a postmortem examination) can deliver a final, accurate diagnosis. And even with imaging and laboratory information, discriminating one cause of NCD from another can be devilishly hard. But here goes.

Sheila has no history of traumatic brain injury, so we can rule out neurocognitive disorder due to trauma. She doesn't have early and prominent difficulties with her memory, so we can put Alzheimer's to the side, though not completely off the table. There is neither hypertension nor stepwise progression of her symptoms, rendering unlikely a vascular cause. History and physical symptoms are inconsistent for Huntington's, Parkinson's, and HIV infection. The criteria for the two types of frontotemporal NCD are infuriatingly complicated, as we'll discover later, but as neither her behavior nor her language appears to have deteriorated enough for a diagnosis of either subtype, we can postpone that annoyance a little longer.

Of course, that still leaves many other disorders that can cause NCD, but our diagnostic foray shouldn't be one exclusively of elimination. There are affirmative reasons to consider NCD with Lewy bodies—in Sheila or in any patient. The main one is that this diagnosis carries an immediate and important implication about treatment. It is the risk that using antipsychotic drugs can lead, as it apparently did with Sheila, to worsening of the cognitive symptoms and to the physical symptoms of neuroleptic malignant syndrome. (That drug reaction is one of the symptoms suggestive of DLB.) In addition, she had the wide fluctuations in alertness and attention and the well-formed hallucinations that constitute core features.

For a diagnosis of probable major NCD with Lewy bodies, Sheila would need at least one core symptom plus at least one other (core or suggestive); Sheila has two core symptoms and one suggestive, more than enough for her working diagnosis. I'd put her current GAF score at 45, but I won't disagree if you argue for a different value. She's been all over the map.

The narrative of Sheila Wilton includes two of my differential diagnosis *bêtes noires*—malingering and schizophrenia. It's not that they never happen; of course they do. But they are two "explanations" that clinicians sometimes use to get themselves off the hook for symptoms that are hard to evaluate, hard to understand, hard to treat, and hard to view optimistically. Each of these diagnoses will only appear late in my evaluative process.

G31.83	Lewy body disease
F02.A2	Major neurocognitive disorder with probable Lewy bodies, mild, with hallucinations

Neurocognitive Disorder Due to Traumatic Brain Injury

Each year in the United States, more than a million people suffer a blow to the head or some other injury that ushers in traumatic brain injury (TBI). Though most cases of TBI are mild, the damage from war and sports injuries can be devastating. And of course, some die of their injuries.

The largest number of patients with TBI are adolescents or young adults (males predominate); older patients, because they injure themselves in falls, are the next most affected age group. Low socioeconomic status is another risk factor, but the biggest risk of all is use of alcohol and drugs—which contribute to nearly half of TBIs. Motor vehicle accidents, including those that involve pedestrians, are the leading proximate cause; falls (especially in older patients) are second. Sports injuries are an important source for younger people; boxing has been famously implicated, but percentagewise, female athletes are the more likely to be affected.

The symptoms of TBI are caused by a disruption of brain structure or physiology that results from violent external force exerted upon the head. Immediate loss of consciousness is typical; after awakening, patients may have trouble focusing and maintaining attention. Delirium is common; even after it clears, deficits in attention are commonplace. Many patients complain of anterograde or retrograde memory loss. Language functions affect about a third of patients with severe TBI. These especially include fluent (receptive) aphasias, though nonfluent (expressive) aphasias are also well represented. Executive functioning is commonly affected. Patients with TBI will also complain of problems with sleep, headaches, and irritability.

Though it can take months, most patients eventually recover. But common sequels include depressive disorders (most frequent), anxiety disorders, and substance misuse. Personality change is sometimes noted. A preinjury mental disorder greatly increases the risk for a postinjury disorder. And TBI, especially if repeated, may increase the likelihood of Alzheimer's—perhaps by as much as fourfold.

Some writers note how challenging it can be to discriminate NCD due to TBI from posttraumatic stress disorder.

Chronic traumatic encephalopathy doesn't fit neatly into the TBI paradigm, caused as it is by *repeated* injury to the brain. It's associated with contact sports such as boxing (then, it's sometimes been called *dementia pugilistica*), American football, soccer, ice hockey, rugby, and even professional wrestling. Symptoms—which include failing memory, aggression, poor impulse control, parkinsonism, depression, and suicide—have been found, tragically, in athletes as young as 17. At least two professional football players, apparently realizing that their brains had been damaged by repetitive playing injuries, have killed themselves, carefully choosing means that would preserve their brains for postmortem examination. The phenomenon makes for riveting scientific studies, television specials, and lawsuits.

Essential Features of **Neurocognitive Disorder Due to Traumatic Brain Injury**

Immediately following head trauma that causes rapid movement of the brain inside the skull, the patient loses consciousness; or may develop amnesia, or disorientation and perplexity, or neurological signs such as seizures, blind spots in the visual field, loss of smell, hemiparesis, or an injury demonstrated by imaging.

Subsequently, the patient's symptoms fulfill criteria for a {mild}{major} neurocognitive disorder (p. 503) and last longer than the immediate postinjury period.

The Fine Print

The D's: • Duration (starts immediately, lasts a week or more) • Differential diagnosis (other medical and mental disorders, factitious disorder, malingering)

Coding Notes

See Table 16.2 (p. 508).

Thornton Naguchi

When Thornton Naguchi arrived home from war, his reception wasn't what he or anyone in his family had imagined. The brass band and confetti (his fantasy) were missing in action; on the other hand, so was the pine box, which had been his mother's fear all along. "She's a firm believer in Murphy's law—if something can go wrong, it will," Thornton tells the interviewer at the VA hospital where he stays for a few days.

Thornton's grandparents had been interned in Idaho during World War II, leaving his grandfather extremely bitter, often railing against the government. Grandpa was something of a tyrant; Thornton got his revenge by enlisting as soon as he was old enough. Within a few months, the Army had posted him to a part of Iraq so remote, he recounts, they'd never heard of tofu.

During Thornton's first week in country, he was riding in the last non-up-armored Humvee in the unit when they hit an improvised explosive device. As he launched into the air, a shard of metal sliced right through his helmet strap; he fell back squarely on his head. When he awakened nearly 24 hours later, he could remember starting off on the mission, but nothing of the actual explosion. It was his sergeant who'd reconstructed those events for him.

After the accident, Thornton was grateful to be alive, but he initially had some trouble focusing—even on watching TV. Though he has always been bright and personable, now he was cross, snapping at a nurse who suggested that he could get up and change the channel for himself.

While still awaiting his discharge papers, Thornton got a job selling cell phones at an electronics outlet near his home. He'd grown up with electronic devices and had kept current with the industry while he was in the Army, so he had little trouble demonstrating the basic features of smart phones.

But keeping in mind the nuances of the different models is a chore—far more so for him than for the other young people who work there. "I need a crib sheet—on my phone—just to keep up," he remarks. "I mean, we're talking 15 or 20 different models here, not to mention the tablets." If a coworker asks an incidental question when Thornton is talking to a customer, he'll lose his train of thought completely. "I'll have to ask the customer where we were. I *know* it's cost me bonus money."

Thornton lives with Yuki, his girlfriend of 4 years. She reports that he seems distracted, "forever drifting out of the picture," as she puts it. He isn't really depressed, she thinks, but he's cranky and impulsive. Occasionally, he'll fling on his clothes and slam out the door. When he returns, he'll say that he only went for a walk. "And he just freaks out at loud noises."

That's apparently what happened one afternoon as he was hanging curtains in their apartment. Yuki dropped a pan lid in the kitchenette, not 10 feet from where Thornton was standing on a ladder. He jerked, overbalanced, and fell hard on the terrazzo floor. "Murphy was an optimist," he tells the paramedics who load him up for his second ambulance ride in 6 months.

Evaluation of Thornton Naguchi

The first step in the diagnosis of any NCD, major or mild, is to demonstrate some decline from previous functioning. This appears to be the case for Thornton, who needs help remembering the different types of cell phone he is supposed to be selling. He manages to avert significant problems with work by keeping a crib sheet—the extra effort required to compensate for his memory problems. He has also been irritable, perhaps a sign of a mild decline in the social cognition domain. And there are also some minor problems with his executive functioning, as suggested by the trouble he has picking up on an interrupted conversation.

Formal testing would probably confirm these modest declines in his cognitive abilities (mild NCD criterion A2), but even without it, a diagnosis of mild NCD can be sustained by a clinical interview and bedside testing. He has continued to support himself (B), isn't delirious (C), and doesn't involve another mental disorder (D).

Now for the TBI bit. Of course, the *sine qua non* of TBI is trauma, which in Thornton's case is well established. After that initial blow to his head, he suffered both unconsciousness and amnesia for the event; either of these would fulfill the diagnostic requirement (criterion B for NCD due to TBI). Long afterward (certainly well past the immediate postinjury period—criterion C), he remains irritable and unfocused, without definite symptoms of a mood disorder. Still, I don't think that his emotional or behavioral sequelae rise to the level of the *with behavioral disturbance* specifier. You may choose to disagree.

Based on how long he was unconscious, the duration of his amnesia, and his disorientation and bewilderment at initial assessment, DSM-5-TR permits us to rate the severity of his TBI. To me this seems, quite frankly, one number too many:* What we really care about is Thornton, not his injury. Prior to his latest fall, his GAF would have been a comparatively robust 71. I hope that he won't now develop chronic traumatic encephalopathy (see the sidebar). Assuming a "no," his diagnosis would be as follows:

S06.2X4S	Diffuse traumatic brain injury with loss of consciousness, 6–24 hours, sequela
F06.70	Mild neurocognitive disorder due to traumatic brain injury, without behavioral disturbance

One more issue. Notice that we have put in the code for Thornton's head injury. Why is this remarkable? When DSM-5-TR first came out, we were told not to. But the rules have changed, and so will we. We're team players. Go Team!

Frontotemporal Neurocognitive Disorder

Once called Pick's disease, frontotemporal NCD—for auld lang syne, I'll use the traditional abbreviation for frontotemporal dementia (FTD)—used to be considered rare. Now, it's known to account for up to 5% of all cases of neurocognitive disorder and perhaps one in six younger patients: Its mean age of onset is somewhere in the 50s. FTD appears to respect neither gender nor race, but it is often familial; about half of cases are transmitted as an autosomal dominant trait related to genes on chromosome 17.

You won't be astonished to hear that FTD affects frontal and temporal lobes of the brain (which lose neurons and accumulate tau protein); in so doing, it can produce diverse clinical pictures. The behavioral variant (frontal lobe involvement) constitutes about 80% of FTD cases. It is characterized either by apathy and social withdrawal or by disinhibition. Apathetic folks basically stay in bed and stop providing their own care. Disinhibited patients behave in socially inappropriate ways—make rude sexual comments, for example, or steal items or otherwise subvert social norms; eating in binges may occur. In both of these subtypes, what you notice is the behavior.

The language variant (temporal lobe lesions) often begins with patients unable to find the right word for a particular object or concept (*anomia*)—though they can point to the correct object when they see it. Understanding spoken language and reading aloud are both initially unimpaired, but with time, these patients may become increasingly unable to produce fluent, meaningful speech. Both the behavioral and the language types begin insidiously and progress slowly, with relative sparing of memory and perceptual–motor skills. Both culminate in compromised activities of daily living. As they progress, the boundaries of the two subtypes become less distinct.

In part because of variability and overlapping features, the syndromes of FTD

---

*Ratings of TBI severity may be helpful in doing research on head injury sequels. If you want to know more, you can turn to page 708 of DSM-5-TR, but I won't discuss it further here. I have my standards.

often go *un*recognized. Final antemortem diagnosis depends heavily on imaging and neuropsychological testing. It is a relatively frequent cause of NCD before age 65, and the behavioral type is somewhat more common than the language type. Here we'll use a couple of vignettes to illustrate what you might expect to confront in patients who haven't yet received the necessary workup.

As Pick's disease, FTD is a venerable diagnosis, dating back to the 1890s. It is remarkable how similar its symptoms resemble what was for many years called *simple schizophrenia,* a term retained in the official nomenclature until 1980. Here is that DSM-II description: It is "characterized chiefly by a slow and insidious reduction of external attachments and interests and by apathy and indifference leading to impoverishment of interpersonal relations, mental deterioration, and adjustment on a lower level of functioning." The entry goes on to explain that there is less in the way of dramatic psychosis than in other subtypes of schizophrenia, yet far more progression than with schizoid personality.

Essential Features of **Frontotemporal Neurocognitive Disorder**

The patient has a {mild}{major} neurocognitive disorder (p. 503). In the face of relatively unimpaired memory and visuomotor function, beginning slowly and progressing gradually, symptoms will be mainly of one of two types. (Some patients will present with features of both types.)

Behavioral variant. The patient has some of these behavior issues: disinhibition (socially inappropriate behavior that may include poor manners, loss of decorum, or rash impulsivity); apathy or inertia; reduced capacity for compassion; compulsive or repetitive behavior; and changes in diet with hyperorality (binge eating, pica, drinking, smoking).

Language variant. There is a gradual but obvious loss of the ability to produce speech, to find the right word, to attach names to objects, and to use grammar and understand the meaning of words.

The Fine Print

The D's: • Duration (chronic) • Differential diagnosis (**physical disease, other mental disorders,** other causes of NCD—especially **cerebrovascular disease,** Alzheimer's, Lewy bodies, **substance use**)

Coding Notes

Specify if:

Probable frontotemporal NCD. An existing pathogenic mutation is known (via

> genetic tests or family history), or imaging shows heavy frontotemporal involvement.
>
> **Possible frontotemporal NCD.** There is no genetic evidence and neuroimaging has not been done.

Record and code as indicated in Table 16.1 (p. 507).

Toby Russo

The telephone request comes from a man in Chicago who is worried about his dad. "When I saw him over the holidays, he wasn't himself," the caller begins. "For a long time, maybe a year, he's been losing interest in things. He's only 56, but he was recently fired from his job; he worked for a package delivery service. I called his former boss, who told me that customers had complained he'd left their packages without ringing, or just dropped them on the steps, not even inside the gate. 'He just didn't seem to give a—to care any longer,' was his exact quote. He said my dad only just shrugged and pocketed his final pay envelope. That was 6 months ago."

Since then, Toby apparently has had several accidents with his car, but he keeps right on driving. The caller ends by asking the clinician to pay a home visit to his dad, who refuses to make an office appointment.

While talking with the clinician, Toby Russo sits in his apartment and stuffs his mouth with Cheetos. He admits that his weight has shot up in the past couple of years, though he doesn't seem much to care. In mute affirmation, about him lie empty Cheetos bags and cereal boxes. His shirt is gray around the neckline and the cuffs are badly frayed; he doesn't appear to have showered recently. But both his recent and remote memory appear intact, and he isn't depressed; he's had no delusions or hallucinations, he says. The driving mishaps? He just ran into a lot of other vehicles, no problem. Maybe he'll get his car fixed, only they've stopped his insurance.

Toby sleeps on a mattress he tossed onto the floor of his living room. Beside it lies a tattered pair of boxer shorts covered in—just what are those spots and blotches, the clinician wants to know. "I smoke, so I have to cough a lot," Toby explains blandly. "In the night, I don't want to get up, so I just spit it there." He guesses the same shorts have lain there, night after night, maybe for weeks. They certainly look it. However, on simple testing (the MMSE), he scores 28 out of a possible 30, missing the day of the week and one of the three objects he is asked to remember.

Within days, Toby slips rapidly downhill. His son, again visiting in town, finds him alone in his apartment. Apparently, he hasn't stirred from his mattress for a day or two. Hospitalized, an MRI revealed marked bilateral atrophy of his frontal and anterior temporal lobes.

Trudy Cantor

At her 60th birthday party, Trudy Cantor's brother, Ted, noticed that she hesitated—maybe *stammered* is a better word—a bit when responding to the toast. She repeatedly struggled to find the right word ("Yes, that's it. *Happy*," she said to her evident relief at the helpful suggestion.) Then she joked, "My senior moments are growing together."

That was 2 years ago. Now, at the clinical appointment Ted finally persuades her to keep, she can read aloud from a printed source, but her spontaneous speech rambles and she never manages to convey her point. Any point.

"Here's the way it's been. I first wanted to get, um, no that's not right, I thought it was another thing. Most of the time, I've been quite, uh, quite, you know, well . . . that's just the way it is. It's been, I mean." She breaks off, with a smile.

By now, she has difficulty identifying a pen by name, yet—it seems a near miracle!—she has continued her part-time employment drafting house plans for a local architect.

Evaluation of Toby Russo

Each of these patients has long-standing cognitive changes that would qualify for a diagnosis of major NCD (frontotemporal NCD criterion A). And each has a personal history of gradually deteriorating (B) cognitive status that, at least initially, isn't remarkable for memory impairment.

Toby shows signs of apathy (criterion C1a-ii), as well as behavioral disinhibition (repeatedly crashing his car and not caring, C1a-i) and hyperorality (stuffing himself on snack food; other patients will smoke or drink to excess, or just put objects into their mouths, C1a-v). From the results on the MMSE, his memory and perceptual–motor functions were probably relatively spared at the time of his initial evaluation (D, though I do wonder about those car crashes). His deteriorating status prompts the definitive MRI (probable frontotemporal NCD criterion 2), and that allows us to state that his diagnosis is, well, probable. DSM-5-TR would allow us to add "with behavioral disturbance" to Toby's diagnosis. That might seem under the circumstance a little silly, but it allows us to note that it's disinhibition and apathy that cause our concern. Because his is a probable case, we list first the medical diagnosis. With a GAF score of 10, Toby's diagnosis will be as follows:

G31.09	Frontotemporal degeneration
F02.C18	Major neurocognitive disorder due to probable frontotemporal degeneration, behavioral variant, severe, with apathy and disinhibition

Evaluation of Trudy Cantor

Over the years, Trudy has experienced a remarkable loss of her language skills, beginning with problematic word finding, gradually (criterion B) progressing to speech that is normally produced but content-free (C2a). The fact that she is still able to work at drafting indicates sparing of perceptual–motor functioning (D). To evaluate whether her ability to learn is spared would require some testing; however, her problems with language are serious, far past the level of mild NCD. Therefore, even with neither testing nor genetic information, on clinical grounds I feel her diagnosis should be possible major frontotemporal NCD. Though she has terrible problems with communication, she doesn't require help with instrumental activities of daily living, so I'd rate her overall severity as mild, and her GAF score somewhere in the 50s.

F03.A0   Major neurocognitive disorder due to possible frontotemporal degeneration, language variant, mild, without behavioral disturbance

---

Wait a minute: There's nothing in Table 16.1 about stating *language variant* or *behavioral variant,* is there? And the answer is, of course, "No, but there should be." It is additional information that may be of value to subsequent clinicians, hence to the patient. So, I went right ahead and put it in. There's no code number attached, so what's the problem?

Vascular Neurocognitive Disorder

Approximately 10% of NCDs have a vascular origin (second only to Alzheimer's). Vascular dementia has also been called *multi-infarct dementia* because its presumed cause is so often a series of strokes. However, some patients are affected by a single event and others may have small vessel disease that doesn't produce infarcts. Whereas patients with Alzheimer's disease deteriorate gradually, many patients with vascular NCD worsen through a series of steps as the strokes occur. Sometimes, however, progression can appear slow and gradual—probably due to the accumulating involvement of multiple small vessels. Vascular NCD is especially likely to develop in a patient who has diabetes or hypertension.

Besides failing memory, patients experience the loss of executive functioning, which can show up as the inability to deal with novel tasks. Apathy, slowed thinking, and deteriorating hygiene are also often noted. Relatively mild stressors may precipitate pathological laughing or crying. These patients are less likely than Alzheimer's patients to have aphasia, apraxia, and agnosia, though any aspect of mental functioning can be affected.

The symptoms of vascular NCD depend on the exact location of brain lesion(s), but several characteristics are typical, especially of what's known as *subcortical ischemic vascular disease*. They include early impairment of executive function and attention, reduced motor performance, and slowed processing of information. Episodic memory (p. 499) is less affected than in Alzheimer's, but mood symptoms (depression, lability) and apathy are especially prominent.

DSM-5-TR notes that for mild vascular NCD, one stroke is adequate, but for major NCD, more than one is needed—unless it is one that is "strategically placed" or other neuroimaging findings apply.

In naturalistic studies, the rate of advance of vascular NCD is about the same as for Alzheimer's; illness in treated patients progresses more slowly.

Some authorities advocate a division of dementias into the *cortical* (or degenerative, such as NCD due to Alzheimer's disease) and *subcortical* (NCD due to most other causes). The subcortical dementias (some texts also call these *secondary* dementias) are allegedly less likely to produce agnosia, apraxia, and aphasia. Other authorities object, pointing out that the pathology of disease is never that neat and that all dementias have some degree of both cortical and subcortical pathology. Because there is so much overlap in symptoms, DSM-5-TR classification seems safer. It categorizes the NCDs much more simply, on the basis of presumed underlying cause.

Essential Features of **Vascular Neurocognitive Disorder**

The patient has a {mild}{major} neurocognitive disorder (p. 503). The symptoms begin after a vascular event and often progress stepwise. There is often prominent decline in complex attention and frontal/executive functioning.

The Fine Print

The D's: • Duration (tends to chronicity) • Differential diagnosis (delirium; **other causes of NCD**—especially Alzheimer's and frontotemporal; other mental disorders; **other physical disorders**)

Coding Notes

Specify:

> **Vascular NCD probably due to vascular disease.** The diagnosis is reinforced by neuroimaging, by proximity (following a cerebrovascular accident), or by both clinical and genetic evidence—for instance, CADASIL.
> **Vascular NCD possibly due to vascular disease.** Neuroimaging isn't available

and there is no established cause–effect relationship with a neurovascular event.

Specify if: {With}{Without} behavioral disturbance.

Record and code as indicated in Table 16.1 (p. 507).

What the heck is CADASIL? The acronym stands for cerebral autosomal dominant arteriopathy with subcortical infarcts and leukoencephalopathy (whew!), a genetic error that causes blood vessel damage, leading to tissue death in various body parts. It is rare (2 or 3 per 100,000 population, and often begins in young adults with migraine with aura. Depression, emotional incontinence, and bipolar symptoms are also found.

Minnie Bell Leach

At their family physician's request, her daughter and son-in-law bring Minnie Bell Leach for consultation. She has lived with them for the past year, since her second stroke. Nearly 5 years earlier, her first stroke left her with a partly paralyzed left leg, but she could care for herself and even do her own grocery shopping. But since the second stroke, she rarely leaves her wheelchair. Flora, her daughter, provides an increasing share of her personal care.

Over the last few months, Minnie Bell has slipped. Even though she keeps her medicine for high blood pressure in a compartmented container, she often forgets to take it. At first, she needed reminding at breakfast, lunch, and bedtime. After a week or two, this improved, and for a while she seemed almost back to her former self. But beginning last Sunday morning, it's clear that she has slipped some more. She neglects to zip her skirt and she buttons her blouse using the wrong holes. She doesn't seem to notice either of these mistakes. She also has trouble expressing herself—at breakfast she asks for "red stuff" for her toast (it's the strawberry jam she and Flora made together last summer). And she's back to taking her medicine only when reminded.

Minnie Bell looks a bit older than her 68 years. She sits quietly in her wheelchair, cradling her left wrist in her right hand. Over her cotton housedress she wears a cloth overcoat that has fallen unnoticed off one shoulder. Although she maintains good eye contact throughout the consultation, she speaks only when directly addressed. In her clear, coherent speech, she denies having hallucinations, delusions, or depression. She does spontaneously complain of a cough, shortness of breath, and numerous aches and pains. She overlooks the fact that she can't walk.

On the MMSE, Minnie Bell scores 20 out of 30. She knows the year but misses the month and date by over 2 months; she can name the city and state, a watch, and a pencil. Although she can repeat the names of three objects (ball, chair, telephone) immediately after hearing them, 5 minutes later she recalls only the ball. She becomes confused when asked to follow a three-part instruction, and she persistently forgets to place the folded paper on the floor. There are no *apraxias:* She can use a pencil to copy a simple figure.

On neurological exam, Minnie Bell's left hand is weak; there is an abnormal Babinski sign (upgoing great toe when the sole of the foot is scratched) on that side.

Evaluation of Minnie Bell Leach

The evidence that Minnie Bell has NCD is as follows: She has increasing difficulty with her memory, as shown by the history of forgetting to take her medication and by the obvious problems with short-term memory (evidence from history and the MMSE). Although she appears to have no agnosias or apraxias (MMSE), her daughter notes the aphasia, substituting "red stuff" for jam—a language problem. There are also increasing problems with executive functioning, as shown by her neglected appearance and her inability to follow a three-step instruction. These problems represent a major decline from her previous level of functioning, and they interfere at least moderately with her everyday life.

The prolonged course of her disease argues against delirium. Minnie Bell denies depression, delusions, and hallucinations, rendering unlikely the diagnosis of a noncognitive disorder such as a pseudodementia (vascular NCD criterion D). A vascular etiology for her disease is suggested by her history of hypertension and by the stepwise progression of her disability following several strokes (B1). Her neurological signs (weakness of her hand, upgoing toe sign) from the start of her decline provide further evidence for a vascular etiology (C). Her clinical course also supports a probable vascular etiology (B2).

I don't see any reports of imaging studies for Minnie Bell; they could be important in determining whether her NCD is *probably* or *possibly* due to vascular disease. However, her difficulties clearly followed in stepwise fashion her series of strokes. That's good enough for DSM-5-TR, and good enough for me. Because Minnie Bell's principal symptom seems to be trouble with executive functioning, she should be diagnosed as follows (with a GAF score of 31):

F01.B0   Major neurocognitive disorder probably due to vascular disease, without behavioral disturbance, moderate

Neurocognitive Disorder Due to Other Medical Conditions

Detailed in DSM-5-TR are several other causes of NCD, each of which is responsible for only a small percentage of total cases. Below, I've summarized the features to look for in those accorded specific criteria in DSM-5-TR. A fuller (though still incomplete) list can be found in the "Physical Disorders . . ." table in the Appendix (p. 661).

Parkinson's disease. The stooped posture, slow movements, rigidity, back-and-forth ("pill-rolling") tremor, and rapid, shuffling gait characteristic of Parkinson's disease are well known and often obvious. Less well known may be the degree to which NCD occurs—affecting a quarter or more of patients with Parkinson's; with advancing age the likelihood of major NCD increases to as high as 80%.

In contrast to dementia with Lewy bodies, the physical aspects of Parkinson's appear first—cognitive features are never the first symptoms to be noticed. That's one of two qualifying factors for a probable or possible diagnosis. The other is that there must be no evidence that another disorder—cerebrovascular disease, Alzheimer's, NCD with Lewy bodies are especially mentioned—or any other mental, neurological, or physical disorder contributes to the development of the NCD. Presence of both factors allows a *probable* diagnosis; presence of only one yields a *possible* diagnosis. See Table 16.1 (p. 507) for details of recording.

Huntington's disease. Age of onset for Huntington's disease averages around 40 years; the first symptoms may be apparently minor changes in personality and executive functioning, followed by deteriorating memory and judgment. A generalized restlessness may precede the characteristic involuntary choreiform movements and slowing of voluntary movements. Prevalence is about 6 per 100,000 in North America and Europe; it is far less frequent in Asia. The cause is an autosomal dominant gene on chromosome 4.

Prion disease. Prion disease is at once miniscule and huge. It accounts for a tiny fraction of all NCDs—perhaps 1 case per million population per year—yet its "mad cow disease" form is so dramatic and unusual that it makes headlines whenever it occurs. The more common type, Creutzfeldt–Jakob disease, is caused by an infectious protein that contains no nucleic acids (that is, neither DNA nor RNA). These particles attack the brain, creating the holes in microscopic sections that account for the collective name *spongiform encephalopathies*. Symptoms include memory loss, hallucinations, personality change, and motor problems. Though the age range is wide, it typically occurs in elderly patients; a few cases are familial. Usually fatal within a year, prion disease is essentially untreatable.

HIV infection. Improvements in antiviral therapy have reduced the various threats posed by HIV infection; yet up to half those infected will have some symptoms of cognitive dysfunction, and up to a third will meet criteria for mild or major NCD. Although HIV infection is not one of the more common causes of neurocognitive disorder, it has rapidly become one of the most important, occurring in young people and laying waste otherwise vigorous lives. That's why I've used it below as the exemplar for this NCD category.

Other causes. The symptoms and course of illness depend heavily on the underlying medical cause. Obviously, so do treatment and prognosis. They might include normal pressure hydrocephalus, hypothyroidism, brain tumor, vitamin B$_{12}$ deficiency, and many others. See the "Physical Disorders . . ." table in the Appendix (p. 661) for more.

Essential Features of **Neurocognitive Disorder Due to Other Medical Conditions**

The patient fulfills criteria for a {major}{mild} neurocognitive disorder.

	Huntington's disease	Parkinson's disease[a]	Prion disease	HIV infection	Other medical condition
Patient has evidence of:	Huntington's disease (family history or genetic testing)	Motor symptoms of Parkinson's disease	Motor features of prion disease (ataxia, myoclonus, tremor)	Documented HIV infection	History, physical exam, or lab evidence of a causative physical disorder
Symptoms not better explained by:	Another mental or medical disorder			Mental, cognitive, non-HIV physical disorders	Another mental disorder or specific NCD
Onset is:	Insidious; gradual progression		Insidious onset; progression is often rapid	—	—

[a]Recorded as probable or possible NCD; see text.

Coding Notes

See Tables 16.1 and 16.2 (pp. 507 and 508) for coding procedures.

Arlen Wing

When he is admitted to the hospital for the third time in 4 months, Arlen Wing has lost 30 pounds—nearly 20% of his body weight. With it seems to have gone much of his will to live: He often neglects to take the cocktail of antiviral medications prescribed to shore up his failing immune system. This and the apathy that is so obvious on admission prompt the request for mental health consultation. Arlen's physician notes that a CT brain scan shows diffuse cortical atrophy; an EEG indicates "nonfocal slowing."

Arlen trained to be a dancer. After he just missed landing a job with the Joffrey Ballet, he joined his long-time companion, Alex, in the business of buying and selling antique dolls. The two made a good living traveling around the country to auctions and doll shows, until Alex rather suddenly died of *Pneumocystis* pneumonia. Arlen soon discovered that he is HIV-positive; he promptly began taking prophylactic medications. He continued to operate his business until the last few months, when his CD4 cell count dropped below 200. That triggered his recent series of hospitalizations.

While the consultant explains the purpose of the visit, Arlen makes eye contact and listens politely. His speech is slow and labored, but there are no abnormalities in its flow. He has no delusions, hallucinations, or other abnormal content of thought. He denies feeling especially sad or anxious—"just tired."

Arlen knows his own name, the name of the hospital, and the month, but he gives the date and year incorrectly. He thinks that he was admitted only yesterday (it was a week ago). He cannot recall the name of the physician who has attended him for the past 3 years. He scores only 14 out of 30 on the MMSE: When asked to pick up a sheet of paper, fold it, and put it on the floor, he twice drops the paper unfolded onto the floor. When asked to tell how an apple and an orange are similar, he can offer no response. He acknowledges being seriously ill and admits that he often neglects to take his cocktail of pills. "I was feeling terrible," he says, "and I thought they might be making me sick."

Evaluation of Arlen Wing

Arlen's history and obvious intellectual decline (major NCD criterion A) point clearly to the NCDs. He is alert, and he adequately focuses his attention on the exam, so a delirium is extremely unlikely (C). His problem with recent memory—especially common in an HIV-related NCD—is obvious. Also typical are his apathy and hesitating speech (slowed-down motor movements in general are also characteristic of this disorder). His impairments represent a significant decline from his previous level of functioning (B). As we'd expect from a non-Alzheimer's dementia, there are no obvious agnosias, apraxias, or aphasias. In all, he clearly conforms to the criteria for an NCD, and his HIV-positive status provides the necessary information as to etiology. We note that Arlen has the behavioral disturbance of apathy.

Informants who know him well will be the most satisfactory source of information about Arlen's executive functioning (has he been having trouble dressing himself, shopping, or taking care of other routine daily tasks?). However, his inability to follow a sequence of events on the MMSE also provides evidence. Discontinuing his medications suggests a lapse in judgment, typical of the later stages of an HIV-related neurocognitive disorder. He denies feeling depressed—evidence (OK, it's not definitive) against a mood disorder with pseudodementia. Because he has given up on important aspects of self-care, I would score his GAF as only 21, though other clinicians might rate him somewhat higher. The severity rating for his major NCD would be less dire; he isn't yet fully dependent on others for all his care.

| B20 | HIV infection |
| F02.B18 | Major neurocognitive disorder due to HIV infection, moderate, with behavioral disturbance (apathy) |

Substance/Medication-Induced Neurocognitive Disorder

NCDs can result from prolonged use of alcohol, sedatives, and inhalants, though in most instances, alcohol will be the main culprit. Patients will have issues with constructional tasks (e.g., drawing), behavior, and memory. These patients are often described as having delusional jealousy or hallucinations. Although the onset is typically gradual, nothing may be noted amiss until the patient has had several days or weeks to dry out.

One form of this disorder is the type variously known as Korsakoff's psychosis or, as it was called in DSM-IV, substance-induced persisting amnestic disorder. (DSM-5 swept the entire former class of amnestic disorders into alcohol-induced major NCD, amnestic–confabulatory type.)

Essential Features of **Substance/Medication-Induced Neurocognitive Disorder**

The use of some substance appears to have caused a patient to have a {major}{mild} neurocognitive disorder (p. 503).

The Fine Print

For tips on identifying substance-related causation, see sidebar, page 95.

The D's: • Duration (endures long after usual course of **intoxication** or **withdrawal**) • Differential diagnosis (**physical disorders, another mental disorder, delirium**)

Coding Notes

When writing down the diagnosis, use the exact substance in the title—for instance, alcohol-induced major neurocognitive disorder. For coding, see Table 15.2 (p. 475).

Specify if:

Persistent. Symptoms of the NCD continue long past the time abstinence begins.

Mark Culpepper

Despite drinking nearly a fifth of bourbon every day until he was 56, Mark Culpepper had avoided consequences. He taught developmental biology for 30 years, but 6 months ago the university offered him early retirement. Soon afterward, his daughter,

Amarette, moved in with him as housekeeper and companion. She provides most of the history for this report.

Amarette could never understand how her father managed to retain his job while drinking as much as he did. Of course, in later years his teaching assignments were always lower-division, and for more than a decade he published no research or scholarly writing at all. He was "COT," as the students put it—"coasting on tenure." Tenure is a powerful influence at the university; it forgave him the occasional missed class he was too hung over to attend, and the fact that he hardly ever graded a paper himself.

By the time his daughter moved in, Mark was fully retired and could devote all of his time to drinking. Amarette quickly put paid to that. She confiscated the contents of his bar and, by combining shame with threats, obtained enough control over his finances to force him into total abstention. She remained steadfast through the week he spent vomiting and "shaking like a mouse on an electric grid," as he put it. At a stroke, she had rid her father of his 30-year habit.

The results were both more and less than Amarette expected. In the next 4 months Mark didn't touch a drop, but neither did he accomplish much of anything else. Even sober, he neglected his appearance, often going for days without shaving. He spent much of his time "working on a paper" that was, as far as she could tell, material recycled from decades-old notebooks. He had simply copied it out unaltered. "Anything there that made any sense at all, you could read in an old freshman biology text. A very old text," she observes while he signs papers to be admitted.

An event the day before precipitated this admission. When she returned from a brief errand, she found him in the living room trying to mop up water from the bathtub he had turned on and apparently forgotten about. The taps were still open full.

Mark is a pleasant man whose rosy nose and cheeks give him a somewhat boyish appearance. He carries a sheaf of papers in a dog-eared manila folder; the title page reads, "Limb Regeneration in the Newt." His speech is normal, and he denies delusions, hallucinations, depression, and suicidal ideas. Although he seems to pay attention during the MMSE, he scores only 19 out of a possible 30. He cannot recall two of three objects after 5 minutes. With difficulty, he correctly spells *world* backward. When asked to follow the three-part instruction (to pick up a piece of paper, fold it, and place it on the floor), he persistently forgets to fold the paper. When asked about this, he brushes it off with, "Well, I was thinking about my research."

Evaluation of Mark Culpepper

Central to many cases of NCD is memory impairment. In Mark's case, this is not so apparent on casual observation. He is pleasant, carries on a conversation in a natural manner, and even appears to be working on a scientific paper. However, with repeated testing, after 5 minutes he can recall only one of the three MMSE objects.

Mark gives no evidence of problems with language, attention, social cognition, or perceptual–motor issues, but Amarette's history suggests that he's developed real problems in caring for himself (neglecting his appearance, flooding the house with bathwater). This loss of executive functioning is reflected in bedside testing by his inability to follow a three-part instruction. It is enough to count as a major NCD (criterion A), though I'd rate it as mild—he still feeds and dresses himself.

Mark focuses attention well, and it doesn't appear to wander during the interview, suggesting that a delirium isn't responsible; persistence of his symptoms past the usual time course for withdrawal fulfills this requirement (B). Heavy, prolonged alcohol use could certainly produce his symptoms (C), which have continued long after Amarette drags him onto the water wagon (D). Other mental pathology is not evident: Mark denies symptoms of depression and psychosis, which are the two principal conditions that might present with neglect and memory loss. Of course, a physical exam, and perhaps some testing, would be needed to rule out other medical illnesses (E). Considering his history, however, an alcohol-induced major NCD seems highly probable.

The matter of Mark's alcohol use disorder requires some thought. At the time he stopped drinking, when he developed shakiness and vomiting, we'd say he was in alcohol withdrawal. That, and the fact that alcohol has clearly affected both his work and his relationship with Amarette, would be enough to diagnose alcohol use disorder. Unaddressed in the vignette are many of the remaining criteria for substance use disorder—craving for alcohol and tolerance, to name just two. A full exploration would probably yield enough symptoms to qualify him for the severest level of involvement. At any rate, we couldn't score it as *mild,* which would be misleading and inconsistent with alcohol withdrawal. OK, perhaps it's going a bit beyond the data, but it seems clinically appropriate to rate Mark's alcohol use disorder as severe; I'll select the appropriate codes from Table 15.2 (p. 475).

Mark's recent retirement leaves him with time on his hands, which could be a problem—or an opportunity. (He might profit from occupational or recreational therapy, or even from referral to day care.) Either way, I'd give him the appropriate Z-code. I can hardly believe that there's nothing to report as regards his medical condition; we should revisit it later. His GAF score right now would be 41.

F10.27	Severe alcohol use disorder in early remission, with alcohol-induced major neurocognitive disorder, nonamnestic–confabulatory type, persistent
Z60.0	Phase of life problem (retirement)

Charles Jackson

A powerfully built 6-footer, Charles Jackson still shows traces of military bearing. Before he left the Army a year ago, he was busted from staff sergeant to buck private; this was the culmination of a string of disciplinary actions for drunkenness. Fortunately, he had served 21 years and did not forfeit his retirement pay.

For over a year, he has had monthly consultations with the current interviewer. On his last MMSE, Charles scored 17: the full 9 points for language, 3 for spelling *world* backward as *drolw*, 3 for registration (immediately repeating three items), and 2 for knowing the city and state.

On this occasion, the interviewer asks when they last met. Charles replies, "Well, I just don't know. What do you think?" To the follow-up question, he says that he guesses he has seen the interviewer before. "Maybe it was last week."

Asking him to remain seated, the interviewer goes into the waiting room to ask Mrs. Jackson how she thinks her husband is doing. She responds, "Oh, he's about the same as before. He sketches some. He can still draw a pretty good caricature of you, as long as you're sitting right in front of him. But mostly he just sits around the house and watches TV. I come home and ask him what he's been watching, but he can't even tell me that."

At any rate, Charles is no longer drinking, not since they moved to the country. It is at least 2 miles to the nearest convenience store, and he doesn't walk very well anymore. "But he still talks about drinking. Sometimes he seems to think he's still in the Army. He tries to give me a direct order to go buy him a quart of gin."

Charles remembers quite a few things, if they occurred long enough ago—the gin, for example, and getting drunk with his father when he was a boy. But he can't remember the name of his daughter, who is 2½ years old. Most of the time, he just calls her "the girl."

The interviewer walks back into the inner office. Charles looks up and smiles. "Have I seen you before?" the interviewer asks him.

"Well, I'm pretty sure."

"When was it?"

"It might have been last week."

Evaluation of Charles Jackson

Charles has not only an especially severe anterograde memory loss (he seems able to form no new memories), but also a considerable degree of retrograde amnesia (he cannot even recall his daughter's name). We hardly need objective testing to conclude that he's suffered a significant cognitive decline (major NCD criterion A). His wife testifies that he just sits around; from that, I'm going to extrapolate that he doesn't pay any of the bills or do household chores (B). We haven't determined, however, the extent to which he is able to provide self-care. Charles shows no evidence of shifting attention or reduced awareness that would indicate a delirium (C).

Given a little rope, Charles appears to confabulate a previous meeting with the examiner. Although confabulation is not a criterion for diagnosis, it is one of the classic symptoms—it even helps make up the named subtype. In alcohol-induced amnestic–confabulatory syndrome, memory is the principal disturbance. However, problems with executive functioning (suggested by Charles's performance on the MMSE) can and do occur.

The main items in the differential diagnosis would include other causes of major NCD and other complications of alcoholism. From the history, we can clear away these sources of confusion. Of course, his geographic isolation assures that his forgetfulness is not due to blackouts associated with alcohol intoxication.

Although elements of history are missing from the vignette, Charles should also receive a diagnosis of alcohol use disorder. Other than the ongoing desire to drink, he has not met the criteria during the past year, so he would earn the qualifier of *in sustained remission*. (I'm almost tempted to add *in a controlled environment*, because of where he lives. Almost tempted, but not quite.) His GAF score will be only 41. His rather complicated, though logical diagnosis comes from Table 15.2 (p. 475):

F10.26	Alcohol use disorder, in sustained remission, with alcohol-induced major neurocognitive disorder, amnestic–confabulatory type, persistent

Neurocognitive Disorder Due to Multiple Etiologies

Whether NCD has one cause or many, the basic symptoms remain the same. Many medical and neurological disorders can be responsible, so the combinations are nearly endless. Any patient's symptoms should be consistent with the underlying pathology, but it may be hard to discriminate the contributing factors on purely clinical grounds.

NCDs with more than one cause are especially common in older people, who are prone to falls and multiple illnesses, and in those whose drinking or drug use puts them at risk for a variety of medical disorders. For example, a patient with alcohol-induced major NCD may also have head trauma, infection, or a degenerative condition such as Marchiafava–Bignami disease (in which the corpus callosum of the brain is affected by chronic alcohol intake).

The symptoms are much the same as with other causes of NCD, so I've given no case example. In fact, I haven't even provided Essential Features; they seem self-evident. Once you've collected the symptoms and made the diagnosis, the remaining problem is this: How the heck do you record it? Basically, here's the plan (from Table 16.2 on p. 508):

First write down the names and codes for each contributing medical condition. Then add the appropriate code for major NCD {with}{without} behavioral disturbance.

Below is the full diagnosis for a moderately ill patient with NCD who has long-established Huntington's disease and who has also suffered a blow to the head and is depressed.

G10	Huntington's disease
S06.2XAS	Diffuse traumatic brain injury with loss of consciousness of unspecified duration, sequela
F02.B3	Major neurocognitive disorder due to Huntington's disease and traumatic brain injury, moderate, with depression

So far, so good. But there's a fly in the ointment. In fact, there's a swarm.

Fly 1. If our patient has a vascular disorder that contributes to, say, a moderately severe major NCD, we need to mention it separately. So, let's say our unfortunate patient with Huntington's has avoided the fall (no TBI) but instead has had a stroke. Here's how the diagnosis would appear:

G10	Huntington's disease
F02.B3	Major neurocognitive disorder due to Huntington's disease, moderate, with depression
F01.B3	Major vascular neurocognitive disorder, moderate, with depression

Note that there's no additional code for the vascular disorder.

Fly 2. OK, suppose instead that our Huntington's patient hasn't had a stroke but has been drinking heavily for several years—though not to the point of confabulation—and we determine that the NCD is partly due to the use of alcohol. Then, with the help of Table 15.2, we'd say:

G10	Huntington's disease
F02.B3	Major neurocognitive disorder due to Huntington's disease, moderate, with depression
F10.27	Severe alcohol use disorder with alcohol-induced major NCD, nonamnestic-confabulatory type, moderate, with depression

Note that although we cannot express the substance use NCD severity in a code number, we can state it in words.

Fly 3. DSM-5-TR criteria state that, in the absence of genetic information (family history or testing), a diagnosis of possible major NCD due to Alzheimer's disease cannot be made if there's evidence of mixed etiology. Specifically mentioned is the example of vascular disease. However, in discussing NCD due to multiple etiologies, DSM-5-TR offers the example of major NCD due to both Alzheimer's disease and vascular disease. I rant about this Catch-22 when discussing Edith Roman's diagnosis. Check there (p. 646) if you'd like another swat at this fly.

Fly 4. Now let's revisit Fly 1. Suppose that our patient has mild NCD with Huntington's and probable cerebrovascular disease. Then we'd say this:

G10	Huntington's disease
I67.9	Cerebrovascular disease

F06.71   Mild neurocognitive disorder due to Huntington's disease and
           cerebrovascular disease, with depression
F06.31   Mood disorder due to Huntington's disease and vascular disease,
           with depressive features

Note that, according to the DSM-5-TR October 2022 update, we only code a vascular etiology when it is probable and the NCD is mild. Go figure.

R41.9 Unspecified Neurocognitive Disorder

The unspecified NCD category includes patients whose cognitive deficits do not fulfill
criteria for delirium or NCD, either mild or major, yet are the dominant apparent cause
of distress or impaired functioning. Because etiology is not known, no other coding will
be possible. You can, however, tack on {with}{without} behavior disturbance—just the
words, no numbers.

CHAPTER 17

Personality Disorders

Quick Guide to the Personality Disorders

DSM-5-TR retains the 10 specific personality disorders (PDs) that were listed in DSM-IV. Of these, perhaps 6 have been studied reasonably well and have a lot of support in the research community. The rest (paranoid, schizoid, histrionic, and dependent PDs), while perhaps less well founded in science, retain their positions in the diagnostic pantheon because of their practical use and, frankly, tradition.

Speaking of tradition, ever since DSM-III in 1980 the personality disorders have been divided into three groups, called clusters. Heavily criticized for a lack of scientific validity, the clusters are perhaps most useful as a device to help us call to mind the full slate of PDs.

Cluster A Personality Disorders

People with Cluster A PDs can be described as withdrawn, cold, suspicious, or irrational.

Paranoid. These people are suspicious and quick to take offense. They often have few confidants and may read hidden meaning into innocent remarks (p. 548).

Schizoid. These people care little for social relationships, have a restricted emotional range, and seem indifferent to criticism or praise. Tending to be solitary, they avoid close (including sexual) relationships (p. 551).

Schizotypal. Interpersonal relationships are so difficult for these people that they appear peculiar or strange to others. They lack close friends and are uncomfortable in social situations. They may show suspiciousness, unusual perceptions or thinking, eccentric speech, and inappropriate affect (p. 554).

Cluster B Personality Disorders

Those with Cluster B PDs tend to be rather theatrical, emotional, and attention-seeking; their moods are labile and often shallow. They often have intense interpersonal conflicts.

Antisocial. The irresponsible, often criminal behavior that defines these people begins in childhood or early adolescence with truancy, running away, cruelty, fighting, destructiveness, lying, and theft. In addition to criminal behavior, as adults they may default on debts or otherwise behave irresponsibly; act recklessly or impulsively; and show no remorse for their behavior (p. 557).

Borderline. These people are impulsive and engage in behavior harmful to themselves (sexual adventures, unwise spending, excessive use of substances or food). Affectively unstable, they often show intense, inappropriate anger. They feel empty or bored, and they frantically try to avoid abandonment. They are uncertain about who they are, and they lack the ability to maintain stable interpersonal relationships (p. 561).

Histrionic. Overly emotional, vague, and desperate for attention, histrionic people need constant reassurance about their attractiveness. They may be self-centered and sexually seductive (p. 564).

Narcissistic. These people are self-important and often preoccupied with envy, fantasies of success, or ruminations about the uniqueness of their own problems. Their sense of entitlement and lack of compassion may cause them to take advantage of others. They vigorously reject criticism and need constant attention and admiration (p. 567).

Cluster C Personality Disorders

Someone with a Cluster C PD will tend to be anxious and tense, often overcontrolled.

Avoidant. These timid people are so easily wounded by criticism that they hesitate to become involved with others. They may fear the embarrassment of showing emotion or of saying things that seem foolish. They may have no close friends, and they exaggerate the risks of undertaking pursuits outside their usual routines (p. 569).

Dependent. These people so need the approval of others that they have trouble making independent decisions or starting projects; they may even agree with others whom they know to be wrong. They fear abandonment, feel helpless when they are alone, and are miserable when relationships end. They are easily hurt by criticism and will even volunteer for unpleasant tasks to gain the favor of others (p. 572).

Obsessive–compulsive. Perfectionism and rigidity characterize these people. They are often workaholics, and they tend to be indecisive, excessively scrupulous, and preoccupied with detail. They insist that others do things their way. They have trouble expressing affection, tend to lack generosity, and may even resist throwing away worthless objects they no longer need (p. 574).

Other Causes of Long-Standing Character Disturbance

Personality change due to another medical condition. A medical condition can affect personality for the worse. This would not qualify as a PD, because it may be less pervasive and not necessarily present from an early age (p. 576).

Other mental disorders. When they persist for a long time (usually years), a variety of other mental conditions can distort the way someone behaves and relates to others, potentially giving the appearance of a personality disorder. Especially good examples include persistent depressive disorder, schizophrenia, social anxiety disorder, and cognitive disorders. Some studies find that patients with mood disorders are more likely to show personality traits or PDs when they are clinically depressed; this may be especially true of Cluster A and Cluster C traits. Personality pathology noted in depressed patients should be reevaluated once the depression has remitted.

Other specified, or unspecified, personality disorder. Use one of these categories for personality disturbances that do not meet the criteria for any of the disorders above, or for PDs that have not achieved official status (p. 579).

Introduction

All humans (and numerous other species as well) have personality traits. These are ingrained ways in which individuals experience, interact with, and think about everything that goes on around them. Personality disorders are collections of traits that have become rigid and work to individuals' disadvantage, to the point that they impair functioning or cause distress. These patterns of behavior and thinking have been present since early adult life and have been recognizable in the patient for a long time.

Personality, and therefore PDs, should probably be thought of as dimensional rather than categorical; this means that their components (traits) are present to a degree in most people but are accentuated in those with the disorders in question. But for good reasons and bad, DSM-5-TR has retained the traditional categorical structure that has been used for many decades.

As currently defined in DSM-5-TR, all PDs have in common the following characteristics.

Essential Features of a **General Personality Disorder**

There is a lasting pattern of behavior and inner experience (thoughts, feelings, sensations) that is clearly different from the person's culture. This pattern will include problems with two or more of *affect* (type, intensity, lability, appropriateness); *cognition* (how the individual sees and interprets self, others, and the environment); *control of impulses;* and *relationships* with other people. The pattern is fixed and maladaptive, and it applies broadly across the person's social and personal life.

The Fine Print

The D's: • Duration (lifelong, with roots in adolescence or even earlier) • Diffuse contexts of life are affected • Distress and disability (work/educational, social, and personal) • Differential diagnosis (**substance use, physical illness, other mental disorders,** personality change due to another medical condition)

The information PDs convey gives the clinician a better understanding of the behavior of patients; it can also augment our understanding of optimal management. As you read these descriptions and the accompanying vignettes, keep in mind the twin hallmarks of the PDs: early onset (typically by late teens) and pervasive nature, such that the maladaptive features affect multiple aspects of work, personal, and social life.

Diagnosing Personality Disorders

The diagnosis of PDs presents a variety of issues. On the one hand, they are often overlooked; on the other hand, however, they are sometimes overdiagnosed—borderline PD has long been, in my opinion, a notorious example. One (antisocial PD) carries a terrible prognosis: Most of these patients, if not all, are hard to treat. The relatively weak validity of PDs suggests that none should be given as the sole diagnosis when another mental disorder can explain the signs and symptoms that make up the clinical picture. For all of these reasons, it is a good idea to have in mind an outline for making the diagnosis of a PD.

1. Verify the duration of the symptoms. Make sure that your patient's symptoms have been present at least since early adulthood (before age 15 for antisocial PD). Interviews with informants (family, friends, co-workers) are especially likely to yield valid material.

2. Verify that the symptoms involve several areas of the patient's life. Specifically, are work (or school), home life, personal life, and social life affected? This step can present real problems, in that patients themselves often don't see their behavior as causing problems. ("It's the world that's out of step.")

3. Check that the patient fully qualifies for the diagnosis in question. This means considering each feature for any of the 10 personality disorders. If you sometimes must make a judgment call, try to be objective. As with other mental disorders, with enough motivation you could force a patient into a variety of unwarranted diagnoses.

4. If the patient is under age 18, confirm that the symptoms have been present for

at least the past 12 months. (And be really sure that they aren't due instead to some other mental or physical disorder.) I prefer not to make such a diagnosis at all in young people.

5. Rule out other mental pathology that may be more acute and have greater potential for doing harm. The flip side is that other mental disorders are also often more responsive to treatment than are PDs.

6. This is also a good time to review the generic features for any other requirements you may have missed. Note that each patient must have two or more types of lasting problem with behavior, thoughts, or emotions from a list of four: cognition, affect, interpersonal relationships, and impulsivity. (This helps ensure that the patient's problems truly do apply broadly across multiple life areas.)

7. Search for other PDs. Evaluate the entire history to learn whether any additional PD is present. Many patients appear to have more than one PD; in such cases, diagnose them all. Perhaps more often, you will find too few symptoms to make any diagnosis. Then you can add to your summary note something on the order of "schizoid and paranoid personality traits."

8. Record all personality and nonpersonality mental diagnoses. Some examples of how this is done are shown in the vignettes that follow.

Although you can learn the rudiments of each PD from the material presented here, it is important to note that these abbreviated descriptions only begin to tap their rich psychopathology. If you want to make a study of these disorders, I strongly recommend that you consult standard texts.

Cluster A Personality Disorders

The PDs included in Cluster A share behaviors generally described as withdrawn, cold, suspicious, or irrational.

F60.0 Paranoid Personality Disorder

What you notice most about patients with paranoid PD (PPD) is how little they trust—and how much they suspect—other people. The suspicions they harbor are unjustified, but because they fear exploitation, they will not confide in those whose behavior should have earned their trust. Instead, they read unintended meaning into benign comments and actions, and they will interpret untoward occurrences as the result of deliberate intent. They tend to harbor resentment for a long time, perhaps forever.

These people tend to be rigid and litigious and may have an especially urgent need to be self-sufficient. To others, they can appear to be cold, calculating, guarded people who avoid both blame and intimacy. They may appear tense and have trouble relaxing during an interview. This disorder is especially likely to create occupational difficulties: Patients with PPD are so aware of rank and power that they frequently have trouble dealing with superiors and co-workers.

Although it is apparently far from rare (it may affect 1–2% of the general population), PPD rarely comes to clinical attention. When it does, it is usually diagnosed in men. Its relationship (if any) to the development of schizophrenia remains unclear, but if you find that it has preceded the onset of schizophrenia, add the specifier *(premorbid)* to the personality disorder.

Essential Features of **Paranoid Personality Disorder**

In many situations, people with PPD demonstrate that they distrust the loyalty or reliability of others. They suspect that others want to deceive, hurt, or exploit them, so they hesitate to share personal information. Unjustified suspicions about the faithfulness of spouse or partner, or even the (mis)perception of hidden content in everyday events or speech, can lead to the bearing of grudges or to rapid response with anger or attacks in kind.

The Fine Print

The D's: • Duration (begins in teens or early 20s and endures) • Diffuse contexts of life are affected • Differential diagnosis (**physical disorders, mood disorders with psychotic features, schizophrenia,** schizotypal and schizoid PDs, substance use disorders, personality change, paranoid traits with physical handicaps, such as deafness)

Coding Note

If paranoid personality disorder precedes the onset of schizophrenia, append to PPD the specifier *(premorbid)*.

Dr. Schatzky

A professor of dermatology at University Hospital, Dr. Schatzky has never consulted a mental health professional. But he is well known to the staff at the medical center and notorious among his colleagues—who mostly refer to him as just "Schatzky." One of them, Dr. Cohen, provides most of the information for this vignette.

Schatzky has been around for several years. He's known as a solid researcher and an excellent clinician. A hard worker, he supervises fellows working on two grants and carries more than his share of the teaching load.

One of the trainees working in his lab, a physician named Masters, is a bright, capable young woman whose career in academic dermatology seems destined to soar. When Dr. Masters gets an offer from an institution in Boston of an assistant professorship and her own lab space, she tells Schatzky that she is sorry, but she will leave at the end of the semester. Furthermore, she wants to use some of their data.

Schatzky is beyond upset. He responds by telling Dr. Masters "What happens in the lab stays in the lab." He won't allow anyone to "rip him off," and he threatens that he will blackball her if she tries to publish papers based on their findings. Furthermore, he tells her she must keep away from students until she leaves. This outrages the other dermatologists. Dr. Masters is one of the most popular young teachers in the department, and the notion that she should have no contact with students seems punitive to all and little short of an assault on academic freedom.

The other dermatologists discuss the situation in a department meeting when Schatzky is out of town. One of the older professors volunteers to try to persuade him to let Dr. Masters teach anyway. Subsequently, Schatzky refuses with the response, "What have I done to you?" He now seems to think that the other professor has it in for him.

This professor tells Dr. Cohen that he isn't really surprised. He's known Schatzky since college, and he's always been a suspicious sort of person. "He won't confide in anyone without a signed loyalty oath," is how the other professor puts it. "Schatzky seems to think that if he says anything nice, it could somehow turn against him. The only person he trusts completely is his wife, a rabbity creature who has probably never in her life disagreed with him."

At the meeting, someone else suggests that the department chairman should talk to Schatzky and try to "jolly him along a bit." But Schatzky has little sense of humor and "the longest memory for a grudge of anyone on the face of the planet."

In the collective memory of all the staff, Dr. Schatzky had never had mood swings or psychosis, and at department dinners, he doesn't drink. "Never out of touch with reality, only nasty," concludes Dr. Cohen.

Evaluation of Dr. Schatzky

Let's begin with a disclaimer: From the information available in this vignette, it appears that Dr. Schatzky has never been interviewed by a mental health professional. Any conclusions must therefore be tentative. We clinicians must be extremely chary of diagnosing patients—or just plain people—for whom we haven't gathered adequate information.

That said, Dr. Schatzky's symptoms have apparently been quite constant and present throughout his entire adult life (at least since college). His issues involve both his thinking and his interpersonal functioning, which in turn lead to problems with work and his personal life.

What symptoms of PPD does Dr. Schatzky have? Without cause, he suspects young Dr. Masters of planning to "rip off" his data (criterion A1). His colleagues note his long-standing concerns about the loyalty of associates (A2). He will never confide in others (A3), and he tries to bar Dr. Masters from teaching, which sounds a lot like holding a grudge (A5). However, he has apparently never questioned the loyalty or fidelity of his wife, which would be another common symptom of this PD. In all, we can find a total of four symptoms, which is what's required for a diagnosis of PPD.

Could a non-PD diagnosis explain Dr. Schatzky's behavior as described? Although the information is incomplete, drug or alcohol use appears unlikely. (It also seems unlikely that anyone of middle age could have been taking a medication long enough to produce character disturbance that had probably lasted his entire adult life.) The vignette provides no evidence of another medical condition. From our available information, Schatzky has never had frank psychosis, such as delusional disorder or schizophrenia, and he has no mood disorder (B).

What about other PDs? Patients with schizoid PD are cold and aloof, and as a result may appear distrustful, but they do not have the prominent suspiciousness characteristic of patients with PPD. Those with schizotypal PD may have paranoid ideation, but they also appear peculiar or odd (not the case here). And Dr. Schatzky doesn't appear to prefer solitude. Those with antisocial PD are often cold and unfeeling, may be suspicious, and have trouble forming interpersonal relationships. However, they are unlikely to have the perseverance required to complete professional training, and Dr. Schatzky has no history of criminal behavior or reckless disregard for the safety of others—only for their feelings.

With a GAF score of 70, Dr. Schatzky's tentative diagnosis (again with the disclaimer that we have no clinical interview with him) would be as follows:

F60.0   Paranoid personality disorder

F60.1 Schizoid Personality Disorder

People with schizoid personality disorder (SzPD) are indifferent to the society of other people, sometimes profoundly so. Typically, they are lifelong loners who show a restricted emotional range; they appear unsociable, cold, and reclusive.

Patients with SzPD may succeed at solitary jobs others find difficult to tolerate. They may daydream excessively, become attached to animals, and often do not marry or even form long-lasting romantic relationships. They do retain contact with reality, unless they develop schizophrenia.

Although it is infrequently diagnosed, SzPD is relatively common, affecting perhaps a few percent of the general population. Men may be at greater risk than women. The case demonstrating SzPD describes Lester Childs, the younger brother of Lyonel Childs, whose history has been presented in connection with schizophrenia (p. 67).

Essential Features of Schizoid Personality Disorder

In many situations, these people remain isolated and have a narrow emotional range. Preferring solitude in their activities, they neither want nor enjoy close relationships, including those with family. They may have no close friends, apart from relatives. Indeed, they enjoy few activities, even showing little interest in sex with other people. Emotionally cold or detached, they seem indifferent to either criticism or praise.

The Fine Print

The D's: • Duration (begins in teens or early 20s and endures) • Diffuse contexts of life are affected • Differential diagnosis (**physical disorders** and substance use disorders, **mood** and **psychotic disorders, autism spectrum disorder,** schizotypal and paranoid PDs, personality change)

Coding Note

If schizoid personality disorder precedes the onset of schizophrenia, append to SzPD the specifier *(premorbid)*.

Lester Childs

"We brought him in because of what's happened with Lyonel. They seem so much alike, and we're worried." Lester's mother sits primly on the office sofa. "After Lyonel was arrested, that's when we decided."

At 20, Lester Childs is in many ways a carbon copy of his older brother. Born several weeks prematurely, he spent his first few weeks of life in an incubator. But he gained weight rapidly and was soon well within the norms for his age.

He walked, talked, and was toilet-trained at the usual ages. Perhaps because they both worked so hard on the farm, or perhaps because there were no other young children for Lester and his siblings to play with, his parents noticed nothing amiss until Lester entered first grade. Within a few weeks, his teacher had telephoned to set up a conference.

Lester was bright enough, they were told; his schoolwork wasn't in question. But his sociability was next to nil. At recess, when the other children played dodge ball or pom-pom-pullaway, he remained in the classroom to color. He seldom participated in group discussions, and he always sat a few inches back from the others in the reading circle. When his turn for show and tell came, he stood silently in front of the class for a few moments, then pulled a length of kite string from his pocket and dropped it onto the floor. Then he sat down.

Most of this behavior seemed familiar—Lyonel hadn't yet begun his deep dive into psychosis—so the parents hadn't been too worried. Even so, they took Lester to their family doctor, who agreed that he was probably normal for their family and that he would "grow out of it." But Lester never did; he only grew older. He even avoided participating in family activities. At Christmas, he would open a present, take it over to a corner, and play with it by himself. Even Lyonel never did that.

When Lester enters the room, he clearly doesn't regard the appointment as much of an occasion. He wears jeans with a hole in one knee, tattered sneakers, and a T-shirt that at one time surely had sleeves. Through much of the interview he continues to leaf through a magazine devoted to astronomy and math. After waiting more than a minute for Lester to say something, the interviewer begins. "How are you today?"

"I'm OK." Lester keeps on reading.

"Your mom and dad asked you to come in to see me today. Can you tell me why?"

"Not really."

"Do you have any ideas about it?"

[Silence.]

Most of the interview goes this way. Lester gives specific information when he is asked directly, but he seems completely uninterested in volunteering anything. Sitting quietly, nose in his magazine, he shows no other abnormalities or eccentricities of behavior. His flow of speech (what there is of it) is logical and sequential. He is fully oriented, and he scores a perfect 30 on the MMSE. He says his mood is "OK"— neither too happy nor too sad. He has never used alcohol or drugs of any kind. He calmly but emphatically denies ever hearing voices, seeing visions, or having beliefs of being watched, followed, talked about, or otherwise interfered with. "I'm not like my brother," he says in his longest spontaneous speech up to that point.

When asked who he is like, Lester says it is Greta Garbo—"she wanted to be left alone." He claims he doesn't need friends; he can also do without his family. Neither does he need sex. He has checked out the sex magazines and anatomy books. Females and males are equally boring. His idea of a good way to spend his life is to live alone on an island, like Robinson Crusoe. "But no Friday."

Tucking his magazine under his arm, Lester leaves the office, never to return.

Evaluation of Lester Childs

Any diagnosis of a PD requires that the characteristics be both pervasive and enduring. Although he is only 20 years old, Lester's issues (they seem problems only to his parents) have certainly been enduring: They were noticeable when he was 6. And as far as we can tell, his rejection of interpersonal contact extends into all facets of his life—family, social, and school.

Lester avoids close relationships, even with his family (criterion A1); he prefers solitary activities (A2); he rejects the notion of having a sexual relationship with anyone (although this could conceivably change with maturity and opportunity—A3); he has always lacked close friends (A5); his affect seems flat and detached (although this could have been an artifact of a reluctant first interview with an unfamiliar interviewer—A7). In any event, Lester meets at least four and possibly five diagnostic criteria (four are required) for SzPD. These symptoms would satisfy three of the areas (cognition, affect, and interpersonal functioning) mentioned in the generic criteria for a PD. His interest in mathematics and astronomy would not be unusual in persons with this disorder, who typically thrive on work that others might find too lonely to enjoy.

Could any other disorder better explain Lester's clinical picture? Patients with depressive disorders are often withdrawn and unsociable, but these conditions seldom persist lifelong. Besides, Lester specifically denies feeling depressed or lonely; any doubts on the point could be explored by asking about vegetative symptoms of depression (changes in appetite or sleep). He also denies having symptoms (delusions and hallucinations) that would suggest schizophrenia; this denial is supported by collateral information from his mother. There are no stereotypies or symptoms of impaired communication, which we would expect from someone with autism spectrum disorder, or disturbance of consciousness or memory, as would be required for a cognitive disorder. From the information we have, he is physically healthy and does not use drugs, alcohol, or medications (B).

What other PDs should we consider? Patients with schizotypal PD can have constricted affect and unusual appearance. Lester's clothing was out of keeping for most visits to a professional office but would be almost expected for someone 20 years old, and he denies having any beliefs that might seem odd. He does not voice any ideas of deep suspicion or distrust, such as might be encountered in paranoid PD. Patients with avoidant PD are also isolated from other people; unlike those with SzPD, however, they don't choose this isolation, and they suffer for it.

If Lester later develops schizophrenia, the qualifier *(premorbid)* would be added at that time to his diagnosis. I find it difficult to place him squarely on the GAF scale. The score of 65 is to some extent a matter of taste. And arguable.

F60.1   Schizoid personality disorder

F21 Schizotypal Personality Disorder

From an early age, patients with schizotypal personality disorder (StPD) have lasting interpersonal deficiencies that severely reduce their capacity for closeness with others. They also have distorted or eccentric thinking, perceptions, and behaviors, which can make them seem odd. They often feel anxious when with strangers, and they have almost no close friends. They may be suspicious and superstitious; their peculiarities of thought include magical thinking and belief in telepathy or other unusual modes of communication. Such patients may talk about sensing a "force" or "presence," or have speech characterized by vagueness, digressions, excessive abstractions, impoverished vocabulary, or unusual use of words.

Some with StPD eventually develop schizophrenia. Many are depressed when they first come to clinical attention. Their eccentric ideas and style of thinking also place them at risk for becoming involved with cults. They get along poorly with others, and under stress they can become briefly psychotic. Despite their odd behavior, many marry and work ordinary jobs. This disorder occurs about as often as schizoid PD.

Essential Features of **Schizotypal Personality Disorder**

Across many social situations, these people tend to be isolated and exhibit a narrow emotional range with others. They will have paranoid or suspicious ideas, even ideas of reference (which, however, are not held to a delusional degree). Their dress or mannerisms may give them an odd appearance; affect may be inappropriate or constricted; speech can be vague, impoverished, or overly abstract. They may report strange perceptions or physical sensations ("someone's tickling me behind my knee"), and their peculiar behavior may be affected by magical thinking, peculiar fantasies, or other odd beliefs (superstitions, a belief in telepathy). With severe social anxiety, which may accompany paranoid ideas and doesn't improve with acquaintance, they tend not to have intimate friends.

The Fine Print

The D's: • Duration (begins in teens or early 20s and endures) • Diffuse contexts of life are affected • Differential diagnosis (physical disorders, **psychotic disorders, mood disorders with psychotic features, autism spectrum disorder** and other neurodevelopmental disorders, paranoid and schizoid PDs, personality change, substance use disorders)

Coding Note

If schizotypal personality disorder precedes the onset of schizophrenia, append to StPD the specifier *(premorbid)*.

Timothy Oldham

"But it's my baby! I don't care what he had to do with it!" Hugely pregnant and miserable, Charlotte Grenville sits in the interviewer's office and weeps with frustration. She is there at the request of the presiding judge in a battle over visitation rights with her yet-unborn child.

The identity of the father has never been in doubt. The week after her second missed period, Charlotte visited a gynecologist and then called Timothy Oldham with the news. She considered threatening to sue him for child support, but that hadn't been necessary. He makes good money installing carpets and has no other dependents. He offered her a generous monthly stipend, beginning immediately. But he wants to help rear their child. Charlotte rejected that idea out of hand and then filed suit. With a crowded court docket, the case has dragged on nearly as long as Charlotte's pregnancy.

"I mean, he's seriously weird!"

"What do you mean, 'weird'? Give me some examples," the interviewer suggests.

"Well, I've known him for the longest time—several years, anyway. He had a sister who died; he talks about her like she's still alive. And he does weird things. Like, when we were making love, right in the middle he started this babble about 'holy love' and dedicating his seed. It put me right off. I told him to stop and get off, but it was too late. I mean, would you want your kid growing up with *that* for a father?"

"If he's so peculiar, how did you get involved with him?"

She looks abashed. "Well, we only did it once. And I might have been a bit drunk at the time."

Timothy isn't just sedate; he's nearly immobile. He sits quietly in the interview chair, a gangly blond whose hair sweeps across his forehead, nearly to his eyebrows. He tells his story in a dull monotone that reveals not the slightest trace of emotion.

Timothy Oldham and his twin sister, Miranda, had been orphaned when they were 4 years old. He has no memory of his parents, other than a vague impression that they might have made their living from a marijuana farm in northern California. The two children were taken in by an aunt and uncle—Southern Baptists who, he says, make the farm couple in Grant Wood's *American Gothic* look cheerful by comparison. "That painting, it's really them. I have a copy of it in my bedroom. Sometimes I can see my uncle moving the pitchfork back and forth to signal me."

"Is it really your uncle? And does the pitchfork really move?" the interviewer wants to know.

"Well, it's more of a feeling I get . . . not really . . . a sign of my Christian endeavor . . ." Timothy continues to gaze straight ahead, but his voice trails off.

The "Christian endeavor," he explains, means that everyone has been put on earth for some special purpose. His uncle always used to say that. He thinks his own purpose might be to help raise the baby growing inside Charlotte. He knows there must be more to life than laying carpets all day.

Timothy has only a few friends, none of them close. He and Charlotte had never spent more than a few hours together. In response to a question, he talks about his sister, Miranda. They had been understandably close; she was the only real friend he had ever had. When they were 16 she died of a brain tumor, and Timothy was devastated. "We were webbed together when we were born. I swore at her graveside it would never be undone."

Still with no inflection in his voice, Timothy explains that being "webbed together" is something you are born with. He and Miranda are webbed yet. It is a Christian endeavor, and she is directing him from beyond the grave to have this baby girl. He says it will be having Miranda back again. He knows that the baby won't actually *be* Miranda, but he knows it will be a girl. "It's just one of those feelings. But I know I'm right."

Timothy responds in the negative to the usual questions about hallucinations, delusions, abnormal moods, substance use, and medical problems such as head injury and seizures. Then he arises from his seat and, without another word, leaves the room.

That evening Charlotte Grenville delivers a healthy baby boy.

Evaluation of Timothy Oldham

Charlotte's testimony suggests that Timothy's peculiarities have been present for years. Although we don't know much about his school career or work, his symptoms would seem likely to affect most areas of his life. This point should be more fully explored.

Timothy's schizotypal symptoms include odd beliefs (his conviction that the baby would be his sister returned to earth; there is no evidence that he comes from a subculture where this sort of thinking is the norm—criterion A2), illusions (the farmer in the painting waving his pitchfork—A3), constricted affect (A6), and absence of close friends (A8). His words ("webbed together," "Christian endeavor") seem metaphorical and stereotyped (A4). Unexplored by the interviewer are the possibility of ideas of reference, paranoid ideas, odd behavior, and excessive social anxiety. Cognitive, affective, and interpersonal symptoms are represented here, however (see the Essential Features for a general PD, p. 546).

This evaluation turns up no indications of another mental disorder. Timothy specifically denies the actual psychotic symptoms necessary to support a diagnosis of delusional disorder or schizophrenia. Other conditions that could entail psychotic symptoms include mood disorders and cognitive disorders, but we've seen evidence against both (B).

Other PDs to consider include schizoid and paranoid PDs. Each of these implies some degree of social isolation, but not the eccentric thinking of StPD. Patients with any of these three Cluster A disorders can decompensate into brief psychoses—a trait held in common with borderline PD. Some patients may qualify for two diagnoses simultaneously: borderline PD and one of the Cluster A PDs. Patients with avoidant PD are socially isolated, but they suffer from it and lack odd behavior and thinking. Of course, a personality change due to another medical condition must be considered in anyone who has a severe or chronic illness; Timothy hasn't.

As of this evaluation, Timothy would receive a GAF score of 75. He hasn't developed schizophrenia, so we won't need the qualifier *(premorbid)*.

F21	Schizotypal personality disorder
Z65.3	Litigation regarding child visitation

Cluster B Personality Disorders

People with Cluster B PDs tend to be dramatic, emotional, and attention-seeking, with moods that are labile and often shallow. They often have intense interpersonal conflicts.

F60.2 Antisocial Personality Disorder

Those with antisocial PD (ASPD) chronically disregard and violate the rights of other people; they cannot or will not conform to the norms of society. This said, people can exhibit ASPD in a number of ways. Some entice us with sweet talk and sweeter deals; they are con artists. Others are, frankly, graceless thugs. Women (and some men) with the disorder may be involved in sex work. In still other individuals, the more traditional antisocial aspects may be obscured by the heavy use—and often purveyance—of illicit drugs.

Although some of these people seem superficially charming, many are aggressive and irritable. Their irresponsible behavior affects nearly every life area. Besides substance use, there may be fighting, lying, and criminal behavior of every conceivable sort: theft, violence, confidence schemes, and child and spouse abuse. They may claim to have guilt feelings, but they don't appear to feel genuine remorse for their behavior. Although they may complain of multiple somatic problems and will occasionally make suicide attempts, their manipulative interactions with others make it difficult to determine whether their complaints are genuine.

DSM-5-TR criteria for ASPD specify that, beginning before age 15, the patient must have a history that would support a diagnosis of conduct disorder (p. 389); as an adult, this behavior must have continued and been extended, with at least four ASPD symptoms.

As many as 3% of men, but only about 1% of women, have this disorder; it is found in about three-quarters of penitentiary prisoners. It runs in families and is more common among lower-socioeconomic-status populations; so, it probably has both a genetic and an environmental basis. Male relatives tend to have ASPD, whereas female relatives may have somatic symptom disorder; both genders are at risk for substance-related disorders.

Although treatment seems to make little difference to patients with ASPD, there is some evidence that the disorder decreases with advancing age, as these people mellow to become "only" substance users. Death by suicide or homicide is the lot of others. Generally, the diagnosis of ASPD will not be warranted if antisocial behavior occurs only in the context of substance abuse. Individuals who misuse substances sometimes engage in criminal behavior, but only when in pursuit of drugs. It is crucial to learn whether patients with possible ASPD have engaged in illicit acts when not using substances.

Although these patients often have a childhood marked by incorrigibility, delinquency, and school problems such as truancy, fewer than half of all children with such a background eventually develop the full adult syndrome. Therefore, we should never make this diagnosis before age 18.

Finally, because ASPD is a serious disorder with no known effective treatment and a dismal prognosis, it must be a diagnosis of last resort. Before making it, redouble efforts to rule out major mental disorders and other PDs.

Essential Features of **Antisocial Personality Disorder**

These people have a history beginning before age 15 of destroying property, serious rule violation, or aggression against people or animals (that is, they fulfill criteria for conduct disorder, p. 389). Since then, in many situations, they lie, con, or give an alias while engaging in behaviors that merit arrest—whether or not they are actually detained. They tend to fight or assault others, and generally fail to plan their activities, relying instead on the inspiration of the impulse. For these behaviors they show no remorse, other than the regret of apprehension. They often do not pay their debts or maintain steady employment, and they may irresponsibly place themselves or other people in danger.

The Fine Print

The D's: • Duration and demographics (diagnosis cannot be made prior to age 18; behavior patterns are enduring) • Diffuse contexts of life are affected • Differential diagnosis (physical and substance use disorders, **bipolar disorders, schizophrenia,** other PDs, ordinary criminality)

Milo Tark

Milo Tark is 23, handsome, and smart. When he works, he earns good money installing heating and air conditioning. He broke into that trade when he left high school, which occurred somewhere in the middle of his 10th-grade year. Since then, he's had at least 15 different jobs; the longest of them lasted 6 months.

Milo's referral for evaluation comes after he is caught trying to con money from elderly patrons at an ATM. The machine is one of two serving the branch bank where his mother works as assistant manager.

"The little devil!" his father exclaims during the initial interview. "He's always been a difficult one to raise, even when he was a kid. Kinda reminds me of me, sometimes. Only, I pulled out of it."

When he was younger, Milo picked a lot of fights. He bloodied his first nose when he was only 5, and the world-class spanking administered by his father taught him nothing about keeping his fists to himself. He later earned a suspension from the seventh grade for extorting $3 and change from an 8-year-old. When the suspension was finally lifted, he ditched class for 47 straight days. Then began a string of encounters with the police, beginning with shoplifting (condoms) and progressing through breaking and entering (four counts) to grand theft auto when he was 15. For stealing the Toyota, he was sent for half a year to a camp run by the state youth authority. "It was the only 6 months we ever knew where he was at night," his father observes.

Milo's time in detention seemed to do him some good, at least initially. Although he never returned to school, for the next 2 years he avoided arrest and intermittently applied himself to learning his trade. Then he celebrated his 19th birthday by getting drunk and joining the Army. Within a few months he was out on the street again, with a bad-conduct discharge for sharing cocaine in his barracks and assaulting two corporals, his first sergeant, and a second lieutenant. For the next several years, he worked when he needed cash and couldn't get it any other way. Not long before this evaluation, he had gotten a 16-year-old girl pregnant.

"She's just a ditsy broad." Milo lounges back, one leg over the arm of the interview chair. He has managed to grow a scraggly beard, and he rolls a toothpick around in the corner of his mouth. The letters H-A-T-E and L-O-V-E are clumsily tattooed across the knuckles of either hand. "She didn't object when she was gettin' laid."

Milo's mood is good now, and he has never had anything that resembles mania. There have been no symptoms of psychosis, except for the time he was coming off speed. He "felt a little paranoid" then, but it didn't last.

The ATM job was a scam thought up by a friend, who had read something like it in the newspaper and decided it would be a good way to obtain fast cash. They never considered that they might be caught, and Milo isn't worried about the effect it could have on his mother.

He yawns and says, "She can always get another job."

Evaluation of Milo Tark

Milo's behavior persistently affects all aspects of his life: school, work, family, and interpersonal relations. By age 15, he easily met criteria for conduct disorder (ASPD criterion C). Afterward, he moved on to full-blown adult criminality that persisted through his early 20s: repeated illegal acts (A1), assaults (on Army personnel—A4), irresponsible work record (A6), impulsivity (no planning about breaking into the ATM—A3), and lack of remorse (toward his mother and the girl he impregnated—A7). His symptoms touch on the areas of cognition, affect, interpersonal functioning, and impulse control (see the description of a general PD). Of course, he is old enough (over 18—criterion B) that we can now consider the diagnosis of ASPD.

People with a manic episode or schizophrenia will sometimes engage in criminal activity, but it is episodic and accompanied by other manic or psychotic symptoms. Milo steadfastly denies any behavior suggesting either a mood or a psychotic disorder (D). Patients with intellectual developmental disorder may break the law, either because they don't realize it is wrong or because they are easily influenced by others. Although Milo didn't do especially well in school, there is no indication this was due to low intelligence.

Because many addicted patients will do nearly anything to obtain money for drugs, substance use disorders are important in the differential diagnosis. Milo has used cocaine and amphetamines (according to him, only briefly), and most of his antisocial behaviors were not associated with drug use. Patients with impulse-control disorders will engage in illegal activities, but this is confined to the context of conduct disorder in younger people and fighting or property destruction in intermittent explosive disorder. Patients with bulimia nervosa sometimes shoplift, but Milo presents no evidence of bulimic episodes. Of course, many of these conditions (as well as the anxiety disorders) can be encountered as associated diagnoses in patients with ASPD.

Career criminals whose antisocial behavior is confined to their "professional" lives may not fulfill all of the criteria for ASPD. They may instead be diagnosed as having adult antisocial behavior, which would be recorded as Z72.811. It constitutes part of the differential diagnosis of the PD.

With a GAF score of 35, Milo's complete diagnosis would be as follows:

F60.2	Antisocial personality disorder
Z65.3	Arrest for ATM fraud

F60.3 Borderline Personality Disorder

Throughout their adult lives, people with borderline PD (BPD) appear unstable. Indeed, the International Classification of Disease calls it emotionally unstable personality disorder (EUPD), and that's the name by which much of the world recognizes it. People with BPD are often at a crisis point as regards mood, behavior, or interpersonal relationships. Many feel empty and bored; they attach themselves strongly to others, then become intensely angry or hostile when they believe they are being ignored or mistreated by those they depend on. They may impulsively try to harm or mutilate themselves; these actions are expressions of anger, cries for help, or attempts to numb themselves against their emotional pain. Although patients with BPD may experience brief psychotic episodes, these resolve so quickly that they are seldom confused with psychoses like schizophrenia. Intense and rapid mood swings, impulsivity, and unstable interpersonal relationships make it difficult for them to achieve their full potential socially, at work, or in school.

BPD runs in families, and it affects perhaps 3% of the general population (with men about equaling women, though women will more likely seek treatment). People with BPD are truly miserable—to such an extent that they can present a serious risk for completed suicide.

The concept of BPD was devised about the middle of the 20th century. These were patients originally (and sometimes still) said to hover between neurosis and psychosis—a "borderline" that is disputed by many clinicians. As the concept has evolved into a PD, it has achieved remarkable popularity, perhaps because so many patients can be shoehorned into its capacious definition.

Although 1–2% of the general population may legitimately qualify for a diagnosis of BPD, it is probably applied to a far greater proportion of the patients who seek mental health care. In my opinion, it may be one of the most overused diagnoses in the DSM. Many of these patients have other disorders that are more readily treatable; these include major depressive disorder, somatic symptom disorder, and substance-related disorders.

Essential Features of **Borderline Personality Disorder**

People with BPD are unstable, existing in a perpetual crisis of mood or behavior. They often feel lonely and bored. Disturbed identity (insecure self-image) can lead them to attach themselves strongly to others whom they later vigorously reject. On the other hand, they may frantically try to avert desertion (which could be actual or fantasied). Pronounced impulsiveness can lead them to engage in other potentially harmful behaviors, such as sexual indiscretions, spending sprees, eating binges, or erratic driving. Stress can cause brief episodes of dissociation or paranoia, but these quickly resolve. Intense, rapid mood swings may yield to anger that is inappropriate and uncontrolled. And, over and over, they may harm themselves or self-mutilate, or threaten (or even attempt) suicide.

The Fine Print

The D's: • Duration (begins in teens or early 20s and endures) • Diffuse contexts of life are affected • Differential diagnosis (mood and psychotic disorders, separation anxiety disorder, other personality disorders)

Josephine Armitage

"I'm cutting myself!" The voice on the telephone is high-pitched and quavering. "I'm cutting myself right now! Ow! There, I've started." The voice howls with pain and rage.

Twenty minutes later, the clinician has Josephine's address and her promise that she will come to the emergency room right away. Two hours later, her left forearm swathed in bandages, Josephine Armitage is sitting in an office in the mental health department. Crisscrossing scars furrow her right arm from wrist to elbow. She is 33, a bit overweight, and chewing gum.

"I feel a lot better," she says with a smile. "I really think you saved my life." The clinician glances at her nonswathed arm. "This isn't the first time, is it?"

"I should think that would be pretty obvious. Are you going to be terminally dense, just like my last shrink?" She scowls and turns 90 degrees to face the wall. "Sheesh!"

Her previous therapist saw Josephine for a reduced fee but couldn't give her more time when she requested it. She responded by letting the air out of all four tires of that clinician's new BMW.

Her current trouble is with her boyfriend. One of her girlfriends is "pretty sure" she saw James with another woman 2 nights ago. Yesterday morning, Josephine called in sick to work and staked out James's workplace so she could confront him. He never appeared, so last evening she banged on the door of his apartment unit until neighbors threatened to call the police. Before leaving, she kicked a hole in the wall beside his door. Then she got drunk and drove up and down the main drag, trying to pick up a date.

"Sounds dangerous," observes the clinician.

"I was looking for Mr. Goodbar, but no one turned up. I decided I'd have to cut myself again. It always seems to help." Josephine's anger has once again evaporated, and she turns back from the wall. "Life's a bitch and then you die."

"When you cut yourself, do you ever really intend to kill yourself?"

"Well, let's see." She chews her gum thoughtfully. "I get so angry and depressed; I just don't care what happens. My last shrink said all my life I've felt like a shell of a person, and I guess that's right. It feels like there's no one living inside, so I might just as well pour out the blood and finish the job."

Evaluation of Josephine Armitage

Early on, this clinician should determine whether the behaviors reported (and observed) have been present since Josephine's late teen years. From her report of the comment made by her "last shrink," this would seem to be the case, but it needs verification.

Josephine has an abundance of maladaptive behaviors, and they are pervasive: Her work is affected (calling in sick on a whim), also her relations with her boyfriend and her previous therapist. The entire episode of staking out James's apartment can be seen as a frantic effort to avoid abandonment (BPD criterion A1). Even her initial moments with her present clinician reveal some swings between idealization and devaluation (criterion A2). She shows evidence of dangerous impulsivity (driving while under the influence of alcohol, trying to pick up a stranger—A4), and she has made repeated suicide attempts—or gestures (A5).

Josephine's mood, even within the limits of this narrative, would seem markedly unstable and reactive to what she perceives to be the clinician's attitude toward her (A6); her anger is sudden, inappropriate, and intense (A8). She agrees with a description of herself as an empty shell (A7). Although patients with BPD are often described as having identity disturbance and occasional, brief psychotic lapses, our view of Josephine provides no evidence for either of these. Even so, she has six or seven BPD symptoms; only five are needed.

A long list of other mental disorders can be confused with BPD; each must be considered before settling on this disorder as a sole (or principal) diagnosis. (This isn't a criterion for BPD, which has no named differential diagnosis, but it is a generic PD criterion as well as one of my personal mantras.) Many patients with BPD also have major depressive disorder or persistent depressive disorder. It's important to establish that suicidal behaviors, anger, and feelings of emptiness are not experienced solely during episodes of depression. Similarly, we need to know that affective instability is not due to cyclothymic disorder. Note that the official criteria don't mention any of these possibilities, though they are featured in the text.

Patients with BPD can have psychotic episodes, but these tend to be brief and stress-related, and they resolve quickly and spontaneously—all of which makes them unlikely to be confused with schizophrenia. The misuse of various substances can lead to suicidal behavior, instability of mood, and reduced impulse control. Substance-related disorders are also often found accompanying BPD and should always be carefully sought. Patients with somatic symptom disorder are often quite dramatic and may misuse substances and make suicide attempts. Although this vignette contains no evidence for any of these (other than getting drunk—was this an isolated event?), the evaluating clinician would need to carefully consider the list just given.

Patients with BPD can also show features of additional PDs. Josephine's presentation is dramatic, suggesting histrionic PD. Patients with narcissistic PD are also self-centered, though they lack Josephine's impulsivity. Those with antisocial PD are impulsive and don't control their anger well; although some of Josephine's behaviors are destructive, she does not engage in overtly criminal activity.

Finally, dissociative identity disorder sometimes accompanies BPD. Further interviewing and observation would be needed to rule out that rare condition. Assuming the verification of Josephine's history, her diagnosis would be as given below. Note that we can identify the injury to her arm as one inflicted without suicide in mind. I would place her GAF score at 51.

F60.3	Borderline personality disorder
R45.88	Nonsuicidal self-injury
S51.809	Lacerations of forearm

There's no such thing as a late-life PD. By definition, the PDs are conditions present, more or less, from the get-go. If you encounter a patient whose character structure appears to have changed during the adult years, search for the cause until you find it. You are likely to turn up a personality change due to another medical condition, a mood or psychotic disorder, something substance-related, a cognitive issue, or a severe adjustment disorder.

F60.4 Histrionic Personality Disorder

Patients with histrionic PD (HPD) have a long-standing pattern of extreme attention seeking and emotionalism that seeps into all areas of their lives. These people satisfy their need to be at center stage in two main ways: (1) Their interests and topics of conversation focus on their own desires and activities; and (2) they continually call attention to themselves by their behavior, including speech. They are overly concerned with physical attractiveness (of themselves and of others, as it relates to them), and they will express themselves so extravagantly that it can seem almost a parody of normal emotionality. Their need for approval can cause them to be seductive, often inappropriately (even flamboyantly) so. Many have normal sex lives, but some will be promiscuous; and still others may be uninterested in sex.

People with HPD are often so insecure, so dependent on the favor of others, that they constantly seek approval; their moods may seem shallow or excessively reactive to their surroundings. Low tolerance for frustration can spawn temper tantrums. Many enjoy talking with mental health professionals (another chance to be the center of attention!), but because their speech is often vague and full of exaggerations, interviewing them can prove frustrating.

Quick to form new friendships, people with HPD also quickly become demanding. Because they are trusting and easily influenced, their behavior may appear inconsistent. They don't think very analytically, so they may have difficulty with tasks that require logical thinking, such as doing mental arithmetic. However, they may succeed in jobs that set a premium on creativity and imagination. Their craving for novelty sometimes leads to legal problems as they seek sensation or stimulation. Some have a remarkable tendency to forget affect-laden material.

HPD has not been especially well studied, but it is not uncommon—it affects over a percent of the general population. It may run in families. The classic patient is female, though the disorder can occur in men.

Essential Features of **Histrionic Personality Disorder**

These people don't just crave the limelight—they are unhappy when not the focus of attention. They actively attempt to draw attention to themselves with their physical appearance and mannerisms. Their manner of speaking may be overly dramatic, but what they say can be nonspecific and vague. They can be gushing or effusive when expressing their emotions, which, however, tend to be superficial and fleeting. These people are too open to suggestion, too readily influenced. They may interpret relationships as being intimate when they're not—even to the extent of behaving in ways that are inappropriately suggestive or seductive.

The Fine Print

The D's: • Duration (begins in teens or early 20s and endures) • Diffuse contexts of life are affected • Differential diagnosis (substance use disorders, somatic symptom disorder, other personality disorders, personality change due to medical condition)

Angela Black

Angela Black and her husband, Donald, have come for marriage counseling; as usual, they are fighting.

"He never listens to me. I might as well be talking to the dog!" Tears and mascara drip across the front of Angela's low-cut silk dress.

"What's there to listen to?" Donald retorts. "I know I irritate her because she complains so much. But when I ask how she'd like me to change, she can never put her finger on it."

Angela and Donald are both 37 years old, and they have been married nearly 10 years. Already they have been separated twice. Donald earns excellent money as a corporate lawyer; Angela has worked as a fashion model. She doesn't work much anymore, but her husband makes enough to keep her well dressed and fashionably shod. "I don't think she's ever worn the same dress twice," Donald grumbles.

"Yes, I have," she snaps back.

"When? Name one time." Donald's question is soft, inviting, like he really wants an answer.

"I do it all the time. Especially recently." For several minutes longer, Angela defends herself, without ever making a concrete statement of fact.

"*Res ipsa loquitur*," says Donald with satisfaction.

"Oh, God! Latin!" She nearly howls. "When he puts in his superior, gratuitous Latin, it makes me want to cut my wrists!"

The Blacks agree on one thing: For them, this is a typical conversation.

He works late most nights and weekends, which upsets her. She spends far too much money on jewelry and clothing. She relishes the fact that she can still attract men. "I wouldn't do it if you'd pay more attention to me," she says with a pout.

"You wouldn't do it if you didn't listen to Marilyn," he retorts.

Marilyn and Angela have been best friends since their cheerleading days in high school. Marilyn is wealthy and independent; she doesn't care what people think and behaves accordingly. Angela typically follows right along.

"Like the pool party last summer," puts in Donald, "when you took off your suits to 'practice cheers' for the races. Or was that your idea?"

"What would you know about it? You were working late. Besides, it was only our tops."

Evaluation of Angela Black

Angela's personality style has a profound effect on her marriage, though the vignette hints that her other social relationships (for example, men at the party) are affected as well. More information would be needed to establish that she has been this way throughout her adult life. However, it seems unlikely that her way of doing business with the world has developed recently.

Angela's symptoms include sexual provocation (inferred from her dancing topless—HPD criterion A2) and a strong need to be the center of attention (A1); excessive concern with physical appearance (A4); dramatic emotional expression (A6); suggestibility (following the lead of her friend Marilyn—A7); and vague speech (commented on by her husband—A5). I thought she might have expressed a touch of rapidly shifting emotional expression (A3), too, but maybe that's just me. Conservatively scored, she has at least six symptoms of HPD (five are required by DSM-5-TR criteria).

Her clinician should gather information adequate to determine that Angela does not have any of the major mental disorders that commonly accompany HPD. These include somatic symptom disorder (does she agree that she's been in good physical health?) and substance-related disorders.

Would Angela qualify for other PD diagnoses? She is certainly focused on herself, and she likes to be admired. However, she lacks the sense of grandiose accomplishment that characterizes patients with narcissistic PD. You can often identify histrionic features in people with borderline PD. Angela's mood is somewhat labile, but she does not report interpersonal instability, identity disturbance, transient paranoid ideation, or other symptoms that characterize borderline patients. Her easy suggestibility might suggest dependent PD but, far from leaning on her husband for support, she routinely fights with him. With a GAF score of 65, I'd diagnose her as follows:

F60.4	Histrionic personality disorder
Z63.0	Relationship distress with spouse

F60.81 Narcissistic Personality Disorder

People with narcissistic PD (NPD) have a lifelong pattern of grandiosity (in behavior and in fantasy), a thirst for admiration, and an absence of empathy. These attitudes permeate most aspects of their lives. They regard themselves as unusually special; they are self-important individuals who commonly exaggerate their accomplishments. (From the outset, however, we need to note that these traits constitute a PD only in adults. Children and teenagers are naturally self-centered; in kids, narcissistic traits don't necessarily imply later pathology.)

Despite their grandiose attitudes, people with NPD have fragile self-esteem and often feel unworthy; even at times of great personal success, they may feel fraudulent or undeserving. They remain overly sensitive to what others think about them and feel compelled to extract compliments. When criticized, they may cover their distress with a façade of icy indifference. As sensitive as they are about their own feelings, they have little apparent understanding of the feelings and needs of others. Any empathy they display may be feigned, just as they may lie to cover their own faults.

Patients with NPD often fantasize about wild success, and they envy those who have achieved it. They may choose friends they think can help them get what they want. Job performance can suffer (due to interpersonal problems), or it can be enhanced (due to their unquenchable drive for success). Because they tend to be concerned with grooming and value their youthful looks, the march of years may yield increasing depression.

NPD has seldom been studied. It appears to occur in around 1% of the general population; most are men. There is no information about family history, environmental antecedents, or other background material that might help us to understand these difficult personalities.

Essential Features of Narcissistic Personality Disorder

People with NPD feel self-important, crave admiration, and lack concern for the feelings of others. They typically exaggerate their own abilities and accomplishments. They tend to be preoccupied with fantasies of beauty, brilliance, perfect love, power, or limitless success, and believe that they are so unusual that they should only associate with people or institutions of rarefied status. Often arrogant or haughty, they may believe that others envy them (though the reverse may be true). Lack of empathy unleashes their feelings of privilege in justifying the exploitation of others to achieve their own goals.

The Fine Print

The D's: • Duration (begins in teens or early 20s and endures) • Diffuse contexts of life are affected • Differential diagnosis (substance use disorders, bipolar disorders, other personality disorders, persistent depressive disorder)

Berna Whitlow

"Dr. Whitlow, you're my backup for emergency clinic this afternoon, and I've got to have some help from you!" Eleanor Bondurak, a social worker at the mental health clinic, is red-faced with anger and frustration. It isn't the first time she's had difficulty working with this clinician.

At the age of 50, Berna Whitlow has worked at nearly every mental health clinic in the metropolitan area. She is well trained and highly intelligent, and she reads voraciously in her specialty. Those are the qualities that have landed her job after job over the years. The qualities that keep her moving from one job to another are known better to her co-workers than to her employers. She is notorious among her colleagues for being pompous and self-centered.

"She said she wasn't going to take orders from me. And her attitude said for her, 'You're nothing but a social worker.'" Eleanor is reliving the moment in a heated discussion with the clinical director. "She said she'd talk to my boss or to you. I pointed out that neither of you was in the building at the time, and that the patient had brought a gun in his briefcase. Then she said I should 'write it up and submit it,' and she would 'decide what action to take.' That's when I had you paged."

With the crisis over (the gun had been unloaded, the patient ultimately deemed not dangerous), the clinical director drops in to chat with Dr. Whitlow. "Look, Berna, it's true that ordinarily the social worker sees the patient and does a write-up before you step in. But this wasn't exactly an ordinary case! Especially in emergencies, the whole team must pull together."

Berna Whitlow is tall, with a straight nose and jutting chin that seems to radiate authority. Her long hair is thick and blond. She raises her chin a bit higher. "You hardly need to lecture me on the team approach. I've been a leader in nearly every clinic in town. I'm a superb team leader. You can ask anyone." As she speaks, she rubs the gold rings that encircle every finger but her thumbs.

"But being a team leader involves more than just giving orders. It's also about gathering information, building consensus, caring about the feelings of oth—"

"Listen," Dr. Whitlow interrupts, "it's her job to work on my team. It's my job to provide the leadership and make the decisions."

Evaluation of Berna Whitlow

From the material we have (which does not include a clinical interview, so our conclusions must be tentative), Dr. Whitlow's personality traits would seem to have caused difficulties for many years. They affect her life broadly, interfering with work (many jobs) and interpersonal relationships. Of course, in a full assessment we'd also inquire about her personality as it affects her family and social life.

Symptoms suggestive of NPD include her haughty attitude (criterion A9), exaggerating her own accomplishments ("I'm a superb team leader"—A1), insisting that she receive orders or requests only from persons of high rank (A3), expecting obedience (from a sense of entitlement—A5), and lacking empathy with fellow workers (A7). And five criteria are what's needed for this diagnosis; affective, cognitive, and interpersonal features are present (see the Essential Features of a general PD).

Several other PDs can either accompany or be confused with NPD. Patients with histrionic PD are also extremely self-centered, but Dr. Whitlow is not as theatrical (although she does wear a lot of rings). As is the case in borderline PD (and most other PDs), patients with NPD have a great deal of trouble relating to other people. But they (including Dr. Whitlow) are not especially prone to unstable moods, suicidal behavior, or brief psychoses under stress. Although there is a hint of the deceitful in narcissistic exaggerations, these people lack the pervasive criminality and disregard for the rights of others that are typical of antisocial PD.

Persistent depressive disorder and major depressive disorder frequently accompany NPD, but there is no evidence in the vignette to support either of those diagnoses. Dr. Whitlow's tentative diagnosis (GAF score of 61) would be as follows:

F60.81   Narcissistic personality disorder

Cluster C Personality Disorders

The characteristics of Cluster C PDs are anxiety, tension, and a superabundance of control.

F60.6 Avoidant Personality Disorder

People with avoidant PD (APD) feel inadequate, are socially inhibited, and are overly sensitive to criticism. These characteristics are present throughout adult life and affect most aspects of daily life. (Like narcissistic traits, avoidant traits are common in children and don't necessarily imply eventual PD.)

Their sensitivity to criticism and disapproval makes these patients self-effacing and eager to please others, but it can also lead to marked social isolation. They may misinterpret innocent comments as implying criticism; often they refuse to begin a relationship unless they are sure they will be accepted. They will hang back in social situations for fear of saying something foolish and may avoid occupations that involve social demands. Other than their parents, siblings, or children, they tend to have few close friends. Comfortable with routine, they may go to great lengths to avoid departing from their set ways. In an interview they can appear tense and anxious.

Although APD has appeared in the DSMs since 1980, relevant research is still sparse. In frequency, it occupies middle ground (about 2% of the general population) as PDs go, roughly equal for men and women. Many such patients marry and work, although they may become depressed or anxious if they lose their support systems. Sometimes this disorder is associated with having a disfiguring illness or condition. APD is not often seen clinically; these patients tend to come to evaluation only when another illness supervenes. There is considerable overlap with social anxiety disorder.

Essential Features of **Avoidant Personality Disorder**

People with APD are socially inhibited, overly sensitive to criticism, and feel generally inadequate. Such patients so fear disapproval that they hold back from intimate relationships; they only become involved with others if they know in advance they will be accepted. Believing themselves inferior, unappealing, or socially clumsy, they are reluctant to risk embarrassment by taking up new activities or assume personal risk. They are deeply concerned about possible criticism or rejection, either in social life or on the job; there, it may cause them to shun assignments that involve personal contact. Indeed, they avoid new personal contacts, which stoke their sense of inadequacy.

The Fine Print

The D's: • Duration (begins in teens or early 20s and endures) • Diffuse contexts of life are affected • Differential diagnosis (substance use disorders, social anxiety disorder, personality change, agoraphobia, other personality disorders)

Jack Weiblich

Jack Weiblich is feeling worse when he ought to be feeling better. At least, that's what his new acquaintances in Alcoholics Anonymous tell him. One reminds him that 30 days' sobriety is "time enough to detox every last cell" in his body. Another speculates that he's having a dry drunk.

"Whatever a dry drunk is," Jack observes later. "All I know is that after 5 weeks without alcohol, I'm feeling every bit as bad as I did 15 years ago, before I'd touched a drop. I've enjoyed hangovers more than this!"

At age 32, Jack has a lot of hangovers to choose from. He had his first drink in his final year of high school. Before that, he'd been a strange, lonely sort of kid for whom meeting other people was torture. While he was still in high school, he had begun to lose his hair; now, except for his eyebrows and eyelashes, he is totally bald. He is also afflicted with a slight, persistent nodding of his head. "Titubation," the neurologist had said. "It's benign—don't worry about it." The sight of his balding, nodding head in the mirror every morning looks grotesque, even to Jack. As a teenager he found it almost impossible to form relationships; he was positive that no one could like someone as peculiar as he was.

Then one evening Jack found alcohol. "Right from the first drink, I knew I'd discovered something important. With two beers on board, I forgot all about my head. I even asked a girl out. She turned me down, but even that was OK. I had found a life."

But the following morning, he still had his old personality. He experimented for months before he learned when and how much he could drink and maintain a glow sufficiently rosy to help him feel well—but not too rosy to function. During a 3-week period in his final year at law school when he sobered up completely, he learned that without alcohol, he still had the same old feelings of isolation and rejection.

"When I'm not drinking, I don't feel sad or anxious," Jack observes. "But I'm lonely and uncomfortable with myself, and I feel that other people will feel the same about me. I guess that's why I just don't make friends."

After law school, Jack took a job with a small firm that specializes in corporate law. They call him "The Mole," because he spends nearly every workday in the law library doing research. "I just don't feel comfortable meeting the clients—I never get along well with new people."

The only exception to this lifestyle is Jack's membership in the stamp club. From his grandfather, he'd inherited a large collection of commemorative plate blocks. When he took these to the Philatelic Society, he thought they'd welcome him ("Well, my collection, anyway") with open arms, and they did. He has continued to build upon his grandfather's collection, and he attends meetings once a month. "I guess I feel OK there because I don't have to worry whether they'll like me. I've got a great stamp collection for them to admire."

Evaluation of Jack Weiblich

Jack's symptoms are pervasive, profoundly affecting his work and social life, and have been present since he was a teenager; that surely qualifies for APD. Other symptoms include the following typical APD features: He avoids interpersonal contact (for example, with clients at the law firm—criterion A1); he feels that he is unappealing (A6); when he joined the stamp club, he was pretty sure that his collection would be accepted (A2). He worries a lot about rejection (A4). Only four criteria are needed; cognitive, occupational, and interpersonal areas are all involved.

Depression and anxiety are both common in patients with APD. Therefore, it is important to search for evidence of mood disorders and anxiety disorders (especially social anxiety disorder) in patients who avoid contact with others. Jack says he feels neither sad nor anxious, but he admits seriously misusing alcohol. The substance-related disorders also commonly bring a patient with APD to the attention of mental health care providers.

In both APD and schizoid PD, patients spend most of their time alone. The difference, of course, is that people with APD are unhappy with their condition, whereas those with schizoid PD prefer it that way. A somewhat more difficult differential diagnosis may be that between APD and dependent PD. (As with Jack, people with dependent PD avoid positions of responsibility.) Note that Jack's avoidant lifestyle may have been bound up in his twin physical attributes—baldness and a nodding head.

Although Jack has an alcohol use disorder (I'll leave the proof of that statement as a take-home exercise), his clinician feels that it is causing him little current difficulty and that the PD is the fundamental problem needing treatment (other clinicians might argue with this interpretation). That's why the PD is listed as his principal diagnosis. Of course, he doesn't qualify for any course modifiers for alcohol use disorder, because he's only been on the wagon for 5 weeks (p. 417); I thought his alcoholism was pretty mild, actually. Also, note that the PD doesn't figure into the coding of the substance use disorder; see Table 15.2 (p. 475). I'd put his GAF score at 61.

F60.6	Avoidant personality disorder (principal diagnosis)
F10.10	Alcohol use disorder, mild
L63.1	Alopecia universalis
R25.0	Nodding of head

F60.7 Dependent Personality Disorder

Much more so than most, patients with dependent PD (DPD) feel the need for someone else to take care of them. Because they desperately fear separation, their behavior becomes so submissive and clinging that other people can take advantage of them—or wound them with rejection. Anxiety blossoms if they are thrust into a position of leadership, and they feel helpless and uncomfortable when they are alone. Because they typically need much reassurance, they may have trouble making decisions. Such people have trouble starting projects and sticking to a job on their own, though they may do well under the careful direction of someone else. They tend to belittle themselves and to agree with people who they know are wrong. They may tolerate considerable abuse (even, sometimes, battering).

DPD is infrequently reported, and it has not been well studied. Some writers believe that it is difficult to distinguish it from avoidant PD. It has been found more often among women than men. Bud Stanhope, a patient with the sleep terror type of non-rapid eye movement sleep arousal disorder, also has DPD; his history is given on page 339.

Essential Features of **Dependent Personality Disorder**

Their need for supportive relationships draws these people into clinging, submissive behavior and fears of separation. Fear of disapproval makes it hard for them to disagree with others; to gain support, they may take extraordinary steps, such as undertaking unpleasant tasks. Low self-confidence prevents them from starting or carrying out projects independently; indeed, they want others to take responsibility for their own major life areas. If they do make even everyday decisions, they require lots of advice and reassurance. Exaggerated, unrealistic fears of abandonment and the notion that they cannot care for themselves will cause these people to feel helpless or uncomfortable when alone; they may desperately seek a replacement for a lost, close personal relationship.

The Fine Print

The D's: • Duration (begins in teens or early 20s and endures) • Diffuse contexts of life are affected • Differential diagnosis (physical and substance use disorders, mood and anxiety disorders, other PDs)

Janet Greenspan

A secretary in a large Silicon Valley company, Janet Greenspan is one of the best workers there. She's never sick or absent, and she can handle any assignment—she's even had some bookkeeping experience. Her supervisor notes that she is polite on the phone, types like a demon, and will volunteer for anything. When the building maintenance crew went out on strike, Janet came in early every day for a week to clean the toilets and sinks. But still, somehow, she just isn't working out.

Her supervisor complains that Janet needs too much direction, even for simple decisions—such as what sort of paper to type form letters on. When asked what she thinks the answer should be, her judgment is good, but she wants guidance anyway. Her constant need for reassurance takes an inordinate amount of her supervisor's time. That's why she has been referred to the company mental health consultant for an evaluation.

At 28, Janet is slender, attractive, and carefully dressed. Her chestnut hair already shows streaks of gray. She appears at the doorway of the office and asks, "Where would you like me to sit?" Once she starts talking, she speaks readily about her life and her work.

She has always felt timid and unsure of herself. She and her two sisters grew up with a father who was affectionate but dictatorial; their mouse of a mom seemed to welcome his tender tyranny. At her mother's knee, Janet learned obedience well. When she was 18, her father suddenly died. Within months, her mother remarried and moved to a far-off city, leaving Janet bereft and panic-stricken. Instead of beginning college, she took a job as a teller in a bank; shortly afterward, she married one of her customers.

He was a 30-year-old bachelor who was set in his ways, and he soon let it be known that he preferred to make all their choices himself. He even began choosing what she would wear. For the first time in a year, Janet relaxed.

But even this security breeds its own anxieties. "He is a lot older, and sometimes at night I wake up, wondering what I'd do if I lost him," Janet tells the interviewer. "It makes my heart beat so fast I think it might quit from exhaustion. I know I could never manage on my own."

Evaluation of Janet Greenspan

Janet has the following symptoms of DPD: She needs considerable advice to make even everyday decisions (criterion A1); she loves it that her husband makes her choices for her (A2); panic-stricken when her father died and her mother left town, she fled into a precipitous marriage (A7); she fears being left to fend for herself, even though she has no indication that this is likely (A8). She even volunteered to clean the office toilet, probably to curry favor with the other staff (A5). We have no evidence that she is reluctant to disagree with others, but otherwise the criteria fit like a rubber glove; five are needed for diagnosis.

Janet reports that she has been this way since childhood; from the history, her character traits have affected both work and personal life. Perhaps it is fortunate (or perhaps not) that she married someone whose need to be in charge complements her dependency. Cognitive, affective, and interpersonal areas are involved (see the Essential Features for a general PD).

Dependent behavior is found in several mental disorders that Janet does not appear to have, including illness anxiety disorder and agoraphobia. The person with the secondary psychosis in what used to be called *folie à deux* (or shared psychotic disorder—now it may be diagnosed as delusional disorder)—often has a dependent personality. Even if Janet had all the required physiological symptoms for generalized anxiety disorder, she would not be given that diagnosis, because her worries were evidently limited to fears of abandonment.

Patients with DPD must be differentiated from those with histrionic PD, who are also impressionable and easily influenced by others, but Janet is not attention-seeking; rather, quite the opposite. Other PDs usually included in the differential diagnosis are borderline and avoidant PD.

With a GAF score of 70, Janet's diagnosis would be a plain vanilla:

F60.7   Dependent personality disorder

F60.5 Obsessive–Compulsive Personality Disorder

People with obsessive–compulsive PD (OCPD) are perfectionistic and preoccupied with orderliness; they need to exert interpersonal and mental control. These traits exist lifelong, at the expense of efficiency, flexibility, and candor. However, OCPD is not just obsessive–compulsive disorder (OCD) in miniature. Many patients with OCPD have no actual obsessions or compulsions at all, though some do eventually develop OCD.

The rigid perfectionism of these people often results in indecisiveness, preoccupation with detail, scrupulosity, and insistence that others do things their way. These behaviors can interfere with their effectiveness in work or with social relationships. Often, they seem depressed, and this depression may wax and wane, perhaps to the point that it drives them into treatment. Sometimes these individuals are stingy; they may be savers, refusing to throw away even worthless objects they no longer need. They may have trouble expressing affection.

Patients with OCPD are list makers who allocate their own time poorly, workaholics who must meticulously plan even their own pleasure. They may schedule a vacation, only to postpone it. They resist the authority of others but insist on their own. They may be perceived as stilted, stiff, or moralistic.

This condition is probably fairly common; prevalence in various studies centers around 5%. It is found about equally in males and females, and it probably runs in families.

Essential Features of **Obsessive–Compulsive Personality Disorder**

These people are intensely focused on control, organization, and perfection. They can become so absorbed with details, organization, and rules of an activity that they lose sight of its purpose. They tend to be rigid and stubborn, perhaps so perfectionistic that it interferes with the completion of tasks. They can be overly conscientious, inflexible, or scrupulous about ethics, morals, and values. Some are workaholics who won't even delegate tasks; others will only work when everyone agrees to do things their way. Some may save worthless items; others are stingy with themselves and with other people.

The Fine Print

The D's: • Duration (begins in teens or early 20s and endures) • Diffuse contexts of life are affected • Differential diagnosis (substance use disorders, OCD, hoarding disorder, other personality disorders, personality change)

Robin Chatterjee

"I admit it—I'm over the top in neatness." Robin Chatterjee straightens a fold in her sari. Born in Mumbai and educated in London, Robin is a graduate student in biology. Now she spends part of her time as a teaching assistant, the rest struggling through her own coursework at a major university. She gazes steadily at the interviewer.

According to her preceptor, a slightly dour Scot named MacLeish who urged her to schedule the mental health interview, the problem isn't neatness. It's completing the work. Every paper she turns in is wonderful—every fact is there, every conclusion well supported, without so much as a misplaced comma in language that sparkles. He asked her why she couldn't learn to let go of them a little sooner, "before the rats die of old age?" She thought it funny at the time, but it's made her think.

Robin has always been orderly. Her mother made her keep neat little lists of her chores, and the habit stuck. Robin admits that she becomes so "lost in lists" that sometimes she hardly has time to finish her work. Her students seem fond of her, but several have said they wished she'd give them more responsibility. One told Dr. MacLeish that Robin seems afraid even to let them do their own dissections; their methods aren't as compulsively correct as hers, so she'll try to do them herself. Finally, she admits that nearly every night, her work habits keep her late in the lab. It's been weeks since she's had a date—or any social life at all. This realization is what spurs her to follow Dr. MacLeish's advice and come for an evaluation.

Evaluation of Robin Chatterjee

Although the prototype for OCPD seems a pretty good fit for Robin, she just barely meets the official criteria. She is workaholic and perfectionistic (OCPD criteria A3 and A2), to the point that these traits interfere with the education of her students. She has enormous difficulty delegating work—even her students' own dissections (A6). And she concentrates so fiercely on her lists of tasks that she sometimes doesn't accomplish the tasks themselves (A1). These tendencies have persisted throughout her young adult life.

Depressed mood is common in such people. Besides OCD itself, the common disorders to consider in a patient with OCPD include major depressive disorder and persistent depressive disorder. Robin is not depressed and, unlike so many patients with OCPD, seems to have no other disorder. Because she barely meets the criteria and is functioning well overall, I would place her GAF score at a relatively high 70.

F60.5   Obsessive–compulsive personality disorder

Other Personality Conditions

F07.0 Personality Change Due to Another Medical Condition

Some medical conditions can cause a personality change, which we'll define as an alteration (typically a worsening) of a patient's previous personality traits. If the medical condition occurs early enough in childhood, the change can last throughout the person's life. Most instances of personality change are caused by an injury to the brain or by some other central nervous system disorder, such as epilepsy or Huntington's disease; however, systemic diseases that affect the brain (for example, systemic lupus erythematosus) are also sometimes implicated.

Several sorts of personality change commonly occur. Mood may become unstable, perhaps with outbursts of rage or suspiciousness; other patients may become apathetic and passive. Changes in mood are especially common when there has been damage to the frontal lobes of the brain. Patients with temporal lobe epilepsy may become overly religious, verbose, perhaps lacking a sense of humor; others may turn markedly aggressive. Paranoid ideas are also frequent. Belligerence can accompany outbursts of temper, to the extent that the social judgment of some patients becomes markedly impaired. Use the type specifiers in the Coding Notes to categorize the nature of the personality change.

If there is a major alteration in the structure of the brain, these personality changes will probably persist. If the problem stems from a correctable chemical issue, they may resolve. When severe, they can ultimately lead to dementia, as is sometimes the case in patients with multiple sclerosis.

Essential Features of **Personality Change Due to Another Medical Condition**

Through physiological means, a medical condition appears to have caused an illness that features lasting change in the person's personality.

The Fine Print

From their *expected* developmental pattern, children will experience a personality change that lasts a year or longer.

The D's: • Duration (enduring) • Distress or disability (work/educational, social, or personal) • Differential diagnosis (**delirium, other physical** or **mental disorders,** substance use disorders, personality disorders)

Coding Notes

Depending on the main feature, specify type:

> **Aggressive type**
> **Apathetic type**
> **Disinhibited type**
> **Labile type**
> **Paranoid type**
> **Other type**
> **Combined type**
> **Unspecified type**

Use the actual name of the general medical condition when you code this disorder, and also code separately the medical condition.

Eddie Ortway

Born in central Los Angeles, Eddie Ortway was raised by his mother—during those periods she was neither hospitalized (for drug or alcohol use) nor jailed (prostitution). Eddie always suspected that his parents had been only briefly acquainted.

Eddie avoided school whenever possible and grew up with no role model in sight. His principal accomplishment was learning to use his fists. By the time he was 15, he and his gang had participated in several turf wars. He made a name for himself as an aggressive enemy.

But Eddie is not a criminal, and the need to earn a living soon set him to work. With little education and no training, he found his opportunities pretty much limited to fast food and hard labor. Sometimes he held several jobs at a time. But, as an old probation report notes, he still had "a raging sense of injustice." Although he gradually stopped associating with his gang, through his middle 20s he continued to deal aggressively with any situation that seemed to require direct action.

His 27th birthday is one of these occasions. Eddie is delivering a pizza to an apartment building in his old neighborhood when he encounters a teenager forcing an old woman into an alley at gunpoint. Eddie steps forward and for his pains receives a bullet that enters his head through the left eye socket and exits at the hairline.

He is admitted to the hospital by way of the operating room, where surgeons debride his wound. He never even loses consciousness and is released in less than a week.

But he doesn't return to work. The social worker's report notes that Eddie's physical condition rebounds within a month, but that he "lacks drive." He appears for every scheduled job interview, but his prospective employers uniformly report that he "just doesn't seem very interested in working."

"I need time to recuperate," Eddie says. He is a good-looking young man whose hair has begun receding from his forehead. An incisional scar runs up onto his scalp. "I still don't think I'm quite ready."

He has been recuperating for 2 years; the purpose of this interview is to learn why. Other than a slight droop to his left eyelid, his neurological examination is completely normal. An EEG shows some slow waves over the frontal lobes; the MRI reveals a localized absence of brain tissue.

Eddie always cooperates with testing procedures, and every clinician he meets notes that he is unfailingly pleasant and polite. However, as one of them writes, "There seems something slightly mechanical about his cooperation. He complies but never anticipates, and he shows little real investment in the proceedings."

Eddie's affect is about medium with almost no lability. His speech is clear, coherent, and relevant. He denies delusions, hallucinations, obsessions, compulsions, and phobias. When asked what interests him, he thinks for a few seconds and then answers that he guesses he is interested in going back home. He earns a perfect score on the MMSE.

In the time since his injury, Eddie admits, he has lived on workers' compensation and spends most of his time watching television. He no longer argues with anyone.

When one examiner asks him what he would do if he again saw someone being mugged, he shrugs and says, "I think people should just live and let live."

Evaluation of Eddie Ortway

The history and examinations clearly substantiate the obvious medical cause for Eddie's persistent personality change (criterion A). Note that it is the physiology of trauma to the brain that produces Eddie's personality change. This is the explicit requirement (B) for this diagnosis, which cannot be made should a change in personality accompany a nonspecific medical condition such as severe pain.

Eddie's normal attention span and lack of memory deficit rule out delirium (D) and major neurocognitive disorder; however, neuropsychological testing should be requested. A PD such as dependent PD could not explain Eddie's condition, because his behavior represents a marked change from his premorbid personality (that is, the way he was until his injury). And the features of Eddie's personality change are not better explained by a different physically induced mental disorder. A mood disorder due to brain trauma would be just one of several possible choices.

Besides head trauma, a variety of other neurological conditions can cause personality change. These include multiple sclerosis, cerebrovascular accidents, brain tumors, and temporal lobe epilepsy. Other causes of behavioral change that could resemble a change in personality include delusional disorder, intermittent explosive disorder, and schizophrenia. But Eddie's personality change began abruptly after he was shot, and he has no prior history that is consistent with any of the other mental disorders mentioned (C). However, many other patients experience apparent personality change associated with mental disorders, including long-term substance use.

Eddie is far from distressed by his condition, but it does impair him both occupationally and socially. That completes the criteria (E) for this diagnosis. In his clinical picture, apathy and passivity clearly stand out as the main features, determining the specific subtype. His GAF score would be a heart-breaking 55.

| S06.330 | Open gunshot wound of cerebral cortex, without loss of consciousness |
| F07.0 | Personality change due to head trauma, apathetic type |

F60.89 Other Specified Personality Disorder

F60.9 Unspecified Personality Disorder

The discussion in DSM-5-TR suggests that patients who have some traits of certain PDs, but who don't fully meet criteria for any of them, could be listed in one of these two categories. Here's my problem with that strategy: We would be branding someone who may be much less impaired than is the typical patient with a PD. My own belief is that it is better just to note in the summary the traits we've identified and avoid making a firm diagnosis—until more data roll in.

CHAPTER 18

Paraphilic Disorders

Quick Guide to the Paraphilic Disorders

The *paraphilias* include a variety of sexual behaviors that most people reject as distasteful, unusual, or abnormal: They involve something other than genital sex with a consenting adult but are not by themselves mental diagnoses. A *paraphilic disorder* is diagnosed when a person feels distressed or is impaired by such behavior. Nearly all of them are practiced largely, perhaps exclusively, by males.

Exhibitionistic disorder. The patient has urges for genital exposure to a stranger who does not expect it (p. 583).

Frotteuristic disorder. The patient has urges related to rubbing his genitals against a person who has not consented to this (p. 588).

Voyeuristic disorder. The patient has urges related to viewing some unsuspecting person disrobing, naked, or engaging in sexual activity (p. 602).

Sexual masochism disorder. The patient has sexual urges related to being injured, bound, or humiliated (p. 594).

Sexual sadism disorder. The patient has sexual urges related to inflicting suffering or humiliation on someone else (p. 596).

Fetishistic disorder. The patient has sexual urges related to the use of inanimate objects (p. 586).

Pedophilic disorder. The patient has urges involving sexual activities with children (p. 590).

Transvestic disorder. An individual has sexual urges related to cross-dressing (p. 599).

Other specified, or unspecified, paraphilic disorder. Quite a few paraphilic disorders are not widely practiced or have received too little clinical attention to warrant codes of their own (p. 604).

Introduction

Defining Paraphilias and Paraphilic Disorders

Literally, *paraphilia* means "improper affection." Paraphilic sexual relationships differ from normal ones with respect to the preferred sexual objects or to how an individual relates to those objects. (We'll take *normal* to mean sex activity that focuses on genital stimulation with a consenting adult partner.) Paraphilic sexual activities revolve around themes of (1) inanimate objects or nonhuman animals; (2) humiliation or suffering of the patient or partner; or (3) nonconsenting persons, including children. DSM-5-TR alternatively divides paraphilias into those that involve anomalous target preferences (children, fetishes, cross-dressing) and those involving anomalous activities (exhibitionism, voyeurism, sadism, masochism, frotteurism). There are many additional paraphilias in the world; DSM-5-TR lists those that are more common and, in some cases, have a greater social impact.

We must further differentiate between a *paraphilia* and a *paraphilic disorder*. The latter is a paraphilia that causes distress to the individual or harm to other people. This distinction fosters parsimony in dispensing mental health diagnoses. For example, we don't have to attach a label of *disorder* to the behavior of a cross-dresser who is comfortable with and in no important way inconvenienced by the behavior. (In a 1991 survey of college students, over half admitted they engaged in some sort of paraphilic behavior.) In short, we identify the paraphilia by the urge, but the paraphilic disorder by the distress or impairment the urge provokes.

Mere desire or fantasy about these sexual activities can upset some people enough to warrant a diagnosis, but for most patients, action upon the desire is usual. (Indeed, DSM-5-TR carefully states that a person who claims to have no distress or disability—work/educational, social, personal, or other impairment—can still receive the diagnosis if the ideas have been repeatedly acted upon.) A person who has thoughts or fantasies about one of these sexual activities but does not act upon them or feel guilty or otherwise distressed would be considered to have the relevant paraphilia but would not be diagnosed with the corresponding paraphilic disorder.

In descending order, the most common paraphilic disorders are pedophilic, exhibitionistic, voyeuristic, and frotteuristic. Those remaining are encountered much less frequently.

Several of these behaviors involve victims who do not consent. Frotteurs, voyeurs, sadists, and exhibitionists are acutely aware of their precarious legal status and usually take pains to avoid detection or to plan their escape. Pedophiles may delude themselves that what they are doing somehow benefits the children they target ("education," perhaps, or "life experience"), but they will nonetheless caution their victims not to tell their parents—or anyone else. Patients who seek clinical help because they have run afoul of the law may not reliably describe the motivation for their activities.

Paraphilic behavior may represent a high percentage of all sexual episodes for many patients, whereas others may only indulge themselves occasionally, perhaps when under stress. Many individuals have multiple, perhaps three or four, paraphilias. They may move from one paraphilic behavior to another and may switch between classes of victim identified by gender, age, touching versus nontouching, and intrafamilial versus extrafamilial status.

Although none of the criteria specify gender, apart from pedophiles almost all patients with paraphilic disorders are male. Most fantasize sexual contact with their victims. And note that a diagnosis does not require that the person admit to experiencing pleasure or other gratification from the behavior: Evidence of the act will do.

A paraphilic disorder is hardly ever due to another medical condition. However, unusual sexual behavior may be encountered in several other mental disorders: schizophrenia, manic episodes, intellectual developmental disorder, and obsessive–compulsive disorder. In addition, personality pathology frequently accompanies paraphilic behavior.

Although none of these criteria sets specify age, most paraphilias begin during adolescence. This is also the time when people begin to discover and explore their sexuality; adolescent boys, in particular, typically experiment with a variety of sexual behaviors. However, any teenager so involved with paraphilic behavior as to meet the diagnostic criteria that appear below should also be considered a candidate for diagnosis.

It should also be noted that the boundaries of what is considered *normal* in human sexual behavior are not sharply drawn. Although pedophilia is universally condemned, even by imprisoned felons, most other paraphilias have parallel behaviors in the general population. Revealing oneself, watching, and touching constitute part of everyday sexual experience. Even coercion and pain (in moderation) figure in the sexual activities of many people whose sex lives would be considered conventional. Cross-dressing has for centuries been an important part of theater. However, I have trouble imagining a normal context for fetishism.

Specifiers for the Paraphilic Disorders

Note that, for each of the paraphilic disorders, there are two specifiers you can use to indicate that the person is no longer pursuing that behavior. Each of these specifiers is more likely to be applied to someone whose behavior can lead to legal difficulties—specifically, patients with exhibitionistic, frotteuristic, pedophilic, voyeuristic, and sometimes sexual sadism disorders.

In a controlled environment is intended for those who are currently living in places that physically prevent pursuit of their paraphilic interests. These would include prisons, hospitals, nursing homes, and other facilities locked against the unsupervised freedom to roam.

In full remission is a less restrictive term you can add to the diagnosis of a person who is not living in a controlled environment yet has had no recurrence of the behavior in question and no distress or impairment from it for at least 5 years.

F65.2 Exhibitionistic Disorder

Although no one knows just how many exhibitionists there are in the world, exhibitionism is a relatively commonplace sexual offense—second only to voyeurism. Even though some women turn up in general population surveys, people who come to clinical or legal attention are almost invariably male, and their victims are nearly always female. In most cases, the victims are unsuspecting strangers; however, a small percentage of exposures are made to people known to the exhibitionist. Men who expose themselves to children may be quite different from those who expose to adults; for example, their recidivism rate is higher.

An exhibitionist tends to follow the same pattern with each offense. He may fantasize while driving around looking for a victim (often he is careful to leave himself an escape route to use if spotted by someone other than the victim). One individual may expose himself with an erection; another may be flaccid. Some are quite aggressive, savoring the look of shock or terror they produce. An exhibitionist may masturbate when he shows himself to the woman or later when he relives the scene in his imagination. Many will fantasize having sex with their victims, but most exhibitionists don't attempt to act upon such fantasies.

Exhibitionism typically begins before the age of 18, but it may persist until 30 or later. Often the urge to exhibit comes in waves: The patient may yield daily for a week or two, then remain inactive for weeks or months. Exhibitionistic behavior most often occurs when a patient is either under stress or has free time. The use of alcohol is seldom a factor.

Many exhibitionists have spouses or partners and pursue relatively ordinary sex lives, though their interest in sex may be greater than average. The behavior has traditionally been regarded as more a nuisance than an actual danger to others, but it can coexist with other paraphilias. Perhaps 15% will have an offense involving contact, such as coercion, pedophilia, or rape. Clearly, a full assessment of paraphilic interests is indicated for any patient involved in exhibitionism.

Essential Features of **Exhibitionistic Disorder**

The person is aroused by genital self-exposure to an unwary stranger and has repeatedly acted on the urge (or feels distress/disability at the fantasy, behavior, or urge).

The Fine Print

The D's: • Duration (6+ months) • Differential diagnosis (physical and substance use disorders, psychotic, and bipolar disorders)

Coding Notes

Specify type:

Sexually aroused by exposing genitals to prepubertal children
Sexually aroused by exposing genitals to physically mature individuals
Sexually aroused by exposing genitals to prepubertal children and to physically mature individuals

Specify if:

In full remission (no symptoms for 5+ years)
In a controlled environment

Ronald Spivey

Ronald Spivey is a 39-year-old attorney who occasionally serves as judge pro tem in the municipal court of his home city. He refers himself when he becomes concerned that a woman might report him for displaying his erect penis at the swimming pool of the apartment complex where they both live.

"I thought she had been looking at me in an interested way," he says, running his fingers through his hair. "She was wearing a very skimpy bikini, and she seemed to be inviting me to reveal myself. So, I sat in such a way that she could look up the leg of my swimming trunks."

Ronald attended law school on a scholarship. He grew up in an inner-city neighborhood that included Hoofer's, a strip-tease joint not far from the Navy recruiting station. When he was in grade school, his friends and he sometimes sneaked in through a side door to watch part of the show. On a dare when he was 15, he pulled down his pants in front of two strippers who were just leaving the building. The women laughed and applauded; later, he masturbated as he fantasized that they were fondling him.

From time to time after that, through college and law school, Ronald would occasionally drive around "trolling," as he calls it—looking for a girl or young woman walking by herself in a secluded area. As he drove, he would masturbate. When he found the right combination of circumstances (a woman he fancied in a secluded location, with no one else around), he'd park his car around a corner, hop out, and confront the woman with his erection. Often, the look of surprise on her face would cause him to ejaculate.

With his marriage, which coincided with his graduation from law school, Ronald's exhibitionistic activity subsided for a time. Although sexual intercourse with his wife was fully satisfactory to both, he continued to imagine showing himself to a stranger, with whom he would then (in fantasy) have intercourse. As a practicing lawyer, he sometimes had afternoons when a continued court case left him at loose ends. Then he might go trolling again, sometimes several times in a month. Or, months might pass with no activity.

About the woman at the swimming pool, Ronald says, "I really think she wanted to." Her bikini had been very revealing, and he'd been thinking for several days about having sex with her. He contrived to sit so that she was virtually sure to glance between his thighs. When she noticed what he had intended her to see, her response was "That confirms what I've always thought about lawyers!" Since then, he has been in near panic at the thought that she might notify the state bar association.

Note that each of the criteria sets for a paraphilic disorder includes in its definition the possibility that a person could qualify for diagnosis by having fantasies about the behavior—as long as these fantasies cause distress. I can find no indication of diagnosis in anyone for any paraphilic disorder that involves fantasy alone, without some other form of activity. I suppose that, out there somewhere, there could be a bloke who is distressed by having fantasies of watching someone else have sex—but it seems unlikely in the extreme that such a person would ever come to clinical attention.

Evaluation of Ronald Spivey

Ronald's history of experiencing excitement from exhibiting himself to a nonconsenting person dates to his teenage years and has persisted for at least 2 decades (criteria A, B). If apprehended, he could lose his livelihood, if not his liberty. The fact that he continues this illegal behavior despite the possibility of dire consequences indicates the strength of his urge. (Note that whereas "trolling" behavior is typical for an exhibitionist, exposing himself to someone he might expect to meet again is not—though it's hardly unheard of.)

Ronald's assumption that the woman wanted him to "reveal" himself illustrates the cognitive distortion to which exhibitionists fall prey. It would be a pretty unusual woman who took any positive interest in a relative stranger who flashed her at a public swimming pool.

Although it is possible that another mental disorder could present together with exhibitionistic disorder, it is unlikely that either schizophrenia or bipolar I disorder would have been present for over 20 years without detection and thus account for the behavior. Of course, intellectual developmental disorder would have prevented Ronald from entering, much less completing, law school. The clinician should take pains to fully evaluate Ronald for additional paraphilic disorders, as well as for substance use, mood, and anxiety disorders. I'd also make a note to self: "Search for personality traits at next interview."

Ronald's exclusive interest in adult women would dictate the specifier; he is not currently in remission, so his complete diagnosis (GAF score of 65) would be as follows:

F65.2   Exhibitionistic disorder, sexually aroused by exposing genitals to physically mature women

F65.0 Fetishistic Disorder

In its original sense (it is derived from Portuguese), a *fetish* was an idol or charm that had magical significance. In the context of sexual activity, it refers to something that excites an individual's sexual fantasies or desires. Such objects can include underwear, shoes, stockings, and other inanimate objects. Bras and panties are probably the most common objects used as fetishes.

The DSM-5-TR definition of fetishistic disorder also includes body parts that aren't integral to the reproductive process. A sexual attraction to feet would be an example of *partialism,* which sometimes occurs along with other fetishes. (There are reports of men who are attracted to women missing body parts, such as a one-legged woman—a sort of fetishistic *jamais vu.*) Cross-dressing that is sexually exciting, as in transvestic disorder, and arousal achieved via objects designed for use during sex, such as dildos or vibrators, are excluded from the definition of fetishistic disorder.

Some people amass collections of their preferred fetishes; some resort to stealing from stores or clotheslines to obtain them. They may smell, rub, or handle these objects while masturbating, or they may ask sex partners to wear them. Without a fetish, such a person may be unable to get an erection.

Fetishism typically begins in adolescence, though many patients report similar interests even in childhood. Some women may show a degree of fetishistic behavior, but nearly everyone with a fetishistic disorder is a male. It tends to be a chronic condition, to the extent that for some people, a fetish may eventually crowd out more traditional love objects.

Essential Features of **Fetishistic Disorder**

The person is aroused by inanimate objects (such as shoes or underwear) or body parts other than genitals (such as feet) and feels distress/disability at the behavior or at the fantasy, idea, or urge).

The Fine Print

The D's: • Duration (6+ months) • Differential diagnosis (transvestic disorder; vibrators and the like)

Coding Notes

Specify type:

> **Body parts**
> **Nonliving objects**
> **Other** (perhaps combinations of the first two types)

Specify if:

> **In full remission** (no symptoms for 5+ years)
> **In a controlled environment**

Corky Brauner

When he was 13, Corky Brauner encountered a pair of his older sister's panties that his mother had accidentally folded into his own underwear. They were embroidered with flowers and the word "Saturday," and he found them peculiarly exciting. He slept with them under his pillow for a couple of nights and masturbated with them twice before sneaking them back into his sister's bureau drawer Friday evening. From time to time throughout the balance of his adolescence, when he was alone in the house, Corky would appropriate items of his sister's underwear.

In college Corky lived alone, so he was able to collect and keep a small wardrobe of lingerie without concern of discovery. Although he had several bras and slips, he liked panties best. By his final year of college, he owned several dozen. Some of these he had purchased, but he preferred those he could persuade a woman to leave behind after a date. He had even stolen one or two pairs from backyard clotheslines, but that was dangerous, and he didn't do it often.

Sometimes, when Corky isn't entertaining company, he will take some panties out of the drawer and play with them. He will sniff them, rub them on his face, and masturbate with them. During these activities, he pretends he is making love to the original owner of the panties. If he doesn't know her, he fantasizes how she might look.

Corky is driven into treatment by the laughter of his most recent girlfriend when he finds that he has to put her underwear under his pillow in order to get an erection when they are making love.

"I've gotten totally fixated on panties," he says during his intake interview. "I seem to prefer them to women."

Evaluation of Corky Brauner

Corky's fascination with panties has persisted for years—far longer than the 6-month requirement (criterion A). Over the years, he has assembled quite a collection, obtained from a variety of sources. Corky's distress (B) stems not from his own perception of his behavior, but from the fact that a girlfriend ridiculed him for it. In this way, he learns that he prefers panties to people—a not infrequent progression for fetishists.

The differential diagnosis of fetishistic disorder includes transvestic disorder, in which men (almost always men) are stimulated by wearing and viewing themselves in women's clothing. Fetishists may put on clothing of the opposite sex, but wearing it is incidental to the sexual gratification they derive from the clothing itself, and they don't fantasize about their own attractiveness when so attired. Corky shows no interest in cross-dressing (C).

Many fetishists have also been involved in rape, exhibitionism, frotteurism, pedophilia, or voyeurism, but none of these behaviors are mentioned in Corky's history (his clinician should ask). Pending the outcome of such an inquiry, Corky's full diagnosis (with a GAF score of 61) will be as follows:

F65.0   Fetishistic disorder, nonliving objects (panties)

F65.81 Frotteuristic Disorder

Frottage (the term derives from the French word *frotter,* meaning "to rub") typically takes place on crowded sidewalks or public transportation. (Ready means of escape is ever a concern for the frotteur.) The perpetrator (invariably a man) selects a victim (usually a woman) who is accessible and whose allure may be enhanced by tight clothing. The frotteur rubs his genitals against her thighs or buttocks, or he may fondle her breasts or genitalia. The process is efficient; on subways, ejaculation usually occurs within the transit time between stops.

The victim typically does not make an immediate outcry, perhaps because she hopes she is mistaken about what appears to be happening. Note that it is the act of touching or rubbing, not the coercion, that is exciting to the frotteur. However, over half have a history of involvement in other paraphilias, especially exhibitionism and voyeurism. A frotteur often fantasizes about an ongoing intimate relationship with the victim.

This condition typically begins in adolescence and is sometimes initiated by observing others engaged in frottage. Most acts occur when the frotteur is between the ages of 15 and 25; frequency gradually declines thereafter. No one appears to know how common this condition is; it may be underreported.

Essential Features of **Frotteuristic Disorder**

Aroused by rubbing against or feeling someone who hasn't consented, the person has repeatedly acted on the urge (or feels distress/disability at the fantasy, behavior, or urge).

The Fine Print

The D's: • Duration (6+ months) • Differential diagnosis (substance use disorders, schizophrenia, manic episode, intellectual developmental disorder, conduct disorder and antisocial personality disorder)

Coding Notes

Specify if:

> **In full remission** (no symptoms for 5+ years)
> **In a controlled environment**

Henry McWilliams

Henry McWilliams was born in London where, dressed in his short pants, white shirt, and school tie, he rode the Underground every day to his exclusive school. One day when he was 9, he saw a man rubbing up against a woman.

Henry was small when he was 9, and even in the crowded subway car he had an excellent eye-level view. The woman (she was an adult, though Henry had no idea how old) was a bit overweight and dressed in a tight-fitting miniskirt. She was facing away from the man, who allowed the weight of the crowd surging through the doors to press him up against her. The man tugged at his crotch, and then, as the train began to move, rubbed himself against her.

"I never saw her face, but I could tell she didn't like it," Henry says. "She tried to push him away, she tried to move, but there was no place for either of them to go. Then the train stopped, and he ran out the door."

When he was 15, Henry and his parents moved to the United States. Now 24, he has referred himself for treatment with this story.

Since his graduation from high school, he has worked as a messenger for a large legal firm. In his official capacity, many days he spends several hours on the subway. In 5 years, he estimates that he has rubbed against 200 women. Now he is seeking help at the insistence of one of the law firm's partners, who the week before happened to ride the same train and had seen him in action.

When Henry is in need, he will go into the men's room and put on a condom so as not to stain his trousers. Then he will roam up and down the outskirts of a crowd on a subway platform until he spots a woman who interests him. This would be someone who is youngish but not young ("They're less likely to scream"), and buxom enough to stretch tight the material of her skirt or slacks. He especially likes it if the material is leather. He will board after she does, and if she doesn't turn around, will rub his erect penis up and down against her buttocks as the train began to roll.

Henry is very sensitive, so it doesn't take much pressure. Sometimes the woman seems not to realize what's happening, or maybe she doesn't want to acknowledge it— even to herself. He usually climaxes within a minute. Then at the next stop he will bolt through the door. If interrupted prior to climax, he may hang around the platform until he locates another woman in another crowd.

"It helps if I imagine that we're married or engaged," he explains. "I'll pretend that she's wearing my ring, and I've come home for a quickie."

Evaluation of Henry McWilliams

Henry's method of operation is typical for frotteurs, most of whom tend to follow the same pattern each time. He has offended on many occasions (criteria A, B), often with romantic fantasies. Henry is not especially upset about his own behavior; he comes for treatment because his employer demands it.

Although patients with schizophrenia or intellectual developmental disorder will sometimes engage in sexual behavior that is inappropriate to the context, Henry bears no evidence of either condition. With a GAF score of 70, his diagnosis would simply be this:

F65.81   Frotteuristic disorder

F65.4 Pedophilic Disorder

Pedophilia is Greek meaning "love of children." In the context of a paraphilia, of course, it means sex with children. Pedophilic disorder is far and away the most common of the paraphilic disorders that involve actual physical contact. Estimates vary, but by the age of 18, up to 20% of American children have in some way been interfered with sexually. Most perpetrators are not strangers but are relatives, friends, or neighbors. The vast majority of pedophiles are men, but women may account for up to 12% of offenders (though some of these involve allowing children to be abused, rather than instigating the act).

The specific act preferred varies with the offender. Some pedophiles seek only to view (child pornography or actual children); others want to touch or undress a child. But most acts involve oral sex or touching of the child's genitals—or of the perpetrator's genitals by the child. In cases other than incest, most pedophiles don't require actual penetration. Those who do, however, may use force to achieve it.

Though some pedophiles do not start offending until midlife, this behavior typically begins in the later teen years. (The definition of pedophilic disorder specifically excludes perpetrators who are adolescents themselves or who aren't at least 5 years older than the victim.) It may be more common among persons who were themselves abused as children. Once pedophilia has begun, it tends to be chronic. Up to 50% use alcohol as a prelude to contact with children. Half or more have other paraphilias.

Many pedophiles limit themselves to children (this type of pedophilia is called *exclusive*); they often further confine themselves to children of a particular sex and age range. However, the majority are also attracted to adults; their pedophilia is called *nonexclusive*. Like other paraphilic individuals, pedophiles may develop a degree of cognitive distortion about their activities: They persuade themselves that children enjoy the sexual experience or that it is important for their development. Most pedophiles do not force their attentions on children, but depend on friendship, persuasion, and guile. A number of studies suggest that children who are lonely or otherwise uncared for may be especially susceptible to the advances of a pedophile.

Overall, perhaps 15–25% of those convicted reoffend within a few years of their release from custody. Alcohol use and trouble forming intimate relationships with adults increase the chances of recidivism. Men who prefer boys are about twice as likely to reoffend as are those who prefer girls.

Some pedophiles limit their attentions to daughters, stepdaughters, or other victims related to them. Then the specifier *limited to incest* can be used, though it isn't clear to me what benefit its use confers. Some perpetrators of incest may be pedophiles, but many men (most incestuous adults are male) only become interested in daughters or stepdaughters who have reached puberty.

Collateral information is especially important in evaluating pedophiles, who have strong reasons to lie about their behavior. And often there's little motivation to tell the truth:

Sentences are long, convicted pedophiles may face a harsh reception in prison, and the prospect of suppressing sex interest with drugs is unappealing to many.

One aspect of the criteria that can be confusing is the required 5-year age difference between perpetrator and victim. As the coding notes indicate, a 15-year-old having a sexual relationship with someone of any age would not be diagnosed as having pedophilic disorder. Someone who is 20 having an affair with a 14- or 15-year-old, however, would.

And that raises another difficult issue. According to DSM-5-TR criteria, the child involved must be prepubescent. If we interpret this strictly, we won't be making the diagnosis in someone whose victim has begun to develop sexually. This has caused a lot of heartburn for clinicians who worry about depathologizing men who prefer children 13 and under who are not prepubertal.

Essential Features of **Pedophilic Disorder**

The person is aroused by the notion of sex with prepubescent children and has acted on the urge (or feels severely distressed or has interpersonal difficulties at the idea or at the fantasies or urges).

The Fine Print

The D's: • Duration (6+ months) • Demographic carve-outs (the patient must be at least 16 years old and at least 5 years older than the victim; do not use this diagnosis for a late adolescent having a relationship with a 12- or 13-year-old) • Differential diagnosis (physical and substance use disorders, psychotic and bipolar disorders, intellectual developmental disorder, criminal abuse of children for profit)

Coding Notes

Specify:

Exclusive type (aroused solely by children)
Nonexclusive type

Specify if:

Sexually attracted to males
Sexually attracted to females
Sexually attracted to both

Specify if:

Limited to incest

There's a bit of an issue here: The criteria for pedophilic disorder are the only ones in this DSM-5-TR chapter that do not expressly allow the specifier *in a controlled environment*. Of course, it also is the only one that doesn't allow *in full remission,* but that is at least logical: Pedophilia has been long established as a lifelong condition. However, who is more likely to do hard time than a pedophile? And just how likely is that person to reoffend while inside? Were I to evaluate such a person again, I'd go right ahead and use the *in a controlled environment* specifier.

Raymond Boggs

At age 58, Raymond Boggs seems an unlikely convict. His orange prison jumpsuit stretches tightly across his pear-shaped body; in contrast to the swagger of younger inmates, he shuffles, head down, along the corridor to the interview room.

Raymond became interested in sex when he was very young. One of his earliest memories was of sex play with a teenage girl who was babysitting him and his infant sister. As an adult, the sight of little girls' bodies particularly fascinates him. He remembers watching his sister having her bath when he was 7 or 8, hanging around until his mother had to shoo him from the bathroom. When they were teenagers, he had watched outside his sister's window at night, trying to get a glimpse of her as she undressed for bed. When she entered puberty, his evening vigils stopped. "It was the body hair. It seemed so coarse and disgusting. That was when I discovered that I only really like girls who are, um, smooth."

Despite these tastes, in his mid-20s Raymond married the daughter of the foreman in the print shop where he worked. During the early years of their marriage, the couple maintained an active sex life. Usually, he would try to fantasize that he was having sex with a young girl. Once he persuaded his wife to shave off all her pubic hair, but she complained that it itched as it grew back and refused to do it again. They had three children, all sons, which in retrospect seemed a minor miracle: Little boys don't tempt him at all.

As the years passed, Raymond acquired a small stack of pornographic magazines that featured children, which he kept hidden under a pile of rags in his tool shed. When his sexual tension became too high, he would masturbate while he imagined himself frolicking with the naked children in the pictures.

By his early 50s, Raymond's life had taken a turn for the worse. His sons had all left home, and a series of pelvic operations caused his wife to reject his sexual advances, sometimes for months at a time. To fill his time, he took up photography. Especially over the long summer months, he found ready subjects in the neighborhood children he befriended. Some of the little girls he could persuade to pose partly or completely disrobed.

He preferred those who are 5 or 6 years old, but on occasion he would photograph a girl as old as 8. (Older children are more independent, harder to persuade.) These sessions occurred principally in a secluded spot behind his tool shed. He used candy and quarters as bait, afterward reminding each child that her parents wouldn't like it if she told.

"I'm not proud of it," he says as he tries to ease the bulging waistband of his prison jumpsuit. "It's just something I couldn't resist. The feeling I'd get when she'd slip down her panties—it was anxiety and ecstasy and butterflies in my stomach. Maybe the way you'd feel if you won the lottery. But I never touched one; all I did was look. And I never thought it might hurt them any."

Raymond had been looking and taking pictures for the better part of 10 years when discovered by a 12-year-old boy who had ventured behind the tool shed to collect native plant specimens for a science exhibit. The boy told his father, who called the girl's mother, who dialed the police. The trial—a 3-week media feeding frenzy—featured the corroborative testimony of no fewer than seven neighborhood girls, now in varying stages of adolescence, who had at one time or another been victimized by Raymond Boggs.

Sentenced to 5–10 years in the penitentiary, Raymond still faces millions of dollars in civil lawsuits. The day after his arrest, his wife filed for divorce and entered therapy, one of his sons broke off contact with him, and another moved out of state.

Evaluation of Raymond Boggs

When the facts of the case are clear, there is little to dispute the diagnosis of pedophilic disorder. Someone with substance intoxication may perpetrate an isolated incident of fondling a child, but then it is usually evident that this is not a frequent sexual outlet. As a result of their overall defective judgment, patients with intellectual developmental disorder or schizophrenia may sometimes fall into this mode of sexual release. Parents (notoriously celebrities) are sometimes accused of child molestation as a part of a messy divorce; frequently the facts do not bear out these allegations. In the case of Raymond Boggs, the legal facts are indisputable. He freely admits to his long-standing interests and behavior (criteria A, B). Of course, his age relative to those of his victims is not in dispute (C). He insists that the acts were never tactile, only visual, which is true of many such pedophiles.

Those with exhibitionistic disorder may show themselves to children, but they don't approach the victims for further sexual activity. Some pedophiles may also have sexual sadism disorder; if so, both diagnoses should be made.

We are asked to choose several specifiers to help pinpoint the patient's pathology. Raymond was sexually attracted only to females, very young ones at that. His GAF score would be about 55. Even though the criteria for pedophilic disorder don't offer the specifier in a controlled environment, I've sneaked in a mention anyway.

F65.4	Pedophilic disorder, nonexclusive type, sexually attracted to females, in a controlled environment
Z65.1	Imprisonment

F65.51 Sexual Masochism Disorder

Many people—perhaps 15% of the general population—derive sexual pleasure from some degree of suffering. However, these behaviors/ideas by themselves are usually benign, and are certainly insufficient for the diagnosis of a disorder. Indeed, most people who engage in masochistic behavior function well, both socially and psychologically. Some women even admit that they like being spanked during sex or that they fantasize about being forced to have sex. Sexual masochism is thus the only paraphilia in which any appreciable number of women appear to participate.

Sexual masochism *disorder* (SMD), however, comprises three principal features: pain, humiliation, and absence of control. This paraphilic disorder typically begins in childhood. The behaviors involved include bondage, blindfolding, spanking, cutting, and humiliation (by defecation, urination, or forcing the submissive partner to imitate an animal). Some form of physical abuse is probably used most often. As time goes on, patients with SMD may require increasing degrees of torture to experience the same degree of sexual satisfaction; in this sense, SMD resembles an addiction.

By choking, pricking, or shocking, some masochists inflict pain upon themselves. Perhaps 30% of them at times also participate in sadistic behavior. A few pursue an especially dangerous behavior called *asphyxiophilia* (or *hypoxyphilia*), in which they induce near-suffocation by means of a noose around the neck, an airtight bag over the head, or the inhalation of amyl nitrite ("poppers"). These people report that the sensation of restricted breathing promotes an especially intense sexual high. Each year, 1 or 2 accidental deaths per million general population occur from these practices.

Although masochists derive sexual gratification from pain or degradation, they do not necessarily surrender complete control. Many sadomasochistic relationships are carefully planned; the partners may agree upon a code word by which the masochist can indicate that it really is time to stop.

Essential Features of Sexual Masochism Disorder

The person is repeatedly sexually aroused by being struck, restrained, humiliated, or in other ways made to suffer and feels distress/disability at these behaviors, fantasies, or urges.

The Fine Print

The D's: • Duration (6+ months) • Differential diagnosis (physical and substance use disorders, spiritual flagellation and other painful rituals)

Coding Notes

Specify if:

   With asphyxiophilia if restricted breathing is involved.

> Specify if:
>
> **In full remission** (no symptoms for 5+ years)
> **In a controlled environment**

Martin Allingham

Martin Allingham comes to medical attention the night he nearly dies. In the apartment he shares with Samuel Brock, the two had devised an elaborate contraption of pulleys, ropes, collars, and shackles that can turn Martin upside down and partly strangle him while Sam applies the whip.

"I get the most beautiful orgasm when I'm about to pass out," Martin reports, much later.

Sam and Martin had been in school together. Sam was a jock; Martin was the class wimp. How perfectly they suited one another they realized one Saturday afternoon when they were 15. The two had argued on the deserted playground, and Sam began sitting on Martin, twisting his fingers into pretzels. Although Martin cried, the growing urgency of his erection was evident as the pain increased. After they parted, Martin had masturbated while recalling the sensation of abject submission.

Without discussing it much, by common consent Sam and Martin met again 2 weeks later. When they were 19, they moved in together, and they have been living together ever since. Now they are 28.

Martin doesn't have to be hurt to enjoy sex, but it greatly enhances the pleasure. He has tried spanking and bondage, but asphyxia is the best. When he was younger, he had played the field and tried other partners. But most of them had hurt him either too much or not quite enough; besides, he and Sam are both afraid of AIDS. For the last several years, they have worked at the same department store and have been faithful to one other.

The night of the accident, Martin got himself into the harness while Sam was at work. He apparently cinched the noose a shade too tight and lost consciousness—though he doesn't remember that. When Sam found Martin, he had no pulse and wasn't breathing. In the Boy Scouts, Sam had learned CPR, which he employed vigorously after calling 911.

A police report was made, and a pair of officers interviewed them both. "We're perfectly suited," Sam explains. "I like to do it; he likes it done." He admits that their sex life had recently become increasingly violent, even death-defying. But that wasn't his idea; it is Martin who needs more to produce the same effects. Sam admits that he "gets off" on pain, but some pain seems to serve about as well as a lot.

"I'd never want to really harm him," he says. "I love him."

Evaluation of Martin Allingham

Martin's sexual behavior includes elements of pain inflicted upon himself (criterion A). Bondage is one of these elements, as well as the practice of asphyxiophilia, with which

Martin enhances his own sexual pleasure. Martin has acted on these urges for years; the impairment it recently caused was nearly terminal (B). He easily fulfills the criteria for SMD.

Note that some sex workers accept pain within limits, because the pay is better than for standard sex. Such individuals should not be diagnosed as having SMD unless they also both derive pleasure from the practice and are distressed or impaired by it.

Masochists will sometimes cross-dress in response to the demands of a sadistic partner. If the act of wearing clothing of the opposite gender also produces sexual excitement (and not just the humiliation of cross-dressing), then transvestic disorder should also be diagnosed. The vignette is silent on the issue, but Martin's clinician should thoroughly explore the possibility of a personality disorder—common among patients with SMD—which could significantly affect therapy. Mention it in the summary. Because his sexual arousal is augmented by the sensation of restricted breathing, Martin's diagnosis (I'd peg his current GAF score at 25) will be as follows:

F65.51   Sexual masochism disorder, with asphyxiophilia

F65.52 Sexual Sadism Disorder

Much of the behavior of sadists complements that of masochists; the difference is that sadists are the perpetrators rather than the recipients. Inflicting pain or humiliation stimulates them sexually. In fact, the suffering of others arouses them sexually, and they fantasize about dominance and restraint. Some women admit to engaging in this sort of activity.

Although early childhood experiences with punishment may prefigure this chronic condition for some, overt behavior typically begins with fantasies during the individual's teen years. The physical methods ultimately employed include bondage, blindfolding, spanking, cutting, and humiliation. Like those with sexual masochism, individuals with sexual sadism may with time need to increase the severity of the torture to produce the same degree of sexual satisfaction.

Most people who engage in sadistic behavior limit themselves to a few partners, most of whom are willing; by definition, these people don't meet DSM-5-TR criteria for sexual sadism disorder unless they are distressed or impaired by their urges. Fewer than 10% of sadists commit rape, but those who do can be even more brutal than other rapists, using more force and inflicting greater pain than is necessary to achieve penetration.

We don't know the frequency of sexual sadism disorder in the general population. In a study of 240 hospitalized sexual offenders, 52 (21%) could be given this diagnosis. Of these, only 16 had been correctly diagnosed before the study.

Essential Features of **Sexual Sadism Disorder**

Another person's suffering, either physical or psychological, provokes sexually arousing fantasies or behaviors that cause the patient to experience distress or impairment or to act upon these sexual urges with someone who hasn't consented.

The Fine Print

The D's: • Duration (6+ months) • Distress or disability (can be work/educational, social, or personal impairment) • Differential diagnosis (physical and substance use disorders, conduct disorder and antisocial personality disorder, personality disorders, nonsadistic rape)

Coding Notes

Specify if:

> **In full remission** (no symptoms for 5+ years)
> **In a controlled environment**

Donatien Alphonse François, the Marquis de Sade

If ever one person has been ineluctably associated with a mental disorder, that would be the Frenchman Donatien Alphonse François, the Marquis de Sade—the patron saint (and etymological père) of sadism. It is both interesting and instructive to explore the degree to which the personal history of this man, who flourished over 2 centuries ago, reflects the condition that bears his name.

Sade (as his biographers call him) was born into a family that was poor but socially prominent, which may help explain his development into a proud, arrogant autocrat. An absent father left the nurturing during his formative years to his libertine uncle.

When he was only 16, Sade entered the army and served with distinction in combat. Forced by his family into a loveless (on his part) marriage, soon after the wedding he demonstrated that his sexual interests could be problematic.

As a child he yearned for his mother's embrace; as an adult he sought solace in the arms of prostitutes. Several of those he hired filed formal complaints that he had tried to whip them; one also claimed he had made her ill by spiking her bourbon with the notorious (and overhyped) aphrodisiac, Spanish fly. He asked many of the prostitutes he frequented to whip *him*—reportedly not so unusual a request among 18th-century Frenchmen, who were known sometimes to address impotence by employing the lash. In prison, he later used huge rectal dildos (which he required his wife, Renée, to procure for him) to gain sexual satisfaction.

What assured his ultimate downfall was neither his passion nor his penury, but the antipathy of his mother-in-law. *Cette dame formidable* reacted to his libertine tendencies by persuading the King to issue a private bill of attainder, then popular among French petitioners. It allowed the authorities to toss Sade into prison and hold him without trial, without end.

In confinement—he spent nearly 29 years either in prison or in the asylum at Charenton and came within a day of execution during the Terror of the French Revolution—he wrote some of the most sexually explicit and violent prose ever composed in any language. His novel *Justine* relates the sexual torture of a young woman at the hands of various men, beginning when she was 12 years old. *The 120 Days of Sodom,* written down in little more than a month while he languished in the Bastille, is a nauseating (pardon my editorial queasy stomach) crescendo of sexual horror that culminates in murder. It is on his writings, rather than his own sexual proclivities, that his reputation rests.

That reputation notwithstanding, Sade's character, at least at this remove, remains to a degree confusing. On the one hand, some regard him as an angry loner with a quick and violent temper who had no true friends. Others describe him as a lifelong charmer who could easily manipulate people, sometimes with threats of suicide.

He was later to develop frequent ideas of persecution that involved Renée. He scrutinized her letters for hidden signals, which he thought contained references to his release date. Yet, during one of his infrequent releases from prison, when he could have exacted revenge on his in-laws, he didn't. His reward was another arrest and, ultimately, incarceration for the rest of his life.

Evaluation of Donatien Alphonse François, the Marquis de Sade

From his own writings and from the work of others, Sade was intensely interested in sexual pleasure derived from inflicting pain and humiliation on other people (criterion A). Although he does not appear to have suffered distress from these desires, he acted upon them repeatedly with nonconsenting individuals when he was quite a young man (B). That qualifies him, even by today's robust standards, for the diagnosis of sexual sadism disorder. (We cannot doubt that the characters described in Sade's *The 120 Days of Sodom* would more than fully qualify for this diagnosis.)

Yet, when we consider the entirety of his life, Sade even better fulfills the definition of sexual masochism disorder: He was much given to receiving the pain of whippings, which contributed to his prolonged incarceration. Yet the power of tradition is such that his name remains firmly attached to behavior that he appears to have pursued personally during a relatively brief chapter in his career.

What other diagnosis might be appropriate? Of course, for anyone with his inclinations we would consider a personality disorder, but it would be in addition to, not instead of, the paraphilic disorder diagnosis. Mention of it belongs in a summary. With only the information given above, the Marquis de Sade's diagnoses (in order of appearance) would read as given below. And I'd give him a GAF score of 71.

F65.51	Sexual masochism disorder
F65.52	Sexual sadism disorder
F52.32	Delayed ejaculation

Leopold von Sacher-Masoch was a 19th-century Austrian writer who enslaved himself to his mistress for 6 months, on the condition that she would wear fur as often as she could and treat him as her servant. He subsequently wrote about the experience in a novel, *Venus in Furs*. This led to the adaptation of his name (along with Sade's) for their respective paraphilias in the 1886 textbook *Psychopathia Sexualis* by Richard von Krafft-Ebing, whose own name, sadly, has not been attached to anything.

Sade and Sacher-Masoch are among the diminishing ranks of individuals whose names are retained as eponyms in DSM-5-TR, and they are the only ones we use as adjectives—as is also the case with the terms *Freudian* and *Jungian*. Disorders using other personal names, such as Münchausen's syndrome, have been rebranded with terms that are more descriptive, though far less colorful.

F65.1 Transvestic Disorder

People with transvestic disorder cross-dress to achieve sexual excitement; they experience frustration when this behavior is thwarted. There is much variability in the amount of cross-dressing. Some will do it occasionally, while alone; others frequently sally forth in public, fully groomed and gowned. Some limit it to underwear; others get completely togged out. Some men (once again, males vastly predominate) spend up to several hours a week donning and wearing women's clothing. Many will masturbate or have intercourse when they cross-dress. They may fantasize about themselves as girls and keep a collection of female clothing, often wearing it under their usual male attire. But only a person who is distressed or impaired in some important way by the pursuit of these behaviors earns the diagnosis of transvestic disorder; those who embrace their own behavior are merely cross-dressers.

Transvestic disorder usually begins during adolescence, or even in childhood. However, most males with transvestic disorder were not effeminate as boys; under 20% of them are gay as adults. As happens with some other paraphilias, the behavior associated with transvestic disorder may gradually replace more traditional modes of sexual gratification. Through videos, magazines, or personal interaction, there may be considerable involvement in the cross-dressing subculture. A small number gradually come to feel increasingly comfortable with their cross-dressing and progress to gender dysphoria, which may provide the final stimulus for them to seek treatment. With age, the sexual excitement attached to cross-dressing may give way to a general sense of well-being.

Some patients have been previously involved in voyeuristic, exhibitionistic, or masochistic behaviors. You can add specifiers for those who are sexually aroused by clothing (*with fetishism*) or by thoughts of themselves as female (*with autogynephilia*). (Too few females with transvestic disorder are reported to justify a parallel, male-denominated term.) In the general male population, the prevalence of cross-dressing to achieve sexual stimulation appears to be just under 3%, though only half of these might qualify for a diagnosis of transvestic disorder.

Essential Features of **Transvestic Disorder**

Arousal by cross-dressing (thoughts, behaviors, or urges) has repeatedly caused the person to feel distressed or to experience work/educational, social, or personal impairment.

The Fine Print

The D's: • Duration (6+ months) • Differential diagnosis (fetishistic disorder, gender dysphoria)

Coding Notes

Specify if:

> **With fetishism** (sexual arousal by clothing or fabrics)
> **With autogynephilia** (sexual arousal by self-visualization as female)

Specify if:

> **In full remission** (no symptoms for 5+ years)
> **In a controlled environment**

Paul Castro

When Paul Castro was 7, his parents employed a teenage neighbor to babysit. Julie was precocious and imaginative; she would persuade Paul to play dress-up in her clothing, which she removed for the occasion. At first Paul only tolerated this, but later he became excited at the sensation of her silky panties as he drew them over his skinny thighs.

When Julie acquired a steady boyfriend and lost interest in Paul, he would sometimes covertly borrow a bra and panties from his mother to dress in. By his late teens, he had collected a small wardrobe of women's underwear, which he would put on as often as once or twice a week. Standing in front of a mirror wearing a bra, its cups attractively padded, he might fantasize himself being embraced—sometimes by a man, sometimes a woman. A time or two he tried on lipstick and an old dress his mother hardly ever wore. But he thought those made him look silly and conspicuous, and he thereafter limited himself to lingerie. However, being male never caused him any doubt or dissatisfaction.

After a year of junior college, Paul got a job as a clerk in a bookstore and moved into his own apartment. Some days he would wear his panties and bra (minus the padding) to work under his sport shirt and slacks. Then, during lunch hour, he might masturbate in the men's room as he imagined himself making love to a beautiful woman, both of them dressed in their silk underwear. If he was otherwise occupied during lunch, throughout the afternoon he would enjoy the delicious sensation of silk next to his skin and the anticipation of release while looking at himself in the mirror that evening.

Paul is thus attired one morning when the paramedics pick him up after a passing bus clips him on his way to work. He awakens to find his right upper arm in a splint, and passersby agog over his size 40C Maidenform bra. His shame over this episode causes him to rethink his behavior and seek treatment.

Evaluation of Paul Castro

Western society encourages some cross-dressing and even considers it normal. Transgender impersonation has had a long and honorable history on the stage and in film; Halloween apparel also comes to mind.

In sexual masochistic disorder, patients may be forced to cross-dress to excite a sadistic lover; if they do not also experience sexual excitement, transvestic disorder would not be diagnosed. Patients with gender dysphoria often dress in clothing appropriate to the opposite sex, but without sexual stimulation. When gay people cross-dress, it is sometimes done to enhance their appeal to other gay individuals; often, however, it is done to be campy or to make fun of society. In any event, something other than sexual stimulation is the goal and transvestic disorder does not apply.

Obviously, Paul's behavior fits none of these alternative explanations. In fact, other than his interest in lingerie, he has conventional heterosexual interests (judged by his fantasies when masturbating; criterion A). He therefore does not earn the specifier *with autogynephilia*. He appears to be aroused by the feel of silk, so we can justify the *with fetishism* specifier. His ultimate distress (GAF score of 71) when he was picked up by the paramedics fulfills criterion B.

F65.1	Transvestic disorder, with fetishism
S42.009	Fractured clavicle

Women can now be diagnosed as having transvestic disorder, which was not the case prior to DSM-5. The change is egalitarian in the extreme: The only study reporting any women seeking sexual stimulation from cross-dressing found just 5 of 1,171 (0.4%), and we don't know whether those few had been distressed or impaired by their behavior. In practical terms, this club remains "for men only."

F65.3 Voyeuristic Disorder

A person with voyeuristic disorder is aroused by watching people engaged in private activities. Of course, many people who do not have a paraphilia also enjoy such viewing—those who patronize pornographic films and websites, for example. The difference consists in the gratification such a patient derives from viewing ordinary people who do not realize they are being watched and would probably not permit it if they did.

In a 2006 Swedish survey, 12% of men (and 4% of women) admitted to at least one incident of voyeuristic behavior. By current standards, most of these individuals would not be diagnosed with a paraphilic disorder. Other surveys find that many people of both sexes would watch others undressing or having sex if they felt they wouldn't be caught. As with other paraphilic disorders, DSM-5-TR requires that the behavior be acted upon repeatedly or cause the individual distress or impairment. The bottom line: Voyeurism is the most commonly reported sexual crime, and nearly all practitioners are men.

Voyeurism typically begins when individuals are in their teens—almost always by age 15. However, it cannot be diagnosed until at least age 18, to set it off from the typical sexual curiosity of adolescents. Once voyeuristic disorder develops, it tends to be chronic. The victims of these "peeping Toms" are almost always strangers. People with voyeuristic disorder will usually masturbate while they are watching. Afterward, they may fantasize about having sex with a victim, though contact with that victim is rarely sought. Some patients prefer this method of sexual gratification, but most also have otherwise unremarkable sex lives. As with exhibitionistic disorder, these patients take precautions to avoid detection.

Essential Features of **Voyeuristic Disorder**

Aroused by watching an unwary person who is undressing or having sex, the person has repeatedly acted on the urge (or feels distress/disability at the fantasy, behavior, or urge).

The Fine Print

The D's: • Duration and demographics (6+ months, age 18+) • Differential diagnosis (conduct disorder and antisocial personality disorder, substance use disorders, traditional sexual interests)

Coding Notes

Specify if:

> **In full remission** (no symptoms, no distress or impairment for 5+ years)
> **In a controlled environment**

Rex Collingwood

The referral came at the request of a Superior Court judge who had been displeased to find Rex Collingwood brought before the bench for his second appearance in less than a year. This time, at age 23, Rex had been caught literally with his pants down, masturbating outside the master bedroom window of a house on a quiet suburban street. He had been so fascinated by the aspect of the woman inside removing her underwear that he failed to notice the approach of her husband, who was walking the dog.

When Rex was growing up in the Midwest, his family had lived near the campus of a small college. He made friends with the caretaker at the student union—a gangly philosophy major named Rollo who, in exchange for minor custodial work, lived rent-free in a room on the second floor. When Rex was 14, Rollo showed him the tiny hole he had discovered in the floorboards immediately above the women's toilet. Intermittently for some weeks, Rex and Rollo squatted in the dark above the peephole, waiting for women to enter. Because they were looking straight down, they couldn't see much, but the images provided plenty of fodder for Rex's fantasy life.

When he graduated from high school, Rex went to work in an auto body shop. The bookkeeper, Darlene, was a year or two older than he, and soon they began living together. Rex and Darlene made love four or five times a week; each expressed satisfaction with the arrangement. Rex sometimes wondered whether he was "oversexed" because he still occasionally had the urge to "go looking." He had tried X-rated videos, but it wasn't the same—those people knew they were being watched, and they were also being paid.

So, every 2 or 3 months Rex would spend a couple of evenings driving on dark, quiet streets, seeking the right venue. Catching a glimpse of naked flesh was titillating, but watching a woman undressing added the delicious suspense of not knowing how much would be revealed. Whatever he saw, Rex would add to the stock of images to conjure up when he made love with Darlene.

Best of all was watching people have sex. He had memorized the locations of several such encounters, and he returned to them again and again when the urge struck. Summertime was best, for then people were less likely to burrow under the covers. He had once or twice stood in the bushes for as long as 2 hours, watching while his targets worked up their passions and his. That was what had drawn him back to the house where he was apprehended—less than four blocks from where he'd been arrested a year before.

"I suppose I should feel ashamed," Rex tells the interviewer, "but I'm not. I think it's normal to be interested. And if they really cared about their privacy, they'd close their curtains, wouldn't they?"

Evaluation of Rex Collingwood

There isn't much of a differential diagnosis in a history like Rex's; he easily fulfills criteria A and B. Had he spent his time watching paid performers on a stage or the Internet, we wouldn't think a thing about it; neither would the judge. Although Rex has acted repeatedly on his urges, the only distress he feels is at the prospect of being punished.

With a GAF score of 61, Rex's complete diagnosis would be:

F65.3	Voyeuristic disorder
Z65.3	Arrest and prosecution

F65.89 Other Specified Paraphilic Disorder

A variety of other paraphilic disorders have been described. As compared to the foregoing disorders, most of these are less common, less well studied, or both. Coded as other specified paraphilic disorder, they include the following:

Paraphilic coercive disorder. An individual enjoys the idea of forcing sex upon an unwilling partner.

Telephone scatologia. As the name implies, this is a preoccupation with talking dirty on the phone. It has been found to be associated with exhibitionism and voyeurism.

Zoophilia. This paraphilia is a preoccupation with having sex with various mammals and other animals. Uncommon in clinical samples, these individuals often report that the attraction is not just sex, but a love for animals.

Necrophilia. Sex with corpses is said to have been the only release available to undertakers in ancient Egypt. Sex with contemporary cadavers, rarely reported, suggests that additional mental or personality diagnoses may be warranted.

Klismaphilia. In this paraphilia, somewhat allied to sexual masochistic disorder, some people achieve sexual pleasure by giving themselves enemas. In some such individuals, klismaphilia is linked with cross-dressing. Though it may be fairly common, this behavior has seldom been reported in the professional literature.

Coprophilia. This is masturbating with feces; it is really uncommon.

Urophilia. Some patients become sexually excited by playing or masturbating with urine. This must be distinguished from the form of sexual masochism in which the person desires to be urinated upon ("golden showers"). Collectively, preoccupations with enemas and urine are termed "water sports" by those who enjoy them.

Infantilism. In this paraphilia, the patient derives sexual satisfaction from being treated like a baby—perhaps wearing diapers and drinking from a bottle.

F65.9 Unspecified Paraphilic Disorder

Use unspecified paraphilic disorder when a paraphilic disturbance does not meet the criteria for any of the disorders described in this chapter, and you decide not to state the reason.

CHAPTER 19

Other Factors That May Need Clinical Attention

You can use the codes provided in this chapter to report certain environmental or other physical or psychosocial events or conditions that might affect the diagnosis or management of your patient. When stating them, be as specific as possible. (Other problems are possible; these are samples.) Many of these were listed on Axis IV of DSM-IV. DSM-5-TR requires that we use ICD-10-CM codes for the problems we identify. Following is a reasonably complete list of those available.

But remember, please, that these behaviors, conditions, and relationships are not mental disorders. I emphasize this point in the attempt to reduce our tendency to carve pathology out of behavior that is, after all, the stuff of everyday human existence.

Suicidal Behavior and Self-Injury

T14.91XA Current Suicidal Behavior, First Encounter

Use if the behavior occurs as part of the patient's initial presentation.

T14.91XD Current Suicidal Behavior, Subsequent Encounter

Use if the behavior occurs during the patient's later treatment for this clinical presentation.

Z91.51 History of Suicidal Behavior

Z91.52 History of Nonsuicidal Self-Injury

R45.88 Current Nonsuicidal Self-Injury

Relational and Family Problems

Parent–Child Relational Problem

Use parent–child relational problem when clinically important symptoms or negative effects on functioning are associated with the way a parent and child interact. The problematic interaction patterns may include faulty communication, ineffective discipline, or overprotection. Various emotional and behavioral problems could ensue. You'd use the following codes:

Z62.820 Parent–Biological Child

Z62.821 Parent–Adopted Child

Z62.822 Parent–Foster Child

Z62.898 Other Caregiver–Child

Z62.898 Child Affected by Parental Relationship Distress

Parents' squabbling or other problems affect the child. Yep, same number as for other caregiver–child relational problem.

Z63.0 Relationship Distress with Spouse or Intimate Partner

Use relationship distress with spouse or intimate partner when clinically important symptoms or negative effects on functioning are associated with the way a patient and spouse/partner interact. The problematic interaction patterns may include faulty communication or an absence of communication. However, this category explicitly excludes problems related to abuse (which are described below).

Z62.891 Sibling Relational Problem

Use this code when clinically important symptoms or negative effects on functioning are associated with the way siblings interact.

Z62.29 Upbringing Away from Parents

This one is for problems that arise because a child is living in foster care or with relatives or friends, but not in residential care or at a boarding school.

Z63.5 Disruption of Family by Separation or Divorce

Z63.8 High Expressed Emotion Level within Family

Lots of yelling and hyperemotional outbursts in the family unit has been linked with relapse in schizophrenia, but it could affect just about anyone.

Z63.4 Uncomplicated Bereavement

It is natural to grieve when a relative or close friend dies. When the symptoms of the grieving process are a reason for receiving clinical attention, DSM-5-TR allows us to code these as uncomplicated bereavement—provided that the symptoms don't last too long and aren't too severe (Table 19.1). The problem is that the sadness of grief can resemble the sadness associated with a major depressive episode.

Certain symptoms can help you decide whether, in addition to being bereaved, the patient is suffering from a major depressive episode:

- Guilt feelings (other than about actions that might have prevented the death)
- Death wishes (other than the survivor's wishing to have died with the loved one)
- Slowed-down psychomotor activity
- Severe preoccupation with worthlessness
- Severely impaired functioning for an unusually long time
- Hallucinations (other than of seeing or hearing the deceased)

TABLE 19.1. Major Depression Compared with Uncomplicated Bereavement

	Major depression	Grief
Expression of mood	Despair and hopelessness	Loss or emptiness
Time course	Steady or waxing	Decrease with time (weeks)
Stability of mood	Persistent	Surges and retreats
Response to humor, distraction	Little or none	May bring relief
Content of thought	Largely unrelieved thoughts of own misery	Memories/thoughts of departed, but some positive thoughts regarding others
Self-esteem	Guilt, blame, worthlessness	"I've done my best"
Passing of time	Time crawls	Time passes as before
Death, dying	Wish for own death, suicidal plans	Life is still worth living
Clinical impairment	Yes	No

In addition, people who are "only" bereaved typically regard their moods as normal. Traditionally, a diagnosis of depressive illness has been withheld in these cases until after the symptoms have lasted longer than 2 months. Now we are encouraged to diagnose major depressive disorder regardless of bereavement, should the symptoms warrant. The table compares the symptoms of major depression with those of uncomplicated bereavement.

Educational Problems

Use educational problems for a patient whose problem is related to scholastic endeavors and who does not have a specific learning disorder or other mental disorder that accounts for the problem. Examples include illiteracy, unavailability of school, poor academic performance, underachievement, or discord with teacher or other students. Even if another disorder can account for the problem, the academic problem itself may be so severe that it independently justifies clinical attention. For example, see the story of Colin Rodebaugh (p. 317).

Z55.0 Illiteracy and Low-Level Literacy

Z55.1 Schooling Unavailable and Unattainable

Z55.2 Failed School Examinations

Z55.4 Educational Maladjustment and Discord with Teachers and Classmates

Z55.8 Problems Related to Inadequate Teaching

Z55.9 Other Problems Related to Education and Literacy

Occupational Problems

Z56.82 Problem Related to Current Military Deployment Status

Don't include psychological reactions here. Rather, use this category when deployment itself is the focus.

Z91.82 Personal History of Military Deployment

Z56.0 Unemployment

Z56.1 Change of Job

Z56.2 Threat of Job Loss

Z56.3 Stressful Work Schedule

Z56.4 Discord with Boss and Workmates

Although, surely this should be "discord with boss or workmates."

Z56.5 Uncongenial Work Environment

Z56.81 Sexual Harassment on the Job

Z56.9 Other Problem Related to Employment

Other problem related to employment could include issues in choosing a career and general dissatisfaction with one's job.

Housing Problems

Z59.01 Sheltered Homelessness

A patient lives in conditions such as a homeless shelter, motel, or other transitional living arrangement.

Z59.02 Unsheltered Homelessness

A patient has no fixed abode, lives in a car, tent, or cardboard box.

Z59.1 Inadequate Housing

Examples: No utilities, overcrowding, vermin, excessive noise.

Z59.3 Problem Related to Living in a Residential Institution

This code is for use with children (or adults) whose problems arise from living away from home in some sort of institution. It does not include emotional responses to the experience of institutional living.

Z59.2 Discord with Neighbor, Lodger, or Landlord

Z59.9 Other Housing Problem

Economic Problems

Z59.41 Food Insecurity

Z58.6 Lack of Safe Drinking Water

Z59.5 Extreme Poverty

Z59.6 Low Income

Z59.9 Other Economic Problem

Problems Related to the Social Environment

Z59.7 Insufficient Social or Health Insurance or Welfare Support

Z60.2 Problem Related to Living Alone

Z60.3 Acculturation Difficulty

For example, postmigration.

Z60.4 Social Exclusion or Rejection

Being a victim of bullying would fit in here.

Z60.5 Target of (Perceived) Adverse Discrimination or Persecution

Examples could include racial or sexual discrimination.

Z65.8 Religious or Spiritual Problem

Patients who require evaluation or treatment for issues pertaining to religious faith (or its lack) may be given the religious or spiritual problem code.

Z65.8 Other Problem Related to Psychosocial Circumstances

This catch-all category could include death or illness of a relative or remarriage of a parent. Yes, I realize that it has the same code numbers as religious or spiritual problem; life's imperfect.

Z60.9 Other Problem Related to Social Environment

Z65.9 Unspecified Problem Related to Unspecified Psychosocial Circumstances

This could cover quite a bit of ground.

Legal/Behavioral Problems

Z65.0 Conviction in Civil or Criminal Proceedings without Imprisonment

Z65.1 Imprisonment or Other Incarceration

Z65.2 Problems Related to Release from Prison

Z65.3 Problems Related to Other Legal Circumstances

Examples include being arrested, suing, being sued.

Z72.811 Adult Antisocial Behavior

If the reason for clinical attention is antisocial behavior that is not part of a pattern (and hence not attributable to antisocial personality disorder, conduct disorder, or a disorder of impulse control), adult antisocial behavior can be coded. Examples would include the activities of career criminals who do not have any of the disorders just mentioned.

Z72.810 Child or Adolescent Antisocial Behavior

Health Care Issues

The labels for many of the codes in the health care category explain themselves.

E66.9 Overweight or Obesity

Z64.0 Problems Related to Unwanted Pregnancy

Z64.1 Problems Related to Multiparity

Z75.3 Unavailability or Inaccessibility of Health Care Facilities

Z75.4 Unavailability or Inaccessibility of Other Helping Agencies

Problems in these two areas could be due to insufficient health insurance or unavailability of transportation to health care services.

Z91.19 Nonadherence to Medical Treatment

Use nonadherence to medical treatment for a patient who requires attention because the patient has ignored or controverted attempts at treatment for a mental disorder or another medical condition. An example would be a patient with schizophrenia who requires repeated hospitalization for refusal to take medication.

Z91.83 Wandering Associated with a Mental Disorder

This code applies especially to patients with major neurocognitive disorders, who are particularly prone to leaving their dwellings and striking off on their own; the negative consequences sometimes make national headlines. Code first the mental disorder, then the Z-code.

Z31.5 Genetic Counseling

Z70.9 Sex Counseling

Z71.3 Dietary Counseling

Z71.9 Other Counseling or Consultation

Other counseling or consultation covers matters such as counseling for weight loss or smoking cessation.

Problems Related to Trauma

Z64.4 Discord with Social Service Provider, Including Probation Officer, Case Manager, or Social Services Worker

Z65.4 Victim of Crime

Z65.4 Victim of Terrorism or Torture

Uh-oh, same number as for crime.

Z65.5 Exposure to Disaster, War, or Other Hostilities

This could only apply if PTSD has been ruled out.

Z91.49 Other Personal History of Psychological Trauma

Z91.89 Other Personal Risk Factors

Problems Related to Abuse or Neglect

The titles of the Z-codes for various types of abuse or neglect are pretty much self-explanatory. Rather than write out every one of them, I've put them into Table 19.2. Also, each of the ICD-10 codes in Table 19.2 should have XA (for initial encounter) or XD (for subsequent encounter) appended. For example, "child neglect abuse confirmed, initial encounter" would be coded T74.02XA). Note that some of the code numbers are the same, though the wording is different. This appears to be intentional, though on whose part I cannot imagine.

Here are three helpful definitions:

Sexual abuse. Any sex act (including those that do not involve contact, such as photography) intended to gratify the perpetrator or others.

Neglect. An act (or omission) that so deprives an individual of basic needs that it could result in physical or psychological harm.

Psychological abuse. Intentional verbal or symbolic acts by a caregiver that could result in psychological harm. Examples include berating, scapegoating, threatening, coercion, and physical confinement.

By the way, there are other codes you can use if the focus of the interview is on the encounter for mental health services for the victim or the perpetrator—different codes if the perpetrator is a parent or not (see Table 19.3). And if the patient has a personal history of abuse or neglect, there are some codes for that, too (see Table 19.4).

TABLE 19.2. Codes for Neglect and Abuse

	Abuse confirmed	Abuse suspected
Child physical abuse [by parent or caregiver]	T74.12	T76.12
Child sexual abuse [by parent or caregiver]	T74.22	T76.22
Child neglect [by parent or caregiver]	T74.02	T76.02
Child psychological abuse [by parent or caregiver]	T74.32	T76.32
Spouse or partner violence, physical	T74.11	T76.11
Spouse or partner violence, sexual	T74.21	T76.21
Spouse or partner neglect	T74.01	T76.01
Spouse or partner abuse, psychological	T74.31	T76.31
Adult physical abuse by nonspouse or nonpartner	T74.11	T76.11
Adult sexual abuse by nonspouse or nonpartner	T74.21	T76.21
Adult psychological abuse by nonspouse or nonpartner	T74.31	T76.31

TABLE 19.3. Codes for Neglect and Abuse When the Emphasis Is on the Encounter for Mental Health Services

Encounter for mental health services for:	Victim	Perpetrator
Child neglect or physical/sexual/psychological abuse by parent	Z69.010	Z69.011
Child neglect or physical/sexual/psychological abuse by nonparent	Z69.020	Z69.021
Adult spouse/partner neglect, physical/sexual violence, or psychological abuse	Z69.11	Z69.12
Adult nonspousal or nonpartner abuse	Z69.81	Z69.82

TABLE 19.4. Codes and Descriptions for a Patient with a Previous History of Neglect or Abuse

Physical or sexual abuse in childhood	Z62.810
Neglect in childhood	Z62.812
Psychological abuse in childhood	Z62.811
Spouse or partner physical or sexual violence	Z91.410
Spouse or partner neglect	Z91.412
Spouse or partner psychological abuse	Z91.411

Medication-Induced Movement Disorders

Medication-induced movement disorders are important in mental health care for two reasons:

- They may be mistaken for mental disorders (such as tic disorders, schizophrenia, or anxiety disorders).
- They can affect the management of patients who are receiving psychotropic medications.

G21.0 Neuroleptic Malignant Syndrome

The use of certain antipsychotic medications (the old term *neuroleptic* has been deemed inaccurate and so is not used in other contexts than those that bear its name), can lead within 3 days to muscle rigidity, fever, and other problems, such as sweating, trouble swallowing, incontinence, and delirium.

G21.11 Antipsychotic Medication– and Other Dopamine Receptor Blocking Agent–Induced Parkinsonism

This used to be called plain vanilla neuroleptic-induced parkinsonism. Oh! for the good old days.

G21.19 Other Medication-Induced Parkinsonism

Many of the antipsychotic agents that have been developed and used over the past 70 years (and a few other medications, too) can induce a frozen face, shuffling gait, and pill-rolling tremor that much resemble naturally occurring Parkinson's disease.

G24.01 Tardive Dyskinesia

After a patient has taken an antipsychotic medication for a few months or more, involuntary movements of the face, jaw, tongue, or limbs may become noticeable. Once begun, these movements can become permanent, even if the medication responsible is discontinued.

G24.02 Medication-Induced Acute Dystonia

Abrupt contracting in muscles of the head, neck, or other portions of the body can produce painful, often frightening spasms. These are due to the use of antipsychotic medications (and others) and occur quite commonly.

G24.09 Tardive Dystonia

G25.1 Medication-Induced Postural Tremor

The use of medications such as antidepressants, lithium, or valproate may cause a fine tremor when the person tries to maintain a position (for example, an outstretched hand).

G25.71 Medication-Induced Acute Akathisia

Shortly after beginning or increasing the dose of an antipsychotic (or other) drug, some patients become acutely restless and unable to remain seated.

G25.71 Tardive Akathisia

G25.79 Other Medication-Induced Movement Disorder

DSM-5-TR suggests that other medication-induced movement disorder may be useful for patients who have symptoms resembling neuroleptic malignant syndrome, but who have used drugs other than antipsychotics.

T43.205 Antidepressant Discontinuation Syndrome

Within a few days of stopping an antidepressant, a patient may develop nonspecific symptoms that can include dizziness, sleeplessness, a peculiar sensation sometimes described as "electric shocks to the brain," nausea, sweating, and many other symptoms. Its incidence is probably proportional to the dose of the antidepressant.

T50.905 Other Adverse Effect of Medication

Other adverse effect of medication can be used for unwanted effects besides movement disorders that become an important focus for clinical attention. Examples include severe hypotension caused by antipsychotic medications and priapism caused by trazodone.

As a seventh digit for either of the two movement disorders mentioned just above, you can tack on further specifiers: A = initial encounter; D = subsequent encounter; S = sequelae.

Miscellaneous Issues That May Be a Focus of Clinical Attention . . .

. . . but are not mental disorders.

R41.83 Borderline Intellectual Functioning

Use borderline intellectual functioning for a patient whose intellect is limited but not so severely as to reach into the mild intellectual developmental disorder range. In concrete terms, that would equate to an IQ within the range of 71–84. The differential between borderline intellectual functioning and mild intellectual developmental disorder can be quite challenging—especially since we no longer define intellectual disability by IQ score.

Z60.0 Phase of Life Problem

Use phase of life problem for a patient whose problem is not due to a mental disorder but to a life change, such as marriage, divorce, a new job, an empty nest, or retirement. It must be discriminated from adjustment disorder.

Z72.9 Problem Related to Lifestyle

Examples include poor sleep hygiene, high-risk sexual behavior.

Z76.5 Malingering

Malingering is defined as the intentional production of the signs or symptoms of a physical or mental disorder. The purpose is some sort of gain: obtaining something desirable (money, drugs, insurance settlement) or avoiding something unpleasant (punishment, work, military service, jury duty). Malingering is sometimes confused with factitious disorder (in which the motive is not external gain, but a wish to occupy the sick role) and with other somatic symptom and related disorders (in which the symptoms are not intentionally produced at all).

Malingering should be suspected in any of these situations:

- The patient has legal problems or the prospect of financial gain.
- The patient has antisocial personality disorder.
- The patient tells a story that does not accord with informants' accounts or with other known facts.
- The patient does not cooperate with the evaluation.

Malingering is easy to suspect and hard to prove. In the absence of a definitive observation (you watch as someone pours sand into a urine specimen or holds a thermometer over a hot light bulb), a resolute and resourceful malingerer can be almost impossible to detect. When malingering involves symptoms that are strictly mental or emotional, detection may be impossible. Moreover, the consequences of this diagnosis are dire: It provides closure in such a way as to totally alienate the clinician from the patient. I therefore recommend that you make this diagnosis only in the most obvious and imperative of circumstances.

Additional Codes

Finally, here are a few additional codes useful for administrative purposes.

Z03.89 No Diagnosis or Condition

This can indicate a patient who has neither a major mental disorder nor a personality disorder. Of course, that won't often be the case, but every mental health practitioner at some time or other will likely encounter patients who have no mental disorder.

F48.9 Unspecified Nonpsychotic Mental Disorder

There are one or two situations in which a diagnosis of unspecified nonpsychotic mental disorder may be appropriate:

- The diagnosis you want to give is not contained in DSM-5-TR.
- You know that a patient has a mental disorder, but you have insufficient infor-

mation to state what it is, and no other unspecified category seems appropriate. Once you have obtained more information, you should be able to change this to a more specific diagnosis. If you cannot even be sure that the patient has no psychotic symptoms, you'd have to use the next code.

F99 Unspecified Mental Disorder

Here is a designation you should hardly ever use—as a final diagnosis—but one that I frequently deploy at first evaluation. It means that you don't even have enough information to be sure what chapter of DSM-5-TR your patient belongs in (if you did, you could use, for example, unspecified depressive disorder). I would most often use this category to describe a patient in an admitting note (which, of course, requires no code numbers at all).

F09 Unspecified Mental Disorder Due to Another Medical Condition

This one pretty specifically tells you when you'd use it.

R69 Unspecified Illness

This one is the least specific of all, but wouldn't you usually have enough information to know that it's *mental?*

CHAPTER 20

Patients and Diagnoses

Clinicians use rules to decide what diagnoses to give their patients. They don't always realize that they are using rules, but they're there, all right.

Throughout my professional life, I've spent a lot of time thinking, talking, and writing about these rules (OK, I usually call them "principles") and how they should be deployed. Here I'm just going to list them, so we can then use them in diagnosing the mental health patients in this chapter. I hope you'll want to know more about how to understand and apply this important part of mental health practice.

Diagnostic Health Care Principles

As you read the patient vignettes that follow, try not to confuse the principles, which are designated with capital letters, with DSM-5-TR criteria, which also have letters. Lots of luck—I've gotten turned around a time or two myself. By the way, I've filched these principles from one of my own books: *Diagnosis Made Easier* (The Guilford Press). Highly recommended.

Create a Differential Diagnosis

A. Arrange your differential diagnosis according to a safety hierarchy.

B. Family history can guide diagnosis, but because you often can't trust reports, clinicians should attempt to rediagnose each family member.

C. Physical disorders and their treatment can produce or worsen mental symptoms.

D. Consider somatic symptom (somatization) disorder whenever symptoms don't jibe or treatments don't work.

E. Substance use can cause a variety of mental disorders.

F. Because of their ubiquity, potential for harm, and ready response to treatment, *always* consider mood disorders.

When Information Sources Conflict

G. History beats current appearance.

H. Recent history beats ancient history.

I. Collateral information sometimes beats the patient's own.

J. Signs beat symptoms.

K. Be wary when evaluating crisis-generated data.

L. Objective findings beat subjective judgment.

M. Use Occam's razor: Choose the simplest explanation.

N. Horses are more common than zebras; prefer the more frequently encountered diagnosis.

O. Watch for contradictory information.

Resolve Uncertainty

P. The best predictor of future behavior is past behavior.

Q. More symptoms of a disorder increase its likelihood as your diagnosis.

R. Typical features of a disorder increase its likelihood as your diagnosis; if you encounter nontypical features, look for alternatives.

S. Previous typical response to treatment for a disorder increases its likelihood as your diagnosis.

T. Use the word *undiagnosed* whenever you cannot be sure of your diagnosis.

U. Consider the possibility that this patient should be given no mental diagnosis at all.

Multiple Diagnoses

V. When symptoms cannot be adequately explained by a single disorder, consider multiple diagnoses.

W. Avoid personality disorder diagnoses when your patient is acutely ill with a major mental disorder.

X. Arrange multiple diagnoses to list first the one that is most urgent, treatable, or specific. Whenever possible, also list diagnoses chronologically.

Case Histories

With experience, sorting through the information from a patient's history and mental status exam becomes gradually easier. After you have evaluated 200 patients or so, you will find that the process has become virtually second nature. In the remainder of this chapter, you'll have an opportunity to try your own diagnostic skills on a variety of patients. Some of them have multiple mental disorders, which may be the norm rather than the exception. A national survey of adults in the general population found that of those who had a lifetime history of at least one disorder, over 60% had more than one. About 14% of all Americans have three or more lifetime diagnoses.

Due to space requirements, these case histories have been somewhat abridged. Other clinicians might disagree with some of my conclusions; my main purpose in presenting them is to demonstrate how a clinician reasons through the facts to arrive at a diagnosis.

Here's one additional suggestion. People learn more rapidly when they are actively involved. So rather than just reading the vignettes and my discussions, I hope you'll try to figure out the diagnoses yourself, using the diagnostic principles and my DSM-5-TR Essential Features. Then compare your answers to mine.

Laura Freitas

Laura Freitas, a 32-year-old divorced woman, is admitted to a mental health unit with this chief complaint: "I'm God." She was referred from an outpatient clinic and serves as her own chief informant.

Laura had her first episode of mental illness at age 19, after her second baby was born. She can remember little about this period, except that it was called a "postpartum psychosis" and she spent some time in isolation for dancing nude in the hospital day room. She recovered and remained well until 3 years ago, when, for reasons she could not remember, she was placed on lithium carbonate. She has taken this medication from then until 7 or 8 days ago, when she stopped because "I felt so well, so powerful that I knew I didn't need it." Over the next several days she became increasingly agitated, slept little, and talked endlessly, until friends finally brought her for treatment.

Laura was born in Illinois, where her father worked as an automobile mechanic. An only child, she often felt that her parents "would have been happier with no children at all." She describes them both as "alcoholics" and notes that she ran away from home overnight on at least one occasion when she was 13. She twice experimented with marijuana as a teenager, but she denies using other drugs, including alcohol.

At 18 Laura was briefly married to a bread salesman, with whom she has two children. The daughter, 13, lives with her father. The son, 14, is hyperactive and was at one time treated with Ritalin; he lives with her.

Laura is a fallen-away Catholic who for the past 2 years has worked at a travel agency. She claims that her health has been "above perfect," meaning that she has no allergies or medical problems. Her only operations were a tonsillectomy when she was 6 and a tubal ligation after the birth of her daughter. Family history is positive for alcoholism in both parents and both grandfathers. A paternal aunt intermittently "went to pieces," becoming excessively religious and imagining various sins for which she felt excessive guilt.

Laura is a somewhat overweight woman who looks about her stated age. She is quite agitated, jumping out of her chair every few moments to pace to the door and back. Given breakfast during a part of this interview, she intentionally smears grape jelly onto the trousers of a passing nurse. Subsequently, she lies down on the floor and kicks her legs in the air in apparent ecstasy.

Laura seems to be struggling to control her verbal output; even so, she skips rapidly from one subject to another. However, the rate at which she speaks is approximately normal. Her affect is clearly elevated, and she declares that she has never felt better in her life. She admits that she might hear voices singing (the interviewer can hear no music); she enjoys singing along with what she hears. She claims that she is "the All-Powerful One" and that she is now "very clear" that she has no need for medication.

Laura is oriented to person, place, and time. She names five recent presidents, and correctly (and with astonishing speed) subtracts serial sevens down, down into the negative numbers. When she finishes, she apologizes for taking so long to complete a task working with numbers. "After all," she remarks, "I created them."

Evaluation of Laura Freitas

Two diagnostic areas stand out in Laura's case—psychosis and mood disturbance. Psychosis can be dealt with summarily: Her delusions were too brief for any of the psychotic diagnoses except brief psychotic disorder or substance-induced psychotic disorder. However, each of these diagnoses requires that a mood disorder not better explain the symptoms, and that, as we will note, is so not the case: Laura's previous manic episodes disqualify her for a psychotic disorder.

Laura's current symptoms strongly suggest a manic episode. It appears that a previous clinician also had thought so: She was successfully treated with lithium (specific for the bipolar disorders) until shortly before this admission. Let us work through the steps necessary to diagnose manic episode (p. 123):

1. *Quality of mood.* Elevated mood is shown in the expansive way Laura expresses herself and in her statement that she has never felt better.

2. *Duration.* Her current symptoms have lasted at least 1 week. Information from informants (principle I) will probably establish that her present episode began even longer ago, perhaps at the point that she started to feel increasingly "well."

3. *Symptoms.* Laura has at least four symptoms (three are required) for manic episode. She is grandiose (she calls herself God and claims that her physical health is "above perfect"). She also is agitated, talks too much, and needs little sleep. I might point out that she has a lot of typical symptoms of mania (principle R).

4. *Impairment.* This is clearly demonstrated by Laura's admission to the hospital, where she smears jelly on a nurse.

5. *Exclusions.* None are noted, including substance use (she had used marijuana only when a teenager) and general medical conditions. However, hyperthyroidism and other endocrine disorders should be ruled out by routine laboratory testing upon admission.

So, Laura fulfills the basic criteria for manic episode. No general medical condition or cognitive disorder seems more likely (diagnostic principle C). If any further confirmation is needed, she had an aunt who might have had a recurrent psychosis. This sort of family history (principle B) better supports a remitting condition such as bipolar I disorder than a chronic psychosis such as schizophrenia. Furthermore, the safety principle (A) demands that we consider more treatable disorders first. And, just to rub it in, reread principle F.

The vignette does not indicate whether Laura has ever had an episode of depression, but for coding purposes, it doesn't matter. Her most recent (current) episode is manic, and she has had at least two prior episodes (one 13 and one 3 years ago when she started lithium). The presence of psychotic features qualifies her for a (not surprising) severity level of severe, with psychotic features. Her delusion that she is God would be mood-congruent for mania.

By the way, in rereading this discussion, I note that I haven't indicated any differential diagnosis—other than giving the back of my hand to psychotic disorders. The symptoms of mania just overwhelmed me, and I didn't think it would add anything to our understanding of this patient with classic bipolar I disorder. Laura would not qualify for any additional episode specifiers (see Table 3.3 on p. 167). The vignette gives no information suggesting that she also has a personality disorder. Her physical health is good. There is no evidence that her divorced status or the treatment of her son for hyperactivity would have any effect on the treatment of her mania, so I won't list any Z-codes for her. I place her GAF score at 25 on the basis that she is currently quite ill, with behavior influenced by delusions, though she does not seem to be in danger of hurting herself or others. Her full diagnosis reads:

F31.2   Bipolar I disorder, current episode manic, severe with mood-congruent psychotic features

KD Riley

"It's been too much, and much too sudden. I so hope you can help."

The student nurse's clip-on nametag says KD Riley, under which it reads "Pronouns: they/their/them."

"I'd just come out as nonbinary and was getting really good acceptance from my friends and a lot of love from both my parents. And then came the fire." A tear escapes and rolls down KD's cheek. "Of course, from the experience of the last few years, we've been expecting a big one. When you live in the forest, you always think, flaming disaster."

The past two summers, KD's part of the forest had barely escaped immolation; but this year, luck ran out. "That Friday afternoon the wind was howling like a banshee, and you could just sense calamity in the air. My dad had cleared a broad fire break around our house, but it wasn't enough. The undergrowth in the surrounding woods was tinder, and once it caught, it set the tall evergreens off like Roman candles. Burning embers sailed right onto the roof. We grabbed our go bags, collected the dog, and jumped into our vehicles with barely enough time before everything blew up."

Located in the center of the city, KD's hospital had escaped unscathed. The services of all student nurses were in strong demand.

"FEMA found us a place to shelter that's dry and safe. And all the bathrooms are unisex and private, so no one's hassling me about whether to use the men's or women's." Another tear. "Everyone's been lovely and kind, so why do I feel so scared? And sad? We're all in the same pickle, yet I'm the only one who feels so stressed? And down? I don't get it!"

Indeed, for the past week, ever since the family escaped the inferno, KD has experienced depression. "Nearly all day long it's there, crushing me. I have a sense that there's no hope for any of us. Logically, I know that none of this seems reasonable. Besides the firebreak, my dad took out a really good insurance policy on the house. And he's got a great job in state government, so we're not going to starve. And my friends have all been lovely, and . . . and . . . " More tears.

Questioning reveals that appetite and weight have remained steady. KD denies thoughts of death or suicide, problems with concentration or interest, and feeling fatigue or guilty. And we find no evidence of panic attacks, obsessional thinking, or phobias. Physical health is "great." Alcohol or street drugs? Scornful denial.

And after a pause: "Look, I know you're going to ask if I have flashbacks or nightmares—I've read about PTSD in my health maintenance class. But I sleep like the dead at night and I don't startle and I'm not irritable or reckless or hypovig—no, *hyper*vigilant. And no dissociation; I remember everything pretty clearly. *Too* clearly. It freaks me out!

"Dad says not to worry; we'll rebuild and life will go on. I know in my heart that we're really lucky. So why don't I feel that way?" And now the trickle of tears becomes a flood that rolls down their cheek.

Evaluation of KD Riley

KD's symptoms were ignited by a horrific fire that consumed the family home and, for a time, threatened all their lives. This natural disaster lines up three stress-related diagnoses for our consideration: acute stress disorder, posttraumatic stress disorder, and adjustment disorder.

Posttraumatic stress disorder and acute stress disorder are defined by the same symptoms; it's how the symptoms are grouped and the time course that make the difference. The short time factor allows us to discard PTSD out of hand, and KD's own reporting (few symptoms of intrusion, dissociation, arousal) puts paid to acute stress disorder. We've not forgotten to consider major depressive disorder (principle F); other than depressed mood, those symptoms are missing in action.

Physical health has been good (principle C) and KD doesn't use substances (principle E), and that brings us to adjustment disorder. The stressor is clearly identifiable and it occurred well within the 3-month window (DSM-5-TR criterion A). KD's distress is greater than circumstances would lead us to expect. Heck, it's even above what KD expected—their siblings, parents, and friends experienced the same stressor but without the same wrenching symptoms of depression and anxiety that have haunted KD (B1). Personal and social functioning have not been affected (B2), but only one of the B's is required for diagnosis. No one died, so bereavement and prolonged grief are not an issue (D), and I don't think we can find symptoms necessary to fulfill criteria for a major depressive disorder (C). Symptoms have been present but a short time, so the specifier of "acute" will be appropriate.

Criterion E says that symptoms must not persist once the stressor has remitted. Clearly, we'll have to revisit KD (who now has a GAF of about 60) in a few months to be sure, but I'm going to confidently state:

F43.23	Adjustment disorder with mixed anxiety and depressed mood, acute

Adrian Branscom

Adrian Branscom is a 49-year-old executive who refers himself to his company's mental health clinician. "I never thought I'd be talking to a shrink," is his first comment upon entering the office.

After serving 2 years as a junior officer in the Army Ordnance Corps, Adrian was recruited by a subsidiary of a large petroleum companies that specializes in oil field development. Bright and energetic, he rapidly climbed the ranks of middle management and was in line for a vice-presidency when a recession hit. Although his share of the restructuring turned out to be no vice-presidency and a 10% pay cut, Adrian feels lucky that he still has a job. His wife's view is less sanguine.

Yoshiko was a Japanese service bride. They had married at the end of a whirlwind romance in Tokyo during a 2-week leave from Adrian's tour of duty in Asia. For the past 20 years, since the births of their daughter and son, she has stayed home with the children.

"She wishes she had stayed home in Japan," Adrian comments wryly. Almost since their wedding, Yoshiko has accused him of taking her away from her people so he could "dump her." In all the years they have lived together, she has never made friends. She spends most of her free time acquiring a collection of Japanese porcelain artifacts. Now she deeply resents her husband's demotion and their loss of income.

"We hadn't been getting along well for years," says Adrian, "but for the last several years we've hit one new low after another. She says if I were a real man, I'd provide better for her."

On many occasions, Adrian has told Yoshiko he thinks they should discuss their problems. Her usual response is "So go ahead and discuss it!" When he tries to state his viewpoint, she will listen for half a sentence; then "She always begins to talk over me. After starting six or eight sentences, I usually give up." Every time Adrian suggests that they seek marital counseling, it provokes a torrent of invective from Yoshiko and a demand for divorce. If he tries to discuss divorce, she cries and says that he is trying to get rid of her and that they'd all be better off if she commits suicide. These tirades make him feel guilty; they have worsened in the past month.

Although Adrian is usually a "happy-go-lucky sort of fellow," for most of the past 6 weeks he has been depressed and anxious. His appetite and energy haven't changed, but he's had trouble sleeping most nights; he often awakens with a pounding heart and the feeling that he is about to smother. His concentration at work and his self-confidence have both plummeted. Increasingly over the past week, he has been thinking about death and the shotgun that still lies somewhere in the attic. Frightened, he has finally decided to seek help.

Adrian was born in West Central Texas, where his father taught school and did a little farming. He was the youngest of three children, all of whom managed to go to college and succeed in business or a profession. "It wasn't until I was out of college that I realized just how dirt-poor my parents were," he says. "I guess we seemed well off because we were all happy."

The family history is negative for substance use and for any other mental disorder. Adrian has never used drugs or alcohol; his moods have never been excessively elevated or irritable. He spends most of his time at work and has very few friends; he has never strayed from the marital bed ("twin beds," he is quick to correct). At home, he enjoys collecting rocks and hiking with his son.

Adrian is a conservatively dressed, somewhat overweight man who looks his stated age. He sits quietly in the office chair during the interview. Once or twice, he reaches for a fresh tissue to wipe his eyes. His speech is clear, coherent, relevant, and spontaneous. His mood is conventionally labile and seems appropriate to his content of thought. He denies having any hallucinations or delusions. He states that he has always been "a fixer"—that he feels it his job to make things work for everyone. He earns a perfect score on the MMSE. His insight and judgment seem unimpaired. "I think we'd all be better off if we lived apart," he concludes. "This is one thing I don't think I can fix."

Evaluation of Adrian Branscom

A rapid reading of Adrian's history suggests three possible diagnostic areas: mood disorder, anxiety disorder, and problems of adjustment. To consider adjustment disorder first, it would be easy to suppose that Adrian's difficulties could be laid completely at the doorstep of his marital strife. After all, he has no history of mental disorder, and his marriage is extremely troubled. But he also has enough symptoms to qualify for a mood disorder (see below), and the criteria for adjustment disorder with depressed mood quite clearly exclude all other mental disorders.

From the information we have, his character structure, though perhaps a bit naïve, reveals none of the interpersonal difficulty we would expect for a personality disorder. However, in a later interview, his clinician should obtain information from informants (principle I); the vignette gives only Adrian's interpretation of his marital situation.

As for the anxiety disorders, Adrian has episodes of awakening from sleep with a pounding heart and shortness of breath, and he has felt anxious for much of the previous few weeks. These symptoms aren't enough to qualify for a panic attack (which can occur during sleep); therefore, we won't diagnose panic disorder. None of his symptoms suggest specific phobia, social anxiety disorder, agoraphobia, or obsessive–compulsive disorder. Although he is a veteran of war, he was evidently not exposed to extremely traumatic events (as would be the case in posttraumatic stress disorder). Generalized anxiety disorder requires a 6-month duration and more symptoms. Although Adrian is overweight, obesity does not have any known relationship to anxiety symptoms; it should be mentioned in his diagnostic summary, however.

Finally, Adrian does have some clear-cut mood symptoms, and when you hear hoofbeats in the street, think of horses, not zebras (principle N). His symptoms include feeling depressed most of the time, insomnia, problems with concentration, feelings of guilt, and an increasing preoccupation with suicide. (DSM-5-TR does not credit low self-confidence and weeping as qualifying depressive symptoms.) His symptoms have been constantly present for over a month and cause him problems with his job. None of the exclusions will apply (general medical condition or substance use), so he will fulfill criteria for a single episode of major depressive disorder.

None of the course or episode specifiers apply (Table 3.3, p. 167). He has only the minimum number of symptoms, but one of these (suicidal ideas) is extremely serious, so his clinician (and I) believe this deserves a severity rating of at least moderate. And that earns him a GAF score of 60. Fortunately, Adrian's suicidal thoughts include no plans; he does not appear to pose a serious imminent risk, though someone should take steps to secure that shotgun still in his attic. His complete diagnosis:

F32.1	Major depressive disorder, single episode, moderate
E66.9	Obesity
Z63.0	Marital discord

Wait a minute! What about Yoshiko? Surely, she deserves some sort of diagnosis. A personality disorder perhaps, you might think.

Of course, Yoshiko's personal characteristics sound pretty alarming, very possibly enough to earn some sort of DSM-5-TR diagnosis. There are just two problems: We haven't nearly enough information, and she isn't our patient. We haven't even interviewed her; all we have is information from her husband. Now, Adrian may well be an acute observer, but he is hardly a disinterested one. We really must have her side of the story before giving her any diagnosis at all. That isn't one of my diagnostic principles, but it's one that every clinician should follow, regardless.

Jeff DeMott

Jeff DeMott is buckled into the back seat of a brand-new all-electric vehicle. Beside him sits his wife, Elaine. They are about to take a demonstration drive with potential customers at the dealership where Jeff works. The Thompsons have come in on the strength of Elaine's friendship with Marty. Roger Thompson is a bit of a smart aleck, but Jeff supposes they can tolerate one another for an hour or so.

Roger tries the self-parking feature, then glides onto the state highway heading away from the city. The cruise control maintains a safe distance from the vehicle in front and the automatic steering keeps the car in its lane. Roger has cranked the speed above the posted limit, and Jeff is about to issue one of his standard cautions—"The collision avoidance sensors don't see everything, so stay alert"—when Roger releases his hold on the wheel and turns around. "Look," he crows, "I don't even need to watch the road! I have my eyes completely closed! And I've surrendered the wheel!" Eyes clamped shut, he giggles as he reaches both hands toward the roof.

Suddenly Marty glances up from her phone and screams.

"Roger, omigod! You're gonna hit—!"

Her sentence hangs, unfinished, as the car plows into an eighteen-wheeler that has just pulled onto the highway. There are sounds of breaking glass and crumpling metal. After that, Jeff loses his bearings. First he is sideways, then upside down, followed by . . . nothing.

In the ER, they X-ray Jeff's chest (two broken ribs, a dislocated shoulder) and tediously insert 18 stitches into his chin. Then they send in the chaplain to inform him, "I'm sorry sir, but you are the only survivor."

After a single night in the hospital, with a heart that's full to breaking, Jeff returns to an empty house. Insurance pays the medical bills and his boss keeps him on the payroll, but Jeff wonders if he can ever return to work and its haunting memories of the worst day of his life.

Sometimes not even sure where he is, for days he sits alone on the sofa and grieves. Twice he fleetingly thinks he sees Elaine standing at the door. He briefly tries to blot out recurrent thoughts of the fatal crash with alcohol, but three days of headache and vomiting persuade him otherwise. Whenever the phone rings, it startles him into a fury, and he answers with angry outbursts. Around midnight, he'll relocate to the bedroom, but for hours he'll stare at the ceiling, unable to dismiss the screaming that ruins his dreams.

With the memorial service looming, for several days Jeff tries to write down his fondest memories of Elaine, but the content will not come—and he lacks the focus for this or any other intellectual task. He refuses the offers of friends to come visit or to go with them—anywhere. He gives wide berth to his own car: Even the thought of its smug, all-electric power train produces nausea so acute that he must dash to the bathroom.

Three weeks in, his experience begins to change. "And not for the better, either," he tells a clinician later. The sudden flashes of enraged horror subside, replaced by a pervasive sadness that, as the weeks drag by, deepens and darkens, filling his day. "The whole world has gone to hell," he repeats to anyone who will listen, "and I'm to blame."

Even his dreams have changed. At first, when Elaine appears to him in the night, her image is achingly sharp and close, almost tangible. Over the next few weeks, with each subsequent dream she seems ever more distant; eventually, only a wisp of her essence touches his sleep. In sorrow, he realizes he has let her go.

But misery hasn't yet released its hold. Now he struggles to get any sleep at all; mealtimes roll past unheeded, and his weight drifts downward. He briefly returns to work, but he has no focus. Although he can get into a car with a customer, the facts and the speeches have deserted him. "It's hopeless; I'm hopeless" he tells his boss. Crushed by fatigue, he wants to be let go, and eventually, he is.

He spends much of the next few months trying to expunge the melancholy with comforting thoughts that he could simply end it all. In the week marking the anniversary of the accident, still living on insurance money and the pitying generosity of neighbors, he finally visits the mental health clinic.

Evaluation of Jeff DeMott

Jeff's diagnosis is complicated, because he has not one disorder, but two. In fact, we'll later ask the question, does he have a third?

The beginning is simple enough, however, for it starts off with the trauma of losing his wife through a horrendous accident that he not only witnesses, but experiences firsthand. His symptom onset—within days, perhaps hours of the accident—directs us not to PTSD but to its early-onset cousin, acute stress disorder. By being both a witness and a victim, Jeff more than fulfills the A criterion for acute stress disorder (in fact, both A1 and A2—directly experiencing the event and witnessing in person the event as it occurred to others), and the time frame is within the 30 days specified by criterion C. Jeff's distress is palpable (D), and substances are not implicated (E).

Now, how many criterion B symptoms can we identify? The vignette is explicit that the horror of that car ride intrudes upon his waking thoughts (B1), and that they influence the content of his dreams (B2). Even his own car sets off abdominal distress, which counts as a physiological reaction to an external cue (B4). Negative frame of mind is demonstrated in his inability to express positive thoughts of Elaine (B5). Initially, he is dazed and unsure even of his surroundings (B6), and he briefly turns to alcohol in an attempt to avoid distressing memories (B8). He avoids the resurgence of feelings a car ride might inflict upon him (B9). His sleep is notably disturbed (B10) and he responds to phone calls with irritation (B11) toward people who are, after all, only trying to help.

Rounding out his rich palette of symptoms is a vigorous startle response to the ringing of the telephone (B14). Count them up: He has one more than the minimum nine symptoms required (and easily fulfills the Essential Features) to complete our diagnosis of acute stress disorder.

The logical extension of that diagnosis—what we kind of expect will happen—would be for Jeff to move on into PTSD. That happens with a substantial percentage of patients with acute stress disorder. But for Jeff, something else happens instead. The trauma-related themes related to the accident gradually drop out and are replaced by issues more associated with a depressive mood disorder. And when we encounter depression, our very early diagnostic efforts should bend toward determining whether the patient qualifies for a major depressive episode (p. 112).

And here's what we can find for Jeff. Jeff's depressive symptoms have indeed been present far longer than the minimum 2 weeks, and they certainly are a change in his previous functioning (major depressive disorder criterion A). The symptoms do cause (overwhelming) clinical distress (B) and we have information that Jeff does not use drugs or alcohol (C). So, let's do our due diligence and count the A criteria. His sadness is pervasive (A1), his interest in nearly everything, as best we can tell, has gone south (A2). His interest in food is nonexistent and his weight plummets (A3), and he suffers nightly from terminal insomnia (A4). He has inappropriate guilt ("I'm to blame," though it was Elaine herself who arranged the car ride, A7), cannot focus his concentration on work (A8), is fatigued (A6), and has death wishes (A9). All in all, not quite a full slate of symptoms, but substantially more than the five required for a diagnosis of major depressive disorder.

But wait a minute, I can almost hear someone exclaim. What about prolonged grief disorder? Shouldn't that enter into Jeff's diagnosis? OK, good idea to take PGD for a spin.

There's no denying, Jeff can present a ticket of admission: the death of a loved one a year or more ago. (Right, it doesn't have to be someone beloved; just someone close, criterion A.) But then, the patient must either dwell on thoughts of the dead person or experience intense longing (B1 or B2). As I read the vignette, after the first month Jeff has bid farewell to Elaine; all his depressive thoughts now are more general.

And so, we come down to the table (on p. 232) that compares symptoms of major depression with those of PGD. A month in, his depressive thoughts are no longer focused on the loss of Elaine ("whole world . . . gone to hell"). He hasn't apparently sought sensory reminders of her, and his desire for death is not so he can be with her but to be shut of his overall misery. He expresses hopelessness and overall seems to experience lack of self-worth. That's several symptoms from the table in favor of major depression. His only symptom that relates to PGD is sleep disturbance, and that is found in both disorders. Finally, PGD criterion F specifically requires that the symptoms must not be better explained by major depression; I hope we'll all agree that Jeff's are.

There! I believe we can now justify two diagnoses for Jeff, given for two different time frames:

For the first month after the accident:

F43.0   Acute stress disorder

And a year (more or less) later:

F32.2   Major depressive disorder, severe

James Chatterton

James Chatterton is 18 when he cuts his wrist on the glass of a window he has just broken; this earns him his first admission to a mental hospital. James's aunt Gertrude is the chief informant on this occasion. "He's always seemed a little cold. Kind of like his cousin, my Betty," she offers.

Even when very young, James was unconventional. He cared so little what other people thought that in fourth grade, when he called the teacher "Gristle Butt," he didn't even acknowledge the suppressed laughter of the other children. "I don't think he had a single friend in school," Gertrude says. "He never cracked a smile, never got angry—not even when he said he thought the other kids were talking about him. He said that quite a lot, as I recall." And as a teenager, he never showed the slightest interest in girls or curiosity about sex.

When James was 14, his mother died suddenly. His father, working in another state, had no time for child care, so James was sent to live with Gertrude. With no friends to speak of, he had plenty of time to study, and he did well during his first years in high school.

He was especially fond of science. Well past the time when most boys give up that sort of thing, he continued to play with the chemistry set he received for Christmas the year he was 9. One day toward spring of his last year of high school, when his cousin Betty was home with her "monthlies," she lifted her skirt and offered to let James touch her. "He came and told me about it immediately," says Gertrude. "He said it made him feel nauseated." The entire family felt relieved when she was hospitalized the following day, her diagnosis of schizophrenia notwithstanding.

For the next several months, James seemed to slip into decline. When his grades fell and his aunt asked why, he only shrugged. He showed no interest in either going to college or getting a job. He spent most of his free time reading chemistry texts, making copious notes in the margins. Some mornings, when his aunt awakened in the early hours, she thought she heard him walking around in his room. Several times she heard him laughing to himself. He took to sleeping late, often past noon; gradually he stopped going to school at all.

That summer Betty returned from the hospital, vastly improved on antipsychotic medication. Within a week she confided to her mother that James had warned her not to take the drug. It was part of a plot by Mormons, he had told her, to make her sterile. Several times during the next 2 months, he lectured her about extraterrestrials.

James stopped eating much of anything and lost at least 20 pounds. Weight loss and sleep disturbance made him look gaunt and older. Then, just before Thanksgiving, he broke the window and cut himself; he was finally admitted to the same hospital where Betty had been a patient.

Apart from his lack of friends and his separation from his parents, James's early life hasn't been remarkable. He experimented with marijuana a few times, but never used other street drugs or alcohol. He smoked about a pack of cigarettes a day. His only medical problem had been an operation for an umbilical hernia when he was 5. Besides Betty, the family history was positive for alcoholism in his paternal grandfather and hyperthyroidism in both his father and an uncle. His mother had been "nervous."

Thin and sallow, James looks several years older than his age. He is dressed in tattered, cut-off blue jean shorts and a T-shirt. In tennis shoes with no laces, he scuffles slowly into the interview room, head down, not even glancing up. Though his facial expression is a blank, he occasionally laughs and cocks an ear to one side. He initially denies that he is hearing voices, but later in the day admits to a different interviewer that a woman keeps telling him to "jack off." He denies having any delusions, including grandeur or persecution. Asked directly about a Mormon conspiracy to sterilize his cousin, he says he isn't at liberty to discuss it.

James claims not to be depressed or suicidal; he says he broke the window and lacerated his arm because he was "upset." He scores 28 out of 30 on the MMSE (he cannot give the name of the hospital and misses the date by several days). Although he agrees that he needs medical attention for his arm, he has no insight about his mental condition.

Evaluation of James Chatterton

James has symptoms in three areas of clinical interest: psychotic thinking, somatic symptoms, and social and personality problems. The somatic symptoms (which include loss of appetite and weight loss), plus a family history of hyperthyroidism, should lead his clinician to consider a general medical condition as a possible cause of his psychosis (principle C). Upon admission, he would receive a complete physical exam and relevant laboratory testing, which would include thyroid tests. For the purposes of this discussion, however, we will assume the absence of thyroid disease.

In this discussion of James's psychotic thinking, I'll follow the outline of the section in Chapter 2 called "F20.9 Schizophrenia" (p. 63). First, we must consider the extent of symptoms: Does James have enough of them to meet criterion A for schizophrenia? His active psychotic symptoms include persecutory delusions (the Mormon plot, extraterrestrials) and the hallucinated woman's voice giving him commands. These two symptoms by themselves would be enough, but he also had the negative symptom of loss of volition (his grades declined, and he showed no interest in work or college).

Although his behavior suggests otherwise, James at first denies hearing voices. This demonstrates the value of principle J (signs beat symptoms), which is confirmed later when he admits that he does in fact have auditory hallucinations. Laughing to himself (possibly responding to something funny his hallucinated voices said?) and having a relative with schizophrenia (principle B) also point strongly to a diagnosis of schizophrenia.

The course of a psychotic disorder is extremely important in determining diagnosis. James's disorder began gradually, without known precipitating factors such as drug use or a traumatic event, and progressed steadily with neither remission nor recovery. That doesn't constitute a criterion, but it sure sounds like a typical story for schizophrenia. Here's the criterion (DSM-5-TR schizophrenia criterion C, actually): Including the prodromal period when he began to withdraw and show lack of volition, he has been ill longer than 6 months—from about April to November. Premorbid personality is discussed below.

The consequences are also severe enough for a diagnosis of schizophrenia: They markedly interfere with James's social life and his attendance at school (criterion B). With this many typical symptoms of schizophrenia, we become increasingly persuaded that this should be the diagnosis (principle Q).

The rest of our job vis-à-vis the schizophrenia criteria is just to rule out other diagnoses. The possibility of another medical condition causing psychotic symptoms has already been discussed and dismissed (DSM-5-TR criterion E for schizophrenia). James has tried marijuana a few times but hasn't used substances enough to account for his remarkable deterioration (also criterion E). He scores 2 points short of perfect on the MMSE, well above the range expected for a cognitive disorder. James has lost weight, sleeps poorly, and cut his wrist on glass, all of which sounds like a mood disorder. However, he denies feeling depressed, his affect at times is inappropriate, and he claims that the wrist cutting was not a suicide attempt. So, I'd dismiss mood disorders, even though, for safety reasons, they should always appear toward the top of a differential diagnoses (principle A).

Finally, we must consider social and personality problems. According to his aunt, from the time he was a little boy, James has been identified by others as "different." He is emotionally distant (schizoid personality disorder criterion A1), doesn't care what others think (A6), has no close friends (A5), shows few expressions of emotion (A7), and prefers solitary activities (A2). We have only Gertrude's perspective on his lack of interest in sex, but even so, he has one symptom more than the required four for schizoid personality disorder. He also has had some ideas of reference (the other children might be talking about him)—a symptom of schizotypal personality disorder—but his aunt does not report other odd beliefs or peculiar speech or behaviors; James is generally more aloof than peculiar. The absence of any other symptoms of suspiciousness also rules out paranoid personality disorder.

James has not yet been ill with active-phase symptoms for a year, so he can receive no course specifier. I have already noted his personality disorder, to which the qualifier *(premorbid)* would be added because it was present long before his schizophrenia became manifest.

James does have a notable problem with sleep, but should it receive an independent diagnosis? He would meet most of the criteria for insomnia disorder with non-sleep-disorder comorbidity (there's a mouthful!), but it was neither the predominant complaint nor a major focus for treatment. Persistent insomnia of this sort tends to normalize once the underlying psychosis has been successfully treated, so it doesn't require special clinical attention and receives no independent diagnosis. With a GAF score of 20, James's full diagnosis is:

F20.9	Schizophrenia
F60.1	Schizoid personality disorder (premorbid)
S61.519A	Laceration of wrist

You may have noticed that at the start of my evaluation of James, I mentioned "areas of clinical interest." Well, what are those?

Many years ago, I thought it would aid explanation to divide all the symptoms you might encounter in patients into groups. I ended up with seven groups, three of which were *psychotic thinking, somatic symptoms,* and *social and personality problems.* Here are the rest: *mood symptoms, anxiety symptoms, cognitive problems,* and *substance use.* I've written much, much more about them in my book *The First Interview,* now in its fourth edition (The Guilford Press).

Gail Downey

"Go ahead, cut!" Gail Downey lies flat on her hospital bed, staring at the ceiling. Her hair is carefully washed and combed, but her expression is stiff. "I want the lobotomy. I'll sign the papers. I can't take this anymore."

A divorcée and mom to three children, Gail looks older than her 34 years. For 5 of those years now, she has had depressions—but no manias or hypomanias. The course of her illness has been marked by frequent suicide attempts and hospitalizations. In her current episode, which has lasted just over a month, she has felt severely depressed throughout nearly every day. She complains that she lies awake each night until the early hours; she has no pep, interest, or appetite. She cries frequently, and she is so distracted by her emotional turmoil that her boss has reluctantly let her go.

Gail has been prescribed at least six antidepressants, often in combination. At first, most of these seemed to help, raising her mood enough that she could at least be discharged from the hospital. She's also responded positively to each of several courses of electroconvulsive therapy. But within a few months of each new treatment, she relapses and must return to the hospital, often with a fresh set of stitches in her wrist. While on a brief pass from the current hospitalization, she has swallowed a nearly fatal overdose of chloral hydrate.

Gail's parents divorced when she was 9; afterward, she lived with her mother. She describes her childhood as "fraught." Beginning at age 13, Gail was arrested three or four times for taking small items such as pantyhose or a tube of lipstick from department and variety stores. Each of these incidents occurred while she was especially stressed, perhaps because of problems at home or a job or personal relationship that was going south. She always notes increasing tension before taking these items and feels "nearly explosive joy" each time she leaves a store with her trophy in the pocket of her overcoat. As a juvenile, whenever she was caught, she had been remanded to the custody of her mother. As an adult, she has been wilier, seldom caught. Only once has she paid a fine. The most recent episode occurred just before the current hospitalization, which may have helped persuade the merchant to drop the charges.

Gail's medical history is a catalog of symptoms. It includes urinary retention, a lump in her throat that at times seems about to strangle her, chest pains, severe menstrual cramps, vomiting spells, chronic diarrhea, heart palpitations, migraine headaches (a neurologist called them "atypical"), and even a brief episode of blindness, from which she recovered after a few days with no special treatment. At the time of the divorce, Gail's husband confided that she had been "frigid" and often complained of pain during intercourse. Starting in her teens, she has taken medicine or consulted a physician for more than 30 such symptoms. The doctors have never found much wrong with her physically; they have either given her tranquilizers or referred her to a succession of psychiatrists.

After several years Gail was evicted from her apartment, and her husband obtained custody of their three children. The only nonmedical person she ever talks to is her mother. Now she is requesting an operation that will permanently sever some of the connections inside her brain.

Evaluation of Gail Downey

Gail has more than enough mood symptoms (low mood, loss of pleasure, insomnia, anorexia, suicidal ideas, loss of energy, trouble thinking) to qualify her current episode as a major depressive episode (you can review the features on p. 112). Any patient who presents with severe depression should be evaluated for major depressive disorder (principle F), which can be potentially life-threatening and often responds quickly to the appropriate therapy.

Gail has had numerous episodes of depression, but no manias or hypomanias and no psychotic symptoms; she has also apparently recovered for at least 2 months between episodes. She therefore qualifies for a diagnosis of major depressive disorder, recurrent. The persistent suicide attempts mark it as severe without psychotic features. The vignette does not give enough information to support other specifiers. But the fact that Gail's depression has been treated so often with such little success is a puzzle. Response to typical treatment for a disorder points in favor of it (principle S), but can we say the inverse? There's no diagnostic principle to that effect, but perhaps there should be: "Repeated failure to respond to typical treatment should prompt consideration of some other condition."

And indeed, since her teens Gail has also had a variety of somatic symptoms, at least some of which (like the migraines) were atypical. We therefore must consider somatic symptom disorder (principle D). We're going to evaluate her somatic symptoms twice; first using official DSM-5-TR criteria (p. 255), then with the old DSM-IV guidelines for somatization disorder (sidebar, p. 256). She adequately fulfills the former: at least one somatic symptom that causes marked distress and causes her to invest a great deal of time into her worries. She has been symptomatic far longer than the 6 months required, and she has experienced a high degree of anxiety relevant to her symptoms.

She also meets DSM-IV somatization disorder criteria, which I believe are far more useful for identifying actual pathology (see the relevant sidebar, p. 259). Gail's symptoms are distributed appropriately across the four groups for that diagnosis. Among the medical and neurological disorders to consider would be multiple sclerosis, spinal cord tumors, and diseases of the heart and lungs. The fact that she had been unsuccessfully treated by so many physicians reduces the likelihood that she has a series of other medical conditions (principle C). The vignette provides no evidence that Gail consciously feigns her symptoms for gain (malingering) or for less concrete motives (factitious disorder).

No additional diagnosis is needed for Gail's anorexia (principle M); any problem with maintaining body weight is not due to refusal of food but to her lack of appetite. Her insomnia could be given a separate diagnosis (insomnia disorder with non-sleep-disorder mental comorbidity) were it serious enough to warrant independent clinical evaluation; it isn't. Similarly, her sexual dysfunction would not be independently coded (even if the vignette gave enough specifics as to its exact nature), because it is easily explained as a symptom of somatic symptom disorder. Oh, and she doesn't abuse substances, so that's one more potential diagnosis to cross off our list.

Finally, Gail's history reveals a pattern of repeated shoplifting (see kleptomania, p. 398) characterized by tension and release. These features cannot be explained by anger, revenge, or some other mental disorder. Hence, we must also give her a diagnosis of kleptomania (principle V).

So, Gail has three codable mental diagnoses. How should we list them? Her major depressive disorder is serious enough that it has been the focus of treatment for at least 5 years; at the beginning of her treatment, that approach was probably sound (principle X). Now, however, that same principle X suggests something quite different: If we make somatization disorder (OK, we can call it somatic symptom disorder for the sake of DSM-5-TR) the focus of her care, it will suggest a common approach to several of her problems. With a great many somatic symptoms causing her to use medications, to experience social consequences (divorce, loss of custody, unemployment), and to suffer from depression culminating in multiple suicide attempts—a full gamut of biopsychosocial complications lasting far longer than the minimum of 6 months—Gail's clinician rates her somatic symptom disorder as both severe and persistent.

The vignette gives little information about her personality; we need to add a note to her diagnostic summary that indicates the need for further exploration. Besides, it's best to avoid diagnosing a personality disorder while depression and other matters are so acute (principle W). Considering all of her recent history, she will earn a low GAF score of 40.

F45.1	Somatic symptom disorder, persistent, severe
F33.2	Major depressive disorder, recurrent, severe without psychotic features
F63.2	Kleptomania
Z56.9	Unemployed
Z65.3	Loss of child custody
Z59.0	Eviction

Reggie Ansnes

At age 35, Reggie Ansnes is admitted to a mental hospital 3,000 miles from home. The admitting note reports that he is agitated, somewhat grandiose, and doesn't even know what city he is in. Although he talks a lot, nothing he says makes much sense. "I have schizophrenia," is one of his few unambiguous statements.

"It must be his schizophrenia," says Faye, his wife, on the telephone to the clinician who admits him. "He tells me he had it once before. We've only been married 3 years."

Five years earlier, Reggie was admitted with psychosis to a mental hospital in Boston. Faye thinks that he then believed he was the son of Jesus, but she doesn't know anything further about his symptoms. The doctor who discharged him said he had paranoid schizophrenia. He had been treated with chlorpromazine; Faye knows that because he was still taking it when they began dating.

For about 2 years after that hospitalization, Reggie was somewhat depressed. He used to complain of trouble concentrating at work, and Faye thinks that not long after the hospital released him, he might have had some suicidal ideas. However, the depression gradually remitted, leaving him relatively mild problems with appetite and sleep. Even those resolved by the time they got married, and he has been just fine ever since. It's now been several years since he took any medication at all.

For several days before Reggie's recent business trip, he had been unusually cheerful. He talked a lot, had loads of energy, and arose early to tackle the work he would miss while he was gone.

Faye says that her husband is in good physical health except for a "slight thyroid condition," for which he takes a low dose of a thyroid medication. She thought it had been checked the last time he visited his doctor, 3 months ago. She is certain that he neither drinks nor uses drugs.

During his first 24 hours in the hospital, Reggie is extremely hyperactive and doesn't sleep at all. His mood is markedly elevated, and he speaks so rapidly that he is often unintelligible. What statements could be understood include, "I am the son of

God," and he shares some ideas for improving the operation of the health care facility. He pays little attention to whatever task might be at hand, so cannot finish the MMSE.

Evaluation of Reggie Ansnes

Thyroid disease is a general medical condition that can cause mood symptoms; however, Reggie's physician recently evaluated his thyroid condition, and it had never before produced symptoms that resembled his current condition. Reevaluation of thyroid function tests would be a reasonable course to follow, in any event (principle C).

As for substance use, Faye's information would militate against substance-induced psychotic disorder, with onset during withdrawal. However, the blood toxicity screen should rule out any possibility of such a psychosis with onset during intoxication (such as phencyclidine intoxication). With the other history available, this is unlikely in the extreme. It is much more usual for patients to use alcohol to attenuate the uncomfortable, driven feeling caused by mania or a psychosis.

A mood disorder is a much stronger candidate. Five years earlier, Reggie had grandiose delusions; afterward, he was depressed for months. After a 2-year period when he seemed completely well, he had once again become psychotic, with elevated mood, hyperactivity, insomnia (decreased need for sleep), and distractibility. Assuming that the tests for thyroid function and toxicity screen come back normal, he will completely fulfill the Essential Features of a manic episode (p. 123), and thus for bipolar I disorder, current episode manic (p. 126). If you like, you can check out these criteria in DSM-5-TR—it's tedious, but great exercise.

The previous history of schizophrenia might appear to provide a readymade diagnosis for this obviously psychotic patient. If Reggie's earlier illness really had been schizophrenia, it would have been in full remission until the current episode. This would be highly unusual, and with mood symptoms as prominent then as they are now, his new history demands a serious rethink (principle H). Furthermore, no matter how psychotic Reggie might appear now, his history of episodic illness with complete recovery virtually compels (principle G) us to diagnose bipolar I disorder. An apparent mood disorder now and schizophrenia years ago would also violate the parsimony rule (principle M), not to mention the basic criteria for schizophrenia.

Reggie's current manic symptoms are markedly disabling; severe is the only appropriate level for him. His psychotic features are completely congruent with manic themes—he thinks he is the son of God—which dictates the code numbers listed below. The other possible specifiers (Table 3.3, p. 167) do not apply. His previous schizophrenia diagnosis was simply wrong and should be expunged (as far as possible) from his records. On admission, his GAF score was a low 30; by discharge, his GAF has rebounded to 90.

F31.2	Bipolar I disorder, current episode manic, severe with mood-congruent psychotic features
E03.9	Acquired hypothyroidism

Reena Walters

Reena Walters is more than happy to tell her story to the handful of students who have gathered around her. In the 4 days she's been hospitalized (this time), she has mainly sat around waiting on many tests.

"It's an aneurysm, I'm afraid," she tells the class with a wry smile. "I had a seizure on Christmas Day, right as we were about to carve the turkey, and instead I ended up here. As a pediatrician, I've got lots better things to do."

"But how did you come to be here, on the locked unit?" the student interviewer wants to know.

Reena settles comfortably into her chair. "It's the only ward in the hospital that has no TVs in the rooms." The students look perplexed. "They're afraid my seizures will be exacerbated by television flicker," she explains patiently. "You're familiar with the phenomenon of induced seizures, right? Good. Over the years, I had a couple of kid patients with the same problem. Never dreamed I'd someday be the one affected." She is controlled pretty well now on medication—the name of which she can't recall right now.

Reena continues her story. She grew up near Modesto, the daughter of itinerant farm workers who made their living picking fruit and hoeing tomatoes. Because the family moved around a good deal, by age 18 she'd attended "literally dozens of different schools." But a scholarship committee at her last high school had plucked her from the fields and sent her off to college. From there, her intelligence and her determination to escape her parents' lifestyle carried her through medical school in southern California and into a career of caring for children. She has been instrumental, she remarks with evident pride, in developing one of the definitive tests for cystic fibrosis in neonates. "I believe it was my finest hour," she almost whispers. Now 59, her chief regret is that a botched D&C and subsequent hysterectomy when she was in her early 30s meant she could never have children of her own.

But now, the student interviewer has bogged down, unsure what to ask next. "Maybe you'd like to hear about my family," Reena prompts with a kind smile. She tells about her father (a quiet, gentle man who never spoke a cross word) and her mother (still living at 97, a saint among women, who still drives her own car). Reena married twice, first to a fellow student who years ago died on a medical mission to Uganda. About 10 years later she married again, this time to a psychiatrist who still practices in the town where they live. Because of his workload, he hadn't yet been able to visit her.

"Could you tell us how you got to the hospital—I mean, what led up to it?"

Reena explains that when she has one of her seizures, she will often behave automatically. "It's called a complex partial seizure. You know? Good. I'll lose track of where I am, but my body plugs right ahead. I can walk and walk, sometimes miles. This time, they found me outside the home of an actor I used to know. The police said I was 'lurking.'" Her laughter is infectious, and after a moment the students join in.

A few minutes later, Reena now departed from the room, the instructor asks the students how they'd evaluate her. Her calm and pleasant demeanor and logical presentation seem highly persuasive to several in the class. "Perhaps, then, we should just take her story at face value," suggested the instructor. That would make hers one of the rarely encountered (on mental health wards) cases of no mental diagnosis (principle U).

On the other hand, one student points out, there was the matter of her medication, the name of which she couldn't recall despite her own status as a medical practitioner. Of course, it could have been just a senior moment, but was it instead the sort of contradictory evidence (principle O) that encourages us to rethink her whole story? Now that they consider it further, wouldn't it be possible just to turn off the television in a room on any medical ward in the hospital? Until they have more data, the students agree to consider her as undiagnosed (principle T).

During the discussion, one student has been sitting back and smiling quietly to herself. She has participated in discussions with the team that cares for Reena; now she offers context.

Yikes! About the only wholly accurate statement Reena made during this interview is her name. None of her three husbands was a physician—she is now once again divorced—and her parents have both been dead for years. She's never been to medical school, never even graduated from college. Reena herself once worked as a medical receptionist; it was there she picked up the jargon she deploys so effectively.

Reena's belief that she has a seizure disorder seems genuine (time after time, she's been closely quizzed on this issue). She can describe the early sensation of a smell of tomatoes ("from the fields of my childhood, I suppose"), followed by the sense of déjà vu that almost always precedes the prolonged periods of unconsciousness, during which she often wanders through strange neighborhoods. Over the years, she's been worked up several times for a seizure disorder, but none of her MRIs and EEGs (some with pharyngeal leads) have revealed pathology. No one has actually seen her having a seizure. (Does she then have factitious disorder, someone asks? But she's only ever been treated in one town, and at one hospital, and she hasn't been observed to manufacture symptoms. Was she malingering? If so, where's the gain?)

On the other hand, she does have a rather long rap sheet with local police. Each contact has been related to her fascination with a local actor who's had occasional success in television. For the years she's followed his career, her desire to be near him has led to half a dozen restraining orders and repeated arrests for stalking. The student ends with, "And if you ask her, she'll be happy to tell you that she's currently pregnant. Never mind her age, and the hysterectomy."

Evaluation of Reena Walters

The presence of multiple delusions for many years (delusional disorder criterion A) without ever fulfilling criterion A for schizophrenia (delusional disorder criterion B) launches this condition to the forefront of our differential diagnosis. (OK, Reena does mention the olfactory hallucination of tomatoes, but this is closely associated with her delusional seizures; this sort of hallucination doesn't really count toward fulfilling criterion A for schizophrenia and is often encountered in delusional disorder.) Outside the context of her specific delusions, her behavior and affect seem rather ordinary (C), and there is no evidence of associated mood episodes (D).

Of course, her personal history presents any number of possible confounds that we have to eliminate before making a definitive diagnosis. We'll need to learn whether she uses substances (F)—and, considering the mendacity of her other statements, that information should come from some source more reliable than she. There is no information to support a different mental condition, specifically body dysmorphic disorder or obsessive–compulsive disorder (D). As to the type of delusions, I'd say they were largely somatic (she believes she has temporal lobe epilepsy). Only hinted at are her possibly grandiose ideas of having a relationship with the actor. If you prefer a more comprehensive (but vague) classification, call the delusions mixed type. I'd rate her GAF as about 35, though I'm happy to entertain arguments. And I'd certainly support something in her summary that points the way to a full evaluation of her personality structure—but later.

F22	Delusional disorder, somatic type
Z65.3	Restraining orders for stalking

Sara Winkler

Before sitting down, Sara Winkler crosses herself three times.

She and her husband—each is 25—have been married 4 years. "I've known her since we were 16," Loren Winkler says, "and she's always been pretty careful. You know, checking the stove to see that it's turned off? Or the doors to make sure they're really locked before we go out? Only, in the last couple of years it's gotten so much worse."

Sara is a college graduate who worked briefly as a paralegal before taking time out to have a family. She is healthy and has no history of alcohol or drug use. When their son, Jonathan, was only 6 months old, she had a terrifying dream in which she plunged a paring knife into the chest of a doll as it lay on the kitchen table. But as the knife entered the plastic body, its tiny arms and legs began to move, and she saw that it was a real child. On the kitchen wall, the word KILL seemed to scroll upward before her eyes, and she awakened screaming. It had taken Loren more than an hour to calm her enough to resume sleeping.

The following evening, while slicing carrots for a salad, she suddenly had this thought: "Would I ever harm Jonathan?" Although the idea seemed absurd, it was accompanied by some of the same anxiety she had felt the night before. She took the baby in to Loren while she finished preparing dinner.

After that, thoughts of knives and of stabbing someone smaller and weaker had increasingly wormed their way into Sara's consciousness. Even if her attention was focused on reading or watching television, she might suddenly visualize the giant block letters *KILL* arising before her eyes.

The idea that she could harm Jonathan seems irrational to her, but the nagging doubt and anxiety torments her daily. She no longer trusts herself in the kitchen with him. Sometimes she can almost feel the muscles of her forearm begin to contract in the act of reaching for a knife. Although she has never followed through on one of these impulses, the thought that she *might* do so terrifies her to the point that she refuses even to open the knife drawer; any cutting must involve scissors, the food processor, or Loren.

Not long after her dream, Sara began trying to ward off her troubling thoughts and impulses. A fallen-away Catholic, she reverted to some of the practices she had known as a child. When she had one of her frightening thoughts, she initially felt comforted if she crossed herself or muttered a Hail Mary. With time, the power of these simple measures seemed to weaken. Then Sara found that if she crossed herself three times or said three Hail Marys (or any combination, in threes), she felt better. Eventually, however, she needed nine of these behaviors before she felt she had adequately protected her son and herself. When she is in public, she can cross herself once and complete the ritual by murmuring Hail Marys under her breath.

With Jonathan now nearly a year old, hours each day are consumed in Sara's repetitive thoughts and activities; Loren cooks nearly all their meals. For several weeks Sara has felt increasingly depressed; she admits that her mood is down nearly all the time, though she's had no suicidal ideas or death wishes. Nothing interests her much, and she is always tired. She has lost over 10 pounds and has insomnia; when she does get to sleep, as likely as not, she'll awaken screaming. When Loren discovers her doing penance 27 times in a row, he insists they come for help.

"I know it seems crazy," Sara says tearfully, "but I just can't seem to get these stupid ideas out of my head."

Evaluation of Sara Winkler

For longer than 2 weeks, Sara has been depressed most of the time. She also has insomnia, fatigue, decreased interest, and weight loss, all symptoms consistent with a major depressive episode. She is physically healthy (principle C) and has no history of substance use (principle E). It is hard to be sure whether she is being impaired by the depression or the symptoms of obsessive–compulsive disorder (OCD); "both" seems a reasonable conclusion. With no prior major depressive, manic, or hypomanic episodes, her diagnosis would be major depressive disorder, single episode. I'd rate the severity specifier as moderate (relatively few symptoms, no suicidal ideas, but considerable distress). There is very little risk that she will actually harm her son.

As for Sara's anxiety, she has neither panic attacks nor generalized anxiety disorder. Rather, her obsessions and compulsions fulfill the criteria for obsessive–compulsive disorder (p. 199). (Although she has another mental disorder, her obsessions are not confined to guilty ruminations related to her major depression.) Her OCD symptoms occupy more than an hour a day (criteria A and B), and she is severely distressed. No other mental or physical disorders would explain her symptoms (D, C). Clearly, Sara's worries are not just an exaggeration of a real-life problem, so her focus of concern is pathological. She recognizes that her fears are unwarranted; we'll grade her insight as pretty good.

In recording of Sara's diagnoses, the depression is listed first to indicate that her clinician regards it as the aspect that most requires clinical attention. (Others might disagree.) The severity of her rituals justifies her GAF score of 45.

F32.1	Major depressive disorder, single episode, moderate
F42.2	Obsessive–compulsive disorder, with good insight

Gemma Livingstone

"I eat, then I throw up." That's how Gemma Livingstone describes her problem during her first interview. Beginning when she was 23, this behavior has been almost continual for 4 years.

Even as a teenager, Gemma worried about her appearance. Along with high school classmates, she crash-dieted from time to time. But her weight seldom varied by more than a few pounds from 116. At 5 feet, 6 inches tall, she had been svelte, but not gaunt. Throughout her adolescence and early adulthood, she had the feeling that if she did not tightly control her eating habits, she would rapidly gain weight—"puff up like a toad," she puts it.

Dealing with the long-ago aftermath of an unwanted pregnancy and subsequent abortion, Gemma had the opportunity to test her theory. Eating what she wanted, she ballooned from a size 8 to a 14 in less than half a year. Once she finally regained control, she vowed she would never lose it again. For 3 years, she's bought nothing larger than a size 4.

Back when Gemma was a teenager, she and her friends simply didn't eat. Whenever dining in a restaurant or with friends, she would push her food around on her plate to disguise how little she was taking in. But when at home she would often consume a full meal, then retire to the bathroom and throw up. At first, this required touching the back of her throat with the handle of a teaspoon she kept in the bathroom for that purpose. With practice, she learned to regurgitate just by willing it. "It's as easy as blowing your nose," she reports.

Gemma's fear of obesity has become the organizing principle of her life. On her refrigerator door she keeps a picture of herself during her "toad" era. She says that every time she looks at it, she loses her appetite. Whereas she previously used laxatives only for constipation, recently she's begun to use them as another means of purging her system: "If I don't have a bowel movement every day, I feel as if I'll burst. Even my eyes get all puffy."

She tried diuretics but threw them out when her periods stopped. She's unsure of the connection, but recently she started to menstruate again. If there's one thing she fears more than getting fat, it is getting pregnant. She has never been very active sexually, but now she and her husband seldom have intercourse more than once a month. Even then, she insists on using both a diaphragm and a condom.

Other than her weight, which has fallen below 90 pounds, Gemma appears to be in good health. A review of systems is positive only for abdominal bloating. Although she occasionally has a day or two when she feels sad and sorry for herself, she laughs this off as "PMS" and adds that it certainly doesn't bother her now. She has never had manic episodes, hallucinations, obsessions, compulsions, phobias, panic attacks, or thoughts about suicide.

Gemma was an only child, born in Virginia Beach, where her father was stationed with the Navy. Subsequently he owned his own heating and air conditioning company; the family was reasonably well off. Gemma has no history of any kind of difficulties with learning or conduct while she was in school. She and her husband were married when she was 21, after she had worked 3 years as a bank teller. They have two children, a son, 7, and a daughter, 5.

Gemma's only brush with the law occurred 2 years ago. She'd forged some prescriptions to obtain amphetamines for dieting, but she copped a plea and rode out the year on probation. She has scrupulously avoided amphetamines since then. She tried marijuana once or twice when she was first out of high school but has never used alcohol or tobacco. Her only surgical procedure was bilateral breast augmentation (using autologous fat, not silicone).

In a separate interview, Gemma's husband states that he thinks his wife feels inadequate and insecure. She frequently dresses in revealing, even alluring clothing; her appearance is less enticing now that she has lost so much weight. When she is denied her way, she will sometimes pout for hours, though he doesn't think there is much real feeling behind this expression of emotion. "She loves to be the center of attention," he says, "but a lot of people don't buy into her act anymore. I think it frustrates her."

Gemma is a dark-haired, slightly built woman who smiles readily and somewhat self-consciously. She wears a V-necked blouse and a very short skirt that she does not try to pull down when she crosses her legs. She speaks with a good deal of eye-rolling and vocal inflections; her answers to the examiner's questions tend to be vague and often discursive. She denies feeling depressed or wishing she were dead; she has never had delusions or hallucinations, but she claims that she is still "fat as a pig." To illustrate, she pinches a fold of skin that sags from her arm. She scores a perfect 30 on the MMSE.

Evaluation of Gemma Livingstone

Gemma's history of disordered eating dates to her high school years. She bears the following features of anorexia nervosa: She is gaunt, yet fearful of gaining weight (AN criterion B), and she perceives herself as fat (C). Through the years she has taken various steps to restrict her intake of food (A). Her current subtype would be binge-eating/purging type; as a teenager, she was of the restricting type. Just how severe do we rate her anorexia? DSM-5-TR criteria grade solely based on body mass index, which in my opinion is an error; surely the type of behavior should count for something. Gemma's weight is under 90 (let's say 89), so for a height of 66 inches, her BMI works out to 14.4, putting her in the extreme category of severity.

Based only on the information she herself provides, we couldn't diagnose Gemma with a personality disorder—that's the usual clinical experience derived solely from a patient's own reports. But from her husband's information (principle I) and from that of the mental status evaluation (principle L), the following criteria for histrionic personality disorder can be established: needing to be the center of attention (1), shifting and shallow emotions (3), drawing attention with physical appearance (4), speaking vaguely (5), and expressing herself dramatically (6). Histrionic personality disorder is often associated with somatization/somatic symptom disorder, but a review of systems reveals minimal symptoms, and she didn't express the disproportionate health concerns often attached to a somatic symptom diagnosis.

Forging prescriptions and using drugs are of course illegal, but Gemma hasn't pursued either behavior since her probation; I don't regard them as evidence of current diagnosable pathology. With a GAF score of 45, her complete diagnosis would read:

F50.02	Anorexia nervosa, binge-eating/purging type, extreme
F60.4	Histrionic personality disorder

Edith Roman

Seventy-six-year-old Edith Roman enters the hospital on this complaint from Sylvia, her daughter: "She's been depressed since her stroke." Beginning about a year ago, Edith has become forgetful. This was first apparent when for 3 weeks out of 4 she neglected to place her Friday night telephone call to Sylvia, who at that time lived several hundred miles away. Each time, when Sylvia made the call herself, Edith seemed surprised to hear from her.

When she finally took a week off work for a visit, Sylvia discovered that Edith had also been neglecting the grocery shopping and housework: The sink was full, the refrigerator nearly empty, and dust blanketed everything. Although Edith's speech and physical appearance had remained about the same, something was clearly wrong. By the end of the week, Sylvia had the answer from a neurologist: early Alzheimer's disease. She stayed over an extra week to move Edith across the state and into her own home. A companion was hired to stay with Edith when Sylvia worked.

This arrangement worked well for several months. Edith's deterioration was gradual and minimal, until the stroke left her limping and unable to remember words. Then her memory was worse than ever; then her depression began. Now, when Edith talks at all, she complains to the companion about how useless and lonely she feels. She sleeps poorly, eats very little, cries often, and says she is a burden.

Edith was born in St. Louis, where until she was 12, her parents ran a small dry-cleaning business. Then her father died and her mother soon married Edith's paternal uncle, who came equipped with two teenagers of his own. They all got along quite well.

Edith graduated from high school, got married, and had her only child. Throughout life, she has been pleasant and spunky, interested in crafts and many other aspects of homemaking. After her husband died, she continued to be active in her social and bridge clubs. Until a year ago, her physical health had been good; she has never used alcohol or tobacco.

An elderly woman dressed in a cotton nightgown and a quilted wrap, Edith sits upright on the edge of her bed, her left hand lying useless in her lap. She makes good eye contact with the examiner; although she doesn't say much spontaneously, she does respond to all questions. Her speech is clear, though she sometimes struggles to find the words she wants. Asked to identify a magazine, she thinks for a moment, then calls it "this papers." She admits to feeling depressed, says that she sees no future for herself, and hopes she can die soon. She denies ever experiencing hallucinations or delusions. On the MMSE, she scores only 16 out of a possible 30.

Evaluation of Edith Roman

The symptoms of Edith's major neurocognitive disorder include failing memory and deteriorating ability to care for herself (p. 503). These symptoms, which began gradually and were gradually worsening, added to the fact (then) of no other cause for her NCD, fulfill criteria for probable Alzheimer's disease (p. 512). But then she had her stroke. At that point, her memory abruptly deteriorated still further, and she developed aphasia (she couldn't think of certain words she wanted to use). She maintained eye contact and appeared to focus her attention on the examiner—evidence against delirium. A neurological exam earlier found no evidence of other medical conditions that might better explain her symptoms.

For far longer than 2 weeks, Edith has also had symptoms of depression. These include constantly depressed mood, loss of appetite and sleep, death wishes, and the feeling of being a burden (more or less equivalent to a sense of worthlessness). Her symptoms would seem to qualify for major depressive episode, which we should diagnose whenever relevant, despite the presence of other disorders (principles F, V). However, because of the presumed etiology (Alzheimer's and neurovascular disease), we will code her depression as due to another medical condition—namely NCD.

Edith's NCD has two causes, each in its own way creating difficulties with communicating and everyday functioning—for Edith and for Sylvia. Because of the peculiarities of the scoring system (ICD-10), we have to record the Alzheimer's and vascular etiologies separately; each earns a severity rating of moderate. (If you thought "severely" affected, I wouldn't fight you on it.) Her depressive symptoms rate the specifier *with behavioral disturbance*. Her GAF score will be 31.

A funny thing happened on the way to Edith Roman's diagnosis: It got tangled in a DSM-5-TR contradiction. The criteria for probable Alzheimer's dementia (p. 690 of DSM-5-TR) state that there must be clear evidence of decline, steady progression, and no evidence of mixed etiology, using cerebrovascular disease as an example. But the criteria for NCD due to multiple etiologies (p. 731 of DSM-5-TR) give as an example vascular NCD plus Alzheimer's! Now that Edith has had a stroke that contributes to her NCD, do we have to reduce her Alzheimer's diagnosis to "possible"? Not to worry; we'll do what's best for the patient and give both diagnoses anyway. Anyone want to complain? See me after class.

G30.9	Alzheimer's disease
F02.B3	Major neurocognitive disorder due to probable Alzheimer's disease, moderate, with depression
F01.B3	Major vascular neurocognitive disorder, moderate, with depression

Clara Widdicombe

Clara Widdicombe has been overweight for a long time, but now, at age 14, she is round-faced and puffy. For all that, she seemed to have been making good progress (with both school and puberty) until one evening when she suddenly began talking, her mother reports, "a blue streak." She insisted that her parents stay up with her to talk about "my agenda." At first, her mood was high, but she became angry when her father said he wanted to go to bed. Within hours, Clara became so agitated that she required hospitalization on a closed ward for adults.

Clara stands 5 feet, 3 inches tall and weighs 211 pounds, which gives her a BMI of 37—well exceeding the level considered obese. Her blood pressure is consistently above 230/110. When she undresses, the hospital staff can see that the skin of her abdomen bears reddened stretch marks they refer to as striae.

For the next several days, Clara's mood is elevated, and she needs little sleep. Even when interrupted, she won't stop talking longer than a few moments. Over and over, she claims to be the mother of Jesus; she's divined the solution to many problems—AIDS, sin, and climate change. She has flight of ideas; she admits that her thoughts race. It is impossible to interrupt her for longer than a moment, and hard to get her attention at all. At one point, she starts to undress in front of visitors—immodest behavior that is completely out of character for her.

Clara has no previous personal history of depression or mania, and her family history is negative for mood disorder. What she does have is an abnormal serum cortisol level. An endocrinologist recommends an MRI, which reveals a pituitary adenoma.

After its surgical removal, she no longer requires psychotropic medications.

Clara becomes euthymic and returns to school.

Evaluation of Clara Widdicombe

Of course, after a successful operation that yields the desired outcome, it's easy to attribute mood symptoms to a tumor. The trick is to make the connection before surgery, and before too many months or years have elapsed. Clara's age at onset (young for bipolar disorder), her appearance (typical "moon" face, marked overweight, classical abdominal striations) are diagnostic giveaways. Other patients have been less fortunate.

During the week of Clara's mental symptoms, she is in turns euphoric and irritable, *and* she has increased goal-directed activity, both of which are required for a manic episode due to another medical condition (criterion A). She has numerous symptoms of mania—she speaks rapidly, needs little sleep, is grandiose, and is even delusional in that she thinks she is Jesus's mother—but a full symptom list isn't required for this diagnosis. Although we might infer from her inability to connect with other people that she is distractible, there isn't enough detail here to diagnose delirium (D). As far as the severity of her symptoms, she suffers from all three consequences mentioned (E): psychosis, hospitalization, and impaired functioning.

Finally, I don't see evidence of another mental disorder (C)—do you? High on the list of her differential diagnoses would be bipolar I disorder, but that requires us first to rule out other medical conditions and substance-induced mood disorders. And this brings us back to her pituitary tumor and Cushing's syndrome, which are well known to produce manic symptoms (B). On admission, I'd give her a GAF score of 25.

Once the final diagnosis is made, her clinicians must determine which (if any) of the possible specifiers she has. Her episode replicates full mania, so I'm going to go with . . .

D35.2	Pituitary adenoma
E24.9	Cushing's syndrome
F06.33	Bipolar and related disorder due to Cushing's syndrome, with manic-like episode

A handful of other medical conditions can produce symptoms of mania (see the chart in Appendix A).

Clara's presentation is perhaps unusual in that she fulfills the DSM-5-TR symptomatic requirements for manic episode. That's unusual? Probably, in that patients who have euphoria and overactivity often lack other qualifying symptoms—grandiosity, decreased need for sleep, pressured speech, flight of ideas, and distractibility. Meeting this need for discrimination, ICD-10 allows us to choose a specifier that reflects the presence (with manic-like episode) or absence (with manic features) of the full diagnostic criteria. This was not possible in DSM-IV, representing another benefit courtesy of the international community.

Jeremy Dowling

"I feel miserable," is the chief complaint of Jeremy Dowling, a 24-year-old graduate student. For this lifelong perfectionist, his thesis deadline a fortnight off isn't improving matters. He is weeks behind schedule, partly because he needs to edit every paragraph into a state of perfection—before he begins to write the next.

Most of the time since his teen years, he has felt "not good enough" and somewhat depressed. He has never had a manic episode. He is socially withdrawn and claims never to take much pleasure in things. "I'm a pessimist, more or less," he says.

Jeremy says his appetite is fine, and he has never had suicidal ideas. His sleep, however, is another matter. With the approaching thesis deadline, he feels he must stay up most nights to complete his work. To that end, he drinks coffee. Lots of coffee. "If I get less than 8 hours sleep a night, I drink a cup every 2 or 3 hours. When I'm up all night, it's four or five cups. Strong coffee." Caffeine aside, he denies ever misusing substances such as alcohol or street drugs.

Jeremy has stayed up all night the last 3 nights, so it's understandable that he always felt tired. He also admits to chronic feelings of guilt and irritability. He has never had crying spells, but his concentration is "a lifelong major problem." For example, while working at the computer, other thoughts and worries intrude, to the point that he has trouble getting his work done.

Jeremy also complains of anxiety. Toward the end of supper, for example, he begins to worry about the amount of work he needs to do. A knot will tighten in his stomach, and the world seems to close in. Time of day little affects how he feels, but he usually improves briefly once he turns in a term paper or other major assignment. He denies ever having problems with shortness of breath, muscle twitching, or palpitations of his heart—unless he's had an extraordinarily large amount of coffee. Then, he will notice that he feels nervous and, often, has an upset stomach. Sometimes, these symptoms keep him home from class. But he has no feelings of impending doom or disaster.

Though Jeremy has always been a list maker, he doesn't describe any obsessional thinking or compulsive behavior. ("I do sometimes straighten out my sock drawer," he is scrupulous to point out.) He describes himself as a person who's always had difficulty making decisions, even to the point that he cannot discard worthless things he no longer needs—even an Easter basket from when he was 10.

Jeremy was born in Brazil, where his father had been studying insects of the rain forest. When he was 4, the family returned to live in southern California. His mother is a professional harpist; she has been in therapy with one counselor or another for 25 years. She has always been somewhat dour, never getting much pleasure out of life. When Jeremy was 16, she obtained a divorce, because, she says, her husband never seemed committed to their relationship. Still later, an antidepressant medication "turned her life around," and now she seemed happy for the first time in her life. It is partly at her urging that Jeremy now seeks treatment.

Several maternal relatives were depressed, including a cousin who'd killed himself by drinking antifreeze. Another relative had also committed suicide, but Jeremy doesn't know the details.

While in high school, Jeremy was "born again"; since then he's attended a fundamentalist church. He so strongly condemns his father for living with another woman without marrying her that, for over 2 years, father and son haven't spoken. Jeremy's only physical problem, he claims, is biting his nails. He has never had any legal difficulties.

He has a serious girlfriend, and they are "trying very hard" to refrain from overcommitting themselves sexually until they can marry.

Jeremy is a tall, rather gangling man whose haggard face and baggy eyes make him look almost aged. Although he moves normally and smiles readily, prominent worry lines are emerging on his forehead. His speech is clear, coherent, and relevant. Most of his spontaneous speech concerns his unfinished thesis; he denies any death wishes or suicidal ideas. He is fully oriented, has an excellent fund of information, and can calculate quickly. His recent and remote memory are unimpaired and his insight and judgment are excellent. "Life is too meaningful," he offers by way of summary, "and I'm wasting it."

Evaluation of Jeremy Dowling

In evaluating mood symptoms, the first business at hand is to determine whether either a major depressive episode or a manic episode has ever been present. Jeremy comes close to satisfying criteria for the former: He has been "somewhat depressed" for a long time, perhaps most of his adult life. This depression is present most of the time, so that he never takes much pleasure in things. He feels chronically guilty and has poor concentration and low self-esteem. However, from history and direct observation he's had no problems with appetite or weight, or any suicidal ideas, and his level of psychomotor activity has never been in question. Although he does complain of fatigue, this symptom appears related to his coffee drinking. His family history is strongly positive for a mood disorder (his mother had been depressed but she improved with treatment, and two relatives committed suicide).

Jeremy has four symptoms (five required) of major depressive episode, and two symptoms (two required) of persistent depressive disorder (PPD). So we have to ask: Is it reasonable to insist that a patient exactly fulfill the criteria? After all, Jeremy nearly meets criteria for major depressive episode, and his family history is strongly positive. A diagnosis of major depressive disorder would point the way to treatment and alert clinicians to possible worsening symptoms (such as suicidal ideas) later. But perhaps it is more important to emphasize the prolonged course of Jeremy's symptoms, which seem almost to shade into a personality disorder (see below). PDD often sets the stage for later major depressive disorder, and DSM-5-TR criteria have blended them anyway, by explicitly stating that even a full major depressive disorder can be diagnosed as a specifier for PDD.

I wouldn't invest a lot of time in this argument—where two excellent diagnosticians may disagree forever, and where you can see the benefits of judging a patient not by (obsessively) counting symptoms but matching to a prototype of an idealized patient. We'll proceed to give him a diagnosis that will promote effective treatment.

There's also the matter of Jeremy's anxiety symptoms. He has never had actual anxiety attacks, phobias, obsessions, or compulsions. But he certainly has been anxious. He worries about a variety of issues—school, his personality, the intensity of his relationship with his girlfriend. He complains of fatigue, troubles with his sleep, and concentration, which would seem (barely) enough to qualify for a diagnosis of generalized anxiety disorder. However, these symptoms have occurred during a mood disorder, leading his clinician to feel that no concurrent anxiety diagnosis is needed. (Jeremy even fails to fulfill the requirements for the mood specifier *with anxious distress;* p. 158). Besides, his anxiety symptoms could be all bound up with his caffeinism, so I'd not add this extra dollop of diagnostic verbiage.

As for substance use, although Jeremy has never used alcohol or street drugs, his high dose of coffee (caffeine intoxication criterion A) on many occasions produces nervousness (B2), upset stomach (B7), palpitations (B10), muscle twitching (B6), and insomnia (B4). These symptoms are sometimes serious enough that he cannot go to school (C). If we can agree that he is otherwise well (D), these symptoms qualify him for a diagnosis of caffeine intoxication. You might wonder about a diagnosis of caffeine use disorder, but that's a step beyond what DSM-5-TR will currently allow. His usage does make one wonder, though.

Finally, self-described as a perfectionistic pessimist who chronically feels he isn't good enough, Jeremy is also a maker of lists and a straightener of drawers who has trouble making decisions and can't discard things. These features, plus his moralistic condemnation of his father, are characteristic of obsessive–compulsive personality disorder. I'll leave the (obsessive) counting of his symptoms as an exercise.

Jeremy's persistent depressive disorder appears to have begun years ago, probably when he was still a teenager. His hypersomnia and increased appetite would qualify him for the specifier *with atypical features* (p. 159), except that I can't identify any evidence of mood reactivity in the vignette. We'll use a Z-code to note a psychosocial/environmental problem, because it could affect management, at least for the next couple of weeks. The GAF score of 65 we'll assign based on his combined disorders.

F34.1	Persistent depressive disorder, early onset, with intermittent major depressive episodes, with current episode
F15.920	Caffeine intoxication
F60.5	Obsessive–compulsive personality disorder
Z55.9	Academic problem (thesis deadline)

Cookie Coates

Upon admission to the mental health unit, Cookie Coates, a 23-year-old single woman, says she is "seeing spiders."

According to old records, the doctor had arrived late for Cookie's birth, which a nurse had tried to hold back by pressure on her head. "I don't know if it would have made any difference, anyway," her mother reportedly told a social worker at the time. "I had measles during my pregnancy."

Whatever the cause, Cookie's development was slow. She walked at 18 months, spoke words at 2 years, and formed sentences at 3. A withdrawn, frightened child, she clung too tightly to her mother even to be left with a babysitter. She didn't start school until she was nearly 7. With an IQ in the low 70s, she attended special classes for her first 2 years. Then special education funds were curtailed in her district, and she was mainstreamed.

In her early school years, Cookie developed a reputation for biting and kicking other children. When she was 11, she was repeatedly disciplined for stealing (and eating) lunches belonging to other children. At about the same time, she began to pull out her hair. Usually, it was only a few strands at a time from the front of her head, but she would work away at it throughout the day. By the end of the school day, there would be little accumulations of hair all around her desk.

However, it was Cookie's persistent tendency to hurt and mutilate herself that first brought her into mental health care. At 9, she bit her lip until it bled. The following year, she gradually fell into the habit of banging her forearms on the edge of a table; this produced chronic swelling and bruising, and eventually a constantly oozing sore. When she was 13, she cut long troughs in her face with a razor and then rubbed dirt into the wounds, producing permanent, hypertrophic scars.

Several of these episodes prompted admission to mental health facilities. Mostly, these were short stays—her behavior usually improved when closely observed—but once, when she was 16 and had set fire to her pantyhose, she was kept for 4 months. During this admission it came to light that from the age of 7, Cookie had been sexually molested almost weekly by her father and two older brothers. She was subsequently admitted to the first in a series of group homes for persons with developmental disabilities.

Cookie's pattern at each of these facilities is to form an immediate, strong relationship with one or more staff members, especially males. Typically, she will call one of them "Daddy." When a staff member disappoints her (as each inevitably does), she proclaims her hatred for that staffer. Her animosity can last for weeks, during which she sometimes sulks and claims to be depressed; at other times, she will become enraged and throw things in her room. Or she might accuse her counselors of conspiring to drive her crazy, so they can return her to the hospital. As she becomes more familiar with a facility, she will request special privileges (extra food at supper, staying up late) and injure herself in some dramatic way when these favors are not forthcoming.

Eventually, Cookie's acting out takes a sexual turn. During parties or other activities with patients from the men's group home, she will lie with her head in the lap of nearly any male patient or run her hand between his thighs. Repeated cautions from her own staff counselors do nothing to eliminate this behavior; she only becomes more cautious about where and when she does it. Most of the men do not complain.

Also in the various group homes, she sometimes eats in binges. Habitually a big eater, at times she will also eat leftovers from the plates of others when they are finished; often she volunteers to clear away the table, even when it is not her turn for KP. None of the staffers who provided information to the admitting clinician is aware of any self-induced vomiting or use of laxatives. And they described her usual activity level as "couch potato."

On admission to the unit, Cookie is an obese woman wearing sweatshirt and sweatpants and no makeup. She fiddles with strands of her hair; although she does not pull any out during the interview, her scalp bears small patches of near-baldness. She denies feeling a sense of either tension or relief as regards her hair pulling, and she doesn't show evidence of distress about it. Displaying no unusual physical movements, she sits quietly and cooperates with the examiner. She says that she feels "hopeless"; her affect is generally appropriate to the content of these thoughts. She speaks slowly and does not volunteer information, but she always responds to questions. Her thinking is sequential and goal-oriented, with no evidence of loose associations.

Cookie reports occasionally seeing "showers of spiders" falling from the ventilator duct in the ceiling of her bedroom. For several years she has intermittently heard voices directing her to harm herself. She tends to notice the voices when she is unhappy. They are quite clearly audible, are not the voices of anyone she knows, and are located within her own head. Upon close questioning, she agrees that they could be her own thoughts. She does not think anyone else can hear them. She talks freely about the sexual abuse she suffered from her father and brothers and describes it in graphic (and seemingly accurate) detail. However, she offers no evidence of either reliving or repressing these experiences.

Cookie scores 28 out of 30 on the MMSE (she remembers only two of three objects at 5 minutes, and she misses the correct date by several days). Although she maintains good attention, she can perform only very simple calculations. She recognizes that there is something wrong with her, but attributes it to others: her parents and a worker at her previous residence who had "dissed" her by laughing when she said she heard voices. She does not believe she needs to be in the hospital and says that she would like to get her own apartment and a job waiting tables.

Evaluation of Cookie Coates

Cookie presents with a wide variety of clinical problems and symptoms, potentially encompassing psychotic, mood, anxiety, impulse-control, eating, and personality disorders, as well as low intellectual functioning. Let's consider that last factor first.

Cookie's IQ scores are consistently in the low 70s. She performs well on the MMSE and has no problems with attention, so she will not qualify for delirium or a major or minor neurocognitive disorder. In her clinician's judgment, the extent of her deficits (problems with self-care, home living, social/interpersonal skills, self-direction, and safety) warrant a diagnosis of mild intellectual developmental disorder.

Cookie also reports feeling hopeless and depressed, but these symptoms appear to be transitory, reactive to her immediate circumstances; to some extent, they seem manipulative. Her psychotic symptoms (seeing spiders, hearing voices) do not carry the conviction of true hallucinations: They often occur when she is unhappy (principle K), and she agrees that the voices could be her own thoughts. She has no loose associations, catatonic behavior, or negative symptoms typical of schizophrenia. In fact, no diagnosis of psychosis appears justified. Although she has abnormal eating behavior, she isn't distressed about it, and she has no history of vomiting or inappropriate use of laxatives or diuretics; her self-evaluation does not overemphasize her weight or body shape. One clinician who reviewed the case felt that her history had some of the features of posttraumatic stress disorder, but she has no history of reliving the sexual abuse she endured as a child.

Cookie's acting out (biting, kicking, hair pulling, and stealing) do not appear to be part of a larger problem with violating societal norms or the rights of others, ruling out conduct disorder. The hair pulling is not associated with stress, and there is no information that she has tried to stop doing it, so we won't diagnose trichotillomania. Self-injury can be encountered in stereotypic movement disorder, but Cookie's behavior doesn't appear to be repetitive and stereotypical. As a small child, she might have qualified for a diagnosis of disinhibited social engagement disorder (because of the excessive readiness to approach strangers), but we don't have information enough for that diagnosis, even in retrospect—and it is no longer a problem.

And so, having ruled out major mental disorders as the cause of these behaviors, we can now consider a personality disorder (principle W). Indeed, most of her self-destructive behaviors seemed well explained by borderline personality disorder (BPD). Beginning in her teens and affecting many life areas, the relevant symptoms include self-harm, intense interpersonal relations (those with various staff members), impulsivity (eating, sexual acting out), reactive mood (temper tantrums), and paranoid ideation. It is a model of instability and suggests the wisdom of the term used in other parts of the world, *emotionally unstable personality disorder.* Although Cookie by no means has every symptom of BPD, those she does report I'd call severe. Her GAF score of 30 reflects an amalgam of all her difficulties.

F70	Intellectual developmental disorder, mild
F60.3	Borderline personality disorder, severe
E66.9	Obesity

Dean Wannamaker

"I keep hearing voices that I can't turn off," Dean Wannamaker complains. They bother him every day, and he isn't sure how much longer he can stand it. Dean is 54, but he first heard voices when he was in his early 40s. In fact, he has been hospitalized on three separate occasions; each time he has been successfully treated with medication. It's now been over 6 years since he was last hospitalized.

"They're in my head, but they sound just as loud and clear as a radio," Dean says. The voices are mostly male, but there are a few women as well; none of them sounds at all familiar. They speak only phrases, not sentences, and they try to order him around. They'll tell him it is time to go home or that it will be OK to have another drink. "Mostly, they seem to be looking out for me." He thinks this time, they've been talking for about 3 weeks.

Dean admits that he's a drinker. He began with sweet wine when 12. In the military he had a few fights that were fueled by beer, and once he was threatened with court-martial. In the end, he managed to "escape with an honorable discharge." Over the years, he's been arrested several times for driving while under the influence of alcohol; the most recent time was 2 weeks ago.

Dean's usual pattern is to drink heavily for several months, then stop suddenly and stay dry for years. His three previous benders occurred 3, 5, and 11 years earlier. The one 11 years ago culminated in his wife walking out on him for good; she was tired of paying his traffic tickets and supporting him when he got fired for missing work. But he had a girlfriend then, Annie—the same woman he's with now—so he didn't mind so much about his wife. What he remembers most vividly is the time he heard voices for nearly 3 months. "It was enough to drive a man to drink," he comments, without a drop of irony.

On the present occasion, the IRS supplied the drive. He makes good money at his trade (he is a meat cutter), and, while he was in the coils of his last bender 3 years earlier, he had apparently neglected to report some of it. Now he is being dunned for back taxes, interest, and penalties, and he doesn't have a single record or receipt to fall back on.

"I didn't intend to start drinking," he says of his current binge. "I only meant to take a drink." Now he has been drinking over a quart of bourbon a day for 2 months. Annie adds that he never looks drunk; and she confirms that he only has these hallucinations after he's quit drinking for "a while."

The middle of three children, Dean was born in Chicago, where his father worked as a meat salesman. His parents divorced when he was 9; his mother remarried twice. During a depression 4 years ago, his older brother shot and killed himself. His sister is a nurse who once was hospitalized for abusing barbiturates.

After the military, Dean attended 2 years of junior college, but he doesn't think it did him much good. "I've never been anything more than a big, dumb city slicker who cuts up dead animals for a living," he says.

Annie reports that Dean has been depressed most of the time for the last month and a half—not quite as long as he's been drinking. He cries some and sleeps poorly, often awakening early in the morning, unable to get back to sleep. His appetite has diminished, and he's lost about 20 pounds. He seems chronically tired, and his sex interest has diminished except when he is drunk, which is most of the time.

Dean looks years older than 60, and he has clearly lost weight. He's over 6 feet tall, but his outsized clothes seem to diminish his stature. He slumps quietly in his chair and speaks only when spoken to, his voice a rumbling monotone. Fully alert, he pays close attention to the conversation and his speech is relevant and mostly coherent. There is very little variation in his affect, and he admits that he feels depressed. He is fully oriented to time, place, and person; he scores 29 out of 30 on the MMSE, failing only to recall a street address after 5 minutes. He says he's never had delusions, but neither does he have much insight into the fact that the voices he hears are not real.

Dean has some thoughts about dying. They began with the depression, and now the voices have jumped on the idea. "They aren't ordering me to do it or anything like that," he explains. "They just think I might be a lot better off."

Evaluation of Dean Wannamaker

To evaluate this complex history, we'll take it in small chunks.

To begin with, what are Dean's diagnosable drinking behaviors? Of course, he has a clutch of indicators for alcohol use disorder (p. 404): There are social symptoms (divorce, arrests). During the current episode of drinking, he demonstrates tolerance (he doesn't appear drunk on a quart per day of hard liquor), continues to drink despite hallucinating (a health issue), and uses more alcohol than he intends ("I only meant to take a drink"). Even if we don't factor in withdrawal symptoms, he qualifies for a diagnosis of alcohol use disorder. He has been actively drinking within the past month, so no course specifier can apply.

Dean's somatic complaints include appetite and weight loss, reduced libido, and insomnia. These represent three separate DSM-5-TR chapters (eating, sleep–wake, and sexual disorders), and a differential diagnosis could be constructed for each. However, to find the resulting collection of independent major mental diagnoses in one patient would be highly unlikely, from either a statistical or a logical viewpoint (principle M—keep it simple). Indeed, these somatic complaints can all be found in patients who have depression, psychosis, or alcohol-related disorders. A mood disorder due to another medical condition must always be considered, especially in someone who has been ignoring health needs (principle F). Although we'd need a physical examination and laboratory tests to be more confident, no information given in the vignette suggests that Dean has any such medical disorder.

Throughout his later adult life, Dean has heard voices intermittently. A principal concern for any patient with psychosis to determine the likelihood of schizophrenia. Although Dean hears voices, that's his only psychotic symptom (OK, his affect is constricted, but I'd chalk that up to the depression). He therefore lacks the "A" portion of the basic criteria, knocking out schizophrenia as well as schizophreniform and schizoaffective disorders. The results of his MMSE would rule out delirium and a major or mild neurocognitive disorder; the history excludes psychotic disorder due to another medical condition. Also, Annie points out that he only hallucinates when he's been drinking. Of course, nearly all psychotic disorders require that the symptoms not be directly related to the use of a substance. That puts the end to any consideration of brief psychotic disorder.

Now, look at the criteria for substance/medication-induced psychotic disorder (p. 93). They require prominent hallucinations or delusions. Inasmuch as the hallucinations never appear unless Dean drinks, and they never last longer than a few weeks after the drinking stops, this history fulfills the criteria for alcohol-induced psychotic disorder, with hallucinations. If this becomes our working diagnosis, we'll add the specifier *with onset during withdrawal*.

As for mood disorder, Dean fulfills the inclusion criteria for major depressive episode: He's had more than 2 weeks of persistent low mood, fatigue, weight loss, insomnia, and thoughts of suicide. His symptoms aren't due to a medical condition, represent a change from his usual self—and they certainly do distress him. However, they did occur after he began drinking, and therefore could be alcohol-related, ruling out major depressive disorder.

The criteria for substance-induced mood disorder are simple, and Dean appears to fulfill them: He is persistently depressed and meets full criteria for a major depressive episode; he has also been drinking for several months, and we know that alcohol can induce severe depression. Although his brother shot himself while depressed, we do not know whether he was also a drinker; a sister had used drugs. OK, family history information isn't a criterion, but as I've noted over and over, it can be a useful guidepost (principle B).

Major depressive disorder is treatable, and it can be lethal. It should be given a high priority for investigation and possible treatment (principle F). However, it should not be automatically diagnosed in every substance-using patient who reports feeling depressed; in many cases, mood symptoms will improve when the patient stops using the substance.

So, how should we regard the relationships of Dean's various diagnoses? Because substance use was surely the first of these symptom groups to appear (principle X)—Dean began drinking at age 12 and had some behavioral problems resulting from it even as a young man in the military—it is reasonable to consider it first. We'll consider two possible scenarios. (1) Alcohol use induces psychosis, and he has an independent major depressive disorder; or (2) alcohol usage induces both a psychosis and a mood disorder. The simplicity of the second formulation, plus our desire not to rush in with possibly unnecessary treatment before it is needed, prompts us to regard the mood disorder as substance-induced—at least until Dean can be withdrawn completely from alcohol. And it follows principle M.

Under ICD-10, where we code the use disorder at the same time as the psychosis or depression, I'd list the psychosis first; it seems to require treatment more urgently. But I'd be happy to entertain arguments. Dean's GAF score would be about 40.

F10.259	Severe alcohol use disorder, with alcohol-induced psychotic disorder, with onset during withdrawal
F10.24	Alcohol-induced depressive disorder, with onset during intoxication

Essential Tables

Global Assessment of Functioning (GAF)

As you will find, you must go fairly far down the list (around 50–70) to reach the point at which most patients described in this book were awarded a diagnosis. Although we can interpolate between these numbers, trying to discriminate a finer degree than 5-unit intervals (65, 25, etc.) is probably futile. As you will notice from the text, on some occasions that hasn't stopped me from trying.

Global Assessment of Functioning (GAF) Scale

Consider psychological, social, and occupational functioning on a hypothetical continuum of mental health-illness. Do not include impairment in functioning due to physical (or environmental) limitations.

Code **(Note: Use intermediate codes when appropriate, e.g., 45, 68, 72.)**

100 | 91	**Superior functioning in a wide range of activities, life's problems never seem to get out of hand, is sought out by others because of his or her many positive qualities. No symptoms.**
90 | 81	**Absent or minimal symptoms** (e.g., mild anxiety before an exam**), good functioning in all areas, interested and involved in a wide range of activities. socially effective, generally satisfied with life, no more than everyday problems or concerns** (e.g. an occasional argument with family members).
80 | 71	**If symptoms are present, they are transient and expectable reactions to psychosocial stressors** (e.g., difficulty concentrating after family argument); **no more than slight impairment in social, occupational or school functioning** (e.g., temporarily falling behind in schoolwork).
70 | 61	**Some mild symptoms** (e.g., depressed mood and mild insomnia) **OR some difficulty in social, occupational, or school functioning** (e.g., occasional truancy, or theft within the household)**, but generally functioning pretty well, has some meaningful interpersonal relationships.**
60 | 51	**Moderate symptoms** (e.g., flat affect and circumstantial speech, occasional panic attacks) **OR moderate difficulty in social, occupational, or school functioning** (e.g., few friends, conflicts with peers or co-workers).
50 | 41	**Serious symptoms** (e.g., suicidal ideation, severe obsessional rituals, frequent shoplifting) **OR any serious impairment in social, occupational, or school functioning** (e.g., no friends, unable to keep a job).
40 | 31	**Some impairment in reality testing or communication** (e.g., speech is at times illogical, obscure, or irrelevant) **OR major impairment in several areas, such as work or school, family relations, judgment, thinking, or mood** (e.g., depressed man avoids friends, neglects family, and is unable to work; child frequently beats up younger children, is defiant at home, and is failing at school).
30 | 21	**Behavior is considerably influenced by delusions or hallucinations OR serious impairment in communication or judgment** (e.g., sometimes incoherent, acts grossly inappropriately, suicidal preoccupation) **OR inability to function in almost all areas** (e.g., stays in bed all day; no job, home, or friends).
20 | 11	**Some danger of hurting self or others** (e.g., suicide attempts without clear expectation of death; frequently violent; manic excitement) **OR occasionally fails to maintain minimal personal hygiene** (e.g., smears feces) **OR gross impairment in communication** (e.g., largely incoherent or mute).
10 | 1	**Persistent danger of severely hurting self or others** (e.g., recurrent violence) **OR persistent inability to maintain minimal personal hygiene OR serious suicidal act with clear expectation of death.**
0	Inadequate information.

Note. From the *Diagnostic and Statistical Manual of Mental Disorders* (4th ed., text rev., p. 34) by the American Psychiatric Association. Copyright © 2000 the American Psychiatric Association. Reprinted by permission.

Physical Disorders That Affect Mental Diagnosis

Medical disorder	Anx	Depr	Mania	Psych	Delir	Dem	Cata	Pers chg	Erect	Ejac	Sex pain	Anorg
Cardiovascular												
Anemia	×											
Angina	×											
Aortic aneurysm									×			
Arrhythmia	×				×							
A-V malformation							×					
Congestive heart failure	×				×				×			
Hyperthyroidism	×				×							
Myocardial infarction	×											
Mitral valve prolapse	×											
Paroxysmal atrial tachycardia	×											
Shock	×				×							
Endocrine												
Addison's (adrenal insufficiency)	×	×			×							
Carcinoid tumor	×											
Cushing's disease	×	×	×		×			×				
Diabetes	×								×			×
Hyperparathyroidism							×					
Hyperthyroidism	×	×	×		×				×			
Hypoglycemia	×	×			×	×						
Hypoparathyroidism	×	×										
Hypothyroidism	×	×		×		×		×	×			×
Inappropriate ADH secretion					×							
Klinefelter's syndrome									×			
Menopause	×										×	
Pancreatic tumor		×										
Pheochromocytoma	×											
Premenstrual syndrome	×											
Hyperprolactinemia												×

(cont.)

Note. Key to column heads: Anx, anxiety; Depr, depression; Psych, psychosis; Delir, delirium; Dem, dementia (major neurocognitive disorder); Cata, catatonia symptoms; Pers chg, personality change; Erect, erectile dysfunction; Ejac, ejaculatory dysfunction; Sex pain, sexual pain syndromes (male or female); Anorg, anorgasmia.

Physical Disorders That Affect Mental Diagnosis (*cont.*)

Medical disorder	Anx	Depr	Mania	Psych	Delir	Dem	Cata	Pers chg	Erect	Ejac	Sex pain	Anorg
Infections												
AIDS	×	×	×			×		×				
Brain abscess					×							
Subacute bacterial endocarditis	×											
Systemic infection	×				×							
Urinary tract infection					×							
Vaginitis											×	
Viral infections		×										
Toxicity												
Aminophylline					×							
Antidepressants	×			×	×				×	×		×
Aspirin intolerance	×											
Bromide				×								
Cimetidine					×							
Digitalis					×							
Disulfiram				×	×							
Estrogens									×			
Fluorides							×					
Heavy metals	×	×										
Herbicides									×			
L-dopa					×							
Steroids	×			×								
Theophylline	×											
Metabolic												
Electrolyte imbalance	×				×							
Hepatic disease		×			×	×			×			
Hypercarbia					×							
Hyperventilation	×											
Hypocalcemia	×											
Hypokalemia	×	×										
Hypoxia					×							
Malnutrition		×			×				×			
Porphyria	×							×				
Renal disease	×			×	×				×			

Medical disorder	Anx	Depr	Mania	Psych	Delir	Dem	Cata	Pers chg	Erect	Ejac	Sex pain	Anorg
Neurological												
Alzheimer's/frontotemporal						×						
Amyotrophic lateral sclerosis						×			×			
Brain tumor	×			×	×	×	×	×				
Cerebellar degeneration						×						
Cerebrovascular accident	×					×		×				
Creutzfeldt–Jakob						×						
Encephalitis	×				×	×	×					
Epilepsy, seizures	×	×			×	×		×				
Extradural hematoma					×							
Head trauma	×				×	×	×	×				
Huntington's	×	×				×		×				
Intracerebral hematoma					×							
Ménière's	×											
Meningitis					×							
Migraine	×											
Multiple sclerosis	×	×	×			×		×	×			
Multi-infarct						×						
Neurosyphilis			×		×	×		×	×			
Normal-pressure hydrocephalus						×						
Parkinson's						×			×			×
Post-anoxia						×						
Progressive supranuclear palsy						×						
Spinal cord disease									×			
Subarachnoid hemorrhage					×		×					
Subdural hematoma					×	×	×					
Transient ischemic attack	×				×							
Wilson's disease	×							×				

(cont.)

Physical Disorders That Affect Mental Diagnosis (*cont.*)

Medical disorder	Anx	Depr	Mania	Psych	Delir	Dem	Cata	Pers chg	Erect	Ejac	Sex pain	Anorg
Pulmonary												
Asthma	×											
Chronic obstructive lung disease	×				×				×			
Hyperventilation	×											
Pulmonary embolus	×											
Other												
Collagen	×											
Endometriosis											×	
Pelvic disease									×		×	×
Peyronie's disease									×			
Postoperative states					×							
Systemic lupus erythematosus	×	×		×	×			×				
Temporal arteritis	×											
Vitamin deficiency												
B$_{12}$ (pernicious anemia)	×	×				×						
Folic acid						×						
Niacin (pellagra)					×	×						
Thiamin (B$_1$) (Wernicke's)					×	×						

Classes (or Names) of Medications
That Can Cause Mental Disorders

	Anxiety	Mood	Psychosis	Delirium
Analgesics	×	×	×	×
Anesthetics	×	×	×	×
Antianxiety agents		×		
Anticholinergics	×	×	×	
Anticonvulsants	×	×	×	×
Antidepressants	×	×	×	×
Antihistamines	×		×	×
Antihypertensives/ cardiovascular drugs	×	×	×	×
Antimicrobials		×	×	×
Antiparkinsonian agents	×	×	×	×
Antipsychotics	×	×		×
Antiulcer agents		×		
Bronchodilators	×			×
Chemotherapeutic agents			×	
Corticosteroids	×	×	×	×
Disulfiram (Antabuse)		×	×	
Gastrointestinal agents			×	×
Histamine agonists				×
Immunosuppressants				×
Insulin	×			
Interferon	×	×	×	
Lithium	×			
Muscle relaxants		×	×	×
NSAIDs			×	
Oral contraceptives	×	×		
Thyroid replacements	×			

Note. From *Diagnosis Made Easier* (2nd ed., p. 116) by James Morrison. Copyright © 2014 by The Guilford Press. Adapted by permission.

Index

Boldfaced page numbers signify Essential Features diagnostic material.
Italicized numbers indicate a definition. The letter *t* after a page number indicates a table.